WOUND CARE ESSENTIALS

Practice Principles

Third Edition

WOUND CARE ESSENTIALS

Practice Principles

Third Edition

Sharon Baranoski, MSN, RN, CWCN, APN-CCRN, DAPWCA, FAAN

President
Wound Care Dynamics, Inc.
Nurse Consultant Services
Shorewood, Illinois

Symposium Director
Clinical Symposium on Advances in Skin &
Wound Care

Editorial Advisory Board
ADVANCES IN SKIN & WOUND CARE

Nursing Advisory Board
Rasmussen College
Romeoville/Joliet, Illinois

Council of Regents & Nursing Advisory Board
Lewis University
Romeoville, Illinois

Elizabeth A. Ayello, PHD, RN, ACNS-BC, CWON, MAPWCA, FAAN

Faculty
Excelsior College School of Nursing
Albany, New York

Clinical Associate Editor
ADVANCES IN SKIN & WOUND CARE

Executive Editor
JOURNAL OF THE WORLD COUNCIL OF ENTEROSTOMAL
THERAPISTS (WCET)

Senior Adviser
The John A. Hartford Institute for Geriatric Nursing

President
Ayello, Harris & Associates, Inc.
New York, New York

 Wolters Kluwer | Lippincott Williams & Wilkins
Health
Philadelphia · Baltimore · New York · London
Buenos Aires · Hong Kong · Sydney · Tokyo

Publisher: J. Christopher Burghardt
Acquisitions Editor: Bill Lamsback
Product Director: David Moreau
Product Manager: Rosanne Hallowell
Editor: Maureen McKinney
Proofreaders: Scotti Cohn and Jerry Altobelli
Editorial Assistants: Karen J. Kirk, Jeri O'Shea, Linda K. Ruhf
Creative Director: Doug Smock
Vendor Manager: Cynthia Rudy
Manufacturing Manager: Beth J. Welsh
Production and Indexing Services: Thomson Digital

The clinical treatments described and recommended in this publication are based on research and consultation with nursing, medical, and legal authorities. To the best of our knowledge, these procedures reflect currently accepted practice. Nevertheless, they can't be considered absolute and universal recommendations. For individual applications, all recommendations must be considered in light of the patient's clinical condition and, before administration of new or infrequently used drugs, in light of the latest package-insert information. The authors and publisher disclaim any responsibility for any adverse effects resulting from the suggested procedures, from any undetected errors, or from the reader's misunderstanding of the text.

Printed in China.

10 9 8 7 6 5 4 3 2 1

Library of Congress Cataloging-in-Publication Data
Wound care essentials : practice principles / editors, Sharon Baranoski,
Elizabeth A. Ayello. — 3rd ed.
    p. ; cm.
  Rev. ed. of: Wound care essentials / Sharon Baranoski, Elizabeth A. Ayello.
2nd ed. c2008.
  Includes bibliographical references and index.
  ISBN 978-1-4511-1304-4 (pbk. : alk. paper)
1. Wounds and injuries–Patients–Care–Handbooks, manuals, etc.   2. Wounds and injuries–
Nursing–Handbooks, manuals, etc.   3. Wound healing–Handbooks, manuals, etc.   I. Baranoski,
Sharon.   II. Ayello, Elizabeth A.   III. Baranoski,Sharon. Wound care essentials.
  [DNLM: 1. Wounds and Injuries–therapy.   2. Wound Healing. WO 700]
  RD94.B374 2012
  617.1—dc23   2011013990

The end to writing this book is the beginning of conveying thanks to those who made the journey with me:

To my husband Jim—spouse extraordinaire for 45 years—I love you. Thanks for helping me be all that I can be.

To my children, Jim, Deb, Jeff, and JR, and their spouses, Tracy, Mark, Kari, and Carissa—thank you for loving and living the word Family and for being such a wonderful part of mine.

To my grandchildren, Madison, Lexi, Brek, Lanie, Brooklyn, and Morgan—you bring laughter, joy, and so much happiness to my life. Someday I hope you can understand why Gramma wrote a book with such "yucky" pictures.

To the authors of this third edition—thank you for your commitment to your profession and for sharing your knowledge and expertise in this book. It is truly appreciated.

To Elizabeth—a dear friend, colleague, and support system. Thank you for the endless hours, long nights, and many trips needed in completing this third edition. It really is the "Book of the Year" in my mind.

With gratitude and love,
Sharon

"Family is everything."

To my parents, Phyllis and Tony, and my brothers, Bob and Ron, and their families for showing me the meaning of a caring family. I am grateful for your sacrifices so I could go to college and become a nurse. You truly taught me that "education changes life."

To my patients, students, and professional colleagues in my global community of wound care. Thank you for the privilege of sharing your journey and for showing me that caring comes in many forms.

To Roberta, thank you for teaching me the power of words.

To Katie, Gary, Courtney, Karen, Carl, Sheila, Teddy, Cara, Paula, Lori, and their families, your friendship brings a welcome balance to my life. As William James said, "Wherever you are, it is your own friends that make your world."

To Sharon, is three times the charm?

To my darling daughters, Sarah and Wendy, your achievements inspire me daily and your smiles bring me joy.

To my husband, A. Scott, as many books say—and they lived "happily ever after." It is our time to sing and dance the night away.

E.A.A.

FOREWORD

In preparation for writing the foreword for the third edition of *Wound Care Essentials*, I did some reading on "knowledge management." While "knowledge management" in a corporate organization differs in many respects from information delivery in the form of a textbook, I found the general concepts interesting and the parallels quite striking. Knowledge management involves gathering data from a variety of sources, organizing it so that patterns become apparent, providing context that is relevant to understanding the principles related to action (in this case, professional practice), and delivering all of these things to the end-user in timely fashion and in a format that expedites rapid assimilation.

These are the "bones" around which this third edition of *Wound Care Essentials: Practice Principles* has been built. It is edited by two of the most respected people in the field of wound care. Sharon and Elizabeth have selected top experts with both scientific knowledge and clinical wisdom who understand the principles behind their practice and can effectively transmit this knowledge to others. Each expert or team of experts has updated their chapter with the latest information. Included in each chapter are relevant portions of the most recent NPUAP/EPUAP clinical practice guideline, up-to-the-minute information on wound treatments and dressings, as well as an entirely new chapter on tubes, drains, and fistulas.

Context is provided with patient scenarios and case discussions as well as an expanded color photo section. The essential context of setting and recent regulatory changes is also interwoven throughout various chapters, including another new chapter on pressure ulcers in neonatal and pediatric populations as well as updates on OASIS-C for home care and MDS 3.0 for long-term care.

The book has been designed with generous use of bulleted points, new icons, and quick-reference charts so that rapid assimilation by the end-user is possible, and chapters have been expanded and reorganized where appropriate to enhance ease of understanding. Finally, the fact that the third edition is being published a scant 3 years after the second edition should give every reader great confidence in the currency of the content and the timeliness of knowledge delivery.

Congratulations to the editors and the authors on producing a book that will help clinicians, whether novices or experts, to manage the complex knowledge surrounding wound care in a truly substantive way.

Barbara Braden, PhD, RN, FAAN
Dean, University College
Creighton University
Omaha, Nebraska

PREFACE

Knowledge is important.

Thank you, dear colleagues, for your enthusiastic support of *Wound Care Essentials*! Your response to our book continues to exceed our expectations. We are delighted to know that our contribution to the wound care literature with this practical compilation of the essential knowledge needed for today's clinicians has helped you. We were honored that our first edition was chosen by our peers as an *American Journal of Nursing* Book of the Year in 2004 and printed in Portuguese as *O Essencial Sobre O Tratamento De Feridas Principios Practicos*.

We are thrilled to know that our book hasn't sat on a shelf unused. Many of you have shared how helpful our book is, whether in studying for certification, writing policies and procedures or, most of all, in your daily patient care. We are especially pleased to learn that many programs and schools have adopted our book as their official textbook for wound care courses. Making a difference in the lives of patients and their families is our ongoing dream. Your comments and encouragement to continue our efforts gave us the impetus to write this third edition.

We have retained the original vision of the book, which was to share what we have learned in the trenches of patient care. We have expanded our vision to include our experience in education because we hold dearly the belief that excellence in practice depends upon excellence in education. Our book continues to combine all that we have learned from our patients, colleagues, research, literature, industry, seminars, and educational programs into one concise wound care resource.

We are doubly honored to create a third edition filled with more chapters, photos, and practical information to guide you in the care of your patients. All chapters have been thoroughly reviewed and updated with the most current information available at the time of writing. One of the things you'll notice about this third edition is that we've added a chapter on tubes, drains, and ostomies. Some content has been reorganized; for example, our venous chapter now has two subsections so that the content on lymphedema is separate. We have integrated patient case scenarios into relevant chapters to help you with the translation of wound knowledge into your everyday practice. You have told us that you value the "Show what you know" questions at the end of each chapter, so we have expanded the explanations of why answers are incorrect. As requested, we've increased the number of color pictures to the maximum that space would allow.

Many people have influenced the content of this book. We would like to acknowledge and thank the contributors to this third edition. We are grateful that most of our previous authors were able to contribute to this edition. We are also honored to welcome several new colleagues to share their expertise with you. We are delighted that once again Barbara Braden has written our foreword! Without the willingness of these wound care experts to share their time, knowledge, and expertise, this book wouldn't be a reality. Thank you all for being part of this third edition.

Just as in practice, teamwork is important in publishing. We continue to be inspired by the memory of our mentor and dear friend, Roberta Abruzzese. We could not have written three books without the wisdom, brilliance, guidance, support, and love of our mentor and dear colleague. While we miss her dearly, we hope that our work reflects the values she held so dear: "Keep the words succinct and clear so to help the clinician by compiling the latest and best information they need in practice."

It takes a village and teamwork to write a book! The diligent editing, meticulous attention to detail, understanding, and flexibility from our Lippincott Williams & Wilkins/Wolters Kluwer Health team made it a much less tenacious experience. We are indebted to the LWW-WKH staff who worked behind the scenes on our behalf. We may not know all of you personally, but your efforts have played an invaluable part in the outcome of this book. Thank you to Rosanne Hallowell and Bill Lamsback for supporting the new additions and changes to our book. To Maureen McKinney, for your laborious task of carefully editing this third edition, we are grateful. It is by far the BEST edition.

To our readers, we hope the pages will be tattered and torn from use and that it doesn't sit on your bookshelf. As once was said, a book is a gift you can open again and again. We hope you open this gift often. For we both believe the old adage, **"Knowledge is important, but what you *do* with the knowledge is *more important*."**

Sharon and Elizabeth

CONTRIBUTORS

Tami de Araujo, MD
Private Practice
Boca Raton, Florida

Mona Mylene Baharestani, PhD, ANP,
  CWON, CWS
Wound Care Program Coordinator
James H. Quillen Veterans Affairs Medical
  Center
Johnson City, Tennessee
Clinical Associate Professor
Quillen College of Medicine
Department of Surgery
Johnson City, Tennessee

Christine Barkauskas, BA, RN, CWOCN,
  APN
Wound, Ostomy Continence Nurse
Wound Healing & Treatment Center
Silver Cross Hospital
Joliet, Illinois

Dan R. Berlowitz, MD, MPH
Director, Center for Health Quality, Outcomes and
  Economic Research
Professor, Boston University School of Public
  Health
Bedford VA Hospital
Bedford, Massachusetts

Joyce M. Black, PhD, RN, CPSN, CWCN,
  FAAN
Associate Professor of Nursing
University of Nebraska Medical Center
Omaha, Nebraska

Steven B. Black, MD, FACS
Director, Wound Healing Services
The Nebraska Medical Center
Omaha, Nebraska

David M. Brienza, PhD
Professor
University of Pittsburgh
Pittsburgh, Pennsylvania

Gregory Brown, RN, ET
Case Manager
Dallas Veterans Medical Center
Dallas, Texas

Janet E. Cuddigan, PhD, RN, CWCN
Associate Professor
Chair, Adult Health and Illness Department
Interim Assistant Dean for Administration
College of Nursing
University of Nebraska Medical Center
Omaha, Nebraska

Linda E. Dallam, MS, GNP-BC,
  CWCN-AP, RN-BC
Pain Management Nurse Practitioner
Department of Anesthesiology
Faculty, Division of Education & Organizational
  Development
Montefiore Medical Center
Bronx, New York

Paula Erwin-Toth, MSN, RN, CWOCN,
  CNS
Director, WOC Nursing Education
Cleveland Clinic
Cleveland, Ohio

Caroline E. Fife, MD, CWS
Associate Professor
University of Texas Health Science Center, Houston
Department of Medicine, Division of Cardiology
Director of Clinical Research
Memorial Hermann Center for Wound Healing
Chief Medical Officer
Intellicure, Inc.
Houston, Texas

Rita A. Frantz, PhD, RN, FAAN
Kelting Dean and Professor
University of Iowa College of Nursing
Iowa City, Iowa

Susan L. Garber, MA, OTR, FAOTA, FACRM
Professor
Department of Physical Medicine & Rehabilitation
Baylor College of Medicine
Houston, Texas

Sue E. Gardner, PhD, RN
Associate Professor
University of Iowa College of Nursing
Iowa City, Iowa

Mary Jo Geyer, PT, PhD, FCCWS, CLT-LANA, CPed
University of Pittsburgh
Rehabilitation Science & Technology Department
Pittsburgh, Pennsylvania

Keith Harding, MB, ChB, FRCGP, FRCP, FRCS
Professor, Sub-Dean of Innovation & Engagement/
  Head of Section of Wound Healing
Department of Dermatology & Wound Healing
School of Medicine
Cardiff University
Cardiff, Wales
United Kingdom

Wendy S. Harris, BSHS
Research Scientist
North Shore LIJ Health System
Manhasset, New York

Samantha Holloway, MSc, PGCE, RN
Senior Professional Tutor
Department of Dermatology & Wound Healing
School of Medicine
Cardiff University
Cardiff, Wales
United Kingdom

Denise Israel-Richardson, MEd, SRN, SCM, (EdD student)
Lecturer, School of Advanced Nursing Education
The Faculty of Medical Sciences
The University of the West Indies
St. Augustine, Trinidad
West Indies

Robert S. Kirsner, MD, PhD
Professor, Vice Chairman & Stiefel
  Laboratories Chair
Department of Dermatology & Cutaneous Surgery
University of Miami Miller School of Medicine
Miami, Florida

Carl A. Kirton, DNP, RN, ANP-BC, ACRN
Chief Nursing Executive & Associate Executive
  Director
Lincoln Medical & Mental Health Center
Clinical Associate Professor of Nursing
New York University
New York, New York

Ronald A. Kline, MD, FACS, FAHA
Arizona Endovascular Center
Chief, Division of Vascular & Endovascular Surgery
Carondelet St. Joseph Hospital
Medical Director, Wound Care
Carondelet St. Joseph Hospital Center for Advanced
  Wound Care
Medical Director, Wound Care
Kindred Hospital
Tucson, Arizona

Steven P. Knowlton, JD, RN
Partner, Locks Law Firm, PLLC
New York, New York

Steven R. Kravitz, DPM, FACFAS, FAPWCA
Executive Director and Founder
American Professional Wound Care Association
Physician Certified in Wound Care-CMET
Richboro, Pennsylvania
Assistant Professor
Department of Podiatric Medicine and Orthopedics
Temple University School of Podiatric Medicine
Philadelphia, Pennsylvania

Diane K. Langemo, PhD, RN, FAAN
Distinguished Professor Emeritus
University of North Dakota College of Nursing
Grand Forks, North Dakota

Lawrence A. Lavery, DPM, MPH
Professor, Department of Plastic Surgery
University of Texas Southwestern Medical Center and
*   Parkland Hospital*
Dallas, Texas

Jeffrey M. Levine, MD, AGSF, CMD,
**   CWS**
Assistant Clinical Professor of Medicine
Albert Einstein Medical College
Bronx, New York
Attending Physician, Beth Israel Medical Center
New York, New York

Courtney H. Lyder, ND, GNP,
**   FAAN**
Dean and Assistant Director, UCLA Health
*   System*
Professor of Nursing & Public Health
University of California, Los Angeles
Los Angeles, California

James B. McGuire, DPM, PT, CPed, CWS,
**   FAPWCA**
Physician Certified in Wound Care-CMET
Director, Leonard Abrams Center for Advanced
*   Wound Healing*
Associate Professor
Temple University School of Podiatric Medicine
Philadelphia, Pennsylvania

Andrea McIntosh, RN, BSN, CWOCN,
**   APN**
Manager, Wound Healing & Treatment Center
Wound, Ostomy & Continence Department
Silver Cross Hospital
Joliet, Illinois

Linda Montoya, RN, BSN, CWOCN,
**   APN**
Clinical Manager
Provena Center of Wound Care & Hyperbaric Medicine
Provena St. Joseph Hospital
Joliet, Illinois

Mary Ellen Posthauer, RD, CD, LD
President
MEP Healthcare Dietary Services, Inc.
Evansville, Indiana

Pamela Scarborough, DPT, MS,
**   CDE, CWS**
Director of Public Relations and Education
American Medical Technologies
Irvine, California

Gregory Schultz, PhD
UF Research Foundation Professor of Obstetrics and
*   Gynecology*
Director, Institute for Wound Research
University of Florida
Gainesville, Florida

R. Gary Sibbald, BSc, MD, MEd,
**   FRCPC (Med Derm), MACP, FAAD,**
**   MAPWCA**
Professor of Public Health Medicine
Director, International Interprofessional Wound Care
*   Course & Masters of Science in Community Health*
Dalla Lana School of Public Health
Physician Certified in Wound Care-CMET
University of Toronto
Toronto, Ontario
Canada

Mary Y. Sieggreen, NP, CNS, APRN,
**   CVN**
Nurse Practitioner
Vascular Surgery/Wound Care
Harper University Hospital
Detroit Medical Center
Detroit, Michigan

Stephen Sprigle, PT, PhD
Professor
School of Applied Physiology
Georgia Institute of Technology
Atlanta, Georgia

Joyce K. Stechmiller, PhD, ACNP-BC,
**   FAAN**
Interim Department Chair, Adult & Elderly Nursing
Associate Professor
University of Florida College of Nursing
Gainesville, Florida

Linda J. Stricker, MSN/ED, RN, CWOCN
Assistant Director, WOC Nursing Education
Cleveland Clinic
Cleveland, Ohio

David R. Thomas, MD, FACP, AGSF, GSAF
Professor of Medicine
Saint Louis University
St. Louis, Missouri

Marjana Tomic-Canic, RN, PhD
Professor of Dermatology
Director, Wound Healing and Regenerative Medicine
Research Program
Department of Dermatology
University of Miami Miller School of Medicine
Miami, Florida

Terry Treadwell, MD, FACS
Medical Director
Institute for Advanced Wound Care
Montgomery, Alabama

David Weinstein, MD
Resident
Department of Internal Medicine
University of Florida College of Medicine
Gainesville, Florida

Gregory Ralph Weir, MB ChB, MMed (Surg), CVS
Vascular Surgeon
Eugene Marais Hospital
Pretoria, South Africa

Karen Zulkowski, DNS, RN, CWS
Associate Professor
Montana State University-Bozeman
Billings, Montana

CONTENTS

I Wound Care Concepts

1. Quality of Life and Ethical Issues 2
—MONA MYLENE BAHARESTANI

2. Regulation and Wound Care 21
—DAN R. BERLOWITZ, DENISE ISRAEL-RICHARDSON, AND COURTNEY H. LYDER

3. Legal Aspects of Wound Care 37
—STEVEN P. KNOWLTON AND GREGORY BROWN

4. Skin: An Essential Organ 57
—SHARON BARANOSKI, ELIZABETH A. AYELLO, MARJANA TOMIC-CANIC, AND JEFFREY M. LEVINE

5. Acute and Chronic Wound Healing 83
—SAMANTHA HOLLOWAY, KEITH HARDING, JOYCE K. STECHMILLER, AND GREGORY SCHULTZ

6. Wound Assessment 101
—SHARON BARANOSKI, ELIZABETH A. AYELLO, AND DIANE K. LANGEMO

7. Wound Bioburden and Infection 126
—SUE E. GARDNER AND RITA A. FRANTZ

8. Wound Debridement 157
—ELIZABETH A. AYELLO, SHARON BARANOSKI, R. GARY SIBBALD, AND JANET E. CUDDIGAN

9. Wound Treatment Options 181
—SHARON BARANOSKI, ELIZABETH A. AYELLO, ANDREA MCINTOSH, LINDA MONTOYA, AND PAMELA SCARBOROUGH

10. Nutrition and Wound Care 240
—MARY ELLEN POSTHAUER AND DAVID R. THOMAS

11. Pressure Redistribution: Seating, Positioning, and Support Surfaces.. 265
—DAVID M. BRIENZA, MARY JO GEYER, STEPHEN SPRIGLE, AND KAREN ZULKOWSKI

12. Pain Management and Wounds 295
—LINDA E. DALLAM, CHRISTINE BARKAUSKAS, ELIZABETH A. AYELLO, SHARON BARANOSKI, AND R. GARY SIBBALD

Color illustration pages C1 through C48 follow page 304.

II   Wound Classifications and Management Strategies

13.   Pressure Ulcers.. 324
—ELIZABETH A. AYELLO, SHARON BARANOSKI, COURTNEY H. LYDER, JANET E. CUDDIGAN,
AND WENDY S. HARRIS

14.   Venous Disease and Lymphedema Management 360

Venous Disease...360
—MARY Y. SIEGGREEN AND RONALD A. KLINE

Lymphedema 379
—CAROLYN E. FIFE, MARY Y. SIEGGREEN, AND RONALD A. KLINE

15.   Arterial Ulcers.. 398
—MARY Y. SIEGGREEN, RONALD A. KLINE, R. GARY SIBBALD, AND GREGORY RALPH WEIR

16.   Diabetic Foot Ulcers.. 420
—LAWRENCE A. LAVERY, JAMES B. MCGUIRE, SHARON BARANOSKI, ELIZABETH A. AYELLO,
AND STEVEN R. KRAVITZ

17.   Sickle Cell Ulcers... 447
—TERRY TREADWELL

18.   Surgical Reconstruction of Wounds 460
—JOYCE M. BLACK AND STEVEN B. BLACK

19.   Tube, Drain, and Fistula Management.................................... 477
—PAULA ERWIN-TOTH AND LINDA J. STRICKER

20.   Atypical Wounds.. 491
—DAVID WEINSTEIN, TAMI DE ARAUJO, AND ROBERT S. KIRSNER

21.   Wounds in Special Populations 511

Intensive Care Population.. 512
—JANET E. CUDDIGAN

Spinal Cord Injury Population... 520
—SUSAN L. GARBER

HIV/AIDS Population 532
—CARL A. KIRTON

Bariatric Population.. 542
—JANET E. CUDDIGAN AND SHARON BARANOSKI

22.   Pressure Ulcers in Neonatal and Pediatric Populations 552
—MONA MYLENE BAHARESTANI

23.   Palliative Wound Care 564
—DIANE K. LANGEMO

24.   Wound Care Perspectives: Present and Future 583
— ELIZABETH A. AYELLO AND SHARON BARANOSKI

Index   *587*

PART I

Wound Care Concepts

CHAPTER 1

Quality of Life and Ethical Issues

Mona Mylene Baharestani, PhD, ANP, CWON, CWS

Objectives

After completing this chapter, you'll be able to:

- describe how wounds and those afflicted by wounds are viewed
- identify quality-of-life impact on patients with wounds and their caregivers
- describe ethical dilemmas confronted in wound care
- identify issues and challenges faced by caregivers of patients with wounds
- describe strategies aimed at meeting the needs of patients with wounds and their caregivers.

TREATING THE PATIENT AS WELL AS THE WOUND

Recent research has given birth to many new wound-healing technologies, including tangential hydrosurgery, tissue-engineered skin substitutes, matrix metalloproteinase modulation, topical growth factors, negative pressure, cell induction, and slow-release antimicrobial therapies. Wound healing is undergoing a broad transformation as research unlocks the mysteries of the multifaceted processes of tissue degradation, regeneration, and repair.

Because wounds affect different patients on different levels, faster, more efficient healing is only one element of providing advanced wound care. Indeed, wounds have financial, psychological, and social implications that must also be addressed. Yet in our fast-paced, stressful clinical practices, do we encourage patients to disavow their wounds?[1] Do we acknowledge the profound life changes and day-to-day challenges faced by chronic wound sufferers?[2] Do we perpetuate patients' fear, shame, and isolation?[1] Do we give patients and their families and caregivers the impression that "wound care is a dehumanizing and reductionist specialty"?[3]

Assessing the meaning and significance of the wound to the patient and his or her caregiver should be as routine as assessing wound size and the percentage of granulation and necrotic tissue, but is it? Hyland et al.[4] report that patients with leg ulcers spend an average of 1.5 to 2 hours per day thinking about their ulcers. Do we know what our patients are thinking? Do we ever ask? The answer to the question, "What impact has your wound had on your quality of life?" posed by a caring and concerned practitioner provides valuable insight into the patient's experience and needs while also setting the stage for mutual goal identification and treatment planning.

Beyond possession of knowledge in basic science, anatomy, pathophysiology, wound-care dressings, drugs, and technologies, advanced wound-care practitioners must be able to deliver care in a compassionate manner, sensitive to the unique impact wounds have on quality of life.

How are wounds viewed?

A wound is defined as a disruption of the integrity and function of tissues in the body. The state of having a wound infers an imperfection, an insult resulting in a physical and emotional vulnerability.[5,6] Wounds and their management are described within a variety of personal, philosophical, and socioeconomic paradigms. (See *Emotional impact of wounds*.)

How are patients with wounds viewed?

Given the negative image by which wounds are viewed, it isn't surprising that patients with wounds are sometimes considered unattractive, imperfect, vulnerable, a nuisance to others and, in some cases, even repulsive.[5-9] Healthcare professionals, in particular, often blame patients and caregivers for the development and recalcitrance of pressure ulcers and venous ulcers, as the following comments reveal.[10,11]

"When I have a pressure ulcer, healthcare professionals ask, 'What happened?' This makes me feel ashamed because I was unable to prevent the pressure ulcer. Why is it that other complications of quadriplegia don't carry this type of stigma? Nobody makes me feel guilty when I have a urinary tract infection."[1]

A 79-year-old caregiver for her bedridden, paralyzed 83-year-old spouse states, "I thought it was nothing." (Referring to nine pressure ulcers.) "The plastic surgeon was quite angry about the sores, asking why I waited so long to bring him to the hospital. I was just dumbfounded. I felt so bad, I said, I just thought it was a sore that would just heal up. I feel so guilty that I didn't do the right thing."[10] According to Charles,[12] patients often feel that they are "relegated to a low priority in terms of medical understanding and delivery of service." Lack of explanation or conflicting information regarding what procedures will entail, results of diagnostic testing, and treatment options and prognosis often results in anger, frustration, resentment, and distrust on the part of patients and their families toward healthcare professionals.[12-16]

Wounds on the face, neck, and hands are obviously the most difficult to conceal, not only from others but also from the patient's own view. The emotional trauma experienced by patients with facial disfigurement requires long periods of adjustment.[17] In fact, one study reports that 30% to 40% of adult burn patients with facial scarring experienced severe psychological problems up to 2 years after discharge from rehabilitation.[18]

Emotional impact of wounds

In addition to the physical discomfort and morbidity associated with wounds, wounds have an inherent emotional effect on the patient as well as the caregivers, family, friends, and strangers he or she may encounter. Even health care professionals aren't immune to an emotional response to a patient's wound.

Wounds are typically perceived as:
- a betrayal of one's own body
- appalling, repulsive
- haunting, scary, associated with horror movies
- nuisance, time-consuming, costly
- smelly, dirty, disgusting
- unpleasant, uncomfortable.
The patient's own perception of his or her wound may include such feelings as:
- embarrassment, humiliation
- guilt, shame
- needing bandages to "hide the evidence" (that is, of imperfection).

For those with visible wounds, even a walk down the street may seem daunting.[19] According to Partridge,[19] disfiguring wounds on the face create a painful double bind of "extreme self-consciousness and self-imposed social isolation." Bernstein[20] describes a "social death" among facially disfigured patients. Social death occurs as the patient's self-consciousness about being in public increases, ties with family and friends are severed and, ultimately, all social interactions cease. Without positive social reinforcement, the patient's self-esteem and self-confidence vanish.[20]

Feelings of shame, embarrassment, powerlessness, and fear can be overpowering for patients during physical examinations. Therefore, as healthcare practitioners, we must be especially aware of the way we touch and dress wounds as well as our posturing and distance from the patient.[19] Partridge[19] emphasizes that we must pay particular attention to the unspoken word conveyed by our communication triangle (from the eyes to the chin).

QUALITY OF LIFE

Unquestionably, wounds have varying effects on the quality of life of those afflicted and on their caregivers. To explore the impact further requires a definition of this complex, multifactorial construct.

Quality of life is a vague and ethereal concept that reflects a patient's perspective on life satisfaction in a variety of situations.[21,22] In an attempt to narrow down the all-encompassing term "quality of life," the term "health-related quality of life" (HRqol) was first used in the late 1980s.[23] In Price's[23] view, "health-related quality of life is defined as the impact of disease and treatment on disability and daily living, or as a patient-based focus on the impact of a perceived health state on the ability to lead a fulfilling life."

Franks and Moffatt[24] add, "The state of ill health may be defined as feelings of pain and discomfort or change in usual functioning and feeling. This is key to the concept of health-related quality of life since it's the patient's own sense of well-being which is important, not the clinician's opinion of [the patient's] clinical status."

Schipper et al.[25] describe the four domains of quality of life as physical and occupational function, psychological state, social interaction, and somatic sensation, with some theorists adding a financial component.

Physical and occupational function

In separate studies by Brod,[26] Ribu et al.,[27] Persoon et al.,[28] and Meijer et al.[29] examining the impact of lower-extremity ulcers on

patients, participants reported feeling drained and fatigued due to sleep disturbances and the high energy expenditure required for mobility. Additionally, antibiotic-related adverse effects of nausea, fatigue, and general malaise were considerable.[26] In Brod's[26] sample, 50% of patients (n = 14) had to retire early or lost their jobs because of an ulcer. Even patients who were still employed experienced decreased productivity, lost time from work due to healthcare appointments, and lost career opportunities.[26]

In a study by Ashford and colleagues[30] of 21 patients with diabetic foot ulcers, 79% of patients reported an inability to maintain employment secondary to decreased mobility and fear of someone inadvertently treading on their affected foot. In another study, all patients interviewed felt that the leg ulcer limited their work capacity, with 50% adding that their jobs required standing for most of their shift.[31] In that same study, 42% of patients identified the leg ulcer as a key factor in their decision to stop working. Even for younger patients, leg ulceration was correlated with time lost from work and job loss, ultimately affecting finances.[31]

Marked restrictions in activities of daily living (ADLs) among those with leg ulcers are also reported in many studies, including those by Hyland et al.,[4] Brod,[26] Phillips et al.,[31] and Walshe.[32] In a study consisting of 88 patients with chronic leg ulcers, 75% reported difficulty performing basic housework.[33] Yet another study by Hyland et al.[4] demonstrated that of 50 patients with leg ulcers, 50% had problems getting on and off a bus and 30% had trouble climbing steps.

In terms of changing one's own clothing and bathing, pain, leg edema, fatigue, and bulky dressings can make such simple acts frustrating, if not impossible.[26,33-35] Phillips et al.[31] conducted personal interviews of 73 patients with leg ulcers, 81% of whom described their mobility and ability to carry out ADLs as adversely affected by their ulcer, with edema being the dominant factor.

Psychological function

Multiple factors affect the psychological response to having a wound or caring for a loved one with a wound. (See *Factors affecting patient response to wounds*.)

ETIOLOGY

According to Magnan,[36] a patient's psychological response to a wound may correlate closely with *how* he or she was wounded. Indeed, imagine the terrifying flashbacks the patient and family caregivers may experience upon viewing open amputation wounds sustained after motor vehicle accidents or burn wounds exposed during whirlpool treatments or the extreme emotions and fears elicited when gangrenous limbs from peripheral vascular disease or necrotic pressure ulcers that extend to the bone are exposed.

▶ PRACTICE POINT

Each dressing change draws attention to the wounded body part and its associated pain, but it also serves as a reminder of the circumstance or disease that resulted in the injury and engenders fears about the future.[36]

PREPAREDNESS

From the onset of hospital, rehabilitation, and home care admission, healthcare professionals plan for a patient's discharge by preparing patients and caregivers for independence. But are we sensitive to the patient's psychological and emotional readiness to deal with the wound? To that end, the patient and family may need to relinquish control to the healthcare provider.[1] The reality is that some patients can't cope with their physical wounds because they're simultaneously struggling with deep emotional wounds. This point is well illustrated by one patient's remarks: "It took everything I had to deal with the reality of having to spend the rest of my life as a quadriplegic" ... "When I have an ulcer (referring to a pressure ulcer), I don't want to see it. I feel like I am in hell and to survive I must separate myself from the wound." ... "I fear the sight of the ulcer."[1]

Factors affecting patient response to wounds

Factors that shape a patient's emotional response to his or her wound include:
- age
- coping patterns
- etiology
- gender
- healing outcomes
  - expectation of healing
  - time to healing
  - acute versus chronic
- impact on activities of daily living
- meaning, significance
- odor, leakage
- pain
- preparedness
- response of others
- social supports
- spirituality
- visibility.

VISIBILITY

As discussed previously, the visibility, severity, and circumstances under which wounding occurred can dramatically affect the patient's acceptance of the wound into his or her altered body image. For some, the wounded body part becomes objectified as though it does not belong to them.[37]

RESPONSE OF OTHERS

Not only is it difficult for patients to view their own wounds, but it is hard for patients to be rebuked by others at the sight of their wounds. Acceptance, pity, dismay, fear, repulsion, and avoidance are the gamut of responses displayed by others to wounds and to those who have been wounded. This can dramatically affect a patient's emotional response to the wound and his or her self-esteem. For patients who must endure the displeasing stares of others to their bandaged wounds, a wound clinic may be the only place where they can receive positive energy and reinforcement.[37]

PAIN

Physical pain associated with wounds is one of the areas in which healthcare professionals are least attentive. Krasner[38] describes pain "as one of those experiences of being that often confounds our understanding, sometimes we may actually flee from facing it." Yet pain is a major factor affecting the HRqol of those with wounds, as we'll see in the section discussing somatic sensation (pain).

MALODOR AND LEAKAGE

The impact of malodor from a fungating breast wound, a necrotic pressure ulcer, or a draining and infected venous leg ulcer can be emotionally and psychologically devastating. A patient may try in vain to mask wound malodor with perfumes and colognes. Their self-image can be crushed by feelings of shame and disgust. Some patients may say that the wound's malodor makes them feel dirty and may apologize to others about the malodor. Some may even limit their social encounters due to fear of offending others. As one patient poignantly describes, "I used to go to church, but the person next to me could smell it (referring to a leg wound) … like rotting flesh, lingering … So I do not go now."[16] Unfortunately, friends and family members may add to these feelings of isolation by avoiding the patient because of the wound's malodor.

Roe et al.[33] reported increased anxiety and depression scores, lower life satisfaction, and decreased social contacts among those with malodorous leg ulcers. Similarly, leakage of highly exudative wounds on to clothing, furniture, and bed linens can lead to feelings of embarrassment and inhibited sexuality and intimacy.[39-42] As women attempt to conceal bulky, saturated dressings with pants, long skirts, or baggy clothing, they become stripped of their feminity.[13,42,43] For palliative care patients and their families, malodor, heavy exudate, and bleeding may further heighten the daily misery of uncontrollable disease.[40,41]

HEALING OUTCOMES

For patients and their caregivers, just hearing that there's hope of healing, that improvement will occur, and that the pain, malodor, and restrictions will one day be gone or lessened can make the situation easier to bear.[7,32]

In clinical practice, the three questions most frequently posed by patients and caregivers are:

- Will this wound heal?
- How long will it take to heal?
- Will the treatment cause pain?

Among patients with chronic leg ulcers and high recurrence rates, healing potential is often viewed with pessimism.[16,32] In interviews of 73 patients with leg ulcers by Phillips et al.,[31] only 3% felt their ulcers would ever heal. This uncertainty toward healing is often echoed by healthcare professionals.[32] Chase and colleagues[37] explain how whole healing from an acute illness for a healthy person has a positive connotation of health and restoration, whereas it may not be the same for those with a chronic illness, such as venous insufficiency ulcers. Indeed, patients describe the healing process as ever present, requiring constant vigilance and need for healthcare follow-up.[37] For patients with chronic ulcers, there are also limitations in mobility, activity, bathing, dressing, and working.[37] This may leave patients feeling powerless, spending more time caring for their ulcers than for themselves.[16,37,43] The uncontrolled nature of the condition often leads to a lack of ownership and a "who cares" attitude.[37] In a sense, freedom is gone and the threat of ulcer recurrence (and possible amputation) is ever present.[37] The fear of recurrence and loss of freedom is vividly portrayed by a patient interviewed by Brown,[11] who stated "the worst thing is knowing there is no cure and they can come back at any time. It's not like a broken arm. It's healed and that's the end of it. I'm scared to get the pain back, so I won't risk it."

Time to healing

Lack of a known time scale for healing is a common complaint from patients, leading to increased frustration, depression, and restricted ADLs by those with leg ulcers,[4,32, 44-47] pressure ulcers,[48] and other types of wounds. Krasner's[49] phenomenological study examined the impact of painful venous ulcers on HRqol and identified frustration as the major theme. In this study, patients suffering with leg ulcers from

2 months through 7 years reported their frustration as stemming from slow healing rates, lower limb swelling, infection, and the formation of new ulcers.[17,49] Other frustrations were related to years of multiple unsuccessful treatments, inadequacy of care from healthcare professionals, or self-blame for the lack of healing.[49]

Although many patients desire wound healing, there are others who use their wounds to get attention or continue healthcare benefits.[50,51] Although it's obvious that most patients desire wound healing, we would be remiss to not ask our patients about their specific goals in relation to their wounds. Wientjes[52] identifies four common behavioral attitudes exhibited by patients whose wounds heal:

- sets attainable goals (for example, to return to work, attend child's wedding)
- receptive to learning
- adherent with treatment
- curious; willingness to see the wound and actively participate in care.

As mentioned earlier, many patients are eager to strive for a goal of wound healing. However, according to Myss,[53] "assuming that everyone wants to heal is both misleading and potentially dangerous. Illness can, for instance, become a powerful way to get attention a patient might not otherwise receive." For some, there can be a manipulative value to keeping a wound, a figurative "street value or social currency." Defining oneself by the wound is an attitude described by Myss as "woundology."[53] For these patients, staying wounded provides benefits, such as continued nursing visits, Meals On Wheels,[53] home health aide services, an excuse to remain unemployed, and/or continued attention by family and healthcare professionals.[52]

ACUTE VERSUS CHRONIC

Some wounds heal quickly and uneventfully, whereas others are present for years or even a lifetime. But are these wounds similarly perceived by those afflicted? Do coping styles vary based on wound chronicity?

Expanding on the works of Parsons,[54] O'Flynn[55] postulates that following an acute minor wound event, the wound and its treatment become the immediate focus of the patient and his or her family. Viewing the wound as deviant, the patient is eclipsed by the wound and readily assumes the role of "sick person." Individual roles and responsibilities are overshadowed and interrupted (to an extent) by the patient's pain and incapacity.[55] During the healing and coping phase the individual continues to be the "patient." Once healing is achieved, however, the individual re-emerges, and normality is regained as good health and quality of life are restored.[55]

How a person reacts emotionally to a wound changes as the circumstances surrounding the wound differ. For example, trauma patients experience extreme emotions and employ various defense mechanisms, such as suppression, regression, denial, distraction, magical thinking, or rationalization.[56] According to Lenehan,[57] the severe injuries endured may open floodgates of suppressed, intense emotions and disturbed images of self. As a result, the patient may present with a rather shallow or blunted affect or "ego constriction" in an attempt to conserve psychological energy.[57] An inner battle occurs between anger, depression, and fear as the patient asks himself or herself, "Will I be treated differently?" and "Will anyone care for me in light of disability and disfigurement?"[57]

Conversely, Phillips et al.,[31] Price and Harding,[58] and Walshe[32] report that patients with chronic wounds cope with the impaired mobility, pain, and sleep disturbances by the process of normalization, by "putting on a brave face."[11] Coping with chronic wounds, according to Dewar and Morse,[59] is accomplished by adaptation, or the untenable process of silent acceptance. Interestingly, Price and Harding[58] found that those who suffered from venous leg ulcers longer than 24 months rated themselves as having less pain and better general health than those with ulcers of less than 24 months.

Neil and Munjas[2] conducted a phenomenological study of 10 patients with chronic non-healing wounds, in which two patterns and six themes emerged. The two identified patterns were contending with the wound and staying home or staying back.[2]

Contending with the wound includes four themes:

- being in pain

- contending with exudate and odor—issues that can cause significant distress, social isolation, and embarrassment
- losing sleep
- noticing; that is, the first time the patient noticed the wound wasn't improving, and other people noticing and caring for the wound.

The second constitutive pattern, staying home or staying back, includes the two themes of isolation and trouble walking. Isolation stems from the patient's fear of going out and acquiring infection and being housebound secondary to immobility (for example, having to stay in bed or with the affected leg elevated). Trouble walking stems from pain or loss of function secondary to the wound. For these participants "the wound becomes the focus of their lives as it makes them immobile or makes walking difficult."[2]

Contrary to other authors who described feelings of normalization among those with chronic wounds, Neil and Munjas[2] found that "chronic wound participants 'became their wound.' The wound is all encompassing. The participant constantly hopes that their wound will get better so that they can resume their former wound-free life. With each passing year, or if the wound worsens despite therapy, hope and compliance may fade."

Beitz[14] conducted a phenomenological study of 16 patients living with chronic wounds and reported similar findings as Neil and Munjas.[2] The themes identified were:

- adapting and maladapting
- altered sleeping habits
- changes in eating patterns
- contending with chronic illness
- dealing with the wound
- explaining causes of wounds
- healing and recuperating
- living and aging
- living with pain
- losing mobility
- meaning and significance of wound
- receiving care.

To better understand how a patient's HRqol is affected, what his or her goals are, and how we can best assist the patient, we must first gain insight into the meaning and significance that the wound holds for the patient. As one patient aptly states, "True understanding

doesn't occur unless we share our strengths, fears, and weakness."[1] Kinmond et al.'s[60] qualitative study examining the HRqol of 21 patients with diabetic foot ulcers identified four major themes:

- living a restricted life—wherein patients lose the freedom to live life as they did before. Mobility is decreased and schedules are now altered by clinic visits and dressing changes.
- existing in social isolation—resulting from restricted mobility, pain, and lack of employment.
- experiencing discredited definitions of self—an inability to shower or bathe, to select one's own shoe styles, to hold a job or even stand long enough to cook results in a deep and compounding loss of self.
- becoming a burden—dependence on others as one's mobility and finances become limited results in whole-family suffering.

Painful venous ulcers have been described as "the literal breakdown of the skin and the figurative breakdown of the embodied self."[61] Pressure ulcer formation has been described by family caregivers as an (unfortunately) normal thing to happen to the bedridden[10,62] and as "truly the worst thing that can happen" by those directly afflicted.[1]

As described in this section, the psychological effects of a wound are deeply ingrained in the patient as a whole. No matter whether the wound is acute or chronic, it is on the mind of the patient at all times. In other words, living with a chronic wound reshapes every aspect of one's life, leaving one subordinate to the wound, the associated pain and, with every dressing change, tension and worry as to how the wound will look … will it be deeper, infected, or gangrenous?[39,63]

IMPACT ON ACTIVITIES OF DAILY LIVING

Physical, somatic, financial, and medical restrictions can result in limitations on a patient's ability to engage in ADLs, further impacting the psychological and emotional ramifications of the wound experience. Hopkins and colleagues[64] describe how pressure ulcers can produce such a restricted life. In their phenomenological study, patients' described how pain from the wound restricted their desire to move and turn or reposition themselves.[64] Similarly, Gorecki and colleagues[65] found that pressure ulcers imposed physical restrictions, lifestyle changes, need for environmental adaptations, intrusive treatments and hospitalizations, and physical dependence contributing to a loss of appetite, insomnia, and a lack of interest in life engagement.

COPING PATTERNS

Breaches in the skin, as with other types of loss, can elicit the process of grieving. Although most patients transcend the continuum from denial, depression, anger, and bargaining to ultimate acceptance, some may become frozen at a certain point or even exhibit regressional behavior about their wound. Walshe,[32] in a phenomenological study examining what it's like to live with a venous leg ulcer from the elderly patient's perspective, identifies four major coping strategies.

- Coping by comparison—by comparing himself or herself with others who have ulcerations, the patient experiences normalization; by comparing himself or herself with patients who have other illnesses (such as stroke), the patient feels more fortunate.
- Feeling healthy—despite the leg ulcerations and the associated debilitating symptoms and restrictions, the patient feels otherwise healthy.
- Altering expectation—the patient reports having reached a point of acceptance, viewing the ulcer as a part of the aging process.
- Being positive—the patient describes himself or herself as lucky and dismisses the symptoms as "not bad at all."[32]

SPIRITUALITY

The power of prayer, hope, and support of a patient's religious beliefs can't be underestimated in providing emotional strength.

SOCIAL SUPPORTS

Many patients with wounds feel pushed to the "side-lines,"[27] seeing a shrinking of their social circle as pain, fears, and physical restrictions increase. The patient with a wound may experience guilt about friends having to change their activities to accommodate his or her limitations and may therefore further limit social interaction.[26] As discussed earlier, malodor, leakage, and wound visibility may also result in decreased social contact. Some patients are over-reliant on a single caregiver, usually a spouse, for physical, emotional, and psychological strength.

Hopkins et al.[64] studied the impact of pressure ulcers not only on the patient but also on the caregiver and found feelings to be conflicted. These feelings were expressed as the burden that the pressure ulcer, and its associated care, places on the caregiver, as well as the feelings of uselessness on the part of the patient receiving the care. Conversely, however, several patients commented that without family, friends and support groups, things would be worse.[64,66] As one patient with a chronic venous ulcer stated, "I used to have lots of friends, was friendly with all the neighbors. Some of them wave at me when they pass my window, but they don't knock or come to see me anymore."[11]

AGE

It appears that age may play a role in wound psychology as well, with younger age having a greater adverse effect on the wound patient's psychological state of mind. For instance, Phillips et al.[31] found that younger patients exhibited greater negativity related to their leg ulcers and greater problems with mobility ($p < 0.001$) than did older patients. Older patients proved more effective in coping with or adapting to their limitations and disability.[31] Franks and Moffatt [67] reported similar findings.

In a cross-sectional study using the Nottingham Health Profile and age- and sex-matched normal scores of 758 patients with leg ulcers, younger males were found to experience the greatest negative impact on HRqol.[68] Among those with diabetes and lower-extremity ulcers, Brod[26] reported that older patients were less affected in the social, employment, and familial arenas. Conversely, in a study measuring HRqol in 63 patients with chronic leg ulcers, age wasn't a statistically significant factor.[58]

GENDER

There's great debate in the literature as to the impact of gender on HRqol in those with wounds. Lindholm et al.[68] report that males have significantly poorer HRqol than females in the areas of pain and physical mobility. Additionally, when compared with the normative scores for males in the areas of sleep disturbance, emotional reaction, and social isolation, males with leg ulcers exhibited increased scores.[68] Price and Harding[58] found poorer HRqol scores in women in the domains of vitality and physical and social functioning. A database of 758 patients with leg ulcers similarly reports women to have a poorer HRqol than males.[24]

But, as Franks and Moffatt[67] point out, in studies of the general population, women score worse on HRqol than males, especially in older age groups. Therefore, the poorer scores among women with leg ulcers may not be related directly to the ulcer.

Social interaction

Limitations in social interactions among those with wounds may stem from the following:

- impaired mobility secondary to pain, causing many patients to become essentially housebound[4,11,32,33,60,64,65,69]
- inability to shower or take baths in order to keep dressings dry[16,28,60,69]
- treatment restrictions, such as the need to stay on bed rest for pressure ulcer management[48,65,70,71]; leg elevation for edema control; and the need to be homebound to receive skilled home care nursing services
- need for an isolation room secondary to neutropenia or multi-drug resistant infection, resulting in increased feelings of loneliness, powerlessness, and social abandonment[71]
- having to schedule "life" around dressing changes and clinic and home care visits[60,72]
- avoidance of social activities where crowds, children, or pets might be encountered, out of fear of injuring the wound site or creating new ulcers[4,32]
- fatigue from disrupted sleep and adverse effects of antibiotics[33,48]
- embarrassment from odor,[64,65,73,74] leakage,[28,42,69,74] and wound visibility

- need to rely on others and assistive devices[22]
- fear of others' response to wounds, orthotic shoes, and bulky dressings[72]
- additional time required to perform dressing changes[4,26]
- difficulty maintaining appearance because shoes and clothing no longer fit over bulky dressings[4,28,33,35,72,75]
- a loss of power and self in selecting the clothes and shoes one wants to wear.[24,28,33,35,72,75]

Patients with wounds may be forced to make significant life changes and find satisfaction in new activities.[61] The ability to participate in such activities as enjoying a sauna, bicycling, running, swimming, or tennis is eliminated because of bulky dressings and compression wraps.

Although healthcare professionals encourage and recognize the value of social interaction to a patient's psychological and emotional function, do we not simultaneously blame patients or label them as nonadherent when they come to our offices with worsening of their edema and deterioration of their leg and foot ulcers secondary to being out and trying to enjoy life? Health-related behaviors need to be considered from the patient's perspective, with the healthcare professional promoting patient empowerment. Adherence requires a partnership between the patient, clinician, and family/significant other.[73]

> ## ► PRACTICE POINT
>
> As healthcare professionals, we must not only acknowledge, but also creatively work with the patient in the challenge of balancing physical wound healing with psychological and emotional healing.

Listen to the words of a patient describing the difficulties of maintaining bed rest to heal his pressure ulcer: "I can remember lying in the hospital ... looking at the paint on the wall. And I could tell you how many little bubbles were in that particular spot.

I memorized them to keep from going mad."[11,48] Another patient with a chronic venous ulcer painfully described his social disconnectedness: "I feel like an island in the middle of a ocean."[11]

Somatic sensation

According to Schipper et al.,[25] the domain of somatic sensation "encompasses unpleasant physical feelings that may detract from someone's quality of life, such as pain." Regardless of the underlying cause of pain, it's one of the most feared sensations in life[76,77] and is the most compelling reason that individuals seek out health care.[78] And, although the threshold of pain varies from patient to patient, making it undeniably subjective, it's an area that's too often neglected in wound care.[78,79]

The devastating impact of painful wounds on all aspects of a patient's HRqol has been the subject of recent numerous studies,[2,11,16,24,28,31,32,34,48,49,61,64,76,77] although incorporation of findings into clinical practice has been slow to follow.

Patients have described pain as the worst thing about having a leg ulcer,[11,16,28,32,69,77,80] with the "first daily act of weight bearing as the most severe pain they experience."[80] The unrelenting, unpredictable nature of the pain frequently makes patients feel as though they aren't in control,[32] but rather the ulcer and its manifestations rule them.[46,63] Leg elevation often makes the burning, stabbing, drilling, throbbing pain worse.[81] Sleep is frequently disrupted by pain,[11,16,28,80] and pain medication is often ineffective.[32] Among those with venous ulcers, pain is often described in three distinct locations: within the ulcer, around the ulcer, and elsewhere in the leg.[80] Additionally, pain for many is felt to be an early warning sign of new ulcers forming or of impending infection.[13]

Krasner's[61] qualitative phenomenological study of 14 patients with painful venous ulcers identifies eight key themes. (See *Painful venous leg ulcers: Key themes*, page 12.)

Participants in Krasner's[61] study vividly described the pain as "the worst thing I have ever gone through in my life" … "like someone is sticking pins in you all the time" … "absolute murder." Pain was described as even worse when the leg was more edematous and during infection. Pain during and after debridement was considered the most intense pain experienced by patients, bringing on a cycle of pain and fear that left many depressed. In a phenomenological study by Langemo et al.,[48] pain is described as "getting a knife and really digging in there good and hard" and "stinging." Yet despite the pain, suffering, and limitations brought on by these ulcers, patients tried to view the pain as an expected (albeit unwanted) occurrence and to "carry on despite the pain."[61]

The duration of pain is also described as an issue most of the time, even during and after closure.[48,70] Indeed, in a Heideggenan phenomenological pilot study, Hopkins et al.[64] found endless pain to be one of the three major themes in their sample of eight pressure ulcer patients. Likewise, among 32 patients with stage III and IV pressure ulcers, Szor and Bourguignon[82] found that 88% experienced pain with dressing changes, although dressings used were consistent with principles of moist healing. Furthermore, 84% of the participants reported pain at rest, and 18% described the pain as horrible or excruciating.[82] In the words of patients, pressure ulcer pain is described as throbbing, burning, unbearable, never-ending, interfering with sleep and making it difficult to find a comfortable position.[65] Among patients with granulating postoperative pilonidal cyst excision and abdominal wounds, Price and colleagues[83] described pain as negatively impacting patients' sleeping patterns and appetite.

Despite the prevalence and intensity of pain among those with wounds, however, Roe et al.[84] found that 55% of community nurses don't include pain as a part of their assessment. Ayello and colleagues[85] found that among patients with chronic wounds in an outpatient clinic, those with pressure ulcers were least likely to be assessed for pain as compared with patients with vascular or neuropathic ulcers. Walshe[32] and Hollinworth and Collier[86] report that patients' descriptions of pain are often devalued and dismissed. In studies by Hollinworth[87] and Dallam et al.,[76] pain medications were seldom administered to manage pain associated with dressing changes, despite the fact that 81% of registered nurses report that patients experience the most pain with dressing changes.[84]

Painful venous leg ulcers: Key themes

Krasner[61] identifies eight key themes in patients with painful venous leg ulcers:

- Being unable to stand
- Expecting pain with the ulcer
- Experiencing pain caused by swelling
- Feeling frustrated
- Having to make life changes
- Interfering with the job
- Starting the pain all over again with painful debridements
- Trying to find satisfaction in new activities

Similarly, Szor and Bourguignon[82] reported that a mere 6% of patients received medication for pressure ulcer pain.

Among patients with diabetic foot ulcers, Ashford and colleagues[30] found that 50% of patients experienced pain during dressing changes, when supine, and during ambulation attempts. However, Ribu et al.[27] found that patients with diabetic foot ulcers fear analgesic dependency.

In their study of 32 patients with a history of intravenous drug abuse and chronic venous ulcers, Pieper and colleagues[88] found that those with larger wounds reported a significantly higher pain intensity than those with smaller wounds.

In patients with malignant fungating wounds, pain was related to nerve or blood vessel damage, exposed dermal nerve endings, or nerve damage resulting in neuropathic pain.[41]

In an attempt to capture nurses' stories about coping with patients' pressure ulcer pain, Krasner[38] conducted a phenomenological study of 42 nurses, identifying three patterns and eight themes:

- Nursing expertly includes the ability to recognize, validate, attend to, acknowledge, and caringly empathize with the patient in pain.
- Denying the pain includes assuming it doesn't exist or failing to hear the patient's complaints or cries. This was described as an effective coping mechanism for healthcare professionals, assisting them in avoiding feelings of failure but obviously at severe detriment to the patient.
- Confronting the challenge of pain occurs when the healthcare professional must come to terms with his or her own feelings of frustration. Negative feelings associated with wound care include anger, helplessness, hopelessness, being upset about performing a procedure that will cause pain, and experiencing pain along with the patient. Perhaps we must, as Krasner[38] states, "take a step back and make a special effort to understand the nearness of the near." By "being with" the patient we may gain insight into the meaning that the pain experience holds for the patient.[38]

Leg ulcer clinics may have a positive impact on HRqol. For example, in a study of 57 patients, of whom 88% had pain at baseline, after 8 weeks of four-layer compression therapy only 60% still had pain.[89] Even more significantly, in another sample of 185 patients with 78% reporting pain prior to entering a community leg ulcer clinic, after 12 weeks of four-layer compression therapy this dropped to 22%.[90]

Financial impact

Time lost from work, missed career opportunities, decreased productivity on the job secondary to pain, early retirement, lost wages, and loss of a job are just a few of the financial stressors affecting the HRqol of the patient with a wound. Too often, patients are faced with having to choose between adherence to medical management (such as keeping one's leg elevated or remaining non-weight bearing) and keeping their job. How does a truck driver, a cashier, or a healthcare professional keep his or her leg elevated and still perform the job? How do wound patients pay their mortgages, pay the bills, and feed their families? What happens when a wound patient loses healthcare coverage after losing his or her job? According to Charles,[12] the financial sequelae of a chronic wound is the societal inheritance of a person who was a positive contributor to one who becomes dependent upon it.

Beyond occupational stressors and dilemmas, patients may also incur additional out-of-pocket expenses for transportation, parking, telephone bills for medical follow-up, home health aide services, dressing supplies not covered by insurance, and drug costs if they have no prescription plan. Those who have no insurance but don't qualify for public assistance may be forced to tap into their savings or refinance their homes. To illustrate this point, listen to the words of wives caring for their bedridden husbands with full-thickness pressure ulcers.

"... all these medical supplies you need to treat these bedsores. I think in the past 2 months, I've spent close to $300 out of my pocket and you're on a fixed income." ... "Thirty-five dollars per month for the hospital bed and $10 for the chair. I paid with our Social Security checks and his pension. Also there were bills and food ... not much was left ... He had a pension and I used to put that aside and we had to live on my Social Security which was $302."[10,62] Concerns about finances may be linked to the healthcare insurance system in the patient's country. For example, finances were not raised as an issue for the European pressure ulcer study by Hopkins et al.[64]

Additional expenses may also be incurred for home modifications, such as wheelchair ramps. Patients with diabetic foot ulcers face the ongoing challenge of affording correctly fitted footwear as their feet are constantly undergoing change with episodes of edema related to diuretics, infection, and the amount of dressing material required. Healthcare professionals, rather than simply dismissing patients as nonadherent, should show empathy toward their patients with regard to these important issues by acknowledging the access and financial hardships faced by patients and their partners.[2,27]

ETHICAL DILEMMAS IN WOUND CARE

No other wound type is fraught with as much ethical dispute as pressure ulcers. Despite major technological breakthroughs in wound healing, the area of pressure ulceration continues to be the "scarlet letter of poor care."[10,62] Pressure ulcers are considered an individual and institutional embarrassment, a point of frustration, failure, and a marker of inferior care

rendered.[10,62] Great expense is incurred in "hiding the ulcer." As Moss and La Puma[91] state, "to hide ugly aesthetics and to unknowingly deny the conditions that contribute to pressure ulcer development, our clinical response may be to cover up or remove the sore, using dressings, skin grafts, myocutaneous flaps, disarticulations, amputations, and hemicorporectomies." But what right do we have as healthcare providers to make such decisions? What gives us the right to exhaust our patients' finances and subject them and their families to spending their lives undergoing aggressive procedures? Decisions for care, and the degree of aggressiveness or lack thereof, must be consistent with the patient's overall physiological status, as well as the patient's and family's "goals of restoration, of function, prolongation of life, or only provision of comfort."[92] It's important to remember that HRqol is the *patient's* perception of well-being, not your opinion of the patient's clinical status.[22] According to Brown,[11] "...until the alleviation of distressing symptoms such as pain and odor with resultant QOL for the patient are formally acknowledged as clinical outcomes, healthcare professionals may continue to pay lip-service to the concept of holistic care." Finding out what the patient wants and what his or her goals are is paramount.[93] Acknowledging this, clinicians must partner with patients and their families in making short- and long-term treatment decisions, regardless of wound etiology. According to Beitz,[94] quality wound care is defined by:

- doing the right things right, which may seem basic but is influenced by multiple variables
- the legal community (inadvertently)
- practice guidelines and standards of care designed by healthcare providers
- the person receiving it and the person perceiving it.

Using general systems theory, Beitz[94] suggests that barriers to quality wound care fall into three general levels: individual, group, and societal.

Individual barriers

Individual barriers to quality wound care include:

- deleterious lifestyle habits, such as drug use, homelessness, or lack of attention to skin hygiene

- fiscal restraints, such as limited healthcare coverage and limited savings
- lack of knowledge regarding preventive measures[94]
- poor health accountability, such as smoking, abusing alcohol, and overeating.

Group barriers

Group barriers to quality wound care include:

- fiscal restraints, resulting in limited home care visits and reimbursement under prospective payment, leading to increased demands placed on family members
- inadequate knowledge of basic wound care on the part of the caregiver
- lack of meaningful organizational partnerships (Although seamless delivery of health care is desired, continuity from acute care to long-term care and home care remains inadequate.)
- lack of well-disseminated, valid wound care guidelines, algorithms, and decision trees[94]
- poor quality improvement processes, wherein data may be collected but outcomes are inadequately analyzed and acted upon.

Societal barriers

Societal barriers to quality wound care include:

- fiscal restraints[95]
- lack of focus on population-based outcomes (An outcomes-based perspective is critical in a fiscally restrained environment. Considering that chronic wounds in some patients won't heal, appropriate goals should be identified and an ethical rationing of resources established.)
- lack of national wound care benchmarks
- national nursing and faculty shortage.

Possible solutions

Systemic solutions to the delivery of cost-efficient, effective chronic wound care as identified by Beitz[94] include:

- access to innovative electronic communication, such as telehealth, image transmissions, less expensive video conferencing, and timely consultation with distant caregivers
- acknowledgement that increasing wound care–related litigation should serve as a

much needed impetus for securing funding for prevention, improved communication, and protocol development
- alternate sites of care such as mobile wound care units
- establishment of a sense of "collective worry" and concern by healthcare professionals, patients, family caregivers, and legislatures regarding chronic wound care and the resources consumed
- healthcare renaissance, which focuses on collaboration and a trans-disciplinary approach to disease prevention and health promotion[94]
- innovative wound care treatments
- new perspective on health, which focuses on promotion and disease prevention
- partnerships between businesses, industry, health care, and academia
- recognition of limited resources
- use of alternative healthcare providers possessing the critical combination of population-based thinking, outcomes assessment, and educational and fiscal abilities.

TRANSITIONING TO HEALTH PROMOTION

In a climate of decreased hospital stays, managed care, and prospective payment with decreased allowances for home visits and supplies, moral and ethical conflicts for community healthcare nurses abound.[95] In fact, community healthcare nurses' focus has had to change from disease prevention and health promotion to the provision of acute care.[95] Documentation of care, limited visits, supply purchasing, and whether the wound care prognosis will better focus on long-term management or short-term cure are ethical concerns and financial realities faced by community care nurses on a daily basis.[95] Community-based ethical concerns in wound care include[95]:

- What kind of wound care is most safe, efficacious, and cost-effective?
- What kind of wound care can be performed at home by trained family members?
- What is the most cost-effective source of wound care supplies?

The new economy is forcing autonomy on vulnerable and often frail elderly patients and family members as never before.[95] Too often, patients and family caregivers are quickly labeled as nonadherent without regard to underlying issues such as[95]:

- confusion over what supplies are needed from medical supply companies
- lack of knowledge
- lack of money to pay for costly drugs, supplies, transportation, office-visit co-pays, and insurance deductibles
- lack of sufficient hospital discharge planning.

In a time of limited healthcare dollars, which patients have access to all available resources, regardless of cost, to close their chronic or complex wounds? We're already seeing the ramifications of the "healthcare cost blindness" described by Bell,[95] where if too much money is spent on some patients' supplies, money will ultimately not be available for others. Will only those with financial means, youth, better health, and more quantifiable productive years be the limited recipients? What choices will be available for elderly patients, those with chronic diseases, and those receiving palliative care? Who will provide care, for how long, and with what resources? Will patients' and their families' concerns, choices, and wishes be heard and acknowledged? For many practitioners the only desirable outcome may be complete healing with best practice being measured against published healing benchmarks, even when healability may not be achievable.[11] Providers must consistently and openly consider the impact of treatment recommendations on patients' overall QOL.[28]

In caring for patients with wounds, a strong patient–provider relationship is critical.[96] Patients want to be seen, to be heard, and to be known.[96] According to Scherwitz and colleagues,[96] the two essential components to healing are the relational joining between a provider devoted to healing and to the patient and the fostering of patients' rights to make choices throughout the healing process.

ISSUES AND CHALLENGES FOR CAREGIVERS

For the family member, the only prerequisite to becoming a caregiver is willingness to take on the role. However, most often, family members are untrained and unprepared for this role.[10,62] Along with the patient, family caregivers also have to deal with their own varying levels of grief. Caregivers' grief is further affected by the patient's overall status, the circumstances leading to the wounded state, and the patient's response to the wound. They also deal with the increased stress and strain of family tension and receive the brunt of the patient's anger and frustration.[26]

As the patient struggles with fears of burdening others, social isolation, loss of control and independence, possible disfigurement, and rejection, the caregiver also struggles. Fears commonly voiced by family caregivers include damaging the wound from a lack of knowledge; development of new wounds; wound recurrence; need for amputation, rehospitalization, emergency room visits, or surgery; disfigurement; reaction of others; possible disability; and fear that the wound may never heal.

Spouses may sleep apart out of fear of dislodging IV lines and wound drainage tubes.[97] Living rooms, dining rooms, and bedrooms may become filled with boxes of antibiotics, IV equipment, and wound dressing supplies, serving as constant reminders of the patient's and family's wounded state, uncertain future, and dwindling resources.[97] The privacy once enjoyed by families is now visibly shaken with visits by medical supply representatives, home care nurses, and possibly care aides.[97]

A recurring fear among caregivers is that they themselves might become ill or disabled and unable to provide care.[10,26,62] Family caregivers are often dealing with disrupted sleep secondary to worrying about the patient and responding to the patient's restlessness.[10,26,62] A general lack of attention to their own health, progressive fatigue, decreased appetite, and decreased nutritional intake may occur as all attention is focused on the patient.[10,26,62]

Caregivers often find their social circle decreasing as they spend increased time providing care.[26] Even time taken for respite may be fraught with feelings of guilt. Emotionally, caregivers may experience deep feelings of fear and loss—fear of losing their loved one, fear of losing the relationship and, possibly, death—as they witness a loved one's bedridden or increasingly debilitated state. Reminiscing about how things used to be may be all that some caregivers have to pull them through. Elderly caregiving spouses usually pursue nursing home placement only as a last resort, holding true to their vows of "till death do us part."[10,62]

Family caregivers also experience financial struggles owing to increased out-of-pocket expenses, decreased productivity in the workplace, unpaid days off due to used vacation and personal time, forced early retirement, and potential job loss.[26] Among elderly caregivers, frustration and confusion regarding reimbursement for needed wound care supplies and drugs and the inability to afford private help in the home are compounded by their meager funds from Social Security and pension checks.[26] In separate qualitative studies by Baharestani[10,62] and Douglas,[16] caregivers voiced the following needs:

• to be able to ask questions of healthcare providers
• to be heard nonjudgmentally
• to have their caregiving role recognized
• to receive information/education in an understandable manner
• to receive support.

SUMMARY

Having a wound or caring for a loved one with a wound can affect multiple facets of a patient's life, possibly unleashing unprecedented fears and vulnerabilities.

In each patient and family caregiver encounter, we as healthcare professionals should ask ourselves, "Do we care enough about the patient's perspective to bear the costs involved to ensure that each person feels that he or she is being treated as a person?"[98] and "Do our actions show that we care?" It is our job as healthcare professionals to care for the whole patient, including the psychological, emotional, and financial issues related to his or her wound care.

PRACTICE POINT

If we as healthcare professionals are to help our patients with wounds and their family caregivers, we need to "... stay connected with our patients; listen, attend ("be with") and comfort; and use a gentler hand."[38]

SHOW WHAT YOU KNOW

1. Those afflicted with wounds are often viewed as:
   A. pleasant and comfortable.
   B. pain-free.
   C. appalling and repulsive.
   D. attractive.

   ANSWER: C. *Those with wounds are often viewed as appalling and repulsive.*

2. Which of the following is one of the four domains of quality of life as identified by Schipper et al.[25]?
   A. Pain-free
   B. Financial freedom
   C. Religious expression
   D. Somatic sensation

   ANSWER: D. *In addition to physical and occupational function, psychological state, and social interaction, somatic sensation is identified as a domain of quality of life.*

3. Wound assessment is commonly lacking in the area of:
A. size.
B. odor.
C. drainage.
D. pain.

ANSWER: D. *Assessment of pain is commonly lacking in wound assessment; size, odor, and drainage are usually assessed.*

4. Quality of life treatment decisions should be based on the:
A. patient's perception of well-being.
B. nurses' perceptions of well-being.
C. family's perception of well-being.
D. physicians' perceptions of well-being.

ANSWER: A. *The patient's perceptions of well-being should direct quality of life treatment decisions.*

REFERENCES

1. van Rijswijk, L., and Gottlieb, D. "Like a Terrorist," *Ostomy/Wound Management* 46(5):25-6, 2000.
2. Neil, J.A., and Munjas, B.A. "Living with a Chronic Wound: The Voices of Sufferers," *Ostomy/Wound Management* 46(5):28-38, 2000.
3. Harding, K. "Complete Patient Care," *Journal of Wound Care* 4(6):253, 1995.
4. Hyland, M.E., et al. "Quality of Life of Leg Ulcer Patients: Questionnaire and Preliminary Findings," *Journal of Wound Care* 3(6):294-298, 1994.
5. van Rijswijk, L. "The Language of Wounds," in *Chronic Wound Care: A Clinical Sourcebook for Health Care Professionals,* 4th ed. Edited by Krasner, D.L., et al. Malvern, PA: HMP Communications, 2007.
6. Husband, L.L. "Venous Ulceration: The Pattern of Pain and the Paradox," *Clinical Effectiveness in Nursing* 5:35-40, 2001.
7. Anderson, R.C., and Maksud, D.P. "Psychological Adjustments to Reconstructive Surgery," *Nursing Clinics of North America* 29(4):711-24, 1994.
8. Faugier, J. "On Being Wounded," *Senior Nurse* 8(1):18, 1988.
9. Hopkins, S. "Psychological Aspect of Wound Healing," *Nursing Times Plus* 97(48):57-8, 2001.
10. Baharestani, M.M. "The Lived Experience of Wives Caring for their Frail, Home-bound, Elderly Husbands with Pressure Ulcers," *Advances in Wound Care* 7(3):40-52, 1994.
11. Brown, A. "Chronic Leg Ulcers, Part 2: Do They Affect a Patient's Social Life?" *British Journal of Nursing* 14(18):986-89, 2005.
12. Charles, H. "Living With a Leg Ulcer," *Journal of Community Nursing* 9(7):22-24, 1995.
13. Hyde, C., et al. "Older Women's Experience of Living with Chronic Leg Ulceration," *International Journal of Nursing Practice* 5(4):189-98, 1999.
14. Beitz, J.M. "The Lived Experience of Having a Chronic Wound: A Phenomenological Study," *Dermatology Nursing* 17(4):272-305, 2005.
15. Hollinworth, H., and Hawkins J. "Teaching Nurses Psychological Support of Patients with Wounds," *British Journal of Nursing* 11(20):S8-18, 2002.
16. Douglas, V. "Living with a Chronic Leg Ulcer: An Insight Into Patient's Experiences and Feelings," *Journal of Wound Care* 10(9):355-360, 2001.
17. Knudson-Cooper, M. "Adjustment to Visible Stigma: The Case of the Severely Burned," *Social Science Medicine* 15B:31, 1981.
18. Wallace, L., and Lees, J. "A Psychological Follow-up Study of Adult Patients Discharged from a British Burns Unit," *Burns* 14:39, 1988.
19. Partridge, J. "The Psychological Effects of Facial Disfigurement," *Journal of Wound Care* 2:168-71, May 1993.
20. Bernstein, N. *Emotional Care of the Facially Disfigured.* Boston: Little, Brown & Co., 1976.
21. Campbell, A., et al. *The Quality of American Life: Perceptions, Evaluations and Satisfaction.* New York: Russell Sage, 1976.
22. Price, P. "Quality of Life," in *Chronic Wound Care: A Clinical Source Book for Health Care Professionals*, 3rd ed. Edited by Krasner, D.L., et al. Wayne, PA: HMP Communications, 2001.
23. Price, P. "Defining and Measuring Quality of Life," *Journal of Wound Care* 5(3):139-40, March 1996.
24. Franks, P.J., and Moffatt, C.J. "Quality of Life Issues in Patients with Chronic Wounds,"

Wounds 10(suppl E):1E-11E, September-October 1998.

25. Schipper, H., et al. "Quality of Life Studies: Definitions and Conceptual Issues," in *Quality of Life and Pharmacoeconomics in Clinical Trials,* 2nd ed. Edited by Spilker, B. Philadelphia: Lippincott-Raven, 1996.

26. Brod, M. "Quality of Life Issues in Patients with Diabetes and Lower Extremity Ulcers: Patients and Caregivers," *Quality of Life Research* 7(4):365-72, May 1998.

27. Ribu L., et al. "Living with a Diabetic Foot Ulcer: A Life of Fear, Restrictions and Pain," *Ostomy/Wound Management* 50(2):57-67, 2004.

28. Persoon, A., et al. "Leg Ulcers: A Review of Their Impact on Daily Life," *Journal of Clinical Nursing* 13(3):341-54, 2004.

29. Meijer, J.W.G., et al. "Quality of Life in Patients with Diabetic Foot Ulcers," *Disability & Rehabilitation* 23(8):336-40, 2001.

30. Ashford R.L., et al. "Perception of quality of life by patients with diabetic foot ulcers," *The Diabetic Foot* 3(4):150-55, 2000.

31. Phillips, T., et al. "A Study of the Impact of Leg Ulcers on Quality of Life: Financial, Social and Psychological Implications," *Journal of the American Academy of Dermatology* 31(1):49-53, 1994.

32. Walshe, C. "Living with a Venous Leg Ulcer: A Descriptive Study of Patients' Experiences," *Journal of Advanced Nursing* 22(6):1092-100, 1995.

33. Roe, B., et al. "Patient's Perceptions of Chronic Leg Ulcers," in *Leg Ulcers: Nursing Management: A Research Based Guide.* Edited by Cullum, N., and Roe, B. Harrow, UK: Scutari Press, 1995.

34. Morton-Fagervik, H., and Price, P. "Chronic Ulcers and Everyday Living: Patient's Perspective in the United Kingdom," *Wounds* 21(12):318-23, 2009.

35. Goodridge, D., Trepman, E., and Embil, J.M. "Health-Related Quality of Life in Diabetic Patients with Foot Ulcers," *Journal of Wound, Ostomy, & Continence Nursing* 32(6):368-376, 2005.

36. Magnan, M.A. "Psychological Considerations for Patients with Acute Wounds," *Critical Care Nursing Clinics of North America* 8(2):183-93, 1996.

37. Chase, S.K., Melloni, M., and Savage, A. "Forever Healing: The Lived Experience of Venous Ulcer Disease," *Journal of Vascular Nursing* 15(2):73-7, 1997.

38. Krasner, D. "Using a Gentler Hand: Reflections on Patients with Pressure Ulcers Who Experience Pain," *Ostomy/Wound Management* 42(3):20-9, 1996.

39. Bland, M. "Challenging the Myths: The Lived Experience of Chronic Leg Ulcer," *Nursing Praxis in New Zealand* 10(1):73-8, 1995.

40. Price, E. "The stigma of smell," *Nursing Times* 92(20):70,72, 1996.

41. Naylor, W.A. "A Guide to Wound Management in Palliative Care," *International Journal of Palliative Nursing* 11(11):572-79, 2005.

42. Benbow, M. "Exploring Wound Management and Measuring Quality of Life," *Journal of Clinical Nursing* 22(6):14-18, 2008.

43. Flett, R., Harcourt, B., and Alpass, F. "Psychosocial Aspects of Chronic Lower Leg Ulceration in the Elderly," *Western Journal of Nursing Research* 16(2):183-92, 1994.

44. Renner, R., et al. "Changes in Quality of Life for Patients with Chronic Venous Insufficiency, Present or Healed Leg Ulcers," *JDDG* 29:339-352, 2009.

45. Morgan, P., et al. "Illness Behavior and Social Support in Patients with Chronic Venous Ulcers." *Ostomy/Wound Management* 50(1):25-32, 2004.

46. Rich, A., and McLachlan, L. "How Living with a Leg Ulcer Affects People's Daily Life: A Nurse-led Study," *Journal of Wound Care* 12(2):51-4, 2003.

47. Neil, J.A. "The Stigma Scale: Measuring Body Image and the Skin," *Dermatology Nursing* 12(1):32-6, 2000.

48. Langemo, D.K., et al. "The Lived Experience of Having a Pressure Ulcer: A Qualitative Analysis," *Advances in Skin & Wound Care* 13(5):225-35, September/October 2000.

49. Krasner, D. "Painful Venous Ulcers: Themes and Stories about Their Impact on Quality of Life," *Ostomy/Wound Management* 44(9):38-49, September 1998.

50. Wise, G. "The Social Ulcer," *Nursing Times* 82(21):47-9, 1986.

51. Augustin, M., and Maier, K. "Psychosomatic Aspects of Chronic Wounds," *Dermatology and Psychosomatics* 4:5-13, 2003.

52. Wientjes, K.A. "Mind-body Techniques in Wound Healing," *Ostomy/Wound Management* 48(11):62-7, November 2002.

53. Myss, C. *Why People Don't Heal and How They Can.* New York: Three Rivers Press, 1997.

54. Parsons, T. "The Sick Role and the Role of the Physician Reconsidered," *MMFQ/Health & Society* 53(3):257-78, Summer 1975.

55. O'Flynn, L. "The Impact of Minor Acute Wounds on Quality of Life," *Journal of Wound Care* 9(7):337-40, July 2000.

56. Schnaper, N. "The Psychological Implications of Severe Trauma: Emotional Sequelae to Unconsciousness," *Journal of Trauma* 15(2):94-98, February 1975.

57. Lenehan, G.P. "Emotional Impact of Trauma," *Nursing Clinics of North America* 21(4):729-40, December 1986.

58. Price, P., and Harding, K. "Measuring Health-related Quality of Life in Patients with Chronic Leg Ulcers," *Wounds* 8(3):91-4, May-June 1996.

59. Dewar, A.L., and Morse, J.M. "Unbearable Incidents: Failure to Endure the Experience of Illness," *Journal of Advanced Nursing* 22(5):957-64, November 1995.

60. Kinmond, K., et al. "Loss of Self: A Psychosocial Study of the Quality of Life of Adults with Diabetic Foot Ulceration," *Journal of Tissue Viability* 13(1):6-16, 2003.

61. Krasner, D. "Painful Venous Ulcers: Themes and Stories about Living with the Pain and Suffering," *Journal of Wound, Ostomy, and Continence Nursing* 25(3):158-68, May 1998.

62. Baharestani, M.M. "The Lived Experience of Wives Caring for Their Homebound Elderly Husbands with Pressure Ulcers: A Phenomenological Investigation" (doctoral dissertation, Adelphi University, 1993). Dissertation Abstracts International (No. 9416018), 1993.

63. Ebbeskog, B., and Eckman, S.L. "Elderly Person's Experience of Living with Venous Leg Ulcers: Living in a Dialectal Relationship Between Freedom and Imprisonment," *Scandanavian Journal of Caring Science* 15:235-43, 2001.

64. Hopkins, A., et al. "Patient Stories of Living with a Pressure Ulcer," *Journal of Advanced Nursing* 56(4)345-53, November 2006.

65. Gorecki, C., et al. "Impact of Pressure Ulcers on Quality of Life in Older Patients: A Systematic Review," *Journal of the American Geriatrics Society* 57(7):1175-83, 2009.

66. Edwards, H., et al. "A Randomized Controlled Trial of a Community Nursing Intervention: Improved Quality of Life and Healing for Clients With Chronic Leg Ulcers," *Journal of Clinical Nursing* 18:1541-49, 2009.

67. Franks, P.J., and Moffatt, C.J. "Who Suffers Most from Leg Ulceration?" *Journal of Wound Care* 7(8):383-85, 1998.

68. Lindholm, C., et al. "Quality of Life in Chronic Leg Ulcer Patients," *Acta Dermato-Venereologica* 73(6):440-43, December 1993.

69. Jones, J., et al. "Depression in Patients with Chronic Venous Ulceration," *Tissue Viability* 15(11):S17-S23, 2006.

70. Fox, C. "Living with a Pressure Ulcer: A Descriptive Study of Patient's Experiences," *Wound Care* 7(6 Suppl):10-22, 2002.

71. Laurent, C. "Beating Bedtime Blues," *Nursing Times* 95(11):61-64, 1999.

72. Foster, A. "Psychological Aspects of Treating the Diabetic Foot," *Practical Diabetes International* 14(2):56-58, 1997.

73. Snyder, R.J. "Venous Leg Ulcers in the Elderly Patient: Associated Stress, Social Support, and Coping," *Ostomy Wound Management* 52(9):58-68, 2006.

74. Hareendran, A., et al. "Measuring the Impact of Venous Leg Ulcers on Quality of Life," *Journal of Wound Care* 14(2):53-57, 2005.

75. Goodridge, D., et al., "Quality of Life of Adults with Unhealed and Healed Diabetic Foot Ulcers," *Foot & Ankle International* 27:274-80, 2006.

76. Dallam, L., et al. "Pressure Ulcer Pain: Assessment and Quantification," *Journal of Wound, Ostomy, and Continence Nursing* 22(5):211-18, September 1995.

77. Hamer, C., and Cullum, N.A. "Patients' Perceptions of Chronic Leg Ulcers," *Journal of Wound Care* 3(2):99-101, 1994.

78. Shukla, D., et al. "Pain in Acute and Chronic Wounds," *Ostomy/Wound Management* 51(11):47-51, November 2005.

79. Price, P. "A Holistic Approach to Wound Care," *WOUNDS* 17(3):55-57, March 2005.

80. Goncalves, M.L., et al. "Pain in Chronic Leg Ulcers," *Journal of Wound, Ostomy, and Continence Nursing* 31(5):275-83, 2004.

81. Hofman, D., et al. "Pain in Venous Ulcers," *Journal of Wound Care* 6(5):222-24, May 1997.

82. Szor, J.K., and Bourguignon, C. "Description of Pressure Ulcer Pain at Rest and at Dressing Change," *Journal of Wound, Ostomy, and Continence Nursing* 26(3):115-20, May 1999.

83. Price, P.E., et al. "Measuring Quality of Life in Patients with Granulating Wounds," *Journal of Wound Care* 3(1):49-50, 1994.

84. Roe, B.H., et al. "Assessment, Prevention and Treatment of Chronic Leg Ulcers in the Community: Report of a Survey," *Journal of Clinical Nursing* 2(5):299-306, September 1993.

85. Ayello, E.A., Wexler, S.S., and Harris, W.S. "Is pressure ulcer pain being assessed?" (In review.)

86. Hollinworth, H., and Collier, M. "Nurses' Views About Pain and Trauma at Dressing Changes: Results of a National Survey," *Journal of Wound Care* 9(8):369-73, 2000.

87. Hollinworth, H. "Nurses' Assessment and Management of Pain at Wound Dressing Changes," *Journal of Wound Care* 4(2):77-83, 1995.

88. Pieper, B., Szczepaniak, K., and Templin, T. "Psychosocial Adjustment, Coping, and Quality of Life in Persons with Venous Ulcers and a History of Intravenous Drug Use," *Journal of Wound and Ostomy Care* 27(4):227-39, 2000.

89. Liew, I.H., et al. "Do Leg Ulcer Clinics Improve Patients' Quality of Life?" *Journal of Wound Care* 9(9):423-26, October 2000.

90. Franks, P.J., et al. "Community Leg Ulcer Clinics: Effects on Quality of Life," *Phlebology* 9:83-86, 1994.

91. Moss, R.J., and La Puma, J. "The Ethics of Pressure Sore Prevention and Treatment in the Elderly: A Practical Approach," *Journal of the American Geriatrics Society* 39(9):905-8, September 1991.

92. La Puma, J. "The Ethics of Pressure Ulcers," *Decubitus* 4(2):43-44, May 1991.

93. Schank, J.E. "Whose Goal of Care Is It? A Colostomy Patient with a Peristomal Lesion of Uncertain Etiology," *Journal of the World Council of Enterostomal Therapists* 27(3), July-September 2007.

94. Beitz, J.M. "Overcoming Barriers to Quality Wound Care: A Systems Perspective," *Ostomy/Wound Management* 47(3):56-64, March 2001.

95. Bell, S.E. "Community Health Nursing, Wound Care, and….Ethics?," *Journal of Wound, Ostomy, and Continence Nursing* 30(5):259-65, 2003.

96. Scherwitz, L.W., Rountree, R., and Delevitt, P. "Wound Caring Is More Than Wound Care: The Provider as a Partner," *Ostomy/Wound Management* 43(9):42-46,48,50, October 1997.

97. Pittman, J. "The Chronic Wound and the Family," *Ostomy/Wound Management* 49(2):38-46, 2003.

98. Price, P. "Health-related Quality of Life and the Patient's Perspective," *Journal of Wound Care* 7(7):365-66, July 1998.

CHAPTER 2

Regulation and Wound Care

Dan R. Berlowitz, MD, MPH
Denise Israel-Richardson, MEd, SRN, SCM (EdD student)
Courtney H. Lyder, ND, GNP, FAAN

Objectives

After completing this chapter, you'll be able to:

- discuss the significance of the U.S. Centers for Medicare and Medicaid Services
- discuss reimbursement issues related to hospitals, skilled nursing facilities, home health agencies, and managed care
- identify quality improvement efforts
- describe essential wound documentation required for reimbursement.

ROLE OF REGULATION IN HEALTH CARE

Regulations are a pervasive feature of the American healthcare system and, not surprisingly, significantly impact the delivery of wound care. Quite often, regulations and reimbursements determine who receives wound care and the level of wound care that's delivered. Thus, knowledge about the regulations that impact wound care in their specific practice setting is essential if clinicians are to provide optimum care.

Although many clinicians may view the current regulatory environment as burdensome and unnecessary, it's essential to recognize the important purpose that regulations fulfill. Quite simply, regulations are the mechanism through which government may promote its interest in the general welfare of society. Experience has demonstrated that government cannot rely solely on conventional market forces, such as the laws of supply and demand, to guide the use of resources to provide optimum care. These market forces, in the absence of the guiding hand of regulations, are often insufficient to ensure that healthcare resources are distributed equitably. In the case of wound care, the goal of current regulations is to ensure access to high-quality wound care, particularly for vulnerable populations such as the elderly and nursing home residents. Wound-care regulations must be viewed from the perspective of how well they are achieving this goal.

At least four types of regulatory instruments are available to the government to help achieve this goal. Government regulations may rely on subsidies or direct payments to providers; they may involve entry restrictions such as licensure and accreditations that seek to limit the ability to offer a particular service; they could use rate-setting or price-setting controls that determine reimbursements for care provided; or they could involve quality controls that seek to improve the care that is provided. Of these different potential mechanisms, the latter two are clearly the major regulatory instruments used in wound care today and are the focus of this chapter. Specifically, we describe the major regulatory organization involved in wound care in the United States—the Centers for Medicare and Medicaid Services (CMS)—including an overview of how wound care is reimbursed by CMS and a description of the organization's efforts in improving the quality of wound care.

CENTERS FOR MEDICARE AND MEDICAID SERVICES

The CMS is a federal agency within the U.S. Department of Health and Human Services. Prior to July 1, 2001, it was called the Health Care Financing Administration (HCFA). The CMS administers the Medicare and Medicaid programs—two national healthcare programs that benefit about 75 million Americans. Moreover, because CMS provides the states with at least 50% of their finances for healthcare costs, the states must comply with federal regulations. The CMS also regulates all laboratory testing (except research) performed on humans in the United States.

Both the Medicare and Medicaid programs are administered through federal statutes that determine beneficiary requirements, what's covered, payment fees and schedules, and survey processes of clinical settings (such as skilled nursing facilities [SNFs] or home health agencies). Both programs have a wide variance on coverage, eligibility, and payment fees and schedules. Therefore, it's important for the clinician to know what's covered and the level of reimbursement prior to developing a treatment plan with the patient. Because CMS remains the largest health insurance agency, many private insurance companies will provide coverage at similar levels.

Medicare

The Medicare program was developed in 1965 by the federal government.[1] In order to qualify for Medicare benefits, a person must be age 65 or older, have approved disabilities if under age 65, or have end-stage renal disease.

In 2008, Medicare provided coverage to 43 million people, spending $764 billion on benefits.[2] These benefit payments are funded from two trust funds—the Hospital Insurance (HI) trust fund and the Supplementary Medical Insurance (SMI) trust fund. Most often these are referred to as Medicare Part A and Medicare Part B, respectively.[3]

The HI trust fund pays for a portion of the costs of inpatient hospital services and related care. Those services include critical access hospitals (small facilities that give limited outpatient and inpatient services to people in rural areas), SNFs, hospice care, and some home healthcare services. The HI trust fund is financed primarily through payroll taxes, plus a relatively small amount of interest, income taxes on Social Security benefits, and other revenues.

The SMI trust fund pays for a portion of the costs of physicians' services, outpatient hospital services, and other related medical and health services. As of 2011, the premium for Medicare Part B is $96.40 per month. In some cases this amount may be higher if the person doesn't choose Medicare Part B when he or she first becomes eligible at age 65 or if the person files taxes greater than $85,000 as an individual or $170,001 as part of a couple. In addition, as of January 2006, the SMI trust fund pays for private prescription drug insurance plans to provide drug coverage under Part D of the program. The separate Part B and Part D accounts in the SMI trust fund are financed through general revenues, beneficiary premiums, interest income and, in the case of Part D, special payments from the States.

By combining both payment sources, the total expenditures from the HI and SMI trust funds are projected to increase at a significant pace in the absence of further reforms. Total Medicare expenditures grew 8.6% in 2008 and now comprise 20% of the $2.3 trillion in national health expenditures; these national health expenditures account for 16.2% of the gross domestic product.[4] These increases reflect growth in medical prices and the volume and intensity of services. In addition, the retirement and aging of the "baby boomer" generation will also increase expenditure growth rates for Medicare. Indeed, Medicare has become the second most expensive entitlement program next to Social Security in the United States.

The Medicare+Choice program was authorized by the Balanced Budget Act of 1997.[5] In this program, beneficiaries have the traditional Medicare Part A and Part B benefits, but they may also select Medicare managed care plans (such as health maintenance organizations [HMOs], preferred provider organizations [PPOs], or private fee-for-service plans). Medicare+Choice plans provide care under contract to Medicare.

They may provide benefits such as coordination of care or reducing out-of-pocket expenses. Some plans may also offer additional benefits, such as prescription drugs.

Prescription drug benefits are available for all Medicare beneficiaries regardless of income, health status, or prescription drug use[6] through Medicare Part D. A range of plans are available, so beneficiaries have multiple options for coverage. Moreover, persons can add drug coverage to the traditional Medicare plan through a "stand-alone" prescription drug plan or through a Medicare Advantage plan, which includes an HMO or PPO and typically provides more benefits at a significantly lower cost through a network of doctors and hospitals. Presently, no wound care products are covered under this benefit.

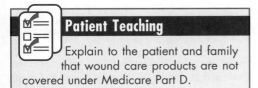

Patient Teaching

Explain to the patient and family that wound care products are not covered under Medicare Part D.

Medicaid

The Medicaid program was developed in 1965 as a jointly funded cooperative venture between the federal and state governments to assist states in the provision of adequate medical care to eligible people.[1] Medicaid is the largest program providing medical and health-related services to America's poorest people. Within broad national guidelines provided by the federal government, each of the states:

- administers its own program
- determines the type, amount, duration, and scope of services
- establishes its own eligibility standards
- sets the rate of payment for services.

Thus, the Medicaid program varies considerably from state to state as well as within each state over time. This wide variance also affects what's covered in wound care. For example, the number of times debridement of a wound is reimbursed differs by state.

REIMBURSEMENT ACROSS HEALTHCARE SETTINGS

Reimbursement directly impacts how clinicians deliver care. Increasingly, third-party payer sources (Medicare, Medicaid, HMOs) are examining where their money is going and whether they're getting the most from providers on behalf of their beneficiaries. Thus, third-party payers are requiring more documentation regarding patient outcomes to justify payment. Clinicians who can document comprehensive and accurate assessments of wounds and the outcomes of their interventions are in a stronger position to obtain and maintain coverage.

Evidence-based wound care should always be the goal of clinicians. However, clinicians are increasingly being challenged to provide optimum wound care based on healthcare setting and third-party payer. This section reviews various healthcare settings and how wound care products and services are reimbursed by CMS.

Hospitals

Hospitals are reimbursed at a predetermined, fixed rate for each discharge under diagnosis-related groups (DRGs) as part of the in-patient prospective payment system (PPS). The payment amount for a particular service is derived based on the classification system of that service. For hospitals, wound care products, devices, and support surfaces are included in the amount. Because the PPS is based on an adjusted average payment rate, some cases will receive payments in excess of cost (less than the billed charges), whereas others will receive payment that's less than cost.[7] The system is designed to give hospitals the incentive to manage operations more efficiently by evaluating those areas in which increased efficiencies can be instituted without affecting the quality of care and by treating a mix of patients to balance cost and payments.

Rehabilitation hospitals and units and long-term-care facilities (defined as those with an average length of stay of at least 25 days) are excluded from the PPS. Instead, they're paid on a reasonable-cost basis, subject to per-discharge limits.[7] They are also paid depending on hospital-specific contracts and different payer sources. Note that CMS doesn't recognize subacute status; rather, subacute facilities are governed by the SNF regulations.

The Deficit Reduction Act (DRA) of 2005 was passed in February 2006 in an effort to limit payments to hospitals for conditions resulting from potentially poor quality of care.[8] Section 5001(c) of the DRA requires the secretary of the Department of Health and Human Services or a designee to identify conditions that (1) are high cost, high volume, or both; (2) result in the assignment of a case to a DRG that has a higher payment when present as a secondary diagnosis; and (3) could reasonably have been prevented through the application of evidence-based guidelines. Section 5001(c) provides that CMS can revise the list of conditions from time to time, as long as it contains at least two conditions.

Stage 3 and 4 pressure ulcers and surgical site infections were identified as two of the initial hospital-acquired conditions (HACs) that met the DRA. (See *The 10 categories of hospital-acquired conditions.*) Thus, if clinicians do not identify and subsequently document the pressure ulcer(s) or specific surgical site infection as present on admission (POA), then the hospital will not be permitted to claim payment either as a primary or secondary diagnosis. The POA Indicator requirement and HAC payment provision only apply to inpatient PPS hospitals. At this time, a number of hospitals are exempt from the POA Indicator and HAC payment provisions, including critical access hospitals, long-term care hospitals, cancer hospitals, children's inpatient facilities, and rural health clinics.

The DRA also directed CMS to develop and standardize patient assessment information from acute and post-acute care settings. This resulted in the development of the Continuity Assessment Record and Evaluation (CARE) Tool. The CARE Tool is intended to measure the health and functional status of Medicare acute discharges as well as changes in severity and other outcomes for Medicare post-acute care patients while controlling for factors that affect outcomes, such as cognitive impairments and social and environmental factors. Many of the items are already collected in hospitals, SNFs, or home care settings, although the exact item form may be different. The tool is being designed to eventually replace similar items on the existing Medicare assessment forms, including the Outcome and Assessment Information Set (OASIS), Minimum Data Set (MDS), Resident Assessment Protocol (RAP), and Inpatient Rehabilitation Facility–Patient Assessment Instrument (IRF-PAI) tools. (See chapter 6, Wound assessment, for more information about the CARE Tool.)

It is anticipated that use of the CARE Tool will help improve the quality of care transitions, leading to a reduction in inappropriate hospital re-admissions. Four major domains are included in the tool: medical, functional, and cognitive impairments, and social/environmental factors. These domains were chosen either to measure case mix severity differences within medical conditions or to predict outcomes such as discharge to home or community, rehospitalization, and changes in functional or medical status. Section G covers skin integrity and is used to assess pressure ulcers, delayed healing of surgical wounds, trauma-related wounds, diabetic foot ulcers, vascular ulcers (arterial and venous), and other wounds (for example, incontinence-associated dermatitis). The CARE Tool is currently in beta testing and can be

---

The 10 categories of hospital-acquired conditions

1. Foreign object retained after surgery
2. Air embolism
3. Blood incompatibility
4. Stage III and IV pressure ulcers
5. Falls and trauma
6. Manifestations of poor glycemic control
7. Catheter-associated urinary tract infection
8. Vascular catheter-associated infection
9. Surgical site infection
10. Deep vein thrombosis/pulmonary embolism

accessed at http://www.cms.gov/DemoProjects EvalRpts/downloads/PACPR_R.

Hospital outpatient centers

The Balanced Budget Act of 1997 provided authority for CMS to develop a PPS under Medicare for hospital outpatient services. The new outpatient PPS took effect in August 2000.[9] All services paid under this PPS are called ambulatory payment classifications (APCs). A payment rate is established for each APC, depending on the services provided. Services in each APC are similar clinically and in terms of the resources they require. Currently, there are approximately 500 APCs. Hospitals may be paid for more than one APC per encounter. Medicare beneficiaries also can pay a coinsurance, which is the amount they will have to pay for services furnished in the hospital outpatient department after they have met the Medicare Part D deductible. A coinsurance amount is initially calculated for each APC based on 20% of the national median charge for services in the APCs. The coinsurance amount for an APC doesn't change until

the amount becomes 20% of the total APC payment. It should be noted that the total APC payment and the portion paid as coinsurance amounts are adjusted to reflect geographic wage variations using the hospital wage index and assuming that the portion of the payment/ coinsurance that's attributable to labor is 60%.

The surgical dressings benefit covers primary and secondary dressings in outpatient acute care clinic settings (for example, a hospital outpatient wound center) and physician offices. (See *Coverage under the surgical dressings benefit*.)[10] Current procedural terminology (CPT) codes are also used in this setting. CPT codes are numbers assigned to every task and service a clinician (for example, physician, nurse practitioner, podiatrist) may provide to a patient, including medical, surgical, and diagnostic services. The codes are then used by insurers (Medicare, state and private) to determine the amount of reimbursement for the clinician. Every clinician uses the same codes to ensure uniformity, but the amount of reimbursement may differ depending on the professional.

Coverage under the surgical dressings benefit

To have the cost of dressings reimbursed under the Medicare/Medicaid surgical dressings benefit, the following criteria must be met:

- The dressings are medically necessary for the treatment of a wound caused by, or treated by, a surgical procedure.
- The dressings are medically necessary when debridement of a wound is medically necessary.

In certain situations, dressings aren't covered under the surgical dressings benefit, including those for:

- drainage from a cutaneous fistula that has not been caused by or treated by a surgical procedure
- first-degree burn
- stage I pressure ulcer

- wounds caused by trauma that don't require surgical closure or debridement (such as skin tears and abrasions)
- venipuncture or arterial puncture site other than the site of an indwelling catheter or needle.

Examples of dressing classifications that are covered under the surgical dressing benefit include:

- foam dressings
- gauze
- nonimpregnated and impregnated dressings
- hydrocolloids
- alginates
- composites
- hydrogels.

Skilled nursing facilities

A patient who is eligible for Medicare may receive Medicare Part A for up to 100 days per benefit period in an SNF.[11] The patient must satisfy specific rules in order to qualify for this benefit. These rules include the following:

- Beneficiary is admitted to SNF or to the SNF level of care in a swing-bed hospital within 30 days after the date of hospital discharge.
- Beneficiary must have been in a hospital receiving inpatient hospital services for at least 3 consecutive days (counting the day of admission but not the day of discharge).
- Beneficiary requires skilled nursing care by or under the supervision of a registered nurse or requires physical, occupational, or speech therapy that can only be provided in an inpatient setting.
- Services are needed on a daily basis.
- Skilled services are required for the same or related health problem that resulted in the hospitalization.

After the SNF accepts a patient with Medicare Part A, all routine, ancillary, and capital-related costs are covered in the PPS. Thus, wound care supplies, therapies, and support surfaces are included in the PPS per diem rate. The Balanced Budget Act of 1997 modified how payments were made for Medicare SNF services.[11] After July 1, 1998, SNFs were no longer paid on a reasonable cost basis or through low volume prospectively determined rates but rather on the basis of a PPS. The PPS payment rates are adjusted for case mix and geographic variation (urban versus rural) in wages. The PPS also covers all costs of furnishing covered SNF services. The SNF isn't permitted to bill under Medicare Part B until the 100 days are in effect.[12]

All SNFs participating in Medicare and Medicaid must also comply with federal and state regulations. In November 2004, CMS released its revised interpretative guidance on pressure ulcers (Federal Tag 314).[13] F-314 is a federal regulation that states that a resident entering a long-term care facility will not get a pressure ulcer or if they have a pressure ulcer it will not worsen. This 40-page document is used by both federal and state surveyors to determine the SNF compliance with F-314. It also provides SNFs with evidence-based approaches to prevent and treat pressure ulcers. SNFs that are found to be noncompliant with the pressure ulcer regulation can receive civil money penalties, which currently range from $500 to $10,000/day, or CMS and the state can withhold payments and close the facility because of system-wide imminent danger to residents. Additional skin or wound regulations include F-309, in which SNFs can be cited for all other ulcers besides pressure ulcers, and F-315, which addresses the need to protect the skin from the effects of urinary incontinence.

RESIDENT ASSESSMENT INSTRUMENT

In order to meet its regulatory role, CMS requires that a Resident Assessment Instrument (RAI) be completed on all SNF residents. The RAI includes the MDS 2.0 RAPs and utilization guidelines that have been in use since 1995. The MDS is a 400-item assessment form that attempts to identify the functional capacity of residents in SNFs. Based on the MDS section, further assessments are triggered by RAPs, which assess common clinical problems found in SNFs, such as pressure ulcers and urinary incontinence. RAPs also have utilization guidelines that assist the healthcare team in planning the overall care of the resident. The comprehensive RAI is completed annually, with quarterly MDS assessments (less comprehensive) completed between the annual assessments. The SNF is required to do another RAI if the resident's health status changes significantly. Only pressure and stasis ulcers are clearly delineated on the MDS 2.0 version; all other ulcers are grouped in the "other" category. Section M of the MDS assesses ulcers by stage, type of ulcer (pressure or stasis), other skin lesions present, skin treatments, and foot problems.[14]

CMS has been using the new MDS version 3.0 since October 1, 2010.[15] This revised version is intended to improve reliability, accuracy, and usefulness; to include the resident in the assessment process; and to use standard protocols used in other settings. These improvements have profound implications for enhanced accuracy, which supports the primary legislative intent that the MDS be a tool to improve clinical assessment. The CMS has adapted the National Pressure Ulcer Assessment Panel's 2007 definition of a pressure ulcer as well as the staging categories of pressure ulcers. One of the new areas in section M (skin) has eliminated the confusion that requires staging of all chronic ulcers.[16,17] Staging of pressure ulcers will involve simply staging the deepest tissue involved and worsening pressure ulcers. Another major change has been the delineation between unstageable pressure ulcers and suspected deep tissue injury.

The RAI is a very useful instrument in planning the care of SNF residents. The RAI User's Manual Version 3.0 no longer uses RAPs to connect MDS data to care planning. Instead of RAPs, there are care area triggers (CATs) and care area assessments (CAAs). MDS 3.0 is tied to care planning first through the CAT grid, which triggers each CAA. Like the prior version, the MDS is only a preliminary screen that will identify potential issues that the interdisciplinary team will further explore. The interdisciplinary team should identify current clinical protocols and resources to guide the CAA, and these resources should be identifiable on request by surveyors.[16]

The CAA is therefore designed to expand the assessment process that begins with the MDS. One area that is beneficial from this expanded assessment is whether the ulcer was avoidable or unavoidable. MDS 3.0 section M does not address unavoidability, but this is an important issue that most if not all facilities would like to incorporate. The CAA allows the interdisciplinary team to identify specific guidelines that can be incorporated into the assessment and care planning process. Because the issue of unavoidability may depend on the presence of multiple comorbidities and physiological disturbances, collaboration with the physician will be an important component of this extended assessment.[16]

CAAs triggered by CATs in section M include pressure ulcers, nutritional status, and dehydration/fluid maintenance. The CAA for pressure ulcers is automatically triggered by any resident considered to be at-risk, any

stage of pressure ulcer, or any worsening ulcer. The net result of these changes is closer linkage of the resident assessment to quality of life, incorporation of updated guidelines for ulcer staging, and broadening of the care planning process to include current clinical protocols and evidence-based standards.[16]

RESOURCE UTILIZATION GROUPS

The RAI is also linked to payment.[18] All Medicare Part A payments are linked to the RAI and, in some states, Medicaid payments are based solely on completion of the MDS. Based on the MDS, each resident is assigned to one of 53 resource utilization groups (RUGs); of note, a version with 66 groups is being tested by CMS on an interim basis. RUGs are clusters of nursing home residents based on resident characteristics that explain resource use.[19] RUG rates are computed separately for urban and rural areas, and a portion of the total rate is adjusted to reflect labor market conditions in each SNF's location. The daily rate for each RUG is calculated using the sum of three components:

- a fixed amount for routine services (such as room and board, linens, and administrative services)
- a variable amount for the expected intensity of therapy services
- a variable amount reflecting the intensity of nursing care that patients are expected to require.

Because of RUGs, it's essential for the SNF to complete the MDS correctly. The SNF must pay close attention to all health problems of the resident because the more intensive the care required, the higher the daily rate will be. Moreover, completing the MDS accurately and in a timely manner will help to ensure correct payments. If an SNF doesn't complete the MDS in a timely manner, it receives a default payment, which is usually significantly lower, or it may not receive payment at all.

Home health agencies

The Balanced Budget Act of 1997 also called for the development and implementation of a PPS for Medicare home health services. On October 1, 2000, home health PPS was implemented.[20] (See *Qualifying for home health benefits*.)

OASIS-C

The process of quality wound management begins on admission. Suggested components of a quality program are assessment (including risk assessment and intervention), documentation and wound measurement, case manager report and collaboration, protocols and physician orders, ulcer care, management of tissue loads, nutrition, and outcomes tracking.[21]

When it's determined that a Medicare patient can receive home health services, an OASIS form must be completed. OASIS is a group of comprehensive assessments that form the basis for delivering patient care, measuring patient outcomes for purposes of outcome-based quality improvement and, since 2000, assisting in the prospective payment system. Revisions to the OASIS tool introduced in late 2002 resulted in a 25% reduction in dataset questions. OASIS-C represents the most comprehensive revision to OASIS since its original release. This revised instrument, which

was rolled out January 1, 2010,[22] better aligns measures in both the MDS 3.0 and the CARE Tool. Major items on the OASIS-C include socio-demographic, environmental, support system, health, and functional status. Based on these assessments, a care plan can be generated. The OASIS-C document specifically classifies stasis ulcers, surgical wounds, and pressure ulcers.[23]

OASIS-C includes data items to measure the use of "best practice" care processes. To that end, data elements were created to measure processes of care in 10 new domains, two of which focus on wound care:

- Pressure ulcer risk assessment, prevention measures, and use of moist healing principles (effective care and prevention)
- Diabetic foot care plan, education, and monitoring (disease specific: high risk, high volume, problem prone)

Payment for home health services is directly linked to the completion of OASIS-C. A case-mix is also applied to calculate reimbursement. The case-mix involves 20 data points to assess three factors: clinical severity, functional status, and service utilization. The system has created 80 home health resource groups (HHRGs).[24] Patients are grouped into the HHRGs based on the OASIS-C results.

Medicare pays home health agencies for each covered 60-day episode of care, and a patient can receive an unlimited number of medically necessary episodes of care. Payments cover skilled nursing and home health aide visits, covered therapy, medical social services, and routine and nonroutine supplies. For each 60-day episode, the payment system can vary, depending on the HHRG, with adjustments to reflect area wage differences.[24]

Home health agencies are required to transmit OASIS-C data electronically to

PRACTICE POINT

Accurate completion of OASIS by clinicians is essential. If you don't answer the questions appropriately, accurately, and completely, your facility won't receive the money and will lose reimbursement.

their state system. Improper completion of OASIS-C can lead to significantly lower payments or no payments at all. Thus, accurate assessments and charting are essential for recouping payments. Some authors[21,25-27] have described innovative ways of teaching staff and ensuring their competency in completing OASIS-C.

DURABLE MEDICAL EQUIPMENT CARRIERS

Implementation of the Medicare program (for instance, eligibility requirements and payments) in home care is handled by numerous insurance companies that are subcontracted by CMS. In 1993, CMS contracted four carriers to process claims for durable medical equipment (DME), prosthetics, orthotics, and supplies (DMEPOS) under Medicare Part B.[28] CMS divided the country into four regions, with each region having its own DME regional carrier. The Healthcare Common Procedure Coding System (HCPCS), an alpha-numeric system used to identify coding categories not included in the American Medical Association's CPT-4 codes, is usually used with DMEPOS.[29]

In January 2006, CMS eliminated fiscal intermediaries who processed Medicare claims (Medicare Part A only) and carriers (Medicare Part B only),[30] eliminated the DME regional carriers, and awarded four specialty contractors through a competitive bidding process. The new DME Medicare administrative contractors (DME MACs) are responsible for handling the administration of Medicare claims from DMEPOS suppliers. The benefit of the new system is a more streamlined process between the beneficiary and the supplier. The DME MACs serve as the point of contact for all Medicare suppliers, whereas beneficiaries can register their claims-related questions to Beneficiary Contact Centers. (See *The four durable medical equipment Medicare administrative contractors*.)

DME MACs clearly define medical coverage policies. The beneficiary usually pays the first $100.00 for covered medical services annually. Once that has been met, the beneficiary pays 20% of the Medicare-approved amount for services or supplies. If services weren't provided on assignment, then the beneficiary pays for more of the Medicare coinsurance plus certain charges above the Medicare-approved amount.

Medicare Part B also provides coverage for Negative Pressure Wound Therapy (NPWT) pumps. In order for an NPWT pump and supplies to be covered, the patient must have a chronic stage III or IV pressure ulcer, neuropathic ulcer, venous or arterial insufficiency

---

The four durable medical equipment Medicare administrative contractors

- *AdminaStar Federal,* serving Illinois, Indiana, Kentucky, Michigan, Minnesota, Ohio, and Wisconsin
- *National Heritage Insurance Company,* serving Connecticut, Delaware, District of Columbia, Maine, Maryland, Massachusetts, New Hampshire, New Jersey, New York, Pennsylvania, Rhode Island, and Vermont
- *Noridian Administrative Services,* serving Alaska, American Samoa, Arizona, California, Guam, Hawaii, Idaho, Iowa, Kansas, Missouri, Montana,

Nebraska, Nevada, North Dakota, Northern Mariana Islands, Oregon, South Dakota, Utah, Washington, and Wyoming
- *Palmetto Government Benefits Administrator,* serving Alabama, Arkansas, Colorado, Florida, Georgia, Louisiana, Mississippi, New Mexico, North Carolina, Oklahoma, Puerto Rico, South Carolina, Tennessee, Texas, U.S. Virgin Islands, Virginia, and West Virginia.

ulcer, or a chronic (at least 30 days) ulcer of mixed etiology. Extensive documentation is required prior to a DME MAC approving coverage for NPWT. Thus, it's important to review the coverage policy prior to applying for coverage.[31]

Support surfaces are also covered under Medicare Part B.[31-33] CMS has divided support surfaces into three categories for reimbursement purposes:

- Group 1 devices are those support surfaces that are static and don't require electricity. Static devices include air, foam (convoluted and solid), gel, and water overlay or mattresses.
- Group 2 devices are powered by electricity or pump and are considered dynamic in nature. These devices include alternating and low-air-loss mattresses.
- Group 3 devices are also considered dynamic in nature. This classification comprises only air-fluidized beds.

Specific criteria must be met before Medicare will reimburse for support surfaces; therefore, it's essential to review the policy before applying for coverage.

Managed care organizations

Manage Care Organizations (MCOs) were developed to provide health services while controlling costs. They combine the responsibility for paying for a defined set of health services with an active program to control the costs associated with providing those services, while at the same time attempting to control the quality of and access to those services. The health benefits, which usually range from acute care services to dental and vision coverage, are usually clearly identified, as are the payment, co-payment, and deductibles that are required for a specific health procedure (for example, compression therapy for chronic venous insufficiency ulcer). Moreover, the MCO usually receives a fixed sum of money to pay for the benefits in the plans for the defined population of enrollees. Typically, this fixed sum is constructed through premiums paid by the enrollees, capitation payments made on behalf of the enrollees from a third party, or both. There are wide variations in MCOs and the services they provide for patients with wounds.

Providing wound care in a complex reimbursement environment

The challenge of providing quality wound care can be magnified when the patient moves from one healthcare sector to another. That's why it's imperative for wound care professionals to understand some of the nuances of the reimbursement agency. A good illustration would be a Medicare beneficiary who was discharged home with a pressure ulcer that had 100% eschar covering the surface. In this scenario, the home care agency would receive no reimbursement for providing wound care until the eschar was removed. However, if the same Medicare beneficiary was discharged to an SNF, the nursing home could receive full CMS payment for the pressure ulcer with 100% eschar. This reimbursement schism can make providing quality wound care extremely challenging.

QUALITY IMPROVEMENT EFFORTS

Regulations related to reimbursements are tightly integrated with efforts in quality assessment and improvement. Indeed, care that's found not to meet quality standards may not be reimbursed. Even appropriate care may not be reimbursed if the condition being treated is the result of a medical error. Moreover, claims for reimbursements for substandard care could be viewed as fraudulent and result in criminal penalties. CMS doesn't rely solely on such punitive methods, however, and various other initiatives exist—most of these efforts center on pressure ulcers and may serve as a model for other wounds.

Role of quality measurement

Measuring quality is central to ensuring quality care. If you don't measure quality, you can't improve it. There are at least three ways in which quality measurement can be used to improve care, and different healthcare settings employ different approaches. Facilitating such quality measurement is the wealth of data available in existing and forthcoming databases, such as MDS 3.0 and OASIS-C, which provide patient-specific information on processes and outcomes of care. ICD-9-CM codes from hospital stays are also now much more informative. Since 2008, they describe pressure ulcer location, stage, and whether the wound was present on admission. These changes may address some of the problems that have been identified when using ICD-9-CM codes to measure rates of pressure ulcers in hospitals.[34]

First, quality measurement is being used to empower consumers of health care. The assumption is that patients and their families, if given information about quality of care, will select those providers offering the best care. Such information then needs to be made available to patients in a timely fashion. Further, providers need to proactively improve their care in order to attract patients. This approach is exemplified by the Home Health Compare and Nursing Home Compare websites maintained by CMS.[35] These sites contain several measures of wound care performance; facility rates of performance on these measures are presented along with national and state-wide rates to permit easy comparisons. To further facilitate use of this information by consumers, Nursing Home Compare employs a rating system that combines information on these quality measures with results from state surveys and staffing levels. Whether this approach will indeed be successful in improving care, however, remains uncertain.[36]

Second, quality measures are being used in quality improvement activities. The systematic use of such data can aid in the identification of quality-of-care problems and help determine the nature of these problems.[37] Nearly all healthcare provider organizations are involved in continuous quality improvement activities, with varying levels of implementation into clinical practice. A central component of such activities is feedback on performance. Indeed, demonstration projects have suggested that providing home care agencies with performance feedback, a process known as outcome-based quality improvement (OBQI), does result in reduced rates of hospitalization. Thus, CMS uses OASIS to determine whether wounds are improving and not only posts these rates on its website but encourages home care agencies to use the data as part of their internal quality improvement program.

Finally, quality measures may help to focus more detailed analyses of the care provided to individual patients. For example, the Agency for Healthcare Research and Quality (AHRQ), as part of its patient safety initiative, has developed a set of indicators based on hospital discharge data. Among the indicators is one for the presence of a pressure ulcer. Patients flagged by the indicator may undergo a more detailed review of the care processes associated with the development and treatment of a pressure ulcer. In nursing homes, state survey agencies are required to conduct annual unannounced surveys at SNFs to determine compliance with federal regulations regarding quality of care. A major focus of these surveys is an evaluation of pressure ulcer prevention and treatment practices and whether the SNF is compliant with care as specified in F-314.[38] Cases reviewed are often identified based on the MDS quality indicators.

Existing quality measures

A wide variety of measures are available to assess the quality of wound care. The Assessing Care of Vulnerable Elders (ACOVE) project, for example, developed a set of 11 indicators that capture different aspects of pressure ulcer care.[39] Each indicator is structured as an *if... then* statement, where the *if* component specifies a specific situation and the *then* component indicates what should be done in that situation. The most widely used measures, though, are those on the Nursing Home Compare and Home Health Compare websites. Nursing homes on Nursing Home Compare are assessed on the prevalence of ulcers, specifically the percentage of high-risk and low-risk long-term residents who have a pressure ulcer. Home care measures on Home Health Compare have recently been expanded. They now capture not only success in wound healing as described by the percentage of patients whose wounds improve or heal after an operation and the percentage of patients who need unplanned medical care related to a wound that is new, is worse, or has become infected, but they also include measures of prevention such as whether risk assessment was performed and whether prevention of pressure ulcers is addressed in the plan of care. While the home care measures generally rely on detailed risk adjustment models that account for a large number of baseline patient characteristics, the measures for nursing homes rely mostly on stratification and exclusion criteria. Concerns have been raised that the nursing home measures may then be biased because differences in facility performance represent differences in resident/patient mix rather than in true facility performance.[40]

While CMS measures of quality are widely available, there are concerns regarding their validity as descriptors of quality. One study compared nursing homes that performed well and poorly on the pressure ulcer measure and found few differences in how care was actually delivered.[41] Another study of a quality improvement program in over 30 nursing homes noted no improvement in their performance on the CMS quality measure but a significant decline in the incidence of stage III and IV pressure ulcers.[42] This suggests that a measure of the incidence of deep pressure ulcers might be a truer measure of quality.

Improving quality of care

CMS also actively promotes quality improvement activities directed toward Medicare beneficiaries. The primary mechanism for this is through quality improvement organizations (QIOs), formerly known as peer review organizations (PROs). PROs initially relied on an "inspect and detect" approach to quality assessment in which medical record reviews would identify problems and be linked to interventions to correct substandard care. The approach was adversarial, penalties for substandard care could be harsh, and few improvements in quality of care could be documented.

In 1992, the Health Care Quality Improvement Initiative significantly changed the role of PROs. Rather than individual case reviews, PROs were to focus now on patterns of care. National guidelines, rather than local criteria, were to be used in evaluating quality of care. Most importantly, PROs were to work collaboratively with providers to improve healthcare delivery. Recognizing this new emphasis on quality improvement, PROs were renamed QIOs in 2001.

QIOs have since developed initiatives in diverse clinical areas and settings. In wound care, most of these efforts have again centered on pressure ulcers. In New York, tool kits have been developed with which hospitals can assess and improve their pressure ulcer prevention and treatment practices. In nursing homes, QIOs from three states developed a strategy to train nursing home teams in quality improvement methods and proper pressure ulcer care. This training was reinforced through the use of outside mentors who regularly met with the teams. As a result of these initiatives and interventions, key processes of care improved dramatically.[42] A particularly impressive quality improvement collaboration within the New Jersey Hospital Association that involved over 150 hospitals and nursing homes resulted in reduction of more than 70% in pressure ulcer rates state-wide.[43]

Pay-for-performance

CMS is increasingly relying on market forces to stimulate improvements in quality of care. Pay-for-performance is viewed as an important way of using reimbursements to improve care. Providers delivering the best care will be reimbursed more than providers delivering poor quality care. While in theory this should be a highly effective mechanism for quality improvement, the data to date, which does not involve wound care, has not been convincing.[44] Basic issues such as the appropriate dollar amount to incentivize care, whether pay-for-performance represents a reward or an agent of change, and how best to measure care have not been completely resolved. While a number of projects have evaluated pay-for-performance in hospital and ambulatory care settings, demonstration projects involving nursing homes are in early stages. The extent to which pay-for-performance will focus on wound care is uncertain.

Documentation

Comprehensive documentation is the critical foundation for successful reimbursement of services and products. Indeed, regulatory agencies, independent of healthcare setting, set forth the requisite documentation for reimbursement, and their requirements for documentation should always be carefully reviewed prior to applying for coverage.

Lastly, thorough documentation justifies the medical necessity of services and products and should reflect the care required in the prevention or treatment of wounds. (See *Essential wound documentation*.)

SUMMARY

Regulatory agencies play a major role in wound care. In March 2010, The Affordable Care Act became law. This law guarantees health insurance for a minimum of 35 million people and will have profound implications for wound care professionals. As the new law is implemented, new regulations will undoubtedly be developed and executed. With the increasing need to evaluate the cost-effectiveness of wound care, regulatory agencies will likely impose further regulations, which will lead to greater complexity in obtaining and maintaining reimbursements. Thus, the key to providing optimum wound care will depend on good documentation that clearly articulates the need for services and products and clearly identifies assessment of the patient, interventions instituted, and outcomes achieved. When this is accomplished, the patient, the provider, and the regulatory agency all benefit.

PATIENT SCENARIO

Clinical Data

Mr. Y, a 72-year-old resident from a long-term care facility, is admitted to the hospital for treatment of pneumonia. He was receiving treatment for a stage III pressure ulcer on his sacrum at the long-term care facility. There is no documentation about the ulcer by the physician in the hospital admission medical record. The nursing admission record documents the presence of a stage III pressure ulcer on the sacrum. Mr. Y is treated successfully for his pneumonia and is returned to the long-term care facility.

Case Discussion

The financial implications regarding use of POA coding have been in effect since October 1, 2008. Under CMS ruling, the practitioner responsible for establishing the medical diagnosis needs to document the diagnosis on admission. In this case, the POA pressure ulcer was not documented by the physician; therefore, the hospital was poised to lose a higher amount of reimbursement for the DRG of a stage III pressure ulcer as a secondary diagnosis. The hospital coder noticed the difference between the physician and nursing documentation and queried the physician. Once it was established that the pressure ulcer was indeed POA, the physician completed his progress note and documented the location and stage of the ulcer. The coder could then submit this secondary diagnosis for billing.

SHOW WHAT YOU KNOW

1. Medicare Part B is a federal program that:
   A. supports state programs to provide services and products to the poor.
   B. reimburses hospitals for wound care services.
   C. reimburses for selected wound services and products in SNFs and home health agencies.
   D. doesn't require co-payment from the beneficiary.

   ANSWER: C. *A is incorrect because it refers to the Medicaid program, which is a collaboration between the federal and state governments to deliver care. B is incorrect because Medicare Part A is for inpatient hospital costs. D is incorrect because Medicare Part B requires the beneficiary to pay a 20% co-payment.*

2. For which one of the following healthcare settings is completion of OASIS-C required?
   A. Hospitals
   B. Home health agencies
   C. Hospital outpatient centers
   D. SNFs

   ANSWER: B. *OASIS-C is only used by home health agencies to assess patients and determine reimbursement.*

3. Which one of the following criteria must a patient with a wound meet in order to qualify for SNF care?
   A. Skilled services must be required for the same or related health problem that resulted in the hospitalization.
   B. The beneficiary must be in the hospital for 2 consecutive days.
   C. Services are needed once per week.
   D. The beneficiary must be admitted to the SNF within 90 days of admission to the hospital.

   ANSWER: A. *B is incorrect because the beneficiary must spend 3 consecutive days in the hospital. C is incorrect because skilled nursing services must be needed on a daily basis. D is incorrect because the beneficiary must be admitted within 30 days of hospitalization.*

4. Which of the following approaches <u>is not</u> being used by CMS to improve the quality of care?
   A. Empower consumers to select high-quality providers through the provision of information on performance.
   B. Increase payments to providers of better care.
   C. Develop computer reminders on when to turn patients.
   D. Work with providers through regional QIOs.

   ANSWER: C. *There are currently no quality initiatives by CMS on turning patients. A, B, and D are all true with regard to CMS. A is true because data on the performance of hospitals, nursing homes, and home health agencies is readily available on the CMS website. B is true because there is tremendous interest at CMS to reward providers of high-quality care, known as pay-for-performance. D is true because QIOs are emphasizing working with providers to improve care rather than just detecting episodes of poor care.*

REFERENCES

1. Centers for Medicare and Medicaid Services. (2010). Overview. Available at: www.cms.hhs.gov/History/. Accessed November 2, 2010.

2. Department of Health and Human Services. (n.d.). Advancing the Health, Safety, and Well-Being of Our People. Available at: http://www.hhs.gov/budget/08budget/2008BudgetInBrief.pdf. Accessed November 2, 2010.

3. Centers for Medicare and Medicaid Services. (2006). 2006 Medicare Trustees Report [Press Release]. Available at: www.cms.hhs.gov/apps/media/press/release.asp?Counter=1846. Accessed November 2, 2010.

4. Centers for Medicare and Medicaid Services. (n.d.). National Health Expenditure Fact Sheet. Available at: https://www.cms.gov/NationalHealthExpendData/25_NHE_Fact_Sheet.asp. Accessed November 2, 2010.

5. Medicare.gov. (2009). Medicare Overview. Available at: www.medicare.gov/Choices/Overview.asp. Accessed November 2, 2010.

6. Centers for Medicare and Medicaid Services. (2006). Fact Sheet: State Reimbursement for Medicare Part D Transition. Available at: http://www.cms.gov/MLNProducts/downloads/Part_D_Resource_Fact_sheet_revised.pdf. Accessed April 25, 2011.

7. Centers for Medicare and Medicaid Services. (2010). Acute Inpatient PPS: Overview. Available at: https://www.cms.gov/AcuteInpatientPPS/. Accessed November 2, 2010.

8. Centers for Medicare and Medicaid Services. (2010). Hospital-Acquired Conditions: Present on Admission Indicator.https://www.cms.gov/Hospital-AcqCond/06_Hospital-Acquired_Conditions.asp. Accessed November 2, 2010.

9. Centers for Medicare and Medicaid Services. (2010). Hospital Outpatient PPS: Overview. Available at: https://www.cms.gov/HospitalOutpatientPPS/. Accessed November 2, 2010.

10. Centers for Medicare and Medicaid Services. (2009). Your Medicare Benefits. Available at: http://www.medicare.gov/publications/pubs/pdf/10116.pdf. Accessed November 2, 2010.

11. Medicare Consumer Guide. (2010). Available at: http://www.medicareconsumerguide.com/medicare-part-a.html. Accessed November 2, 2010.

12. Centers for Medicare and Medicaid Services. (2007). Medicare Coverage of Skilled Nursing Facility Care. Available at: http://www.medicare.gov/publications/pubs/pdf/10153.pdf. Accessed November 2, 2010.

13. Centers for Medicare and Medicaid Services. (2004). CMS Manual System: Guidance to Surveyors for Long-Term Care Facilities. Available at: http://hsag.com/App_Resources/Documents/PrU_LS1_F_314.pdf. Accessed April 5, 2011.

14. Roberson S., and Ayello, E.A. "Clarification of Pressure Ulcer Staging in Long-term Care under MDS 2.0," *Advances in Skin and Wound Care* 23(5), 206-10, 2010.

15. Centers for Medicare and Medicaid Services. (2010). Nursing Home Quality Initiatives: MDS 3.0 Training Materials. Available at: https://www.cms.gov/NursingHomeQualityInits/45_NHQIMDS30-TrainingMaterials.asp#TopOf Page. Accessed November 2, 2010.

16. Levine, J.M., Roberson, S., and Ayello, E.A. "Essentials of MDS 3.0 Section M: Skin Conditions," *Advances in Skin and Wound Care* 23(6):273-84, 2010.

17. Ayello, E.A., Levine, J.M., and Roberson, S. "Late breaking CMS Update on MDS 3.0 Section M: Skin Conditions—Changes in Coding of Blister Pressure Ulcers," *Advances in Skin and Wound Care* 23(9), 2010. In press.

18. Fries, B.E., et al. "Refining a Case-Mix Measure for Nursing Homes: Resource Utilization Groups (RUG-III)," *Medical Care* 32(7):668-85, July 1994.

19. Rantz, M.J., et al. "The Minimum Data Set: No Longer Just for Clinical Assessment," *Annals of Long Term Care* 7(9):354-60, September 1999.

20. Centers for Medicare and Medicaid Services. (2010). Home Health PPS Overview. Available at: http://www.cms.gov/homehealthpps/. Accessed November 2, 2010.

21. Johnston, P.J. "Wound Competencies and OASIS-One Organization's Plan," *The Remington Report* 10(3), 5-10, May-June, 2002.

22. Centers for Medicare and Medicaid Services. (2010). Home Health Quality Initiatives: OASIS User Manuals. Available at: https://www.cms.gov/HomeHealthQualityInits/14_HHQIOASISUserManual.asp. Accessed November 2, 2010.

23. Centers for Medicare and Medicaid Services. (2010). OASIS Overview. Available at: http://www.cms.gov/oasis/01_overview.asp. Accessed November 2, 2010.

24. Centers for Medicare and Medicaid Services. (2010). Available at: http://www.cms.gov/Home-HealthPPS/01_overview.asp#TopOfPage. Accessed July 23, 2010.

25. Wright, K., and Powell, L. "Wound Competencies and OASIS-One Organization's Plan," *Caring Magazine* XXI(6):10-13, June 2002.

26. Cullen, B., and Parry, G. "Wound Competencies and OASIS-One Organization's Plan," *Caring Magazine* XXI(6):14-16, June 2002.

27. Everman, R., and Ferrell, J. "Wound Care Case Management Influences Better Patient Outcomes," *The Remington Report* 10(3):36-37, May-June 2002.

28. The Federal Register. (2005). Medicare Program: Changes in Geographical Boundaries of Durable Medical Equipment Regional Service Areas. Available at: http://www.thefederalregister.com/d.p/2005-02-25-05-3729. Accessed November 2, 2010.

29. Centers for Medicare and Medicaid Services. (2010). HCPCS Coding Questions. Available at: https://www.cms.gov/MedHCPCSGenInfo/20_HCPCS_Coding_Questions.asp. Accessed November 2, 2010.

30. Centers for Medicare and Medicaid Services. (2010). FY2011 Online Performance Appendix. Available at: http://www.cms.gov/Performance Budget/Downloads/CMSOPAFY2011.pdf. Accessed November 2, 2010.

31. The Federal Register. (2006). Medical Program: Competitive Acquisition for Certain Durable Medical Equipment, Prosthetics, Orthotics, and Supplies (DMEPOS) and Other Issues. Available at: www.cms.hhs.gov/quarterlyproviderupdates/downloads/cms1270p.pdf. Accessed November 2, 2010.

32. Medicare.gov. (2009). Your Medicare Coverage. Available at: http://www.medicare.gov/coverage/home.asp. Accessed November 2, 2010.

33. Newby, J. (2008). Get Ready for the 2009 *ICD-0* Coding Changes. Available at: http://www.in-afp.org/clientuploads/CodingBillingPDFs/2009_Update.pdf. Accessed April 5, 2001.

34. Polancich, S., Restrepo, E., and Prosser, J. "Cautious Use of Administrative Data for Decubitus Ulcer Outcome Reporting," *American Journal of Medical Quality* 21(4):262-268, 2010.

35. Harris, Y., and Clauser, S.B. "Achieving Improvement Through Nursing Home Quality Measurement," *Health Care Financing Review* 23(4):5-18, 2002.

36. Mukamel, D.B., and Spector, W.B. "Quality Report Cards and Nursing Home Quality," *Gerontologist* 43(special issue II):58-66, 2003.

37. Karon, S.L., and Zimmerman, D.R. "Using Indicators to Structure Quality Improvement Initiatives in Long-term Care," *Quality Management in Health Care* 4(3):54-66, 1996.

38. Lyder, C.H. "Pressure Ulcers in Long-Term Care: CMS Initiatives," *ECPN*, January 2005.

39. Bates-Jensen, B.M. "Quality Indicators for Prevention and Management of Pressure Ulcers in Vulnerable Elders," *Annals of Internal Medicine* 135(8 Part 2), 2001.

40. Li Y., et al. "The Nursing Home Compare Measure of Urinary/Fecal Incontinence: Cross-Sectional Variation, Stability over Time, and the Impact of Case Mix," *Health Services Research* 45(1):79-97, 2010.

41. Baier, R.R., et al. "Quality Improvement for Pressure Ulcer Care in the Nursing Home Setting: The Northeast Pressure Ulcer Project," *Journal of the American Medical Directors Association* 4(6):291-301, November-December 2003.

42. Lynn, J., et al. "Collaborative Clinical Quality Improvement for Pressure Ulcers in Nursing Homes," *Journal of the American Geriatrics Society* 55(10):1663-69, 2007.

43. Holmes, A., and Edelstein, T. "Envisioning a World Without Pressure Ulcers," *Extended Care Product News* 122:24-9, 2007.

44. Petersen, L.A., et al. "Does Pay-for-Performance Improve the Quality of Health Care?" *Annals of Internal Medicine* 145(3):265-72, 2006.

CHAPTER 3

Legal Aspects of Wound Care

Steven P. Knowlton, JD, RN
Gregory Brown, RN, ET

Objectives

After completing this chapter, you'll be able to:
- identify and describe the major litigation players and their roles in a lawsuit
- define the four elements of a malpractice claim
- describe the general rules for proper wound care charting
- identify and describe the ways the medical record, standards, or guidelines can be used in a malpractice case
- state documentation practices that predispose the medical record to legal risks
- describe strategies to improve consistency and accuracy of medical record documentation that minimize potential litigation risk.

THE CURRENT CLIMATE

In recent years, the concept of patients as "consumers of health care" has risen to the forefront. Rather than blindly trusting clinicians, the consumer-patients of today are better educated and more aware of healthcare issues and more willing to make use of legal resources when treatment goes awry. Although wound care generates no more litigation than many areas of healthcare practice, and arguably less than some others, the threat of litigation still affects the way clinicians approach the delivery of care.

Clinicians need to protect themselves while ensuring evidence-based, high-quality care to their consumer-patients. This chapter sets forth basic legal principles and suggests practice strategies that protect clinicians *and* advance patient care.

LITIGATION

Over the course of human history, it became apparent that some nonviolent means of settling disputes must be developed. The law and

the legal process, including litigation, were and continue to be one of civilized society's experiments at achieving nonviolent resolutions to disputes. The success of this experiment is itself the source of much dispute, to which no resolution (nonviolent or otherwise) is currently in sight.

Contrary to television and film portrayals, the real-life litigation process is arduous and time-consuming. While fictitious television and film lawsuits resolve in a matter of weeks or months, usually ending with a dramatic trial resulting in a stunning jury verdict, most real-life cases take years to get through the legal system. In some jurisdictions with crowded dockets, they can take as long as 5 years to resolve. Those that require appeals can take considerably more time before all issues are finally put to rest. Trials (dramatic or not) are few and far between, as nearly all lawsuits are settled before trial. When trials do happen, they're usually slow-moving, uninteresting affairs that tax the patience and attention of jurors. Litigants expecting "Perry Mason" moments from their attorneys are sure to be disappointed and, as anyone who has ever served on a jury knows, closing arguments by attorneys are never, ever over in the 5 minutes before the final commercial.

Despite the difficulties and drawbacks, the litigation process does afford citizens an impartial forum for dispute resolution grounded in the law. And the law, as Plato stated, is "a pledge that citizens of a state will do justice to one another."

The discussion in this chapter is limited to *civil litigation;* that is, litigation in which citizens have a dispute with each other—rather than *criminal litigation,* in which the state or a government seeks to prosecute a party for the violation of law. There are significant differences between the two forms of litigation (standards of proof, for example). The remedy sought in civil litigation is monetary damages. In contrast, only the prosecuting state or government may seek to deprive the alleged lawbreaker of his or her liberty by incarceration.

HOW IS A MEDICAL MALPRACTICE LAWSUIT BORN?

Litigation begins the moment a person believes he or she has been wronged by another and seeks the advice and counsel of an attorney in an effort to "right the wrong" or "get justice." During the initial interview between the prospective client and the attorney, the attorney makes a number of preliminary judgments usually based solely on the client's presentation:

• Is this the type of case the attorney is capable of handling? Does it fall within his or her expertise and practice experience? Does the attorney have the time to handle the matter?
• Is the client's story credible?
• Will the client make a good witness?
• Are the damages, if proven, sufficient to warrant entering into the litigation process?
• Is there a party responsible (liable) for the client's injuries?
• How likely is it that both liability and damages can be proven?
• Are there any glaring problems or difficulties with the case?

If the answers to these questions are satisfactory and the client wishes to retain the attorney, a lawsuit has then been conceived.

Before filing the legal documents that start the litigation process in a medical malpractice case, most attorneys perform an intensive investigation in order to definitively answer questions concerning liability and damages. Medical records and other information must be obtained and examined by an expert to determine whether a malpractice claim can be made, information related to the identities of potential defendants must be analyzed, and strategic legal issues related to jurisdiction (which court can the case be brought in) must be thought through. If after this investigation the attorney still believes the case has merit, legal papers starting the actual lawsuit will be filed, and a lawsuit will be born. (See *Players in the litigation process.*)

THE PRETRIAL LITIGATION PROCESS

The pretrial litigation process consists of several steps: complaint and answer, discovery, and motion practice.

Complaint and answer

The initial legal paper that gives rise to a lawsuit is called the *complaint.* While procedural requirements vary between jurisdictions, generally the complaint is a document that sets out the claims made by the plaintiff against the defendant, the basis of the jurisdiction of the court, the legal theories under which the plaintiff is making the claims, and in some jurisdictions, the amount of damages claimed.

The defendant must then file an *answer* within the permitted time that responds on a count-by-count basis to the plaintiff's complaint and that, depending again on jurisdictional rules, may also include claims against the plaintiff. These two basic *pleadings* initiate the formal lawsuit.

Discovery

Discovery is the process by which the parties find out the facts about each other, about the incidents that have given rise to the claims of malpractice alleged by the plaintiff, and the defenses to those claims asserted by the defendant. In order to obtain discovery, the law has provided discovery devices—procedural mechanisms by which the parties ask for and receive

Players in the litigation process

The litigation process is initiated and enacted by people with a dispute to resolve and those whose task it is to aid in resolving that dispute.

The parties

The principal parties involved in litigation are the *litigants*—the individuals on either side of the dispute. The *plaintiff* is the person who initiates the lawsuit and who claims he or she has suffered injury due to the actions of another. A lawsuit may be filed by multiple plaintiffs.

The plaintiff sues the *defendant*—the person or organization alleged to have injured the plaintiff by his/her or its actions. In most cases the parties are individuals, but parties can be corporations, companies, partnerships, government agencies or, in some cases, governments themselves.

The judge

The *judge* is an individual, usually an attorney, who has been appointed or elected to oversee lawsuits on behalf of the state or government under whose jurisdiction the lawsuit is brought. The judge acts as referee during the pretrial phase of the case and decides legal issues that arise as the lawsuit progresses toward trial. In a trial, the judge's responsibility is *to interpret the law*.

The jury

The *jury* is a panel of citizens chosen by the attorneys for the litigants to hear evidence in the case and render a decision or verdict. The jury's responsibility is *to determine the facts* in a trial. It's up to the jury to decide whether the plaintiff and his or her attorney proved their case, thereby rendering a decision about the defendant's liability and the amount of damages the defendant should pay to the plaintiff.

---

information. Demands are routinely made for documents and other tangible items related to the lawsuit's claims, for statements made by the parties to others, and for witnesses to the incidents. Then, pretrial testimony (*deposition*) is taken of the parties to the lawsuit. This testimony, while out of court, is sworn testimony transcribed by a certified court reporter and can be used for any purpose in the lawsuit, including for purposes of *impeachment*—the demonstrating of prior untruthful or inaccurate testimony, or a challenge to the credibility of a witness—at trial.

Finally, *expert discovery*—information about the opinions of experts retained by the parties—is usually permitted. Experts are individuals accepted by the court to assist the finder of fact—the jury—in understanding issues that commonly fall outside of the experience of the typical juror. In medical malpractice cases, as you will read later, the plaintiff must prove that there was a deviation from the standard of care that resulted in an injury. Expert testimony related to the field of medicine, treatments, and standards of care at issue in the case is usually essential to successfully meet proof requirements for each element of a malpractice claim brought by a plaintiff. Likewise, the defense of such claims nearly always mandates opposing expert testimony—in essence, an explanation by a credentialed individual supporting the actions taken by the defendant from which the claim of malpractice stems.

Motion practice

Disputes over discovery often arise in the context of a lawsuit, and those disputes that can't be resolved by the parties require court intervention. Formal resolution of these disputes usually requires an application to the court—a *motion*—setting forth the dispute and the position of the party making the application (the moving party, or *movant*) and requesting certain *relief* or results to be *ordered* by the court. Naturally, this requires a response from the other party—the *opposition*—that sets out the reasons why the court shouldn't grant the relief requested.

Some motions can be decided by the court *on the papers*, that is, without a formal oral presentation (*oral argument*) by the parties before the judge is assigned. More complicated motions, especially those seeking to eliminate or modify legal claims, almost always require argument before the presiding judge or court.

The trial

While the vast majority of lawsuits settle sometime before trial ("out-of-court settlements"), some cases do proceed to trial. Medical malpractice trials are almost without exception jury trials. Once it's determined that settlement isn't an option, a trial date is set and the attorneys begin to prepare. In federal jurisdictions and many state courts, litigants are required to prepare pretrial statements and submissions. They also disclose exhibit lists (materials and documents the attorneys anticipate they will use at trial). Furthermore, they designate deposition testimony to be read or, if the testimony was videotaped, to be shown at trial. The pretrial submission and disclosure process helps to ensure that the trial is as fair as possible and eliminates the possibility of "trial by ambush"—thus, the "Perry Mason" moments of television and film renown are relatively few and far between.

On the day of the trial, the attorneys for the parties proceed with jury selection. Each attorney tries to select jurors that he or she believes will decide in favor of (*find for*) his or her client. Procedurally, the jury selection process varies widely by jurisdiction. In some courts, the trial judge will take an active role by questioning the jurors. The fight over selection is then left to the attorneys. Other jurisdictions permit the attorneys to question jurors directly without court supervision and the trial judge becomes involved only when a dispute arises. As you can imagine, jury selection in a jurisdiction with strong judicial control is a much briefer process than in those jurisdictions where the attorneys are left to their own devices. No matter what the individual procedure, once the jury is chosen (*empanelled*), the trial begins.

At trial, the parties each give an opening statement, one of the two times in the entire trial that the attorneys are permitted to speak directly to the jurors. After opening statements, the plaintiff's attorney states the plaintiff's case. Because the burden of proof is on the plaintiff, the plaintiff's attorney goes first. After the plaintiff's direct case is finished, the plaintiff "rests," and the defendant's attorney presents the defendant's case. The *direct case* consists of factual testimony from witnesses (the plaintiff and others) as well as expert testimony, deposition testimony, and demonstrative evidence, such as charts, medical records, graphs, photographs, and drawings.

The opposing party has the right to cross-examine each witness after the direct examination, and then redirect examination and recross-examination may follow as necessary. After all the evidence has been presented by both sides, the parties make closing statements (*summations*), which is the last time the attorneys are permitted to speak directly to the jurors.

Once summations are completed, the judge then instructs the jurors on the appropriate law that they're to apply to the facts of the case. Remember that the jury is the *finder of fact*—it determines what happened, when it happened, who did it, where it happened, and how it happened—and the judge is the *interpreter of the law*. After the jurors receive the judge's instructions, they leave the courtroom and begin deliberations.

Every trial attorney hopes to be lucky enough to serve on a jury that goes to deliberations. For trial lawyers, understanding what happens inside the jury room during deliberations is the Holy Grail of trial practice. In jurisdictions that permit attorneys to interview jurors after verdict, attorneys often spend many hours with the jurors who are willing to discuss the case in order to determine what did—and what didn't—work during the trial. It's often surprising to find that what the lawyer thought was of prime importance wasn't so important to the jury. The jury room in our legal system is sacrosanct, and, no matter how it happens, the jury will eventually arrive at a verdict that will be delivered to the parties in open court. Once the verdict is read and the jury excused, the trial is over.

APPEALS

Each jurisdiction has an appellate process, of which the litigants may take advantage. Depending on the jurisdiction, appeals may add years (and many dollars) to the resolution of claims and lawsuits.

LEGAL ELEMENTS OF A MALPRACTICE CLAIM

A medical malpractice claim is made up of four distinct elements, each of which must be proven to the applicable standard of proof in the jurisdiction of the case. The usual standard of proof for civil cases is a *preponderance of the evidence*. The preponderance standard can be best described as a set of scales that represent the plaintiff on one side and the defendant on the other, which are evenly balanced at the start. In a trial, the party that wins is the one on the side of the scale that dips lower at the end. In other words, in order to prevail, plaintiffs need to show by only 50.0000001%—just a bit more than one-half—that they've proven each of the elements that make up a malpractice claim.

The four general elements that make up a malpractice claim are:

- existence of a duty owed to the plaintiff by the defendant
- breach of that duty
- injury that's causally related to that breach of duty
- damages recognized as law.

Duty

In general, there is no duty to protect a person endangered by the actions or omissions of another if there is no special relationship between the two persons. The patient–physician relationship is the basis for the claim of duty between the plaintiff-patient and the defendant-healthcare professional in medical malpractice cases because that relationship permits the patient to rely on the physician's knowledge, expertise, and skill in treatment. Thus, the allegations of medical negligence arise within the course of that professional relationship. Translating that definition into healthcare terms, some examples of a duty may be the obligation of a healthcare practitioner to give patients care that is:

- consistent with the level of his or her experience, education, and training
- permitted under the applicable state practice act
- authorized or permitted under the policies and procedures of the institution that are applicable to the position.

> **PRACTICE POINT**
>
> *Duty:* In negligence cases, *duty* may be defined as obligation, to which the law will give recognition and effect, to conform to a particular standard of conduct toward another. The word *duty* is used throughout the Restatement of Torts to denote the fact that the actor is required to conduct himself in a particular manner at the risk that if he doesn't do so, he becomes subject to liability to another to whom the duty is owed for any injury sustained by such other, of which that actor's conduct is a legal cause. (Restatement, Second, Torts, Section 4.)[1]

Breach of duty

In addition to proving the existence of a duty, the plaintiff must also prove the defendant breached that duty. Breach of duty can result from commission, omission, or both. Most often, to establish this element of the claim, the plaintiff in a medical malpractice case must also show that the defendant healthcare practitioner deviated from an accepted standard of care or treatment. The practitioner isn't required to provide the highest degree of care, but only the level and type of care rendered by the average practitioner. What the standard of care is, and whether and how it was deviated from, must be established for the jury, and this is most often the province of expert testimony.

Breach of duty in the healthcare setting may be illustrated in the following ways:

- failure to give care within the applicable practice act

- failure to perform professional duties with the degree of skill mandated by the applicable practice act
- failure to provide care for which the circumstance of the patient's condition warrants.

> ### ☞ PRACTICE POINT
>
> #14 _Breach:_ The failure to meet an obligation to another person that's owed to that person; the breaking or violating of a law, right, obligation, engagement, or duty by commission, omission, or both.[1]

Injury causally related to a breach of duty

In a medical malpractice case, proof of an injury isn't enough unless that injury can be causally linked to a breach of duty by a healthcare practitioner. That breach of duty is then considered the proximate cause. Without the breach of duty, the injury wouldn't have occurred. (See _Proving proximate cause._)

Proximate cause in the healthcare setting can be illustrated by the following examples:

- fractured hip due to a fall because of failure to raise the side rails of the bed
- decreased total protein due to failure to provide nutrition (either failure to provide actual nourishment or failure to call a consult)

> ### Proving proximate cause
>
> While standards of proof related to proximate cause may vary among jurisdictions, one of two questions is almost always used to determine this issue:
>
> - Was the healthcare practitioner's negligent conduct a "substantial factor" in causing the injury?
> - Would the injury not have happened if the healthcare practitioner hadn't been negligent?

- osteomyelitis resulting in limb amputation following failure to call an infectious disease consult and provide antibiotic therapy.

> ### ☞ PRACTICE POINT
>
> #14 _Proximate cause:_ That which, in a natural and continuous sequence, unbroken by any efficient intervening cause, produces injury, and without which the result wouldn't have occurred and without which the accident couldn't have happened, if the injury be one that might be reasonably anticipated or foreseen as a natural consequence of the wrongful act.[1]

Damages

Finally, the fourth element that makes up a malpractice claim is damages. A healthcare practitioner may be held liable for damages when the jury finds that the practitioner deviated from the applicable standard of care in treating the plaintiff-patient and, as a result, caused injury resulting in legally recognized damages. In most jurisdictions, a plaintiff may recover for proven monetary losses (lost wages and unreimbursed medical expenses) and for pain and suffering that result from the proven injury. As noted previously, it's the jury—the finder of fact—that sets the monetary award to the plaintiff.

> ### ☞ PRACTICE POINT
>
> _Damage:_ Loss, injury, or deterioration caused by the negligence, design, or accident of one person or another, with respect to the latter's person or property.
>
> #14 _Damages:_ A pecuniary compensation or indemnity that may be recovered in the courts by any person who has suffered loss, detriment, or injury, whether to his or her person, property, or rights, through the unlawful act or omission or negligence of another.[1]

As we have shown, in order for a plaintiff to prevail in a medical malpractice claim, all four of the elements discussed above must be satisfied. Three of four won't do. They must score perfectly on all four to prevail before a jury.

THE MEDICAL RECORD IN LITIGATION

The medical record is arguably the single most important piece of evidence in a medical malpractice case. It serves as a crucial tool for the delivery of science-based care. It is also:

- a legal document
- a communication tool
- the supporting basis for treatment decisions and modifications
- one of the primary tools for the evaluation of treatment modalities.

At one time or another in the education of a healthcare practitioner, whatever the specialty or discipline, this directive is taught: "If it wasn't written down, it didn't happen." Nowhere does this statement ring more true than in a medical malpractice case. (See *Effects of incomplete charting*.) Before we consider the role documentation plays in the medico-legal world, let's first consider for a moment how important the medical record is in the care and treatment of patients.

Communication tool

The medical record is the primary method of communication between members of the healthcare team. Oral report and rounding are essential communication devices, but it's impractical and unrealistic to expect that every healthcare team member be present during report or rounds. Such disciplines as physical therapy, occupational therapy, and respiratory therapy are rarely present for report or rounds. The myriad medical specialists available to the primary physician (infectious disease consultants, for example) are also rarely present during rounds, yet it's imperative for the delivery of good science-based care that every healthcare team member have the most current and up-to-date patient information. The medical record is the only way to accomplish this. It's available 24 hours per day to any practitioner who can utilize it to stay informed about the patient's progress.

Effects of incomplete charting

What happens when charting is incomplete? In addition to providing a poor medical record of a patient's care to help jog the practitioner's memory if a lawsuit occurs, it can create other problems. Competent attorneys can create havoc when gaps exist in the record. Nothing makes proving the plaintiff's case easier than such gaps, especially near or around the time of the alleged malpractice if the claim revolves around a single incident. If the claim concerns a continuous or extended course of treatment, the absence of documentation related to treatment outcomes, observations, and the basis for the treatment is strong evidence of negligence. Where the record contains gaps, you can be certain that the plaintiff's attorney will be happy to suggest to a jury what happened during those undocumented times, and those suggestions won't be of benefit to the healthcare facility or the individual practitioner.

Treatment evaluation and support

Documenting patient treatment outcomes and responses in the medical record is a key method for evaluating treatment modalities and therapies. The typical patient with pressure ulcers will undergo an extended course of treatment that will change over the course of time. In order to establish a basis for treatment and modification, there must be well-documented observations and evaluations of the patient. Upon initiation of treatment, careful observation and documentation of the patient's condition is critical in order to establish a baseline for initial treatment and care and to measure treatment against. Without a carefully documented record, treatment, evaluation, patient outcomes, and treatment modifications are impossible to justify—in court

General documentation guidelines

Listed here are some general rules for documentation that serve your patient's needs and can help in the defense of a lawsuit.

- Be thorough—record the date and time for each entry.
- Be accurate—use units of measure instead of estimates (for example, "patient had a 6-oz cup of ice chips" instead of "patient had some ice chips").
- Be factual—think of yourself as a newspaper reporter and answer the following questions: who, what, when, where, why, and how.
- Be objective—record only the facts. Remember that you're communicating information that others will rely on. If your patient is to benefit from your professional training, judgment, and observational

skills, your colleagues must have objective, factual information to rely upon.
- Write legibly—print if necessary.
- Only use approved abbreviations.
- Make contemporaneous entries—finish your documentation before you leave work for the day. Don't add notations days later unless your facility permits such additions—and even then, adhere strictly to your facility's policy governing such additions.
- Be truthful—don't fake, misrepresent, exaggerate, or misstate the facts in the medical record.
- Most importantly, don't assign blame. While it's important to relate the facts completely and accurately, assigning blame in the medical record is fodder for malpractice actions and does nothing to advance the care of your patients.

or at the bedside. (See *General documentation guidelines*.)

PRACTICE POINT

Accurate and complete patient outcomes and responses to treatment and care must be documented in the record, as they're the basis for care decisions and legal defense.

LEGAL ASPECTS OF WOUND DOCUMENTATION

Wound assessments are some of the most detailed and time-consuming documentation a healthcare provider will perform. Radiologists can view internal organs with a variety of internal imaging techniques and generate detailed, consistent reports. Myriad laboratory values are also available to monitor internal organ system functions. Wounds,

however, are not yet amenable to sophisticated imaging techniques and many accepted laboratory values cannot monitor their healing objectively. Wound assessment and documentation is still mostly a subjective, visual, pen-and-paper exercise that requires a good base of knowledge to perform accurately. Wound assessment and monitoring are typically left to the staff nurse or wound specialist. Wounds require an intricate, multi-faceted assessment of their many attributes. (See chapter 6, Wound assessment.) Different levels of knowledge among caregivers can result in inaccurate, inconsistent, and erroneous wound documentation. Multiple areas of documentation for wound issues can make quick access to this information difficult. Multiple wounds on a single patient add even more of a documentation burden. Such complexity can lead to inconsistent documentation—and treatment—and may leave a provider or facility open to legal liability.

The medical record serves several purposes. First and foremost it is a communication tool that allows real-time coordination of care by multiple disciplines. It also acts as a historical record to determine the efficacy of past interventions and guide future care. The medical record is also a factual record utilized in lawsuits to determine the quality of care rendered, the occurrence of physical harm, and other legal issues. Most state nursing and medical boards and federal regulatory agencies require "timely and accurate" documentation of findings in the medical record. Due to the wide range of specialty care areas and ever-changing rules, regulations, and laws, state and federal boards offer little guidance on *how* to meet this documentation standard. It's left to the individual facility or provider to determine the appropriate standards. The absence of standards has resulted in a wide range of documentation practices.

The American Nurses Association[2] has clarified that nurses are expected to record their assessments and diagnoses of the patient's skin integrity in the medical record. Staging of pressure ulcers and differentiating them from other wounds is within the scope of nursing practice.

We recommend the following processes and procedures to improve the consistency and documentation of care for pressure ulcers, acute and chronic wounds, or any other untoward event that occurs while a patient is under care. These recommendations are not designed to promulgate or establish a particular standard of care for wound documentation but rather to make providers aware of the common difficulties that may occur with wound documentation and to propose solutions.

The flow of information

To find the latest laboratory value in a chart you go to the lab section. To find the latest chest X-ray result you go to the radiology section. To find the latest wound description you go to…? Wound documentation is often found scattered throughout the chart in activity of daily living (ADL) forms, nursing assessments, narrative notes, wound assessment forms, and many other sections. The organization and composition of the medical record in any given facility often evolves over the years with no real appreciation for how one would look at the chart globally. This is especially true of nursing documentation forms as they are added to and modified over time. In such situations duplication of information becomes increasingly common. Consistent documentation by nursing staff then becomes much more difficult to provide and to review at a later date.

In order to evaluate the effectiveness of the medical record as a communication tool, one should critically examine from an outsider's perspective just how information flows within the record. A medico-legal reviewer attempting to determine if care was accurately and consistently provided can sometimes be stymied by a poorly structured chart whose organization makes sense to the facility—yet to no one else. Information that cannot be found readily will often be ignored. If the appropriate form or the proper location in the chart cannot be found easily, certain information may not be documented. If wound care documentation can take place in multiple areas of the chart, it may be documented multiple times—or not at all—because of the uncertainty as to where the information should be properly entered. The medical record is a documentation system. If documentation is inconsistent, a systems approach may be applied in order to evaluate and improve the structure and flow of documentation, rather than actually getting staff to just "document more."

Admission assessment

Both the medical and nursing admission assessments provide a "snapshot" of the patient's status at the time of admission. The admission assessment is an area where one cannot over-document. The more information that's documented about the patient at the time of admission, the better informed the healthcare team will be, and thus decisions can be made based on the best information available. Discovery and description of any lesion during admission assessment are critical in determining the course of care and, in a lawsuit, in determining the ultimate liability for any wounds that develop or deteriorate during the patient's stay. Preexisting lesions should be documented carefully and thoroughly with regard to size, location, and characteristics. A detailed description of the wound is more important than an actual wound diagnosis during admission assessment. The chart should reflect what interventions were taken and who was notified of the existence of the wound and any other findings.

A general rule often heard in nursing and wound care circles is that any pressure ulcer that develops after 24 hours of admission is considered to be acquired at the facility rather than inherited. However, the definition of suspected deep tissue injury (DTI), a deep tissue discoloration under intact skin or a blood-filled blister that may ultimately evolve to a full-thickness lesion—as further defined in 2009 by the National Pressure Ulcer Advisory Panel (NPUAP)–European Pressure Ulcer Advisory Panel (EPUAP)[3] Pressure Ulcer Prevention and Treatment guidelines—makes this general rule difficult to defend. For example, the patient may be admitted with an inconspicuous-looking skin discoloration in the sacral area or other bony prominence that ultimately evolves into a full-thickness pressure ulcer. The process of tissue ischemia and necrosis can take several days to become visible to the naked eye when all that was observed and documented on admission was a sacral discoloration. Therefore, nursing and medical staff should be made aware of this new NPUAP-EPUAP definition[3] and incorporate it into their assessments. (For more information, see Chapter 13, Pressure ulcers).

Because pressure ulcers are a frequent reason for litigation in health care, they will be highlighted as a key exemplar in the remainder of this chapter.

Pressure ulcer risk assessment

All patients should be assessed for pressure ulcer risk. A pressure ulcer risk assessment can include any validated scale, such as the Braden or Norton scale. Risk scales are tools that quantify risk factors associated with pressure ulcer development, such as nutrition, moisture, and mobility, among others. A pressure ulcer risk assessment scale can provide detailed insight into the care needs of the patient far beyond skin protection. The frequency of risk assessment is open to debate and is based primarily on the guidelines or custom of the individual nursing unit.

Ideally, every patient admitted to a healthcare facility should be assessed upon admission to identify individuals at risk for pressure ulcer development. Those at risk should then have routine follow-up assessments during their stay. A risk assessment is also recommended when the patient is transferred to another unit or whenever there is a significant change in the patient's condition. The nursing admission and/or daily assessment is a logical chart area in which to document risk assessment. The most important aspect with any risk assessment is: What is done with the information? Validated risk assessment tools are powerful and accurate predictors of pressure ulcer development but are useless if the information they provide is not acted upon. Each risk factor is ideally suited as an individual plan to prevent, mitigate, or improve a decline in the level of functioning.

Pressure ulcer development

Sometimes the underlying problems that result in the development of pressure ulcers can be managed, healed, or avoided altogether. In other instances the disease burden can be so great that ulcers will occur or fail to heal despite the best of care. Indeed, the Centers for Medicare and Medicaid Services (CMS) recognizes that pressure ulcers are unavoidable in long-term care if the facility had (1) evaluated the resident's clinical condition and pressure ulcer risk factors, (2) defined and implemented interventions that are consistent with resident needs, goals, and recognized standards of practice, (3) monitored and evaluated the impact of the interventions, and (4) revised the approaches as appropriate.[4] In 2010, the NPUAP hosted a consensus conference and modified this definition to make it applicable to other care settings. The revised definition of "unavoidable" in reference to pressure ulcer development is "that the individual developed a pressure ulcer even though the provider had evaluated the individual's clinical condition and pressure ulcer risk factors; defined and implemented interventions that are consistent with individual needs, goals and recognized standards of practice; monitored and evaluated the impact of the interventions; and revised the approaches as appropriate."[5] Any documentation system regarding pressure ulcer prevention should be able to clearly and efficiently outline these criteria.

PRACTICE POINT

Consider the following NPUAP consensus conference statement that there are patient situations that could lead to unavoidable pressure ulcers[5]:

- skin failure
- hemodynamic instability that may preclude turning or repositioning
- patient refusal to reposition.

Nursing units where the disease burden of patients is extremely high include intensive care units (ICUs), long-term care units, and hospice. For ICU patients, frequent and consistent monitoring should be performed on the high-risk areas of the sacrum, heel and trochanter, and the occipital area. We frequently find in chart reviews that dynamic, pressure-distributing mattresses are obtained *after* the development of a pressure ulcer. While this may be a logical and justifiable escalation of care and intervention for a general medical–surgical population, it's important that special emphasis be placed on these high-risk populations.

The infamous "Turn Q 2" check box

Many nursing patient-care flow sheets have "Turn Q 2" (turn every 2 hours) on their checklist of pressure ulcer prevention strategies. The presence or lack of a check in this box on these flow sheets is often used by attorneys to undermine or paint a negative picture of the quality and consistency of care delivered by nursing staff. The origins of the requirement to reposition patients every 2 hours for pressure ulcer prevention are obscure and not well grounded in science. The 1994 Agency for Health Care Policy and Research (AHCPR) guidelines specifically recommended repositioning every 2 hours.[6] Such an absolute time requirement for repositioning or other inter-

ventions does not permit individual clinical judgment. Patient care should be based on the dynamic evaluation of a patient's status by qualified personnel and not on a single, fixed point. Some patients may require more frequent repositioning and some less as a result of the use of a pressure-distributing mattress[7] or the need for uninterrupted sleep. Some may be unable to turn due to critical illness. Some may have undergone diagnostic procedures, thereby precluding staff from attending to them every 2 hours. There are simply too many variables that determine when and how a patient is positioned to require a rigid timetable that likely bears little or no resemblance to the patient's actual needs. The NPUAP-EPUAP Prevention and Treatment Guidelines state that repositioning frequency should be influenced by the support surface used (Strength of evidence = A).[3]

We recommend removing the "Turn Q 2" check box from nursing forms, admission order templates, pressure ulcer prevention orders, and other areas. The check box could be replaced with a statement such as "reposition according to patient needs as determined by pressure ulcer risk assessment" or some other language determined to better meet patient care needs and risk-management requirements for proper documentation. We note, however, that this more flexible standard requires a more rigorous approach to documentation of the actions taken by healthcare personnel. Many staff members are accustomed to the check-off system and may fail to adequately document interventions without such a system. Management should consider training and monitoring to ensure compliance with documentation standards. This new method connects the risk assessment to the intervention and allows much more flexibility for staff to deliver timely and effective care rather than basing care on a single number.

Discovery of a pressure ulcer

The initial discovery of a pressure ulcer is typically documented in the nursing narrative note section. Any ongoing assessments (and actions, including notification of appropriate medical personnel) should then be documented per facility policy in a wound care form, ADL form, or narrative notes, but preferably in just one place in the chart for easy access. The response to the discovery of the lesion is just as critical as documenting the lesion itself. Documentation should include what immediate interventions were taken; who was notified (the charge nurse, the incoming staff, the physician, the wound care specialist, and/or the family), what topical care was provided to the lesion (ointments or creams, hydrocolloids, or other dressings); and any actions that were taken to minimize further damage (an air mattress, heel suspension boots, lowering the head of bed, repositioning, and other interventions). Such documentation demonstrates that your facility has a system in place to act quickly and appropriately to changes in the patient's condition.

Correct identification of the lesion

The etiology of the lesion must be correctly identified in order to provide the most appropriate and effective care. Examine the wound for yourself, review the patient's medical history, make your own judgment, and if it differs with others discuss your concerns with the team. When in doubt about the etiology or progress of a wound, don't make a speculation in the chart; simply document what you observed. Remember, objective description beats subjective guessing every time.

Differentiating between a pressure ulcer and an ischemic ulcer in the lower extremity can be particularly difficult. For example, is the development of a wound on the lateral aspect of the foot in a person with peripheral vascular disease the result of pressure or arterial insufficiency? The argument could be that "but for" the pressure, the lesion would not have occurred. The counterargument could be that "but for" the arterial insufficiency, the tissue could have easily tolerated the pressure exerted on the foot. Objective data are required to solve this dispute. In this case, formal vascular laboratory studies are needed to determine the extent of ischemia and the avoidability of such lesions. Most chronic wounds have distinctive locations, sizes, and presentations and can be easily differentiated by trained personnel. However, some wounds will defy easy categorization or diagnosis. All lesions require as much objective data as possible to establish the correct diagnosis and appropriate care plan.

Notification and participation of the physician

The patient's primary physician must be notified of any untoward event in a timely manner, including development of a pressure ulcer or other wounds. Good practice requires documentation of when the physician was notified, the response to the notification, any orders given, and the plan for examination and follow-up. Physicians must also meet the standard care (what a reasonable and prudent provider would do in the same or similar situation) when managing a patient's wound. In facilities with an active wound care department, the routine management of the lesion is often handed to staff by the primary physician. The physician typically signs verbal orders that are written by these specialists. This allows interdisciplinary care and provides maximum potential to heal or mitigate the wound. This does not, however, relieve the physician of the responsibility to monitor the condition of the wound.

Physicians should arrange to examine the wound on a routine basis, have a good understanding of the rationale behind the wound care orders being signed, and be involved in consulting other specialties as needed to maximize healing. Physicians should take the lead in notifying the patient's family about the development of any lesion, just as they would any other negative event that occurs under their care. Pressure ulcers are symptoms of underlying medical, physical, and psychosocial problems. They are therefore a multidisciplinary issue involving nursing, nutrition, social work, physical therapy—and medicine—among many other specialties.

Notifying the patient and family

Prompt and thorough notification of the patient and family of any new wound or other adverse event is critical to ensure full understanding and participation in care.

In some states, such as New Jersey, this is required by law.[8] Full disclosure of all facts related to the development of the wound should be provided: When was it discovered? How was it discovered? What interventions were being taken to prevent the wound? What interventions are being taken now? Give plenty of time for the information to be absorbed, and allow for questions. Many in the lay community believe that pressure ulcers or "bedsores" are the result of negligence. An initial negative reaction to an adverse event may be expected, but prompt and full disclosure of the situation will go a long way toward minimizing lingering doubts and suspicions about the adequacy of care in your facility. When discussing the situation with the patient and family, use explanations, not excuses. While the patient's health status may have played a significant role in the development of the adverse event (for example, a pressure ulcer, dehisced surgical incision, or other chronic wound) it is probably best not to dwell on this topic initially as it may be interpreted by family members as "blaming the patient." Follow-up conversations and briefings with the patient and family may serve as a better time to discuss the realistic goals of healing, once they digest the initial information and the effects of the care plan are better known. More in-depth information about communicating with the family regarding pressure ulcers can be found elsewhere in the literature.[9]

The patient and family should also be educated that new wounds, especially pressure ulcers, are likely to look worse before they look better. A suspected deep tissue injury (DTI) may look rather innocent to the family as a "simple deep bruise" (discoloration) with maybe a little torn skin. The suspected DTI may evolve through a course that can include tissue ischemia, tissue necrosis, necrotic tissue separation, and even ultimate cavitation or ulceration. Lay persons could easily and incorrectly construe such a change in the wound as substandard care. Preparing the family in advance and setting expectations will reduce the shock of seeing a wound go through this natural process. Any conversations with family members and their response to the information should be promptly documented.

Ongoing wound documentation

Wound documentation places a significant burden on the healthcare provider due to the intricate nature of wound assessments. One way to ease this burden is to use logical, well-structured wound documentation forms or computer templates. Check boxes or drop-down lists are recommended for efficient documentation and to limit erroneous entries. Wound assessment forms can be structured in many different ways and will almost always improve the accuracy and consistency of documentation. Such forms can be created easily with word-processing or spreadsheet software. A glossary of terms should also be developed for the more obscure terminology used on the wound care form. Drop-down menus, forms, and check boxes, however, are no substitute for narrative nursing assessments when required, and space must be provided in the medical record for such notes as needed.

Frequency of assessment will depend on the wound type, its phase of healing, the resources available to the wound care specialist, and other factors. CMS recommends a weekly thorough assessment with daily monitoring of the dressing and wound to assess for complications in long-term care patients.[4] Weekly assessments by a wound specialist allow subtle changes to be noticed that would ordinarily be missed with more frequent inspection. Daily monitoring can be noted in the narrative notes, on treatment sheets, or on a wound assessment form per facility policy, but preferably in just one location for ease of reference. Wound documentation should be consistent and concise. Frequent brief, but thorough, notes indicate consistent care.

Wound photography... or wound imaging?

Wound photography has become more popular with the advent of inexpensive, quality digital cameras. Three national organizations have position statements about the use of wound photography in wound care.[10-12] What is the rationale behind wound photography? Is it for assessment and diagnosis or just an attempt to mitigate legal liability? Consider *wound imaging* as an assessment and diagnostic tool just like an X-ray or magnetic resonance imaging. If thought of in this manner, wound imaging might be obtained routinely and consistently (per your facility policy and procedure) as with any other assessment and diagnostic imaging. A series of wound images will allow for more efficient and informed interventions and may assist in a legal defense should one become necessary. This regular, methodical approach is in contrast to taking one or two photographs during an inpatient stay to "cover ourselves legally"; taking this approach often backfires. What would any individual, and especially a juror, react more positively to: A series of detailed photographs showing progress of the wound or one or two photographs taken at odd intervals throughout the patient's stay? One reveals consistency; the other does not.

Wound imaging supplements—but does not replace—the need for written documentation. Each image should have accompanying text discussing what is observed in the photograph. This is similar to obtaining a radiologist's report after medical imaging. Consent for noninvasive medical imaging is rarely required, and the same should also be true for wound imaging as long as the patient cannot be readily identified. Management should clear the consent issue with legal counsel and risk managers. (See Chapter 6, Wound assessment.)

Collaboration, coordination, and communication

Collaboration, coordination, and communication of all specialty services are essential in maximizing the potential for wound healing. Documentation of "the three C's" may also demonstrate to the medico-legal expert—and ultimately to a jury—that coordinated, consistent, interdisciplinary care was provided. Most facilities with a wound care team have policies that specify consultation for certain types of lesions. Many wound, ostomy, and continence (WOC) nurses provide both consult services and hands-on care at their facility.[13] If the WOC nurse acts in a consultant role, he or she should examine how consults by other facility services are structured and document in a similar manner. Consultants not only provide recommendations

or establish a care plan, but they also educate other providers on their specialty and the rationale for their recommendations.

Wound care services are also provided by physical therapists in many facilities. As with WOC nurses, consults ideally should be based on the format at their facility and include a care plan and follow-up. Adequate follow-up by either a WOC or staff nurse should be ensured prior to the patient being discharged from physical therapy services. In addition, consults to plastic surgery, vascular surgery, or other surgical specialties are also part of interdisciplinary care. Because there are wide variations in approaches to chronic wound care by these specialties, disagreements can arise. Therefore, consistent documentation of communication among the specialties will resolve any differences and is an indicator of quality, interdisciplinary care.

Policies and procedures: normative or positive?

Policies and procedures (P&Ps) establish standards of care within the facility. In any legal proceeding, P&Ps will be scrutinized and compared with the care that is documented in the chart. P&Ps are typically divided into two types of philosophies: normative and positive. A normative P&P describes what care *can* realistically and consistently be provided. A positive P&P describes what care *should* ideally be provided. P&Ps with a positive, ideal focus can cause great trouble in legal proceedings because they set unrealistic and unattainable goals that often exceed a reasonable standard of care.[14]

When establishing P&Ps in your facility, avoid using absolute terms like "will" and "must" and specifying exact time frames for routine nursing interventions unless absolutely necessary. For example, a P&P that states "All patients will have a pressure ulcer risk assessment every Tuesday and Friday" sets an unrealistic expectation. Missing 1 day or doing the assessment on a Saturday instead of Friday is a violation of your own standard of care. Rewording the P&P to read "All bedfast or chairfast patients should have a pressure ulcer risk assessment twice a week" gives nursing staff more leeway in their care and documentation. In a lawsuit, "violations" of P&Ps are not always a liability in the defense of such actions. Departures that are explained by and supported by science-based care—and that are fully and completely documented contemporaneously—can often be used to the advantage of the defense. Sometimes P&Ps must spell out exactly when and where something will or must be done, but mostly they should focus on guiding and educating staff members rather than enforcing strict rules and timelines for care. (See *Preventative legal care: Eight key areas of vulnerability for institutions*.)

Preventative legal care: Eight key areas of vulnerability for institutions

1. Words have meaning— Assessing the legal implications of healthcare facility "policies and procedures"

KEY CONCEPT: Healthcare facility policies and procedures are "guidelines," not rules or regulations—and should be created and treated as such. These guidelines should be carefully crafted and periodically reviewed with regard to their clinical currency as well as their legal and healthcare implications. Words such as "never," "must," "shall," and "immediately" should be rigorously avoided.

2. Assessing compliance with prescribing rules

KEY CONCEPT: Healthcare organizations and clinicians should review standing orders to ensure that they are in compliance with prescribing regulations.

3. Changing and practicing within scope of practice

KEY CONCEPT: Healthcare institutions should ensure that caregivers are practicing within their scope of practice with regard to pressure ulcer assessment and documentation.

4. Managing expectations and communicating carefully

KEY CONCEPT: The people most likely to be asked difficult questions (regarding why, how and when pressure ulcers develop) by patients and their families are not always in the best position to provide an accurate big-picture response. Front-line staff should be trained in how to delegate questions professionally and with compassion.

5. Clinical documentation

a. Skin assessments

KEY CONCEPT: Skin assessments should be conducted regularly and in accordance with the guidelines of a particular institution. Note that the skin assessment is different from the risk assessment and both must be performed.

b. Risk assessments

KEY CONCEPT: Pressure ulcer risk assessment guidelines for an organization should be worded in ways that are compatible with federal terminology.

c. Pressure ulcer assessment

KEY CONCEPT: The importance of reasonably complete documentation cannot be overemphasized. Medical record documentation from any provider involved in the care and treatment of the patient may be used to support the determination of whether a condition was present on admission. A "provider" means a physician or any qualified healthcare practitioner who is legally accountable for establishing the patient's diagnosis.[12]

d. Charting

KEY CONCEPT: Good pressure ulcer documentation should include a wound description, measurement and wound care treatments, as well as documentation of

(continued)

Preventative legal care: Eight key areas of vulnerability for institutions (continued)

pressure redistribution devices and techniques, including support surfaces and turning schedules.

e. Electronic health records (EHRs)

KEY CONCEPT: Electronic record systems may not accommodate the documentation needs of pressure ulcer patients.

f. Photography

KEY CONCEPT: Photography has advantages and drawbacks in terms of litigation; know the guidelines set forth by the organization.

g. Staging

KEY CONCEPT: Training in the use of NPUAP pressure ulcer staging is recommended for all healthcare professionals, including physicians. When in doubt about a pressure ulcer's stage, all clinicians are encouraged to "describe what they see." Careful attention should be given to the discharge ulcer assessment.

6. Preventability—Avoidable, unavoidable, preventable or never events?

KEY CONCEPT: Government regulations and governmental language can be used to help juries decide healthcare malpractice and wrongful death cases. Understand these documents and how

reimbursement terminology maps onto clinical practice.

7. Education—The need for learning never ends

KEY CONCEPT: Since clinician knowledge of pressure ulcers has been linked to pressure ulcer incidence, initial and ongoing education about best practices is essential. Patient education should do more than address the basics of skin care; it should help patients formulate realistic expectations about their treatment, risks, and recovery.

8. Preventive clinical care

KEY CONCEPT: "Bundles" work and should be implemented when appropriate. While there may be insufficient data for evidence-based product and device selection in pressure ulcer care, evidence-guided selections can be made.

© Copyright 2009 International Expert Wound Care Advisory Panel.
Ayello, E.A., Capitulo, K.L., Fife, C.E., Fowler, E., Krasner, D.L., Mulder, G., Sibbald, R.G., Yankowsky, K.W. "Legal Issues in the Care of Pressure Ulcer Patients: Key Concepts for Healthcare Providers. A Consensus Paper from the International Expert Wound Care Advisory Panel." *World Council of Enterostomal Therapists* 29(9):8-22, July-September 2009.

Pressure ulcer prevention and treatment[6] practices have undergone significant revisions and changes since the first AHCPR guidelines were released almost 20 years ago. In addition to these recommendations, guidelines from NPUAP-EPUAP (2009) and the Wound, Ostomy and Continence Nurses Society (2010) incorporate the latest research and recommendations.[3,13] The CMS guidelines[4] in particular are thorough, complete, and easy to read by a wider range of healthcare providers. While developed for long-term care, they are easily adaptable to acute care and other settings and provide compre-

hensive education and guidance while avoiding "absolute" terminology. Incorporation of these guideline recommendations into your practice indicates that your facility is up-to-date on the latest changes that impact pressure ulcer care.

Discharge—to home or another facility

The patient and caregiver should have adequate resources to manage the wound upon discharge to the home or another facility.[14] Documentation of this coordination should include teaching strategies and the patient/caregiver response to them, consults with social work or home care, and any equipment or supplies sent home with the patient. Ensure that the patient has adequate follow-up for medical and wound issues.

The discharge assessment should be a thorough and complete "snapshot" of the patient before leaving your facility. As with the admission assessment, you cannot over-document in this area. Thoroughly assess and document any wounds and the condition of high-risk pressure ulcer areas. Document any communication with the receiving facility. Alert the receiving facility to any wounds and describe them in detail. The medical discharge summary typically does not go into significant detail about wound therapy, and thus the onus for this communication is placed on nursing. List all previous and current wound therapies, which will avoid wasted time in trying therapies that have already yielded little or no results. List all previous and current preventive measures and equipment, such as air mattresses, seat cushions, and heel protectors.

SUMMARY

The patient's chart is an important legal document because it provides a written record of the care provided. It also serves as a means of communication among healthcare professionals about the patient's responses to care. Complete and accurate documentation is not only essential for good patient care, but it is also the basis for mounting a defense in the event of legal action. Make your entries in the patient's record legible, thorough, professional, and factual. Ensure that all information is correct and accurate.

Consistent documentation is a reflection of the quality, interdisciplinary care provided to an individual. Chronic wounds are often symptoms of many underlying medical, physical, and psychosocial problems. Documentation of these multiple issues requires a well-structured documentation system. Ensure your documentation system allows healthcare providers to consistently and concisely communicate and access their findings. Policies and procedures should be updated as new research and practices appear. The documentation system should incorporate and reflect these new practices. Such interventions will maximize communication among the interdisciplinary team and help to improve patient outcomes.[14]

PATIENT SCENARIO

Clinical Data

A 66-year-old woman presented herself and was admitted to the emergency department with complaints of headache, nausea, and right upper extremity weakness for 24 hours. Physical examination showed the patient's blood pressure to be 140/86 mm Hg, heart rate 64 bpm, and temperature 100.2°F. Her right extremity grip strength was diminished. Blood test results revealed a decreased leukocyte count and mild hypokalemia.

The patient's prior medical history included a myocardial infarction, hypertension (treated with medication), type 2 diabetes mellitus, and a questionable history of transient ischemic attack.

Before the patient could be sent to radiology for routine X-rays, she suffered precipitous cardiovascular collapse requiring intubation, pressor support, and admission to the ICU. Borderline perfusion was achieved with large doses of pressors (dopamine, norepinephrine) and intravenous fluids. Urine output was diminished but acceptable.

The provisional diagnosis was idiopathic cardiovascular collapse/compromise; sepsis was ruled out.

Hospital Course

The patient remained in the ICU for 24 days. She suffered a cerebral infarct (requiring no surgical intervention) on day 3. Hemodynamic instability lasting 12 days required pressor support and intubation. Total parenteral nutrition was begun on day 7.

On day 24, the patient was transferred to a step-down unit with a sacral pressure ulcer that measured 5.6 × 11.2 cm with an average depth of 0.5 cm and significant undermining. Necrotic tissue was evident at the deepest parts of the wound and on some edges.

(continued)

Surgical, nutritional, and neurologic consults were provided on admission to the step-down unit. A stepwise debridement plan was put into place. The patient subsequently underwent three surgical procedures to close the wound.

The ICU nursing notes 72 hours after admission included the formation of a sacral blister; progress of the wound was documented subsequently. Treatment orders were for saline and other moist dressings. A pressure redistribution bed was not ordered or provided until day 16.

The physician notes clearly indicate that the patient was critically unstable through day 12, maintaining only borderline perfusion. Concern for potential digit loss secondary to tissue hypoxia/coagulopathy/hypotension was noted by the ICU physician and in notes by the vascular consultant until day 12.

Case Discussion

This case was reviewed independently by three law firms, all of whom turned the case down. Expert review uniformly cited the critical, unstable nature of the first 12 days of hospitalization and the critically compromised perfusion as the reason for the ulcer. The experts also opined that while the ulcer was clearly a bad result, it was not an unacceptable result of the risk–benefit analysis performed by the caregivers in light of the patient's critically compromised circulatory status. While some experts privately opined that in a perfect world all sacral pressure ulcers would be preventable, in the real world, as in this case, they would not opine that the formation of this ulcer was the result of medical or other negligence.

From a practice point of view, if a patient's condition is such that the caregivers conclude that measures ordinarily sufficient to delay or prevent tissue breakdown cannot be utilized, clear documentation of the decision-making process and conclusions should be made. In this case, the documentation was inadequate in this regard.

1. In a medical malpractice trial, what's the role of the jury and the judge?
   A. Interpreter of the law; finder of fact
   B. Finder of fact; finder of fact and interpreter of the law
   C. Finder of fact; interpreter of the law
   D. Both judge and jury find fact and interpret the law

   ANSWER: C. *The jury determines who, what, when, why, where, and how—in other words, what happened. The judge interprets the law by instructing the jury about the law to be applied to the facts as it has determined them. The other options are incorrect.*

2. At trial, how many of the four elements of a medical malpractice claim must a defendant convince a jury that the plaintiff has failed to prove in order to successfully defend against a claim of medical malpractice?
   A. One
   B. Two
   C. Three
   D. Four

   ANSWER: D. *The plaintiff must prove all four elements in order to prevail at trial.*

3. The medical record is:
   A. a communication tool.
   B. destroyed after 1 year.

C. a tool to communicate opinions related to a patient's care.

D. an optional part of health care.

ANSWER: A. *Opinions related to patient care aren't proper entries in a medical record. The medical record is a communication tool among practitioners, and is best used for the transmittal of factual information. The other options are incorrect.*

4. Which one of the following statements about standards of care, practice guidelines, and policies and procedures is <u>false</u>?

A. They should be reviewed at regular intervals but never amended.

B. They should be reviewed at regular intervals and amended to reflect new information and research.

C. They should be based on research and practice experience.

D. They should be patient-outcome oriented and quantifiable.

ANSWER: A. *Standards must be reviewed and amended to reflect the latest research and practice experience in a treatment area. Standards based on practice experience only and not supported by research may not survive judicial scrutiny at trial and don't offer the patient the best care.*

5. Given the new definition and understanding of suspected deep tissue injury (DTI) from NPUAP, an area of purplish discoloration on an immobile patient's sacrum that was not documented on admission but appears 24 hours later would:

A. be classified as an acute medical wound.

B. be documented as a stage IV pressure ulcer.

C. have occurred prior to admission.

D. be documented as a stage III pressure ulcer.

ANSWER: C. *Suspected DTI damage may occur days before it is visibly evident on the patient. The other options are incorrect.*

6. Which of the following exemplifies the best way to document frequency of turning a patient in the medical record?

A. A 2-hour check box

B. Regular turning q 2 hours

C. q 4-hour turning

D. Individualized turning schedule based on patient assessment q 4-hour turning

ANSWER: D. *An individualized turning schedule based on patient assessment q 4-hour turning is the best way to document the frequency of turning in the medical record. The other options are incorrect because they are rigid and inflexible and do not allow for individualized patient care. Too many variables can impact repositioning to mandate an absolute time frame for all patients.*

7. Normative policies and procedures describe care that can be:

A. realistically and consistently provided.

B. used for normal staffing situations only.

C. ideally strived for.

D. exceeded to achieve magnet status.

ANSWER: A. *Normative policies and procedures describe care that can be realistically and consistently provided. The other options are incorrect. Answer B is the definition of positive policies and procedures; C, policies are not based on staffing ratios; and D, has nothing to do with normative policies.*

REFERENCES

1. *Black's Law Dictionary*, 5th ed. New York: West Publishing Company, 1979.
2. Patton, R.M. "Is Diagnosis of Pressure Ulcers Within an RN's Scope of Practice?" *American Nurse Today* 5(1):20, 2010.
3. National Pressure Ulcer Advisory Panel (NPUAP) and European Pressure Ulcer Advisory Panel (EPUAP). Prevention and treatment of pressure ulcers: clinical practice guideline. Washington DC: National Pressure Ulcer Advisory Panel, 2009.
4. Centers for Medicare and Medicaid Services (CMS) Tag F-314. Pressure Ulcers. Revised guidance for surveyors in long term care. Issued November 12, 2004. Available at: *http//new.cms.hhs.gov/manuals/download/som107ap_pp_guidelines_ltcf.pdf*. Accessed October 11, 2010.
5. National Pressure Ulcer Advisory Panel (NPUAP). Not all pressure ulcers are avoidable. Press Release. Available at: *www.npuap.org/A_UA%20Press%20Release.pdf*. Accessed September 22, 2010.
6. Bergstrom, N., et al. *Treatment of Pressure Ulcers.* Clinical Practice Guideline. No. 15 AHCPR No. 95-0652. Rockville, MD: Agency for Health Care Policy and Research; December 1994.
7. Defloor, T., Grypdonck, M., and De Bacquer, D. "The Effect of Various Combinations of Turning and Pressure Reducing Devices on the Incidence of Pressure Ulcers." *Int J Nurs Stud* 42(1):37-46, 2005.
8. New Jersey Department of Health and Senior Services. March 3, 2008. The Department of Health and Senior Services published in the New Jersey Register (40 N.J.R. 1094(a)) final rules implementing the Patient Safety Act (n.J.S.A.26:2H-12.23to12.25). Available at: *http://www.njha.com/LibrarySection/pdf/Patient_Safety_Regulations*. Accessed September 22, 2010.
9. Ayello, E.A., Capitulo K.L., Fife, C.E., Fowler, E., Krasner, D.L., Mulder, G., Sibbald, R.G., Yankowsky, K.W. Legal issues in the care of pressure ulcer patients: Key concepts for healthcare providers. A consensus paper from the International Expert Wound Care Advisory Panel. *WCET* 29(3):8-22, July/September 2009.
10. National Pressure Ulcer Advisory Panel Photography FAQ. Available at: *http://www.npuap.org.DOCS/PhotographyFaq.doc.* Accessed June 22, 2010. (Revision pending 2011.)
11. Wound, Ostomy and Continence Nurses Society (WOCN). Professional Practice Series. Photography in Wound Documentation. Available at: *http://www.wocn.org/WOCN_Library/Position_Statements/.* Accessed April 5, 2011.
12. American Professional Wound Care Association (APWCA). Resources, Photographic guidelines. Available at: *http://www.apwca.org.* Accessed June 22, 2010.
13. Wound, Ostomy and Continence Nurses Society. Guideline for Prevention and Management of Pressure Ulcers. Mount Laurel, NJ: Author, 2010
14. Brown, G. "Wound Documentation: Managing Risk," *Adv Skin Wound Care* 19(3):155-65, March 2006.

CHAPTER 4

Skin: An Essential Organ

Sharon Baranoski, MSN, RN, CWCN, APN, CCNS, DAPWCA, FAAN
Elizabeth A. Ayello, PhD, RN, ACNS-BC, CWON, MAPWCA, FAAN
Marjana Tomic-Canic, PhD, RN
Jeffrey M. Levine, MD, AGSF, CMD, CWS

Objectives

After completing this chapter, you'll be able to:

- discuss the different layers of the skin
- state the functions of the skin
- list skin changes associated with the aging process
- differentiate between skin assessment and wound assessment
- describe risk factors and treatments for skin tears
- identify and classify common skin conditions
- define the emerging concepts of skin failure and skin changes at the end of life.

SKIN ANATOMY AND PHYSIOLOGY

The skin is the largest external organ of the body. Human skin is composed of two distinct layers: the epidermis, the outermost layer; and the dermis, the innermost layer. (See *Layers of the skin,* page 58.) The dermal-epidermal junction, commonly referred to as the basement membrane zone (BMZ), separates the two layers. Under the dermis lies a layer of loose connective tissue, called subcutaneous tissue, or hypodermis. (See *Skin layer functions,* page 59.)

The epidermis is a thin, avascular layer that regenerates itself every 4 to 6 weeks. It's divided into four layers or strata (presented in order from the outermost layer inward). (See *Layers of the epidermis,* page 60.)

- *Stratum corneum*—consists of dead keratinocyte cells; flakes and sheds; is easily removed during bathing activities and more efficiently by scrubbing the surface of the skin.
- *Stratum granulosum*—also contains Langerhans cells in addition to keratinocytes.[1]

- *Stratum spinosum*—contains keratinocytes and Langerhans cells.
- *Stratum basale or germinativum*—single layer of epidermal cells (keratinocytes); contains melanocytes; can regenerate.

A fifth layer, the *stratum lucidum,* lies between the stratum corneum and the stratum granulosum. This packed translucent line of cells is found only on the palms and soles and is not seen in thin skin.

The epidermis is composed of keratinocyte cells. Basal keratinocytes (stratum basale) have the capacity to divide, giving rise to suprabasal layers of epidermis. Once basal keratinocytes leave the stratum basale, they start the process of differentiation, during which they die. This process involves making insoluble proteins and their crosslink, which, along with lipids and membrane components, form the insoluble, horny stratum corneum layer.[2-5] In order to maintain the barrier, keratinocytes have the capacity to completely regenerate the epidermis. If damaged (such as with wounds,

Layers of the skin

Two distinct layers of skin, the epidermis and dermis, lie above a layer of subcutaneous fatty tissue (also called the hypodermis). The dermal-epidermal junction (also called the basement membrane zone) lies between the dermis and epidermis.

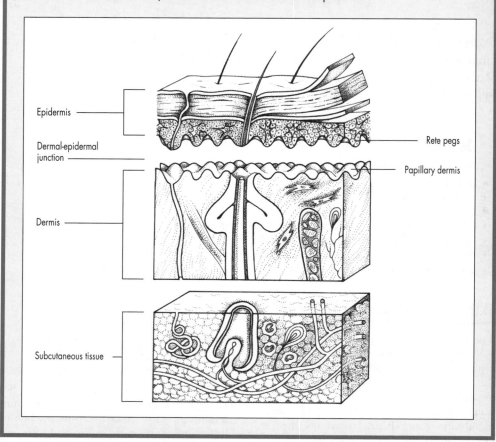

Epidermis

Dermal-epidermal junction

Dermis

Subcutaneous tissue

Rete pegs

Papillary dermis

burns, or exposure to UV light or chemicals), keratinocytes change their biology in order to repair the damage. Instead of differentiating, they become "activated" and start to divide rapidly and, in the case of a wound, they migrate over the gap to repair the damage.[3] They also signal to other neighboring cell types, such as fibroblasts, Langerhans cells, and melanocytes, that the skin barrier is compromised and that they're needed to help repair the damage. Once the damage is repaired, the keratinocytes cease their activation and resume their normal differentiation process.[6]

The BMZ separates the epidermis from the dermis. It contains fibronectin (an adhesive glycoprotein), type IV collagen (a non–fiber-forming collagen), heparin sulfate proteoglycan, and glycosaminoglycan.[7] The BMZ has an irregular surface—called rete ridges or pegs—projecting downward from the epidermis that interlocks with the upward projections of the dermis. The two interlocking sides resemble the two sides of a waffle iron coming together. This structure anchors the epidermis to the dermis, preventing it from sliding back and forth. As skin

Skin layer functions

The chart below shows characteristics and general functions of each layer of the skin.

Skin layer	Characteristics	General function
Epidermis	• Outer layer of skin • Consists of five layers (or strata): corneum, lucidum, granulosum, spinosum, and basale (or germinativum) • Repairs and regenerates itself every 28 days	• Protective barrier (sun damage, transepidermal water loss) • Organization of cell content • Synthesis of vitamin D and cytokines • Division and mobilization of cells • Maintaining contact with dermis • Pigmentation (contains melanocytes) • Allergen recognition (contains Langerhans cells) • Differentiates into hair, nails, sweat glands, and sebaceous glands
Dermis	• Consists of two layers—papillary dermis and reticular dermis—composed of collagen, reticulum, and elastin fibers • Contains a network of nerve endings, blood vessels, lymphatics, capillaries, sweat and sebaceous glands, and hair follicles	• Supports structure • Mechanical strength • Supplies nutrition • Resists shearing forces • Inflammatory response
Subcutaneous tissue (hypodermis)	• Composed of adipose and connective tissue • Contains major blood vessels, nerves, and lymphatic vessels	• Attaches to underlying structure • Thermal insulation • Storage of calories (energy) • Controls body shape • Mechanical "shock absorber"

ages, the basement membrane flattens, and the area of contact between the epidermis and dermis decreases by 50%, thus increasing the risk of skin injury by traumatic, accidental separation of the epidermis from the dermis. (See *Effects of aging on the BMZ*, page 60.)

The dermis is an essential part of the skin and is commonly referred to as the "true skin."[8] As the second layer, it's the thickest layer and is composed of many cells. The major proteins found in this layer are collagen and elastin, which are synthesized and secreted by

Layers of the epidermis

The epidermis consists of four layers, as illustrated below.

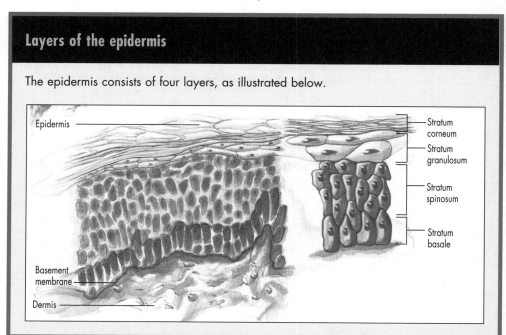

Epidermis

Stratum corneum

Stratum granulosum

Stratum spinosum

Stratum basale

Basement membrane

Dermis

Effects of aging on the BMZ

The illustrations below show the effects of aging on the basement membrane zone (BMZ). Specifically, the basement membrane flattens, reducing the area of contact between the epidermis and the dermis by 50%.

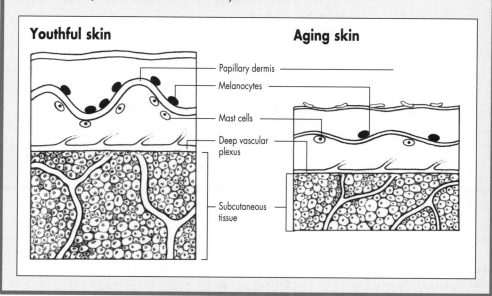

Youthful skin

Aging skin

Papillary dermis

Melanocytes

Mast cells

Deep vascular plexus

Subcutaneous tissue

fibroblasts; collagen forms up to 30% of the volume or 70% of the dry weight of the dermis.[7-9] The dermis is a matrix that serves to support the epidermis. It's divided into two areas, the papillary dermis and the reticular dermis.[7]

- The *papillary dermis* is composed of collagen and reticular fibers. Its distinct, unique pattern allows fingerprint identification for each individual. It contains capillaries for skin nourishment and pain touch receptors (pacinian corpuscles and Meissner's corpuscles).
- The *reticular dermis* is composed of collagen bundles that anchor the skin to the subcutaneous tissue. Sweat glands, hair follicles, nerves, and blood vessels can be found in this layer.

The main function of the dermis is to provide tensile strength, support, moisture retention, and blood and oxygen to the skin.[8] It protects the underlying muscles, bones, and organs. The dermis also contains the sebaceous glands that secrete sebum, a substance rich in oil that lubricates the skin. Furthermore, it also contains hair follicles that are the source of multipotent stem cells, which have the capacity to restore the epidermis.[6]

The subcutaneous tissue, or hypodermis, attaches the dermis to underlying structures. Its function is to promote an ongoing blood supply to the dermis for regeneration. It's primarily composed of adipose tissue, which provides a cushion between skin layers, muscles, and bones. It promotes skin mobility, molds body contours, and insulates the body.

SKIN FUNCTION

Skin is an important organ whose diverse functions are not always appreciated. (See *Skin functions.*) In adults, the skin weighs between 6 and 8 lb (2.7 and 3.6 kg) and covers more than 20 ft² (1.9 m²). Skin thickness varies from 0.5 to 6 mm according to its location on the body; for example, skin can be as thin as $1/_{50}$" on the eyelids and as thick as $1/_3$" on the palms and soles, where greater protection is needed. The skin receives one-third of the body's circulating blood volume—an oversupply of blood compared with its metabolic needs.

Skin functions

Functions of the skin include:
- protection from:
  - fluid and electrolyte loss
  - mechanical injury
  - ultraviolet injury
  - pathogens
- temperature regulation
- metabolism
- sensation
- synthesis
- communication.

The normal range of skin pH is 4 to 6.5 in healthy people.[10,11] This "acid mantle" helps to maintain a normal skin flora by serving as a protective barrier against bacterial and fungal infections. It also supports the formation and maturation of epidermal lipids and assists in maintaining their protective barrier function. The acid mantle also provides indirect protection against invasion by microorganisms and protection against alkaline substances.[10] If the acid mantle loses its acidity, the skin becomes more prone to damage and infection. Frequent use of soap products and over-washing can alter the stratum corneum and its ability to serve as a protective barrier. Alternatively, several skin conditions can *increase* the skin's surface pH, including eczema, contact dermatitis, atopic dermatitis, and dry skin.[12,13] Systemic diseases may also increase the skin's surface pH, such as diabetes, chronic renal failure, and cerebrovascular disease.[14]

The skin's major functions are protection, sensation, thermoregulation, excretion, metabolism, and communication.[15] Skin protects the body by serving as a barrier from invasion by organisms such as bacteria. The epidermis synthesizes natural antimicrobials called defensins.[16,18,19] Because staphylococcal species (such as *Staphylococcus aureus* or *Staphylococcus epidermidis*) tolerate salt, they are present in large numbers as resident bacteria on the skin.[15,16] Another organism found on the skin is yeast, which is commonly seen on the trunk and ears and as fungus between the toes.[15,17]

Sensation is a key function of the skin. Areas that are most sensitive to touch have a greater number of nerve endings.[17] These include the lips, nipples, and fingertips. In humans, the fingertips are the most sensitive touch organ and enable us to correctly identify objects by touch (stereognosis) rather than by sight. Many tactile corpuscles lie at the base of hair follicles, and shaving reduces the tactile sensibility of that skin area. In hairless body regions, the tactile corpuscles are called Meissner's corpuscles.[17] Pleasurable, firm touching sensations, such as from a massage or hugs of affection, are transmitted via the skin as they generate nerve transmissions through these tactile corpuscles.

Itch is one of the alarm sensations of the skin and serves as a defense mechanism. Chemicals that are released after skin injury may promote the inflammatory process and can also induce itch or pain. Itch and pain are in close regulatory relationship—for example, central pain inhibition may enhance the act of itching while also inhibiting the act of itching.[20]

Somatic pain (from the outer body surfaces and framework) is also communicated through the skin. Superficial (acute) pain to a local area is usually transmitted by very rapid nerve impulses through A-delta fibers.[17] Superficial pain tends to be sharp but ceases when the pain stimulus stops. Deep (chronic) pain impulses are transmitted slowly over the smaller, thinly myelinated C fibers. In contrast, this type of pain tends to spread over a more diffuse area, lasts for longer periods of time, and remains even after the pain stimulus is gone.[17] As a sign of possible skin injury, pressure also serves as a protective warning sensation.

Temperature regulation and fluid and electrolyte balance are achieved in part by the skin. Thermoregulation is controlled by the hypothalamus in response to internal core body temperature. Peripheral temperature receptors in the skin assist in this process called *temperature homeostasis*.[21] By losing a copious amount of water—for example, sweating—through the skin, lungs, and buccal mucosa, homeostasis of body temperature is maintained. Skin temperature is controlled by the dilation or constriction of skin blood vessels. When core body temperature rises, the body will attempt to reduce its temperature by releasing heat from the skin. This is accomplished by sending a chemical signal to increase blood flow in the skin from vasodilation, thus increasing skin temperature.

> ### ▶ PRACTICE POINT
>
> Increased temperature → Skin blood vessel vasodilation → Heat loss from epidermis → Body maintains temperature homeostasis.

In contrast, the opposite occurs when the body's core temperature is reduced; the chemical signal causes decreased blood flow from vasoconstriction, thus lowering the skin's temperature.[21,22]

> ### ▶ PRACTICE POINT
>
> Decreased temperature → Skin blood vessel vasoconstriction → Heat conservation → Body maintains temperature homeostasis.

The skin also aids in the excretion of end products of cell metabolism and prevents excessive loss of fluid. Other important functions of the skin include its manufacturing ability and immune functions.[23] For example, when exposed to ultraviolet light, the skin can synthesize vitamin D[24] and, although the skin's hypersensitivity responses in allergic reactions are commonly seen, the skin's role in immune function isn't always fully appreciated. Indeed, Langerhans cells and tissue macrophages, which play an important role in digesting bacteria, as well as mast cells, which are needed to provide proper immune system functioning, are all present in the skin.[1,7,15] In addition, keratinocytes are very powerful in generating a rapid inflammatory response because they contain pre-stored, pro-inflammatory signals, such as interleukin-1, which is released the moment the barrier is broken and is considered the first signal of wounding.[25]

AGING AND THE SKIN

Changes in aging skin

Age-related changes in the dermis are numerous, but the most striking is the approximately 20% loss in dermal thickness that probably accounts for the paper-thin appearance of aging skin.[26,27] This decrease in dermal cells and proportional reduction in collagen fibers, blood vessels, nerve endings, and collagen lead to altered or reduced sensation, thermoregulation, rigidity, moisture retention, and sagging skin.[26,28] Flattening of the dermal-epidermal junction decreases nutrient transfer and increases the fragility of aging skin.

A decrease in differentiation and formation of the stratum corneum is also detected in aging skin. Reduced collagen deposition in elderly skin could explain the development of dermal atrophy and might relate to poor wound healing.[29] The subcutaneous fat below the dermis consists primarily of adipose tissue and provides mechanical protection and insulation. Its loss during aging results in parallel reductions in these protective functions. Subcutaneous tissue undergoes site-specific atrophy in such areas as the face, dorsal aspect of the hands, shins, and plantar aspects of the foot, increasing the energy absorbed by the skin when trauma occurs to these areas.[30]

Many of the changes in aged skin are linked to the hormones estrogen and androgen. Decreased estrogen in menopausal women, similar to ovariectomized mice, leads to a decrease in collagen deposition, slower epithelialization, and delayed wound healing. These effects may be reversible by hormone replacement therapy (HRT).[31] In addition, a genetic polymorphism in estrogen receptor-beta has been linked to a predisposition to venous ulcerations in both male and female patients.[32] In contrast to estrogen, which is beneficial for wound healing, androgens are implicated in the etiology of venous ulcerations. In addition, use of inhibitor (antagonist of androgen) or castration in mice leads to increased collagen deposition and acceleration of wound healing.[33]

A decrease in pain perception may make elderly people more vulnerable to traumatic environmental insults such as wearing tight shoes, stepping on an object, or hitting legs on the side of a chair. Aging skin is also less able to manufacture vitamin D when exposed to sunlight.[26,27] The number of Langerhans cells and mast cells diminishes in aging skin, translating into decreased immune function.[26,30,34] Medications also have adverse effects on the skin's immune function. For example, steroids cause thinning of the epidermis.[28,35]

Skin changes seen with aging are accelerated by sun exposure, specifically due to ultraviolet (UV) radiation.[26,36] UV irradiation causes local inflammation and local immunosuppression with DNA damage. Changes induced by photoaging are superficially similar but differ slightly under the microscope. Photodamaged skin looks coarse, rough, and wrinkled and is prone to developing malignancy.

Skin integrity

Alteration in skin integrity is a clinical practice issue in every continuum of care. Because of the anatomic and physiologic changes that occur with aging, elderly people are especially vulnerable to alterations in skin integrity.[34,37] (See *Hallmarks of aging skin*, page 64.) As skin ages, the epidermis gradually thins. The dermal-epidermal junction flattens and dermal papillae and epidermal rete pegs are effaced, making the skin more susceptible to mild mechanical trauma. A decrease in the number of sweat glands and their output explains some of the dry skin seen in elderly people.[26]

Aging skin is less able to retain moisture due to a decrease in dermal proteins, which leads to oncotic pressure shifts and diminished fluid homeostasis, thereby putting elderly people at risk for dehydration. Normal water content of the skin is 10% to 15%. Below 10%, the skin becomes dry and is more vulnerable to damage.[28] Because soap increases the skin's pH to an alkaline level, using emollient soap and bathing every other day, instead of every day, can decrease the incidence of skin injury, such as skin tears, in elderly patients.[10]

Hallmarks of aging skin

The following changes in skin can occur due to the normal aging process.

Decreased
- Dermal thickness, causing thinning of the skin (especially over the legs and forearms)
- Fatty layers (leaving the bony prominences less protected)
- Amount and flexibility of collagen and elastin fibers (leaving the elastin unable to recoil and causing skin wrinkling)
- Size of rete ridges (making the basement membrane flatter, which allows the epidermis and dermis to separate more easily, increasing the risk for injury such as a skin tear)
- Sensation and metabolism
- Sweating due to atrophy of sweat glands (leading to dry skin)
- Subcutaneous tissue (leading to less padded protection over bony prominences)
- Vascularity and number of capillaries (leaving the elderly more prone to heat stroke)

Increased
- Time for epidermal regeneration (leading to slower healing)
- Damage to skin from the sun

An elderly person's skin is less stretchable due to a decrease in elastin fibers.[26,29,34] Because of the thinning of the epidermal layer, the skin becomes a less-effective barrier against water loss, bruising, and infection; this thinner epidermis also impairs thermal regulation, decreases tactile sensitivity, and diminishes pain perception.[26,27,30,38] Due to a decreased amount of dermal proteins, the blood vessels become thinner and more fragile, thereby leading to a type of hemorrhaging known as senile purpura. Hematomas can dissect into surrounding skin, usually over the extensor surfaces of the hands and forearms, resolving to leave brownish discoloration caused by hemosiderin deposits. The appearance of dissecting hematomas can mimic the dermal changes associated with bleeding diathesis or an impaired clotting system. According to Selden and colleagues,[30] the pathophysiology of skin tears parallels that of senile purpura.

Patient Teaching

Alert the patient/family/caregiver that skin tears often occur over areas of senile purpura in the elderly. (See *color section, Senile purpura, page C2.*)

SKIN ASSESSMENT VS. WOUND ASSESSMENT

Although not always given the priority in clinical practice, the skin or integumentary system should be part of the routine head-to-toe assessment of all patients.[39] A skin assessment should include an actual observation of the entire body. A skin assessment differs from a wound assessment in that the former looks at the patient's entire body and not just open wounds.

PRACTICE POINT

Factors affecting skin resilience[28]
- Aging of skin
- Critical illness
- Malnutrition and dehydration
- Excess moisture
- Skin conditions that cause dryness

Lacking consensus in the literature as to what constitutes a minimal skin assessment, the U.S. Centers for Medicare & Medicaid Services (CMS) nevertheless recommend the following five parameters as a minimal skin assessment

Elements of a basic skin assessment

To perform a basic skin assessment you must, at a minimum, assess its temperature, color, moisture, turgor, and integrity.

Temperature
- Normally warm to the touch
- Warmer than normal could signal inflammation
- Cooler than normal could signal poor vascularization

Color
- Intensity: paleness may be an indicator of poor circulation
- Normal color tones: light ivory to deep brown, yellow to olive, or light pink to dark, ruddy pink
- Hyperpigmentation or hypopigmentation reflect variations in melanin deposits or blood flow

Moisture
- Dry or moist to the touch
- Hyperkeratosis (flaking, scales)
- Eczema (endogenous or exogenous)
- Dermatitis, psoriasis, rashes
- Edema

Turgor
- Normally returns to its original state quickly
- Slow return to its original shape (dehydration or effect of aging)

Integrity
- No open areas
- Type of skin injury (Use the appropriate classification system to identify and record injury type.)

Elements of a comprehensive skin assessment

Consider the following when performing a comprehensive skin assessment.

Inspection
- Normally smooth, slightly moist, and same general tone throughout
- Tone depends on patient's melanocytes. Skin pigmentation varieties include light ivory, light pink, dark ruddy pink or red, yellow, olive, light brown, deep brown, and black.
- Pigmentation can exhibit:
  - pallor: mucosa, conjunctivae
  - cyanosis: nail beds, conjunctivae, oral mucosa
  - jaundice: sclerae, palate, palms

  - hyperpigmentation: increase in melanin deposits or blood flow;
  - hypopigmentation: decreased vascular/venous patterns, usually symmetric
  - scars and bruises for location, color, length, and width

Palpation
- Moisture: perspiration
- Edema: extremities, sacrum, eyes
- Tenderness
- Turgor, elasticity
- Texture

Olfaction
- Normal body odor

- Absence of pungent odor
- May indicate presence of bacteria or infection
- Poor hygiene

Observation of hair and nails
- Hair
  - Hirsutism: excessive body hair
  - Alopecia: hair loss
- Nails (can reflect the patient's overall health)
  - Color, shape, contour
  - Clubbing, texture, thickness

Skin alterations
- Previous scars
- Graft sites
- Healed ulcer sites

in long-term care settings: temperature, color, moisture, turgor, and intact skin or presence of open areas.[40-42] (See *Elements of a basic skin assessment*, page 65.) However, some patients may require more comprehensive assessment, which would include looking for and documenting any lesions, scars, bruising, or hemosiderin deposits. (See *Elements of a comprehensive skin assessment*, page 65.)

Once skin integrity is lost and the epidermis is no longer intact, a thorough wound assessment with documentation is required. (See chapter 6, Wound assessment and documentation, for more information.) The first step is to identify the type or etiology of the wounded skin—for example, differentiate a skin tear from a pressure ulcer. Next, a wound assessment should minimally describe the following characteristics: location, size, exudate, and type of tissue. Remember the phrase frequently heard in wound care: "Look at the whole patient, not just the hole in the patient."

IMPLICATIONS FOR PRACTICE

Alterations in skin integrity, perhaps due to skin trauma or other skin conditions, may cause undue pain and suffering for patients. Health care professionals should have up-to-date information about prevention techniques, the appropriate use of dressings and tapes and, most importantly, the prevention of skin integrity injuries.

Skin trauma
SKIN TEARS

Skin tears, sometimes called *skin* or *epidermal skin stripping injuries*, are a clinical challenge, especially among older patients.[43] Payne and Martin define a skin tear as "a traumatic wound occurring principally on the extremities of older adults. Skin tears are a result of friction alone or shearing and friction forces that separate the epidermis from the dermis (partial-thickness wound) or that separate both the epidermis and the dermis from underlying structures (full-thickness wound)."[44] Although the Payne-Martin definition is often cited, there is no universally agreed upon skin tear definition worldwide. Highlights of the

Canadian[45] and Australian[46] skin tear initiatives are described later in this chapter.

Maintaining skin integrity in patients who have frail skin first requires awareness of the severity of the problem. In addition, in the case of injury and tear, documenting and reporting such occurrences is of utmost importance and may save lives because early detection halts progression. The friction and shear that may occur with turning or lifting an elderly patient can injure the skin. Ambulating or transferring patients may also present a problem if they bump into objects, such as chairs, beds, or tables. Removing adhesive dressings or tape can shear delicate skin. However, skin stripping is a potential problem for any person regardless of age when adhesive dressings or tape is incorrectly removed or vulnerable skin isn't adequately protected. Despite the frequency with which skin tears are seen in practice, the literature contains limited information about these wounds.

Prevalence
Skin tears are perceived to be common in elderly patients in all healthcare settings. Although they are seen in practice, the prevalence of skin tears may be unreported, especially in the community.[46] Prevalence is unknown in Canada, and various rates are reported in different care settings in the United States.[45] Long-term care residents have one to three skin tears per year.[47] A wide range of prevalence rates—14% to 24%—have been reported in long-term care settings in the United States.[47] Hanson and colleagues reported prevalence rates of 6.3% and 6.4% in two rural U.S. nursing homes.[48] In another study,[49] skin tear incidence was reported as an average of 18 skin tears per month.

Skin tears occur most commonly in the upper extremities.[47,48] In a retrospective study, almost one-half of skin tears were found to have occurred without any apparent cause. When the cause is known, approximately one-quarter resulted from wheelchair injuries, and one-quarter were caused by accidentally bumping into objects. Transfers and falls accounted for 18% and 12.4%, respectively.[47]

Although nearly 70% to 80% of skin tears occur on the arms and hands,[44,48] these wounds may occur on other areas of the body as well. Skin tears that occur on the back and buttocks are commonly mistaken for stage II pressure ulcers. Pressure may be a related cause in skin tears, but the etiology of skin tears differs from that of pressure ulcers.[30] Skin tears need to be documented as separate occurrences and not grouped into pressure ulcer categories. (See chapter 13, Pressure ulcers.)

Risk factors

According to a retrospective review by White and colleagues,[50] the patients most at risk for sustaining skin tears are those who require total care for all activities of daily living. Skin tears in these patients frequently result from routine activities, such as bathing, changing clothing, or being repositioned or transferred.

Independent ambulatory residents sustained the second highest number of skin tears, primarily on the lower extremities. Many of these patients had edema, purpura, or ecchymosis. Slightly impaired residents made up the third highest risk category. These patients sustained injury from hitting stationary equipment or furniture as well as the reasons just described in the dependent and independent ambulatory patients.[50]

In 59 hospitalized patients, Meuleneire[51] found an increased risk of skin tears in patients with cardiac, pulmonary, and vascular disorders. The risk was further complicated if patients had dementia, visual or balance problems, or were receiving steroid therapy.[51] In 1994, White and colleagues developed a skin integrity risk assessment tool that highlights

Evidence-Based Practice
Skin Integrity Risk Assessment Tool

White, et al. (1994)[50] recommend implementing a skin-tear risk prevention care plan for patients who meet any of the criteria in group I below, for patients who meet four or more criteria in group II, for patients who meet five or more criteria in group III, and for patients who meet three criteria in group II and three or more criteria in group III.

Group I
- History of skin tears within past 90 days
- Actual number of skin tears

Group II
- Decision-making skills impaired
- Vision impaired
- Extensive assistance/total dependence for activities of daily living (ADLs)
- Wheelchair assistance needed
- Loss of balance
- Bed or chair confined
- Unsteady gait
- Bruises

Group III
- Physically abusive
- Resists ADL care
- Agitation
- Hearing impaired
- Decreased tactile stimulation
- Wheels self
- Manually or mechanically lifted
- Contracture of arms, legs, shoulders, hands
- Hemiplegia or hemiparesis
- Trunk: partial or total inability to balance or turn body
- Pitting edema of legs
- Open lesions on extremities
- 3 to 4 senile purpuric lesions on extremities
- Dry, scaly skin

three groups of patients at risk for skin tears.[50] (See *Evidence-Based Practice: Skin Integrity Risk Assessment Tool*, page 67.) Awareness of the existence and use of this tool varies worldwide.

Classification

As mentioned earlier, the initial classification system for skin tears evolved in the late 1980s thanks to the work of Regina Payne and Marie Martin.[52] Their pilot research study led to the development of the Payne-Martin Classification System for Skin Tears.[44,52] This useful tool provides healthcare professionals with a method to enhance documentation and track outcomes of care in the assessment of skin tears. Several researchers have used this new taxonomy in their studies as tool validation continues.

The revised 1993 Payne-Martin classification system for skin tears is divided into three categories based on whether tissue is lost in the skin tear.[44] Best practice recommendations using this classification system have been proposed by Canadian authors LeBlanc and colleagues.[45] Because the Payne-Martin system was not widely used in Australia, Carville and associates launched the Skin Tear Audit Research (STAR) study.[46] This study resulted in a modified skin tear classification system with new descriptors.[46] (See *color section, Classification of skin tears*, page C1.)

Prevention protocols

Although little has been written about the prevention of skin tears, best practice protocols gleaned from the literature may prevent many skin tears.[53,54] If the patient is at risk, consider these preventive measures:

- Encourage your colleagues and the patient's family members to use proper positioning, turning, lifting, and transferring.
- Promote the use of long sleeves and pants to add a layer of protection.
- Secure padding to bed rails, wheelchair arm and leg supports, and any other equipment that may be used.
- Use paper tape or nonadherent dressings on frail skin. Always remove these products gently to prevent skin injury.
- Use skin sealants, liquid bandage, or soft silicone or foam dressings to protect vulnerable skin from adhering tapes and dressings.

- Use stockinettes, gauze wrap, or a similar type of wrap rather than tape to secure dressings and drains.
- Use pillows and blankets to support dangling arms and legs.
- Move and turn the patient with a lift sheet.
- Minimize the use of soap and alcohol solvents; consider the use of no-rinse, waterless, or liquid-gel cleansers.
- Avoid scrubbing skin when bathing; pat skin dry rather than rubbing it dry.
- Apply a moisturizing or emollient agent to dry skin.
- Provide a well-lit environment to prevent falls.
- Educate staff on the importance of gentle care.

Additional best practice recommendations from Le Blanc et al.[45] with level of evidence can be found in *Evidence-Based Practice: Quick Reference Guide: Prevention and Treatment of Skin Tears*.

Patient Teaching

Advise the patient/family/caregiver to avoid using soap and instead use skin protectant and hydrating products.

Research[54] has shown that skin tears can be reduced in nursing homes when skin care protocols are used.[48,49,55,56] In a 4-month prospective study in a 173-bed long-term care facility, the use of emollient soap was associated with a lower incidence of skin tears than non-emollient soap.[57] Skin tears in a long-term care facility declined from 23.5% to 3.5% with the implementation of a no-rinse, one-step, bed bath protocol rather than soap and water.[55] Likewise, Hanson and colleagues[48] found that skin tears were significantly decreased in two different rural nursing homes when skin care protocols were introduced. Specifically, skin tear prevalence was reduced from 6.3% to 1.4% in one nursing home and 6.4% to 3.3% in another.[48] In another study, Bank found that by educating staff and implementing the above-mentioned skin care protocols, skin tears were reduced from a monthly average of 18 to 11.[49]

Evidence-Based Practice
Quick Reference Guide: Prevention and Treatment of Skin Tears

Interpretation of evidence: The framework depicts the levels of evidence that are used to classify the research behind the development of this quick reference guide by the authors, based on the Registered Nurses' Association of Ontario (RNAO) and the National Guidelines Clearinghouse (NGCH).

Ia. Evidence obtained from meta-analysis or systemic review of randomized controlled trials (RCTs)

Ib. Evidence obtained from at least one RCT

IIa. Evidence obtained from at least one well-designed controlled study without randomization

IIba. Evidence obtained from at least one other type of well-designed quasi-experimental study

III. Evidence obtained from well-designed non-experimental descriptive studies, such as comparative studies, correlation studies, and case studies

IV. Evidence obtained from expert committee reports or opinions and/or clinical experiences of respected authorities

Recommendations	Level of evidence
Identify and treat the cause.	
1. Obtain a complete patient history that includes general health status and identifies risk factors that may put the patient at risk for a skin tear as well as factors that may affect the healing of existing skin tears.	IV
2. Identify persons at high risk for skin tears	IV
3. Support the prevention of skin tears through skin hygiene, hydration, responsible bathing, good nutrition, appropriate clothing, removal of environmental risk factors, and correct turning, positioning, and transferring.	IV
Address patient-centered concerns.	
4. Assess and assist with psychological needs in the development of a patient-centered plan (pain and quality of life).	IV
Provide local wound care.	
5. Classify and document skin tears according to the degree of trauma.	III–IV
6. Provide and support an optimal wound-healing environment.	III
7. Determine the effectiveness of interventions.	IV
8. Consider the use of adjunctive therapies for non-healing but healable skin tears.	Ia–IV
Provide organizational support.	
9. Develop an interprofessional team with flexibility to meet the patient's needs.	IV
10. Educate the patient, caregiver, and healthcare professional on the prevention and treatment of skin tears.	IV

Education of nurses and nursing assistants is another key to reducing skin tears in long-term care facility residents. In a 10-month descriptive study of 30 patients with Alzheimer disease in which nurses and nursing assistants were educated on skin tear prevention, 26 of 30 patients remained free of skin tears using a preventive skin program.[58] In a separate study, 416 registered nurses in two affiliated hospitals demonstrated an increased ability to identify and assess skin tears, differentiate skin tear categories, and better understand treatment protocols after using a Web-based educational program.[59]

Management

The management or treatment of skin tears varies according to institution, and little has been published regarding the preferred treatments for skin tears. However, the basic goals of care should be to control bleeding, realign any skin or flap, assess degree of tissue loss and fragility of surrounding skin, prevent infection, control pain, restore skin integrity, and promote patient comfort.[44,46,53,54]

Many types of skin and wound care products are used to promote a healing environment. In fact, a review of the literature reveals that the following methods are used to treat skin tears[41,45,51, 60-67]: soft silicone dressings, liquid bandage/skin glue, petrolatum ointment and nonadherent dressings; hydrogels, Telfa, foams, and transparent films; and adhesive strips. Hanson and colleagues found that skin tear healing time was reduced from 39.07 days (SD +38.26) to 30.16 days (SD +26.19) following implementation of a skin care protocol using skin protectants on the dry skin of the upper extremities of nursing home residents.[48] In a non-randomized study of 20 institutionalized adults, using liquid bandage resulted in complete healing within 7 days in 18 of 20 patients (90%).[63] In a study of 88 category I and II skin tears in 59 patients treated using a soft silicone net dressing, 83% of the wounds healed within 8 days.[51] Many clinicians recommend the use of soft silicone dressings, hydrogels, foams, skin glue, and petroleum-impregnated gauze.[45,59] Recommendations for skin tear management also include cleansing the skin tear with normal saline and preserving rather than removing the skin flap when present (for example, categories

I and II).[51] The previous practice of closing category I and II skin tears with sutures[61] is now believed to cause additional trauma and is not generally advocated.[51]

Important skin conditions in the elderly

Although many skin conditions warrant attention in clinical practice, two leading skin conditions seen in elderly people, xerosis and pruritus, aren't always given the importance and priority they deserve. These seemingly minor skin problems cause the skin to dry, itch, and crack; without effective recognition and intervention, the skin continues to deteriorate, leading to more chronic skin conditions that include fissures, infection, and cellulitis. Because there are many other skin conditions that are beyond the focus of this chapter, the authors recommend consulting the dermatology literature.

PRACTICE POINT

Skin assessments are required in all healthcare settings.

XEROSIS

Xerosis is the medical term for dry skin.[68] In xerosis, the skin appears dry, scaly, and flaky. (See *Xerosis.*) Although there is a xerosis scale, it's not widely used in clinical practice. Clinicians generally classify xerosis as mild, moderate, or severe. (See *Xerosis terminology.*)

The term *xerosis* has no particular diagnostic implication. Xerosis can be caused by environmental factors or can be a symptom of an underlying disease. For this reason, a patient's complaint of "dry" skin needs to be explored further. Skin exposure to a dry environment, such as central heating, wind, temperature extremes, or air conditioning, can all lead to xerosis.

Management

The goal in treating xerosis is to protect the skin from excessive transepidermal water loss and return the natural moisturizing factors

Xerosis

This photo depicts xerosis—also known as *dry skin*—of the foot.

(NMF) to the stratum corneum. This is best accomplished by using moisturizing agents that contain lipids—an essential component in forming an impervious barrier, or seal, on the stratum corneum, thus preventing further water loss. (See *Moisturizer functions and ingredients*, page 72.) As water is retained, the skin surface is flattened and scaling is reduced.[68] Instructing the patient, family, and caregiver on cleansing, environmental fac-

tors, and hydration is also important. (See *Patient Teaching: Patient Education to Avoid Xerosis*, page 73.)

PRACTICE POINT

Skin can become dry when transepidermal water loss drops below 10%.

PRACTICE POINT

Stop the Xerosis Cycle!
• Dry skin (xerosis)
• Pruritus
• Scratching

Because many moisturizers dissipate after 3 to 4 hours, we recommend using long-lasting moisturizers to cool, soothe, and restore barrier function. The goal is to break the itch-scratch-itch cycle, which happens because dry skin is often itchy, causing patients to

Xerosis terminology

Mild

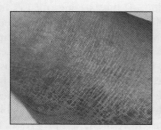

Dry skin with minimal flaking

Treatment: Hydrate the skin frequently using a moisturizing agent.

Moderate

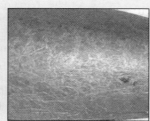

Dry skin with a scaly, fish-like appearance that's easily rubbed off the skin surface

Treatment: Use an exfoliating emollient moisturizing agent.

Severe

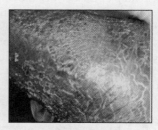

Cracking, parched appearance of skin that resembles dry earth

Treatment: Use moisturizer with urea, alpha-hydroxy acid, or lactic acid to exfoliate calloused dry skin.

Moisturizer functions and ingredients

Moisturizer functions
- *Humectants* promote water retention within the stratum corneum.
- *Occlusives* minimize water loss to the external environment.
- *Emollients* contribute to stratum corneum hydration.

Moisturizer ingredients (main types)
- Humectants
  - glycerin
  - urea
  - hydroxy acids (lactic acid)
  - propylene glycol
  - protein rejuvenators
- Occlusives and emollients
  - petrolatum
  - mineral oil
  - lanolin

scratch their skin. In turn, excessive scratching can ultimately lead to a break in the skin. Once the skin barrier is broken, it becomes a portal of entry for bacteria, which can lead to infection. This repetitive scratching causes chronic thickening of the dermis known as *lichenification*. Therefore, prompt identification of the itch-scratch-itch cycle as well as teaching the patient about skin damage (from scratching) is extremely important in helping the skin to heal and reducing the occurrence of lichenification. (See *Itch-scratch-itch cycle*, page 74.)

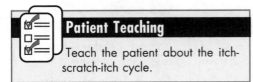

Patient Teaching

Teach the patient about the itch-scratch-itch cycle.

PRURITUS

Pruritus is the medical term for itchy skin and is a common symptom for several dis-

eases.[5] Therefore, taking a detailed patient history aids in determining whether the cause of pruritus is an underlying disease or if it's simply untreated xerosis. For example, pruritus may be a symptom of renal or liver disease, scabies, or dry skin from aging. (See *Pruritus*, page 74.) Helping patients understand the itch-scratch-itch cycle and their own behavioral pattern is important to successful management. (See *Treatment plan for pruritus*, page 75.[5])

MOISTURE-ASSOCIATED SKIN DAMAGE

Just as dry skin can be a problem, exposure to excessive moisture can also cause skin damage. Common causes of moisture-associated skin damage (MASD) include incontinence, wound exudate, fistula or stoma effluent, and perspiration.[69] Skin damage from moisture is distinct from pressure damage, and differentiating the correct etiology between these two types of skin injuries is important for appropriate treatment and prevention.[69-72] (See *Differentiating between MASD and pressure ulcers in the perineal and genital area*, page 75.) It is not clear whether it is moisture alone or a combination of wetness coupled with irritants within the moisture source that causes MASD.[6]

INCONTINENCE-ASSOCIATED DERMATITIS

The remainder of this section focuses on MASD caused by incontinence of urine, stool, or both. Incontinence-associated dermatitis (IAD) is sometimes referred to as perineal dermatitis or, in infants, "diaper dermatitis." Recent publications[69-71] have advocated for the use of the term MASD to identify these skin lesions. IAD is believed to be reversible, begins as persistent redness, and progresses to partial-thickness skin injury but not full thickness wounds.[69] Although there are three IAD instruments discussed in the literature, they are not yet widely used in practice.[70]

Gray and colleagues[70] summarized several research studies about the prevention of IAD and concluded that routine perineal skin protocols that avoided soap and incorporated cleansing products with a pH range of normal skin

Patient Teaching
Patient Education to Avoid Xerosis

To avoid xerosis, patients should be given clear instructions regarding cleansing, their environment, and remaining hydrated.

Cleansing

- Avoid long baths; limit baths to 15 minutes or consider showering instead.
- Bathe every other day rather than daily.
- Use tepid water rather than hot water when bathing.
- Use pH-balanced soaps (4.0 to 6.5), avoid excessive use of deodorant soaps, and rinse well.
- Avoid vigorously cleaning the skin with a washcloth.
- Pat or blot the skin, rather than rubbing with a towel, so some water is left on the skin.
- Apply moisturizers *immediately* after bathing or showering.

Environment

- Use a humidifier during the winter months when central heating is being used.
- Drink plenty of water.
- Wear a sunscreen with a sun protection factor (SPF) of 15 or higher that contains a moisturizer.
- Use non-fragrant laundry detergents, fabric softeners, and similar products.
- Implement fall safety precautions because bathing surfaces may be slippery if using bath oils.

Hydration

Apply moisturizers frequently and with the correct gentle application technique for the specific product being used (check product directions).

---

were effective along with reducing skin scrubbing and friction. Use of products that moisturize and protect the skin was recommended.[70] Holistic care also requires interventions to address and minimize episodes of incontinence, such as a scheduled toileting program.[70] Other strategies to prevent skin exposure to urine or stool include use of containment devices such as condom catheter, anal pouch, or bowel management system. If absorptive products are used, they should wick urine or stool away from the skin. Recommendations for a structured skin care regimen include cleaning the skin daily and after each incontinence episode using a no-rinse cleanser (not scrubbing the skin); applying humectants or an emollient

moisturizer; barrier creams; ointments with petroleum, zinc oxide or dimethicone; or skin sealant products.[70-72] If a fungal infection is also present, antifungal products will be required.[70,72]

Skin failure

As discussed at the beginning of this chapter, the skin is the largest organ of the body. Can the skin as an organ fail? The literature supporting skin failure is very limited. The concept was first discussed in 1989 by Goode and Allman, who noted that "multiple/multiorgan failure is a terminal stage of many diseases that occurs as the body wastes away."[73]

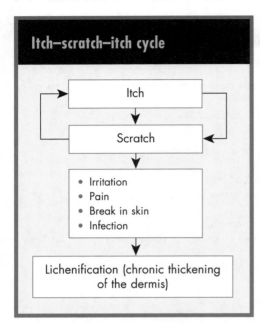

Itch–scratch–itch cycle

Itch → Scratch →

- Irritation
- Pain
- Break in skin
- Infection

↓

Lichenification (chronic thickening of the dermis)

These authors concluded that the skin's susceptibility to failure and death must be considered in multiorgan death syndrome.[73] The term *skin failure* was again supported in the literature in 1991 by LaPuma.[74] Patients at the end stages of life and in the intensive care setting were the focus of an editorial in 1993 regarding skin and underlying tissue damage.[75] In 1996, Leijten et al. discussed chronic skin failure in older adults with multiple comorbidities that can lead to pressure ulcers, especially at the end of life.[76] Hobbs and coworkers discussed the condition of skin failure in an abstract at a national program in 2000.[77]

The term *skin failure* has not been clinically defined or well accepted in the healthcare setting. The first written definition of skin failure was presented in 2006 by Langemo and Brown,[78] who defined it as an event in which the skin and underlying tissue die as a result of hypoperfusion that occurs concurrent with severe dysfunction or failure of other organ systems. They further break this definition down into three types of events that trigger skin failure: acute skin failure, chronic skin failure, and end-stage skin failure.[78]

- Acute skin failure is an event in which skin and underlying tissue die due to hypoperfusion concurrent with a critical illness.
- Chronic skin failure is when skin and underlying tissue die as a result of hypoperfusion concurrent with an ongoing chronic disease state.
- End-stage skin failure is when skin and underlying tissue die as a result of hypoperfusion concurrent with the end of life.
- Diagnostic testing is currently not available to detect tissue necrosis in its decisive stages.

Pruritus

Pruritus is frequently seen in the following conditions and diseases:
- Brain tumor
- Biliary cirrhosis
- Diabetes mellitus
- Drugs
- Idiopathic (has no diagnostic cause)
- Liver disease
- Malignancies
- Multiple sclerosis

- Polycythemia (itch occurs after a hot bath)
- Psychological (anxiety disorders)
- Renal failure
- Senile pruritus (idiopathic pruritus in the elderly)
- Thyroid disorders (improves with treatment)
- Topical infections

Adapted with permission from Tomic-Canic, M. "Keratinocyte Cross-Talks in Wounds." *Wounds* 17:S3-6, 2005.

Treatment plan for pruritus

- Manage the underlying disease that causes the pruritus.
- Use topical emollients and bathing strategies as outlined in the xerosis care plan.
- Implement behavior modification (stopping scratching and breaking the itch-scratch-itch cycle).
- Keep nails short.
- Wear gloves at night to decrease skin damage.

- Use cotton sheets, which may be more soothing to itchy skin.
- Help the patient avoid wearing clothing that can irritate the skin, such as wool or other "scratchy" fabrics.
- Limit the indiscriminate use of topical steroids and antihistamines as their effectiveness needs further investigation.

Adapted with permission from Gilhar, A., et al. "Ageing of Human Epidermis: The Role of Apoptosis, Fas and Telomerase," *British Journal of Dermatology* 150:56-63, 2004.

Skin changes at life's end© (SCALE©)

The literature on skin changes at life's end is limited. Key opinion leaders convened in 2008 to discuss this important topic. According to Sibbald and Krasner,[79] "General agreement was reached that like any other organ of the body, skin is subject to a loss of integrity due to internal and external insults." Contrary to popular myth, not all pressure ulcers are avoidable. The panel concluded that our current appraisal of the complex skin changes at life's end and terminal pressure ulcers (including the Kennedy Terminal Ulcer) is limited. Additional scientific research and the consensus of expert knowledge is necessary to assess the important etiological factors of SCALE, to clinically describe and diagnose the conditions, and to recommend appropriate pathways of care. Knowledge transfer into

Differentiating between MASD and pressure ulcers in the perineal and genital area

Characteristic	Moisture-associated dermatitis (MASD) or incontinence-associated dermatitis (IAD)	Pressure ulcer
Location	Often in skin folds; diffuse	Usually over bony prominences; well circumscribed
Color	Red or bright red	Red to bluish-purple
Depth	Intact skin to partial-thickness wound	Intact skin to partial- or full-thickness wound
Necrosis	None	May be present
Pain and itching	May be present	May be present

Adapted with permission from Gray, M., Bohacek, L., Weir, D., Zdanuk, J. "Moisture vs Pressure. Making Sense out of Perineal Wounds. *JWOCN* 43(2):134-42, 2007.

practice techniques must then be implemented for improved patient outcomes. This process must include clinicians, laypeople and policy makers concerned with the care of people at life's end to adequately address the medical, social, legal and financial ramifications of SCALE."[79] SCALE will be discussed further in Chapter 24, Palliative care.

SUMMARY

The skin is the largest organ of the body and commonly the most forgotten. Skin is exposed daily to environmental irritants and chemicals as well as physical and mechanical injury, any of which may lead to impaired skin integrity.

This chapter provided an overview of skin structure and criteria for a skin assessment vs. a wound assessment. Identification and classification of skin tears as an exemplar for acute traumatic skin injury were also presented, including skin tear risk factors and prevention opportunities as well as treatment strategies. The importance of identifying common skin conditions in the elderly, specifically xerosis, pruritus (including the role of breaking the itch-scratch-itch cycle), and MASD, is described. The use of moisturizers in the treatment of these conditions was also highlighted. Skin failure and SCALE©, two multifaceted subjects regarding dysfunctional skin processes, were also introduced.

PATIENT SCENARIO

Clinical Data

Mr. TA is an 89-year-old, newly admitted resident of a long-term care facility. He is recently widowed and can no longer live alone at home. He has mild dementia and needs assistance with ambulation and activities of daily living. Because he did not always make it to the bathroom in time, his son suggested that he wear an adult containment brief/diaper. The adult briefs were not changed regularly, nor was a protective barrier lotion applied. As can be seen in Figure 4-1A, Mr. TA has moisture-associated skin damage (MASD), or incontinence-associated dermatitis (IAD), as a result of urinary and fecal incontinence. On his initial skin assessment, a skin tear is noted on his left forearm over an area of senile purpura (Figure 4-1B). As you recall, the upper extremities are the most common place for skin tears. Because part of the epidermal skin flap is missing but more than 25% of the flap is still present, the tear is documented as a Payne-Martin category II skin tear.

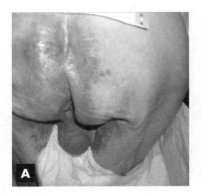 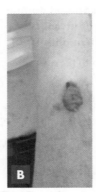 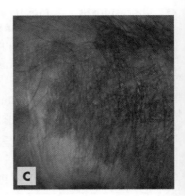

Figure 4-1. (A) Incontinence-associated dermatitis. (B) Skin tear. (C) Senile purpura. (Views A and B, E.A. Ayello. View C, Courtesy B. Beck, RN, WOCN. See *color section, Patient scenarios,* page C40, for the color versions of these images.)

Case Discussion

Mr. TA has several skin care problems that need to be addressed. Because he already has a skin tear, Mr. TA is assessed as being in group I using the Skin Integrity Risk Assessment Tool developed by White and colleagues; this means that his skin is vulnerable to developing additional tears. Implementing strategies to prevent further injury include protecting other areas of senile purpura (Figure 4-1C) on his arms by encouraging him to wear long sleeves to add a layer of "padding" to protect his skin. This also has the added benefit of helping him feel more comfortable as he often complained of feeling cold.

Staff is reminded to implement the facility's skin tear guidelines, which include attention to transfer techniques such as not grabbing Mr. TA's arms when assisting him to get out of bed or up from a chair and providing adequate lighting so he does not bump into furniture. Using a no-rinse product rather than soap and hot water for bathing, as well as not rubbing the skin during cleansing, are also part of safe skin handling.

Local care of Mr. TA's skin tear was also required. After cleansing with normal saline, a soft non-adherent silicone dressing was placed over the skin tear so that no additional tearing of the skin would occur during dressing removable. The dressing was held in place with a gauze wrap. Skin sealants were used over the other areas of senile purpura that were thought to be at risk. Three weeks after presentation, his skin tear had healed.

The skin damage from incontinence required other interventions as well. First, a toileting assistance program was initiated. Skin surrounding the reddened area was protected with skin sealant that had no alcohol to prevent any discomfort or pain from product application, and skin barrier cream was applied. The use of adult briefs was discontinued. No incontinence pads were used on his bed because moisture-damaged skin may be more prone to pressure ulcer development. Mr. TA was turned and repositioned every 3 hours, and daily skin assessment was conducted.

Mr. TA required frequent skin care to his sacral area due to his IAD, but after 2 months the skin healed and a prevention protocol using skin barrier lotion was initiated. Due to the frequent turning and repositioning as well as ambulation schedule with physical therapy, Mr. TA remained pressure ulcer free.

SHOW WHAT YOU KNOW

1. While bathing a patient, you notice some flakes of skin on the washcloth. Which layer of the skin is this?
    A. Stratum granulosum
    B. Stratum spinosum
    C. Stratum lucidum
    D. Stratum corneum

    ANSWER: D. *The cells of the stratum corneum can shed and look like flakes during routine cleaning activities such as bathing.*

2. Which of the following is a normal function of the skin?
    A. Synthesis of vitamin K
    B. Elimination of carbon dioxide
    C. Regulation of glucose levels by Langerhans cells
    D. Thermal regulation by skin blood flow dilation or constriction

    ANSWER: D. *Upon stimulus from the hypothalamus, skin blood vessels will either vasoconstrict (heat needs to be conserved to elevate temperature) or vasodilate (heat needs to be eliminated to lower temperature) depending on specific needs. Skin can synthesize vitamin D, not vitamin K. Carbon dioxide is eliminated via the lungs. Glucose levels are regulated by the islets of Langerhans in the pancreas, not the Langerhans cells in the skin.*

(continued)

3. What is the role of keratinocytes in skin?
   A. Differentiation
   B. Cross-talk to fibroblasts
   C. Participating in BMZ
   D. Maintenance and repair of the barrier

   ANSWER: D. *The entire biology of keratinocytes is dedicated to barrier formation and maintenance.*

4. Which of the following is NOT considered part of a routine skin assessment?
   A. Color
   B. Turgor
   C. Temperature
   D. Ankle-brachial index (ABI)

   ANSWER: D. *ABI is a test used for peripheral vascular disease; it does not tell you about skin assessment. Answers A, B, and C should all be part of a skin assessment.*

5. Which of the following patients is most at risk for skin tear injury?
   A. A 22-year-old male following surgery for an inguinal hernia repair
   B. A 37-year-old male with a fractured humerus
   C. A 64-year-old female 3 days post cataract extraction
   D. A 72-year-old female with rheumatoid arthritis on steroid therapy

   ANSWER: D. *A 72-year-old female is the oldest and least mobile and is receiving steroids, which are known to further cause thinning of the skin, so she is at highest risk.*

6. A partial-thickness skin tear with less than 25% of epidermal flap loss using the Payne-Martin method would be classified as category:
   A. I.
   B. II.
   C. III.
   D. IV.

   ANSWER: B. *Answer A is incorrect because there is no tissue loss in category I. C is incorrect because in category III there is complete loss of the tissue flap. D is incorrect because the Payne-Martin classification system contains no category IV.*

7. Which of the following interventions for a resident in a long-term care facility with a skin tear on the lower right leg should you question?
   A. Clean the patient daily using detergent.
   B. Pad the wheelchair arm and leg supports.
   C. Apply a non-adherent dressing to the skin tear.
   D. Encourage the patient to wear soft, fleece-lined pants.

   ANSWER: A. *Nonemollient soaps should be used instead of detergent, which dries the skin. The literature suggests that routine every-other-day bathing for elderly people is adequate (unless the skin is soiled) and can reduce skin tear injury. Answers B, C, and D are all interventions to consider as part of a skin tear protocol.*

8. Which of the following should be included in the care plan of a person with xerosis?
   A. Have the patient shower daily.
   B. Use a deodorant soap.

C. Dry the skin completely with vigorous rubbing.
D. Apply an emollient immediately after bathing.

ANSWER: D. *Emollient moisturizers are a cornerstone in the treatment of xerosis. Answer A is incorrect because daily cleaning of the skin either by showering or bathing is not recommended as it further dries the skin. Answer B is incorrect because a low pH soap needs to be used as deodorant soaps have a high pH that makes the skin alkaline. Answer C is incorrect because rubbing can irritate dry skin.*

9. Which of the following best defines pruritus?
   A. Multiple blisters on the skin
   B. Traumatic open area on the skin
   C. Itchy skin
   D. Weepy skin

   ANSWER: C. *Pruritus is the medical term for itchy skin.*

10. _____ is defined as an event in which the skin and underlying tissue die due to hypoperfusion that occurs concurrent with severe dysfunction or failure of other organ systems.
    A. Xerosis
    B. Skin failure
    C. Skin tear
    D. Pruritus

    ANSWER: B. *is the correct definition; Answers A, C, and D refer to other skin injuries or conditions. Xerosis is dry skin, and pruritus is itchy skin. Skin failure is a new concept in which the skin dies due to hypoperfusion.*

REFERENCES

1. Koch, S., et al. "Skin Homing of Langerhans Cell Precursors: Adhesion, Chemotaxis, and Migration," *J Allergy Clin Immunol* 117: 163-68, 2006.
2. Blumenberg, M., and Tomic-Canic, M. "Human Epidermal Keratinocyte: Keratinization Processes," *EXS* 78:1-29, 1997.
3. Freedberg, I.M., et al. "Keratins and the Keratinocyte Activation Cycle," *J Invest Dermatol* 116:633-40, 2001.
4. Tomic-Canic, M., et al. "Epidermal Repair and the Chronic Wound," in *The Epidermis in Wound Healing*. Edited by Rovee, D.T., and Maibach, H.I. Boca Raton, Fla.: CRC Press; 2004: pp 25-7.
5. Tomic-Canic, M. "Keratinocyte Cross-Talks in Wounds," *Wounds* 17:S3-6, 2005.
6. Morasso, M.I., and Tomic-Canic, M. "Epidermal Stem Cells: The Cradle of Epidermal Determination, Differentiation and Wound Healing," *Biol Cell* 97:173-83, 2005.
7. Habif, T.P. *Clinical Dermatology: A Color Guide to Diagnosis and Therapy.* Philadelphia: Mosby, 2004.
8. Kanitakis, J. "Anatomy, Histology and Immunohistochemistry of Normal Human Skin," *Eur J Dermatol* 12:390-99; quiz 400, 2002.
9. Eckes, B., and Krieg, T. "Regulation of Connective Tissue Homeostasis in the Skin by Mechanical Forces," *Clin Exp Rheumatol* 22:S73-76, 2004.
10. Yosipovitch, G., and Hu, J. "The Importance of Skin pH," *Skin and Aging* 11:88-93, 2003.
11. Waller, J.M., and Maibach, H.I. "Age and Skin Structure and Function, A Quantitative Approach (I): Blood Flow, pH, Thickness, and Ultrasound Echogenicity," *Skin Res Technol* 11:221-35, 2005.
12. Rippke, F., et al. "Stratum Corneum pH in Atopic Dermatitis: Impact on Skin Barrier Function and Colonization with *Staphylococcus Aureus*," *Am J Clin Dermatol* 5:217-23, 2004.
13. Yilmaz, E., and Borchert, H.H. "Effect of Lipid-Containing, Positively Charged Nanoemulsions on Skin Hydration, Elasticity and Erythema-An In Vivo Study," *Int J Pharm* 307:232-38, 2006.

14. Kurabayashi, H., et al. "Inhibiting Bacteria and Skin pH in Hemiplegia: Effects of Washing Hands with Acidic Mineral Water," *Am J Phys Med Rehabil* 81:40-46, 2002.

15. Damjanov, I. *Pathology for the Health-Related Professions.* Philadelphia: W.B. Saunders, 2000.

16. Yamasaki, K., Gallo, R.L. "Antimicrobial Peptides in Human Skin Disease," *Eur J Dermatol* 2008 Jan-Feb;18(1):11-21.

17. Hughes, E., and Van Onselen, J. *Dermatology Nursing: A Practical Guide.* London: Churchill Livingstone, Inc, 2001.

18. Bardan, A., et al. "Antimicrobial Peptides and the Skin," *Expert Opin Biol Ther* 4:543-49, 2004.

19. Niyonsaba, F., and Ogawa, H. "Protective Roles of the Skin Against Infection: Implication of Naturally Occurring Human Antimicrobial Agents Beta-Defensins, Cathelicidin LL-37 and Lysozyme," *J Dermatol Sci* 40:157-68, 2005.

20. Stante, M., et al. "Itch, Pain, and Metaesthetic Sensation," *Dermatol Ther* 18:308-13, 2005.

21. Charkoudian, N. "Skin Blood Flow in Adult Human, Thermoregulation: How It Works, When It Does Not, and Why," *Mayo Clin Proc* 78:603-12, 2003.

22. Minson, C.T. "Hypoxic Regulation of Blood Flow in Humans. Skin Blood Flow and Temperature Regulation," *Adv Exp Med Biol* 543:249-62, 2003.

23. Kupper, T.S., and Fuhlbrigge, R.C. "Immune Surveillance in the Skin: Mechanisms and Clinical Consequences," *Nat Rev Immunol* 4:211-22, 2004.

24. Wolpowitz, D., and Gilchrest, B.A. "The Vitamin D Questions: How Much Do You Need and How Should You Get It?" *J Am Acad Dermatol* 54:301-17, 2006.

25. Barrientos, S., Stojadinovic, O., Golinko, M.S., Brem, H., Tomic-Canic, M. "Growth factors and cytokines in wound healing." *Wound Repair Regen* Sep-Oct;16(5):585-601, 2008.

26. Venna, S.S., and Gilchrest, B.A. "Skin Aging and Photoaging," *Skin and Aging* 12:56-69, 2004.

27. Gilhar, A., et al. "Ageing of Human Epidermis: The Role of Apoptosis, Fas and Telomerase," *Br J Dermatol* 150:56-63, 2004.

28. Dealy, C. "Skin Care and Pressure Ulcers," *Advances in Skin and Wound Care* 22(9):421-8, quiz 429-30, 2009.

29. Waller, J.M., and Maibach, H.I. "Age and Skin Structure and Function, a Quantitative Approach (II): Protein, Glycosaminoglycan, Water, and Lipid Content and Structure." *Skin Research and Technology* 12:145-54, 2006.

30. Selden, S.T., et al. "Skin Tears: Recognizing and Treating This Growing Problem," *Extended Care Product News* 113(3):14-15, May-June, 2003.

31. Ashcroft, G.S., Dodsworth, J., et al. "Estogen Accelerates Cutaneous Wound Healing Associated with an Increase in TGF-ß₁ Levels," *Nature Medicne* 3:1209-1215, 1997.

32. Ashworth, J.J., Smyth, J.V., Pendleton, N., et al. "Polymorphisms Spanning the *0N* Exon and Promoter of the Estrogen Receptor-Beta (ERB) Gene *ESR2* Are Associated with Venous Ulceration," *Clin Genet* Jan;73(1):55-61, 2008.

33. Gilliver, S.C., and Ashcroft, G.S. "Sex Steroids and Cutaneous Wound Healing: The Contrasting Influences of Estrogens and Androgens," *Climacteric* 2007 Aug;10(4):276-88, 2007.

34. Fletcher, K. "Skin: Geriatric Self-Learning Module," *MEDSURG Nursing* 14(2):138-142, 2005.

35. Lee, B., and Tomic-Canic, M. "Tissue Specificity of Steroid Action: Glucocorticoids in Epidermis," in *Molecular Mechanisms of Action of Steroid Hormone Receptors.* Edited by Krstic-Demonacos, M., and Demonacos, C. Kerala, India: Research Signpost, 2002.

36. Matsumura, Y., and Anathaswamy, H.N. "Toxic Effects of Ultraviolet Radiation on the Skin," *Toxicology and Applied Pharmacology* 195(3):298-308, 2004.

37. Fisher, G.J. "The Pathophysiology of Photoaging of the Skin," *Cutis* 75:5-8; discussion 8-9, 2005.

38. Geriatric Nursing Resources for Care of Older Adults. *Normal Aging Changes.* Available at: GeronurseOnline.org. Accessed June 6, 2006.

39. Wysocki, A.B. "Skin Anatomy, Physiology, and Pathophysiology," *Nurs Clin North Am* 34 (5): 777-97, 1999.

40. Holloway, S., and Jones, V. "The Importance of Skin Care and Assessment," *Br J Nurs* 14: 1172-1176, 2005.

41. Baranoski, S. "Skin Tears: Staying on Guard Against the Enemy of Frail Skin," *Nursing* 33(Suppl):14-20, 2003.

42. Centers for Medicare and Medicaid Services (CMS). "Guidance to Surveyors for Long Term Care Facilities," *Pressure Sores* Revised Tag F 314:144, November 2004.

43. Baranoski, S. "Meeting the Challenge of Skin Tears," *Advances in Skin & Wound Care* 18:74-75, 2005.

44. Payne, R.L., and Martin, M.L. "Defining and Classifying Skin Tears: Need for a Common Language," *Ostomy/Wound Management* 39(5): 16-20, 22-24, 26, 1993.

45. LeBlanc, K., Christensen, D., Orsted, H.L., Keast, D.H. "Best Practice Recommendations for the

Prevention and Treatment of Skin Tears," *Wound Care Canada*. 6(1):14-30, 2008.

46. Carville, K., Lewin, G., Haslehurst, P., Michael, R., Santamaria., N, Roberts, P. "STAR: A Consensus for Skin Tear Classification," *Primary Intention* 15(1), 18-28, 2007.

47. Malone, M.L., et al. "The Epidemiology of Skin Tears in the Institutionalized Elderly," *J Am Geriatr Soc* 39:591-95, 1991.

48. Hanson, D.H., et al. "Skin Tears in Long-Term Care: Effectiveness of Skin Care Protocols on Prevalence," *Advances in Skin & Wound Care* 18:74, 2005.

49. Bank, D. "Decreasing the Incidence of Skin Tears in a Nursing and Rehabilitation Center," *Advances in Skin & Wound Care* 18:74-75, 2005.

50. White, M.W., et al. "Skin Tears in Frail Elders: A Practical Approach to Prevention," *Geriatr Nurs* 15(2):95-99, 1994.

51. Meuleneire, F. "Using a Soft Silicone-Coated Net Dressing to Manage Skin Tears," *Journal of Wound Care* 11(10):365-69, 2002.

52. Payne, R.L., and Martin, M.L. "The Epidemiology and Management of Skin Tears in Older Adults," *Ostomy Wound Manage* 26:26-37, 1990.

53. LeBlanc, K., and Baranoski, S. "Prevention and Management of Skin Tears," *Advances in Skin and Wound Care* 22(7):325-32, quiz 333-4, 2009.

54. Ratliff, C.R., and Fletcher, K.R. "Skin Tears: A Review of the Evidence to Support Prevention and Treatment," *Ostomy Wound Management* 53(3):32-42, 2007.

55. Birch, S., and Coggins, T. "No-Rinse, One-Step Bed Bath: The Effects on the Occurrence of Skin Tears in a Long-Term Care Setting," *Ostomy Wound Management* 49:64-7, 2003.

56. Bank, D., and Nix, D. "Preventing Skin Tears in a Nursing and Rehabilitation Center: An Interdisciplinary Effort," *Ostomy Wound Management* 52(9):38-46, 2006.

57. Mason, S.R. "Type of Soap and the Incidence of Skin Tears among Residents of a Long-term Care Facility," *Ostomy Wound Management* 43(8): 26-30, 1997.

58. Brillhart, B. "Pressure Sore and Skin Tear Prevention and Treatment during a 10-Month Program," *Rehabilitation Nursing* 30(3): 85-91, 2005.

59. McTigue, T., D'Andrea, S., Doyle-Munoz, J., Forrester, D.A. "Efficacy of a Skin Tear Education Program. Improving the Knowledge of Nurses Practicing in Acute Care Settings," *JWOCN* 36(5):486-92, 2009.

60. Baranoski, S. "Skin Tears: The Enemy of Frail Skin," *Advances in Skin & Wound Care* 13:123-26, 2000.

61. O'Regan, A. "Skin Tears: A Review of the Literature," *WCET Journal* 22:26-31, 2002.

62. Cuzzell, J. "Wound Assessment and Evaluation: Skin Tear Protocol," *Dermatology Nursing* 14:405-16, 2002.

63. Milne, C.T., and Corbett, I.O. "A New Option in the Treatment of Skin Tears for the Institutionalized Resident: Formulated 2-Octycyanacylate Topical Bandage," *Geriatric Nursing* 26(5):321-5, 2005.

64. Edwards, H., Gaskill, D., and Nash, R. "Treating Skin Tears in Nursing Home Residents: A Pilot Study Comparing Four Types of Dressings," *International Journal of Nursing Practice* 4(1): 25-32, 1998.

65. Thomas, D.R., Goode, P.S., LaMaster, K., Tennyson, T., Parnell, L.K. "A Comparison of an Opaque Foam Dressing versus a Transparent Film Dressing in the Management of Skin Tears in Institutionalized Subjects," *Ostomy Wound Management* 45(6):22-8, 1999.

66. Groom, M., Shannon, R.J., Chakravarthy, D., Fleck, C.A. "An Evaluation of Costs and Effects of a Nutrient-based Skin Care Program as a Component of Prevention of Skin Tears in an Extended Convalescent Center," *JWOCN* 37(1):46-51, 2010.

67. Lukas, M. "Management of Multiple Skin Tears in a Patient with Chronic Liver and Renal Disease," *Advances in Skin & Wound Care* 18:75, 2005.

68. Lebwohl, M., et al. *Treatment of Skin Disease: Comprehensive Therapeutic Strategies*. London: Harcourt Publishers Limited (Mosby), 2002.

69. Gray, M., Bohacek, L., Weir, D., Zdanuk, J. "Moisture vs Pressure. Making Sense out of Perineal Wounds," *JWOCN* 34(2):134-42, 2007.

70. Gray, M., Bliss, D.Z., Doughty, D.B., Ermer-Seltun J., Kennedy-Evans, K.L., Palmer, M.H. "Incontinence-associated Dermatitis— A Consensus," *JWOCN* 34(1):45-54, 2007.

71. Defloor, T. Schoonhoven, L., Fletcher, J., et al. "Statement of the European Pressure Ulcer Advisory Panel— Pressure Ulcer Classification. Differentiation between Pressure Ulcers and Moisture Lesions," *JWOCN* 32(5): 302-6, 2005.

72. Zulkowski, K. "Perineal Dermatitis versus Pressure Ulcer: Distinguishing Characteristics," *Advances in Skin & Wound Care* 21(4)382-8; quiz 389-90, 2008.

73. Goode, P.S., and Allman, R.M. "The Prevention and Management of Pressure Ulcers," *Med Clin North Am* 73:1511-24, 1989.

74. LaPuma, L. "The Ethics of Pressure Ulcers," *Decubitus* 4(2):43-4, 1991.

75. Witkowski, J.A., and Parish, L.C. "Skin Failure and the Pressure Ulcer," *Decubitus* 6(5):4, 1993.
76. Leijten, F.S., DeWeerd, A.W., Poortvliet, D.C., et al. "Critical Illness Polyneuropathy in Multiple Organ Dysfunction Syndrome and Weaning from the Ventilator," *Intensive Care Med* 22: 856-61, 1996.
77. Hobbs, L., Spahn, J.G., Duncan, C. "Skin Failure: What Happens When This Organ System Fails." Poster presented at the WOCN Society 32nd Annual Conference, Toronto, Ontario, Canada; June 2000.
78. Langemo, D.K., and Brown, G. "Skin Fails Too: Acute, Chronic, and End-stage Skin Failure," *Advances in Skin & Wound Care* 19:206-11, 2006.
79. Sibbald, R.G., and Krasner, D.L. "SCALE: Skin Changes at Life's End," *Wounds* 21(12):329-36, 2009.

Acute and Chronic Wound Healing

Samantha Holloway, MSc, PGCE, RN
Keith Harding, MB, ChB, FRCGP, FRCP, FRCS
Joyce K. Stechmiller, PhD, ACNP-BC, FAAN
Gregory Schultz, PhD

Objectives

After completing this chapter, you'll be able to:
- describe the physiology of wound healing
- discuss the cascade of wound healing events
- compare acute and chronic wound healing
- discuss the role of biofilms in wound healing.

WOUND HEALING EVENTS

When a patient experiences tissue injury, it's essential that hemostasis is rapidly achieved and tissue is repaired to prevent invasion by pathogens and restore tissue function. The process of wound healing is a complex sequence of events that starts when the injury occurs and ends with complete wound closure and successful, functional scar tissue organization. Although tissue repair is commonly described as a series of stages, in reality it's a continuous process during which cells undergo a number of complicated biological changes to facilitate hemostasis, combat infection, migrate into the wound space, deposit a matrix, form new blood vessels, and contract to close the defect.

However, wound closure isn't a marker of healing completion; the wound continues to change, in a process called remodeling, for up to 18 months post closure. During this prolonged phase of remodeling and maturation, the closed wound is still quite vulnerable.

Patient Teaching

Remind your patient that the process of wound healing can take up to 18 months. Although the wound may appear to be closed, changes are occurring in the underlying tissue. This means that the wound is still vulnerable to damage. Tell the patient to seek professional advice if he or she has any concerns about the wound.

WOUND HEALING CASCADE

The process of healing is usually divided into four phases—hemostasis, inflammation, proliferation/repair, and maturation/remodeling—each of which overlaps the others while remaining distinct in terms of time after injury. (See *Sequence of molecular and cellular events in skin wound healing*, page 84.)

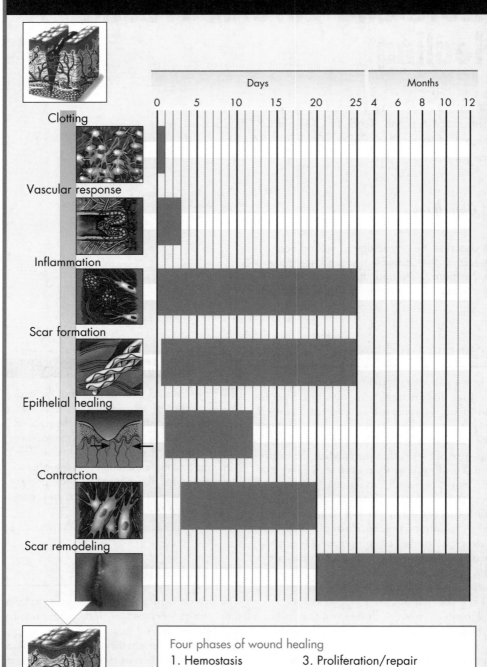

Sequence of molecular and cellular events in skin wound healing

Days — Months

Clotting

Vascular response

Inflammation

Scar formation

Epithelial healing

Contraction

Scar remodeling

Four phases of wound healing
1. Hemostasis
2. Inflammation
3. Proliferation/repair
4. Maturation/remodeling

Hemostasis

The disruption of tissue following injury causes hemorrhage, which initially fills the wound and exposes the blood to various components of the extracellular matrix (ECM).[1] Platelets aggregate and degranulate, which activates factor XII (Hageman factor), resulting in clot formation and hemostasis. Hemostasis stops hemorrhage at the site of blood vessel damage. This is essential as it preserves the integrity of the closed and high-pressure circulatory system to limit blood loss. A fibrinous clot forms during coagulation, acting as a preliminary matrix within the wound space into which cells can migrate.

After the fibrin clot forms, another mechanism is activated as part of the body's defense system—fibrinolysis—in which the fibrin clot starts to break down. This process prevents clot extension and dissolves the fibrin clot to allow ease of further cell migration into the wound space,[2] allowing the next stage of healing to proceed.

Inflammatory phase

As the fibrin clot is degraded, the capillaries dilate and become permeable, allowing fluid into the injury site and activating the complement system. The complement system is composed of a series of interacting, soluble proteins found in serum and extracellular fluid that induce lysis and the destruction of target cells. C3b, a complement molecule, helps bind (opsonize) neutrophils to bacteria, facilitating phagocytosis and subsequent bacterial destruction.

Cytokines and some proteolytic fragments that are hemoattractive are also found in the wound space.[2] Their abundance and accumulation at the site of injury initiate a massive influx of other cells. The two main inflammatory cells—neutrophils and macrophages—are attracted to the wound space to mount an acute inflammatory response.[3]

Neutrophils appear in a wound shortly after injury and reach their peak number within 24 to 48 hours; their main function is to destroy bacteria by the process of phagocytosis. Neutrophils have a very short life span: After 3 days without infection, their numbers reduce rapidly.

Tissue macrophages are derived from blood monocytes and arrive approximately 2 to 3 days after injury, followed by lymphocytes. Like neutrophils, macrophages also destroy bacteria and debris through phagocytosis; however, macrophages are also a rich source of biological regulators, including cytokines and growth factors, bioactive lipid products, and proteolytic enzymes, which are also essential for the normal healing process.[2,4]

CYTOKINES, GROWTH FACTORS, AND CHEMOTAXIS

Cytokine is a broad term that includes such molecules as growth factors, interleukins, tumor necrosis factors, and interferons. These molecules act on a variety of cells by exerting a wide range of biological functions by means of their specific receptors on target cells or proteins. Pathogens, endotoxins, tissue degradation products, and hypoxia are all factors that stimulate cells to produce cytokines following injury. The main cellular sources for these cytokines are platelets, fibroblasts, monocytes and macrophages, and endothelial cells. These cells are involved in physiological as well as pathological conditions (for example, tumors), although in wound healing they play an important role as mediators. Cytokines regulate cell proliferation, migration, matrix synthesis, deposition and degradation, and inflammatory responses in the repair process. (See *Major cytokines involved in wound healing*, page 86.)

Immediately after injury, platelet degranulation releases numerous cytokines, including platelet-derived growth factor (PDGF), transforming growth factor (TGF), and epidermal growth factor (EGF). These cytokines,

Major cytokines involved in wound healing

Cytokine	Cell source	Biological activity
Pro-inflammatory cytokines		
Tumor necrosis factor (TNF-α)	Macrophages	↑ PMN margination and cytotoxicity ↑ MMP synthesis
Interleukin-I (IL-1)	Macrophages, keratinocytes	↑ Fibroblast and keratinocyte chemotaxis ↑ MMP synthesis
Interleukin-6 (IL-6)	Macrophages, keratinocytes, PMNs	↑ Fibroblast proliferation
Interleukin-8 (IL-8)	Macrophages, fibroblasts	↑ Macrophage and PMN chemotaxis ↑ Collagen synthesis
Interleukin-γ	Macrophages, T-lymphocytes	↑ Macrophage and PMN activation ↓ Collagen synthesis ↑ MMP synthesis
Anti-inflammatory cytokines		
Interleukin-4 (IL-4)	T-lymphocytes, basophils, mast cells	↓ TNF-α IL-1, IL-6 synthesis ↑ Fibroblast proliferation, collagen synthesis
Interleukin-10 (IL-10)	T-lymphocytes, macrophages, keratinocytes	↓ TNF-α, IL-1, IL-6 synthesis ↓ Macrophage and PMN activation

together with other chemotactic agents, such as tissue debris and pathogenic materials, attract neutrophils and, later, macrophages. In time these cells contribute to a larger number and variety of cytokines, which participate in the healing process.[4] (See *Patient Teaching: Normal and abnormal signs of the inflammatory process.*)

Cytokines have diverse effects on the healing process, interacting in additive, synergistic, or inhibitory ways. (See *Major growth factor families*, page 88.) For example, keratinocyte growth factor enhances the stimulation of collagenase synthesis exerted by insulin-like growth factor. TGF is inhibitory to fibroblast growth in the presence of EGF but stimulates cell division when PDGF is present.

Proliferation phase

The proliferation phase usually begins 3 days after an injury and lasts for a few weeks. This phase is characterized by the formation of granulation tissue in the wound space. The new

Patient Teaching
Normal and abnormal signs of the inflammatory process

Discuss the *normal signs* of the inflammatory process with your patient: ✓ #30

- Redness
- Swelling

- Heat
- Pain

Clarify that in the early stages of the healing process you would expect the wound to exhibit these signs. However, advise the patient to *seek urgent medical attention* if any of the signs listed below are present, as these may be *signs of infection:*

- Wound breakdown
- Bleeding
- Increased pain

- Pus or unusual drainage
- Spreading redness around the wound
- Flu-like symptoms

PRACTICE POINT

Keep in mind that the induration, heat, discomfort, redness, and swelling experienced during the inflammatory phase are part of the normal wound healing processes and aren't, at this stage, likely to be due to wound infection. Remember to share this information with your patients.

tissue consists of a matrix of fibrin, fibronectin, collagens, proteoglycans, glycosaminoglycans (GAGs), and other glycoproteins.[5] Fibroblasts move into the wound space and proliferate. Because the type III collagen in the wound has

PRACTICE POINT

During the first 3 weeks after surgery, the patient is at high risk for wound dehiscence and evisceration. Advise the patient that he or she should follow any postsurgical advice very carefully as the repaired tissue will not regain its full strength. The wound is at risk of breakdown if undue pressure is exerted on the area. For instance, patients who have undergone an abdominal procedure should support their abdomen with a soft pillow if they need to cough. They should also avoid any heavy lifting or exertion as designated by their physician.

decreased tensile strength, the patient is at risk for such abnormalities as wound dehiscence or opening of wound edges in a previously closed wound that healed by primary intention. If organs are protruding from the now opened wound, it's called *evisceration*, which is a medical emergency that requires immediate surgery.

ROLE OF FIBROBLASTS

Fibroblasts play a key role during the proliferation phase, appearing in large numbers within 3 days of injury and reaching peak levels on the 7th day. During this period they undergo intense proliferative and synthetic activity. Fibroblasts synthesize and deposit extracellular proteins during wound healing, producing growth factors and angiogenic factors that regulate cell proliferation and angiogenesis.[6]

Granulation tissue is comprised of many mesenchymal and non-mesenchymal cells with distinct phenotypes, inflammatory cells, and new capillaries embedded in a loose ECM composed of collagens, fibronectin, and proteoglycans.

ROLE OF ECM PROTEINS

ECM consists of proteins and polysaccharides and their complexes produced by cells in the wound space. The two main classes of matrix proteins are fibrous proteins (collagens and

Major growth factor families

Growth factor family	Cell source	Actions
Transforming growth factor (TGF) β TGF-β1 TGF-β2 TGF-β3	Platelets Fibroblasts Macrophages	Chemotactic for fibroblasts Promotes extracellular matrix formation ↑ Collagen and tissue inhibitors of metalloproteinase (TIMP) synthesis ↓ Matrix metalloproteinase (MMP) synthesis Reduces scarring ↓ Collagen ↓ Fibronectin
Platelet-derived growth factor (PDGF) PDGF-AA; PDGF-BB; VEGF	Platelets Macrophages Keratinocytes Fibroblasts	Activates immune cells and fibroblasts Promotes extracellular matrix (ECM) formation ↑ Angiogenesis ↑ Angiogenesis
Fibroblast growth factor (FGF) Acidic FGF, Basic FGF, KGF	Macrophages Endothelial cells Fibroblasts	↑ Angiogenesis ↑ Keratinocyte proliferation and migration ↑ ECM deposition
Insulin-like growth factor (IGF) IGF-I, IGF-II, Insulin	Liver Skeletal muscle Fibroblasts Macrophages Neutrophils	↑ Keratinocyte and fibroblast proliferation ↑ Angiogenesis ↑ Collagen synthesis ↑ ECM formation ↑ Cell metabolism
Epidermal growth factor (EFG) EGF, HB (Heparin-binding), TGF-α, Amphiregulin, Betacellulin	Keratinocytes Macrophages	↑ Keratinocyte proliferation and migration ↑ ECM formation
Connective tissue growth factor (CTGF) CTGF	Fibroblasts Endothelial cells Epithelial cells	↑ Collagen synthesis Mediates action of TGF-βs on collagen synthesis

→ #31

elastin) and adhesive proteins (laminin and fibronectin). In addition, the ECM contains polysaccharides called proteoglycans and GAGs.

Collagen is the most abundant protein in animal tissue and accounts for 70% to 80% of the dry weight of the dermis.[7] The collagen molecule consists of three identical polypeptide chains bound together in a triple helix. Made mainly by fibroblasts, at least 19 genetically distinct collagens have been identified. Collagen synthesis and degradation are finely balanced.[4]

Elastin is a protein that provides elasticity and resilience.[7] It is composed of fibrous coils that stretch and return to their former shape, much like metallic coils. Because of these properties, elastin helps maintain tissue shape. Elastin represents only 2% to 4% of the human skin's dry weight; it's also in the lungs and blood vessels. It's secreted into the extracellular space as a soluble precursor, tropoelastin, which binds with a microfibrillar protein to form an elastic fiber network.

Laminin and fibronectin are two fiber-forming molecules. Their function is to provide structural and metabolic support to other cells. Fibronectin is found in plasma and contains specific binding sites on its molecular wall for cells, collagens, fibrinogens, and proteoglycans. It plays a central role in tissue remodeling, acting as a mediator for physical interactions between cells and collagens involved in ECM deposition, thereby providing a preliminary matrix.

Proteoglycans consist of a central core protein combined with a number of GAG chains that may be one or several types. GAGs consist of long, unbranched chains of disaccharide units that can range in number from 10 to 20,000.[8] A highly complex group of molecules, proteoglycans are characterized by their many diverse structural and organizational functions in tissue. Forming a highly hydrated gel-like "ground substance," they can contain up to 95% (w/w) carbohydrates. Originally, however, they were thought to contribute to tissue resilience due to their capacity to fill much of the extracellular space.

ANGIOGENESIS

Angiogenesis is the formation of new vessels in the wound space and is an integral and essential part of wound healing.[9] The vascular endothelial cell plays a key role in angiogenesis and arises from the damaged end of vessels and capillaries. New vessels originate as capillaries, which sprout from existing small vessels at the wound edge. The endothelial cells from these vessels detach from the vascular wall, degrade and penetrate (invade) the provisional matrix in the wound, and form a knob-like or cone-shaped vascular bud or sprout. These sprouts extend in length until they encounter another capillary, to which they connect to form vascular loops and networks, allowing blood to circulate. This pattern of vascular growth is similar in skin, muscle, and intestinal wounds.

EPITHELIALIZATION

Epithelial healing, or epithelialization, which begins a few hours after injury, is another important feature of healing. Marginal basal cells, which are normally firmly attached to the underlying dermis, change their cell adhesion property and start to lose their firm adhesion, migrating in a leapfrog or train fashion across the provisional matrix. Horizontal movement is stopped when cells meet. This is known as contact inhibition.

WOUND CONTRACTION

The final feature of the proliferation phase is wound contraction, which normally starts 5 days after injury. Wound contraction appears to be a dynamic process in which cells organize their surrounding connective tissue matrix, acting to reduce the healing time by reducing the amount of ECM that needs to be produced. The contractile activity of fibroblasts and myofibroblasts provides the force for this contraction. These cells may use integrins and other adhesion mechanisms to bind to the collagen network and alter its motility, bringing the fibrils and, subsequently, the wound edges closer. Such contraction may not be important in a sharply incised, small, and noninfected wound; however, it's critical for wounds with large tissue loss.[10]

Although several theories exist to explain the wound contraction process, its exact mechanism remains unclear. In particular, the type and origin of fibroblasts that appear in the wound haven't yet been determined.[1,3,11-13]

The myofibroblast theory suggests that the contraction force occurs when the movement of microfilament (actin) bundles (also termed *stress fibers*) contracts the myofibroblast in a muscle-like fashion. Because the myofibroblast displays many cell:cell and cell:matrix (fibronexus) contacts, the cellular contraction pulls collagen fibrils toward the body of the myofibroblast and holds them until they're stabilized into position. This gathering of collagen fibers toward the myofibroblast cell "body" leads to the shrinkage of granulation tissue. The ECM of the wound is continuous with the undamaged wound margin, enabling the granulation tissue shrinkage to pull on the wound margin, leading to wound contraction. The myofibroblast theory further proposes that the coordinated contraction (cellular shortening) of many myofibroblasts, synchronized with the help of gap junctions, generates the force necessary for wound contraction.[13]

The traction theory proposes that fibroblasts bring about a closer approximation of matrix fibrils by exerting "traction forces" (analogous to the traction of wheels on tarmac) on extracellular matrix fibers to which they're attached. This theory proposes that fibroblasts neither shorten in length nor act in a coordinated multicellular manner (as proposed by the myofibroblast theory); rather, a composite force, made up of traction forces of many individual fibroblasts, is responsible for matrix contraction. Such traction forces act as shearing forces tangential to the cell surface generated during cell elongation and spreading. According to the traction theory, the composite effect of many fibroblasts gathering collagen fibrils within the wound is thought to bring about wound contraction.[14]

network. Other components include hyaluronic acid and proteoglycans. The network has two main roles: as a substratum for the migration and growth of cells and as a template for subsequent collagen deposition. Collagen deposition becomes the predominant constituent of the matrix and soon forms fibrillar bundles and provides stiffness and tensile strength to the wound.

Collagen deposition and remodeling contribute to the increased tensile strength of skin wounds. Within 3 weeks of injury, the tensile strength is restored to approximately 20% of normal, uninjured skin. As healing continues, the skin gradually reaches a maximum of 70% to 80% tensile strength. Different organs regain tensile strengths to differing degrees. The remodeling process involves the balance between the synthesis and degradation of collagen. A range of collagenases regulates the latter. This process is also characterized by a gradual reduction in cellularity and vascularity. Differentiation of fibroblasts into myofibroblasts with resultant apoptosis (programmed cell death) are also features of tissue remodeling.[13]

Patient Teaching

Teach your patient who has a wound left open to heal (secondary intention) that clinicians will be looking for indications that wound healing is progressing normally:

• Healthy pink tissue in the wound bed
• Signs of new tissue growth at the wound edges
• Decreasing wound size over time

PRACTICE POINT

A patient history should always include information about prior wounds. Healed wounds never achieve the same tensile strength as uninjured skin, thereby increasing the potential for reinjury.

Patient Teaching

Remind the patient that the wounded area is never as strong as uninjured tissue so it is always vulnerable to damage. Simple measures such as keeping the scar tissue moisturized will help to optimize the condition of the tissue. Advise the patient to seek help if the scar begins to break down.

Maturation phase

The maturation phase normally starts 7 days after injury and may last for 1 year or more. The initial component in the deposited ECM is fibronectin, which forms a provisional fiber

The scar is the final product of wound healing and is a relatively avascular and acellular mass of collagen that serves to restore tissue continuity and some degree of tensile strength and function. However, the strength of the scar remains less than that of normal tissue, even many years following injury, and it's never fully restored. (See *Summary of wound healing*.)

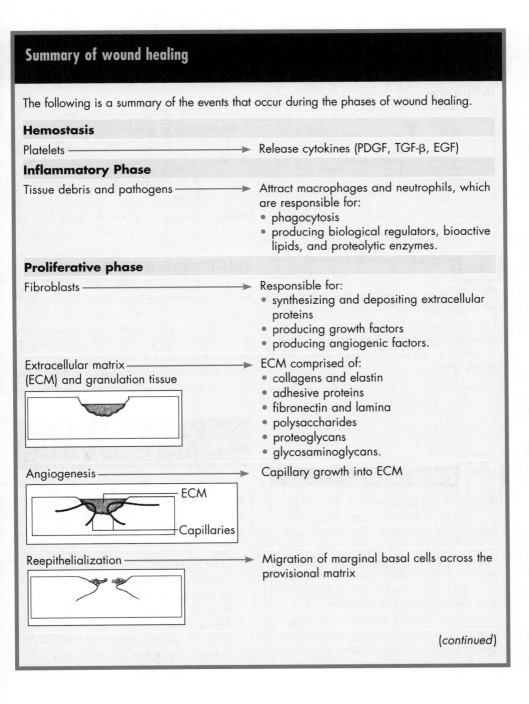

Summary of wound healing

The following is a summary of the events that occur during the phases of wound healing.

Hemostasis

Platelets ⟶ Release cytokines (PDGF, TGF-β, EGF)

Inflammatory Phase

Tissue debris and pathogens ⟶ Attract macrophages and neutrophils, which are responsible for:
- phagocytosis
- producing biological regulators, bioactive lipids, and proteolytic enzymes.

Proliferative phase

Fibroblasts ⟶ Responsible for:
- synthesizing and depositing extracellular proteins
- producing growth factors
- producing angiogenic factors.

Extracellular matrix (ECM) and granulation tissue ⟶ ECM comprised of:
- collagens and elastin
- adhesive proteins
- fibronectin and lamina
- polysaccharides
- proteoglycans
- glycosaminoglycans.

Angiogenesis ⟶ Capillary growth into ECM

ECM
Capillaries

Reepithelialization ⟶ Migration of marginal basal cells across the provisional matrix

(continued)

Summary of wound healing (continued)

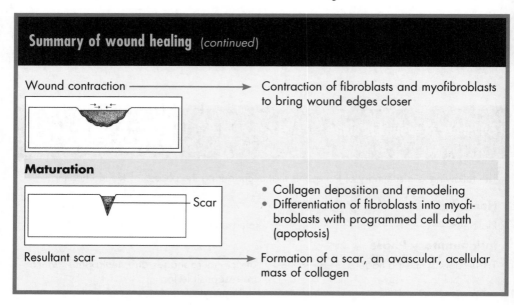

Wound contraction ⟶ Contraction of fibroblasts and myofibroblasts to bring wound edges closer

Maturation

Scar

• Collagen deposition and remodeling
• Differentiation of fibroblasts into myofibroblasts with programmed cell death (apoptosis)

Resultant scar ⟶ Formation of a scar, an avascular, acellular mass of collagen

PRACTICE POINT

The width of the resultant scar of a wound healing by secondary intention is about 10% of the original defect, primarily due to the process of wound contraction, working in conjunction with proliferation.

Patient Teaching

Inform the patient of the changes that occur to scar tissue over time. Initially, the scar may be red and raised but over time will become paler and flatten out. This process may take up to 2 years. Occasionally there may be signs of abnormal healing, such as a scar remaining raised or swollen. If this occurs, the patient should seek further advice from a healthcare practitioner as this may indicate hypertrophic or keloid scarring.

ROLE OF MATRIX METALLO-PROTEASES IN WOUND HEALING

Proteases, especially the matrix metalloproteinases (MMPs), play essential roles in all phases of normal wound healing. (See *Role of MMPs in wound healing*.) For example, during the inflammatory phase, damaged extracellular matrix proteins (such as collagen) must be

Role of MMPs in wound healing

Proteases (especially matrix metalloproteinases [MMPs]) play important, beneficial roles in normal wound healing. They perform the following functions:

• Contract wound matrix through use of myofibroblasts
• Implement angiogenesis (breakdown of capillary basement membrane)
• Migrate cells (epidermal cells, fibroblasts, vascular endothelial cells)
• Remodel scar extracellular matrix (ECM)
• Remove damaged ECM (especially during the inflammatory phase of healing)

removed so that newly synthesized collagen molecules can correctly align with collagen molecules in the wound matrix, permitting migration of epidermal cells and fibroblasts into the wound bed. (See *Extracellular matrix proteins and MMPs: Critical factors for epithelial migration, angiogenesis, and contraction,* page 94.) To remove damaged collagen molecules, collagenases (see *Families of MMPs, TIMPs, and ADAMs,* page 94), make a single cut in collagen molecules, which permits the gelatinases to further degrade collagen molecules into small fragments that are then removed from the injury area by neutrophils and macrophages. MMPs also play a key role in angiogenesis by first degrading the basement membrane that surrounds vascular endothelial cells (VECs). This causes new capillary buds to sprout and "channels" to erode the ECM, through which the VECs migrate, eventually creating new capillary arcs. Furthermore, MMPs are required for myofibroblasts to contract ECM during the maturation or remodeling phase. The actions of MMPs are controlled by their natural inhibitors, the tissue inhibitors of metallproteinases (TIMPs).

ACUTE vs. CHRONIC WOUND HEALING

Molecular and cellular abnormalities in chronic wounds

There would appear to be little consensus regarding the definition of acute and chronic wound etiologies. Chronicity implies a prolonged or lengthy healing process, whereas acute implies uncomplicated, orderly or organized, or rapid healing. Bates-Jensen and Wethe[15] define an acute wound as "a disruption in the integrity of the skin and underlying tissues that progresses through the healing process in a timely and uncomplicated manner." Typically, surgical and traumatic wounds, which heal by primary intention, are classified as acute.

On the other hand, Sussman[16] defines a chronic wound as "one that deviates from expected sequence of repair in terms of time, appearance, and response to aggressive and appropriate treatment." The Wound Healing

Society uses the definition of chronic wound as proposed in 1992 by Lazarus and colleagues: Chronic wounds are wounds that "fail to progress through a normal, orderly, and timely sequence of repair or wounds that pass through the repair process without restoring anatomic and functional results."[17] Such wounds usually heal by secondary intention and are associated with pathology; for example, diabetes, ischemic disease, pressure damage, and inflammatory diseases.

Patient Teaching

- Teaching patients the words used to describe the types of wound healing (acute, chronic, primary, secondary) may help them appreciate the time it may take for their wound to heal.
- Discuss the importance of moist wound healing to your patients, and inform them of what factors have been taken into consideration when deciding the most appropriate treatment for their wound.

The physiological differences between wounds that heal slowly and those that heal rapidly have been studied in a variety of ways. (See *Imbalanced molecular environments of healing and chronic wounds,* page 95.) One experiment explored the effect of chronic wound fluid on cell function.[18] Researchers cultured fibroblasts from human neonatal foreskin to use as a laboratory model of acute wounds. They then exposed the model to either chronic wound fluid or a control and found that chronic wound fluid dramatically inhibited the growth of the fibroblasts. According to Phillips et al.,[18] these results indicate that the microenvironment of chronic wounds impairs wound healing.

Other researchers[5,19] theorize that prolonged inflammation is the most significant factor in delayed healing. Indeed, Hart[5] proposes that the prolonged inflammatory phase is due to the presence of inflammatory

Extracellular matrix proteins and MMPs: Critical factors for epithelial migration, angiogenesis, and contraction

Epithelial migration

Epidermal cells at the leading edge of migrating sheets secrete several types of matrix metalloproteases (MMPs); fibroblasts migrating through provisional wound matrix also secrete MMPs.

Angiogenesis

Endothelial cells secret MMPs that degrade the basement membrane surrounding capillaries, allowing endothelial cells to proliferate and migrate toward angiogenic factors produced by cells in ischemic areas.

Contraction

Fibroblasts transform into myofibroblasts, which express contractile fibers and MMPs, and as myofibroblasts contract, force is applied to collagen fibers that reduces the size of the wound.

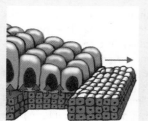
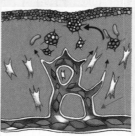
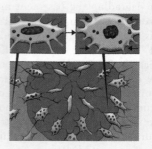

Families of MMPs, TIMPs, ADAMs

Collagenases
- Matrix metalloproteinase (MMP)-1, MMP-8, MMP-13, MMP-18
- Cut native type I collagen at one site

Gelatinases
- MMP-2, MMP-9
- Cut type collagen after collagenses make initial cut
- Cut native type IV collagen in basement membranes

Stromelysins
- MMP-3, MMP-10, MMP-11, MMP-19
- Cut core protein of proteoglycans

Metalloelastase/ matrilysin
- MMP-7, MMP-12
- Cut multiple substrates, including type IV collagen

Membrane-type MMPs (MT-MMPs)
- MT-MMP1 (MMP-14), MT-MMP2 (MMP-15), MT-MMP3 (MMP-16), MT-MMP4 (MMP-17)
- Attached to plasma membrane, active pro-MMPs

Tissue inhibitors of metalloproteinases (TIMPs)
- TIMP-1, TIMP-2, TIMP-3, TIMP-4
- Specific inhibitors for MMPs

A disintegrin and metalloproteinase (ADAM)
- Aggrecanase-1 (ADAM-1)

Tumor necrosis factor–α (TNFα) converting enzyme (TACE)

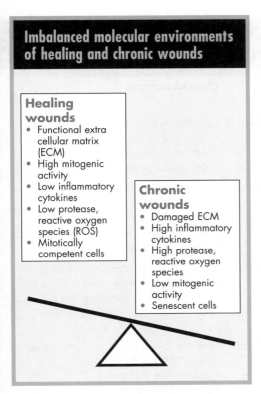

Imbalanced molecular environments of healing and chronic wounds

Healing wounds
- Functional extra cellular matrix (ECM)
- High mitogenic activity
- Low inflammatory cytokines
- Low protease, reactive oxygen species (ROS)
- Mitotically competent cells

Chronic wounds
- Damaged ECM
- High inflammatory cytokines
- High protease, reactive oxygen species
- Low mitogenic activity
- Senescent cells

Wound biofilms

Bacterial biofilms are known to contribute to numerous chronic inflammatory diseases, and recent evidence suggests that biofilms also play an important role in impairing healing in chronic skin wounds.[20-24] Wound bacteria that grow in clumps embedded in a thick, self-made, protective, slimy barrier of sugars and proteins are called a wound biofilm. Biofilms are defined as complex, dynamic microbial communities made up of microorganisms (bacteria and fungi) that synthesize and secrete a protective matrix that attaches the biofilm firmly to the wound surface.[25] They consist of a single bacterial or fungal species or, more commonly, may be polymicrobial, that is, they contain multiple diverse species that are continuously changing.[26]

Biofilms trigger a chronic inflammatory response that results in the accumulation of neutrophils and macrophages surrounding biofilms. The neutrophils and macrophages secrete high levels of reactive oxygen species (ROS) that affect the biofilm and the surrounding tissue. Inflammatory cells also secrete high levels of proteases (MMPs and elastase) that can help to break down the attachments between biofilms and the tissue, dislodging the biofilms from the tissue.[27] However, the ROS and proteases also damage normal surrounding tissue, proteins, immune cells, and tissue cells, impairing healing.

leukocytes, typically neutrophils and their production of proinflammatory cytokines that perpetuate inflammation. He also argues that the release of tissue-damaging proteinases, which degrade newly formed tissue, delay or prevent normal wound healing processes. In addition to prolonged inflammation, Hart[5] suggests several other factors that may induce chronicity, including recurrent physical trauma, ischemic reperfusion injury, subclinical bacterial contamination, and foreign bodies.

Because chronic wounds are typically characterized by full-thickness tissue loss, reepithelialization is prolonged due to the loss of appendages.[3] Normally, epithelial cells require the smooth, moist surface of the basement membrane to move across the wound. In chronic wounds, epithelial cells latch onto and pull themselves across the scaffolding of macromolecules of the provisional matrix, such as laminin and fibronectin.

PREDISPOSING FACTORS FOR DEVELOPMENT OF WOUND BIOFILMS

In vulnerable tissue, biofilms arise from planktonic bacteria attaching and forming a protective community before they are killed by the patient's immune system, by antibiotics, or by debridement. Thus, general conditions that impair the immune system or reduce the effectiveness of antibiotic drugs favor the development of biofilms in wounds. These conditions include ischemia or necrosis of tissue; poor patient nutrition; co-morbidities that impair immune function, such as HIV, diabetes, major trauma, radiation treatment; or treatment with immune-suppressing drugs.

TIME: Principles of wound bed preparation

Clinical observations	Molecular and cellular problems	Clinical actions
Tissue Nonviable or deficient	Defective matrix and cell debris impairing healing	Debridement (episodic or continuous) • Autolytic, sharp, surgical, mechanical, or biological • Biological agents
Infection or inflammation	*High bacteria counts or prolonged inflammation* ↑ Inflammatory cytokines ↑ Proteases ↓ Growth factor activity	*Remove infected foci* *Topical/systemic* Antimicrobials Anti-inflammatories Protease inhibitors
Moisture imbalance	Dessication slowing epithelial cell migration Excessive fluid causing maceration of wound	Apply moisture-balancing dressings Compression, negative pressure, and other methods of removing fluid
Edge margin non-advancing or undermined	Epidermal margin not migrating Nonresponsive wound cells and abnormalities in protease activities	Reassess cause, refer, or consider corrective advanced therapies: • Adjunctive therapies • Bioengineered skin • Debridement • Skin grafts

© International WBP Panel.

ASSESSMENT OF BIOFILMS

In chronic wounds, it can be difficult to distinguish biofilms from slough. Wound slough has been described as a viscous, yellow, and relatively opaque layer on wound beds, while biofilm found in wounds can appear more gel-like and shiny.[28] There is an important link between biofilms and slough. Biofilms stimulate inflammation, which increases vascular permeability and the production of wound exudate and buildup of fibrin slough.[29] Therefore, slough may indicate that biofilm is present in the wound. Unfortunately, chronic skin wounds are frequently assessed with standard clinical microbiology laboratory assays that are designed to culture single, planktonic bacteria, and they do not adequately measure biofilm bacteria. Currently, the most reliable method to confirm the presence of microbial biofilm is specialized microscopy.[30-34] Recently, an analysis using special cultivation techniques of biopsies from chronic wounds found that 60% of the specimens contained biofilm structures in

Effects of clinical actions	Clinical Outcome
Restoration of wound base and functional extracellular matrix proteins	Viable wound base
Low bacteria counts or controlled inflammation ↓ Inflammatory cytokines ↓ Proteases ↑ Growth factor activity	Bacterial balance and reduced inflammation
Restore epithelial migration, desiccation avoided Edema, excessive fluid controlled, maceration avoided	Moisture balance
Migrating keratinocytes and responsive wound cells Restoration of appropriate protease profile in wound	Advancing epithelial margin

comparison with only 6% of biopsies from acute wounds.[24]

MANAGEMENT OF BIOFILMS

Antibiotics and antiseptics kill single bacteria very easily, but the biofilm barrier blocks most antibiotics and antiseptics from reaching the bacteria, particularly in the center of the wound matrix. Wound biofilms are resistant to antibodies, antibiotics, disinfectants, and phagocytic inflammatory cells. Wound biofilms

can be effectively treated by a combination of debridement and/or cleansing to remove the biofilms, followed by application of dressings that block new bacteria from reaching the wound and killing bacteria left in the wound bed. These treatments can heal wounds, but patients must comply with the treatment plan because biofilms can re-form within a day and the wound will not heal.

Wound bed preparation

Wound bed preparation (WBP) is a systematic approach to correcting the molecular and cellular abnormalities, which is critical to promoting healing of chronic wounds. Recently, the concept of WBP has emerged in a systematic, comprehensive approach to wound care management that addresses four key aspects of practice principles: tissue debridement, inflammation/infection, moisture balance, and edge of the wound (TIME).[35] (See *TIME: Principles of wound bed preparation*.) In some WBP models, the letter T (for tissue—nonviable or deficient) has been replaced with a letter D, for debridement. The four principles are then known as DIME[36,37] instead of the TIME.

SUMMARY

The molecular and cellular environment of chronic wounds differs substantially from that of acute healing wounds. Specifically, non-healing wounds have chronically elevated pro-inflammatory cytokines, which lead to chronically elevated levels of proteases (MMPs and neutrophil elastase) and reactive oxygen species (ROS) that degrade the components that are essential to healing, such as ECM components, growth factors, and receptors. Cells in the base of non-healing wounds often become insensitive to growth factors resulting in senesent cells. Clinical studies using topical application of protease or dressings that bind proteases or use vacuum-assisted closure dressings have shown that reversing these molecular and cellular abnormalities promotes healing of chronic wounds.

PATIENT SCENARIO

Clinical Data

Mrs. B is 68 years old. She underwent a total abdominal hysterectomy (TAH) for underlying fibroids. The patient is generally fit and well and other than a high body mass index (>30) has no underlying health problems. The wound was initially closed by primary intention with subcuticular sutures. However, 14 days after surgery the wound began to shows signs of breakdown (dehiscence) (Figure 5-1A). Five days later, the wound dehisced (Figure 5-1B).

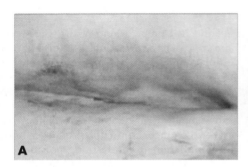 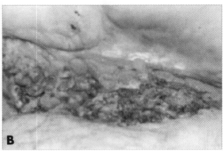

Figure 5-1. **(A)** Wound appearance 2 weeks post surgery. **(B)** Wound appearance at week 3. (See also *color section*, *Patient Scenarios*, page C41, for the color versions of these images.)

The wound would be described as an acute wound because it is a surgical wound. However, because the wound has decreased tensile strength (approximately 20% of normal, uninjured tissue) due to the laying down of collagen in the healing process, the wound has broken down or dehisced. There are no signs of protrusion of any internal organs (evisceration), so there is no need for immediate surgery. In addition, there is no excessive bleeding so hemostasis has been established. There are signs of fibrin clots in the wound that may delay healing. Through the inflammatory process, cells such as neutrophils and macrophages are attracted to the wound site to try and destroy bacteria and remove debris such as the dead tissue shown here. In combination with cytokines, these cells assist with the wound healing process. As healing progressed, new tissue was laid down (known as granulation tissue); this process relies on having an adequate blood supply, so the wound bed and surrounding skin were monitored for signs of sufficient perfusion.

Case Discussion

Over the next several weeks, the wound decreased in size through the action of both fibroblasts and myofibroblasts. This process, known as wound contraction, helps to reduce the amount of new tissue that is laid down in the wound. To assist in the healing process, the wound required a moist environment to aid in the debridement of devitalized tissue and to ensure the ideal medium for cells to be active. Measures were also taken to prevent excess moisture and maceration, which may lead to further breakdown. An appropriate moisture-balancing dressing was chosen and the wound observed for signs of healing at the margins as well as the base. The surrounding skin was protected with a skin barrier to prevent maceration from wound exudate. In addition to local wound management, Mrs. B was referred to a dietitian for nutritional advice and a physical therapist for guidance on appropriate activity levels.

The wound did heal but took much longer than normal. The patient was advised that the resultant scar was vulnerable and may be at risk of breakdown, so careful monitoring of the wound would be required.

SHOW WHAT YOU KNOW

1. Immediately following tissue injury, the priority is to:
   A. modify the immature scar tissue.
   B. achieve rapid hemostasis.
   C. rapidly fill the wounded area with granulation tissue.
   D. destroy bacteria.

   ANSWER: B. *Rapid hemostasis is essential as it preserves the integrity of the closed and high-pressure circulatory system to limit blood loss.*

2. The main mechanism by which chronic wounds fail to heal is believed to be:
   A. too rapid progress from hemostasis to maturation.
   B. a failure of fibroblasts and myofibroblasts to facilitate wound contraction.
   C. a dysfunction of collagen remodeling.
   D. a prolonged inflammatory phase.

   ANSWER: D. *Because chronic wounds contain abnormally high levels of proteinases and proinflammatory cytokines, prolonged inflammation is believed to be the most significant factor in delayed healing.*

3. During the proliferative phase, the framework that new tissue grows into is commonly called:
   A. the extracellular matrix.
   B. the complement system.
   C. chemotaxis.
   D. apoptosis.

   ANSWER A. *New tissue, or granulation tissue, grows into the extracellular matrix, which is composed of neovascular tissue, collagens, fibronectin, and proteoglycans.*

REFERENCES

1. Witte, M., Barbul, A. "General Principles of Wound Healing," *Surgical Clinics of North America* 77:509, June 1997.
2. Steed, D. "The Role of Growth Factors in Wound Healing," *Surgical Clinics of North America* 77:575, June 1997.
3. Martin, P. "Wound Healing: Aiming for Perfect Skin Regeneration," *Science* 276:75, April 1997.
4. Slavin, J. "Wound Healing: Pathophysiology," *Surgery* 17(4):I-V, April 1999.
5. Hart, J. "Inflammation 2: Its Role in the Healing of Chronic Wounds," *Journal of Wound Care* 11:245-49, July 2002.
6. Stephens, P., Thomas, D.W. "The Cellular Proliferative Phase of the Wound Repair Process," *Journal of Wound Care* 11:253-61, July 2002.
7. Wysocki, A.B. "Anatomy and Physiology of Skin and Soft Tissue," *Acute and Chronic Wounds: Nursing Management.* Edited by Bryant, R.A. St. Louis: Mosby–Year Book, Inc., 2000.
8. Clark, R.A.F. *The Molecular and Cellular Biology of Wound Repair,* 2nd ed. New York: Plenum Publishing Corp., 1996.
9. Neal, M. "Angiogenesis: Is It the Key to Controlling the Healing Process?" *Journal of Wound Care* 10(7):281-87, July 2001.
10. Calvin, M. "Cutaneous Wound Repair," *Wounds* 10(1):12, January 1998.
11. Rohovsky, S., D'Amore, P. "Growth Factors and Angiogenesis in Wound Healing," in Ziegler, T., et al., eds. *Growth Factors and Wound Healing: Basic Science and Potential Clinical Applications* (pp. 8-26). New York: Springer-Verlag New York, Inc., 1997.
12. Berry, D.P., et al. "Human Wound Contraction: Collagen Organisation, Fibroblasts and Myofibroblasts," *Plastic and Reconstructive Surgery* 102(1):124-31, July 1998.
13. Tejero-Trujeque, R. "Understanding the Final Stages of Wound Contraction," *Journal of Wound Care* 10(7):259-63, July 2001.
14. Ehrlich, P. "The Physiology of Wound Healing: A Summary of the Normal and Abnormal

Wound Healing Processes," *Advanced Wound Care* 11(7):326, November-December 1998.

15. Bates-Jensen, B.M., Woolfolk N. "Acute Surgical Wound Management," in Sussman, C., and Bates-Jensen, B.M., eds. *Wound Care: A Collaborative Practice Manual for Health Professionals* (pp. 322-335). Baltimore: Lippincott Williams and Wilkins. 2007.

16. Sussman, C., Bates-Jensen, B.M. "Wound Healing Physiology: Acute and Chronic," in Sussman, C., and Bates-Jensen, B.M., eds. *Wound Care: A Collaborative Practice Manual for Health Professionals* (pp. 21-51). Baltimore: Lippincott Williams and Wilkins. 2007.

17. Lazarus, G.S., et al. "Definitions and Guidelines for Assessment for Wounds and Evaluation of Healing," *Archives of Dermatology* 130(4):489-93, April 1994.

18. Phillips, T.J., et al. "Effect of Chronic Wound Fluid on Fibroblasts," *Journal of Wound Care* 7(10):527-32, November 1998.

19. Yager, D.R., Nwomeh, B.C. "The Proteolytic Environment of Chronic Wounds," *Wound Repair and Regeneration* 7(6):433-41, November-December 1999.

20. Costerton, J.W., Stewart, P.S., Greenberg, E.P. "Bacterial Biofilms: A Common Cause of Persistent Infections," *Science* 284(5418):1318-22, 1999.

21. Costerton, J.W. "The Etiology and Persistence of Cryptic Bacterial Infections: A Hypothesis," *Review of Infectious Diseases* 6(Suppl 3):S608-16, 1984.

22. Hall-Stoodley, L., Stoodley, P. "Evolving Concepts in Biofilm Infections," *Cell Microbiology* 11(7):1034-43, 2009.

23. Wolcott, R.D., Rhoads, D.D., Bennett, M.E., et al. "Chronic Wounds and the Medical Biofilm Paradigm," *Journal of Wound Care* 19(2):45-50, 52, 2010.

24. James, G.A., Swogger, E., Wolcott, R., et al. "Biofilms in Chronic Wounds," *Wound Repair and Regeneration* 16(1):37-44, 2008.

25. Stoodley, P., Sauer, K., Davies, D.G., Costerton, J.W. "Biofilms as Complex Differentiated Communities," *Annual Review of Microbiology* 56:187-209, 2002.

26. Hall-Stoodley, L., Stoodley, P. "Evolving Concepts in Biofilm Infections," *Cell Microbiology* 11(7):1034-43, 2009.

27. Gibson, D., Cullen, B., Legerstee, R., Harding, K.G., Schultz, G. "MMPs Made Easy," *Wounds International* 1(1):1-6, 2010.

28. Hurlow, J., Bowler, P.G. "Clinical Experience with Wound Biofilm and Management: A Case Series," *Ostomy Wound Management* 55(4):38-49, 2009.

29. Wolcott, R.D., Rhoads, D.D., Dowd, S.E. "Biofilms and Chronic Wound Inflammation," *Journal of Wound Care* 17(8):333-41, 2008.

30. Dowd, S.E., Sun, Y., Secor, P.R., et al. "Survey of Bacterial Diversity in Chronic Wounds Using Pyrosequencing, DGGE, and Full Ribosome Shotgun Sequencing," *BioMed Central Microbiology* 8(1):43, 2008.

31. Edwards, R., Harding, K.G. "Bacteria and Wound Healing," *Current Opininion in Infectious Diseases* 17(2):91-6, 2004.

32. Costerton, W., Veeh, R., Shirtliff, M., et al. "The Application of Biofilm Science to the Study and Control of Chronic Bacterial Infections," *Journal of Clinical Investigation* 112(10):1466-77, 2003.

33. Kaeberlein, T., Lewis, K., Epstein, S.S. "Isolating 'Uncultivable' Microorganisms in Pure Culture in a Simulated Natural Environment," *Science* 296(5570):1127-9, 2002.

34. Bjarnsholt, T., Kirketerp-Moller, K., Jensen, P.O., et al. "Why Chronic Wounds Will Not Heal: A Novel Hypothesis," *Wound Repair and Regeneration* 16(1):2-10, 2008.

35. Schultz, G.S. "Wound Bed Preparation, A Systemic Approach to Wound Bed Management," *Wound Repair and Regeneration* 11(Suppl1):S1-28, 2003.

36. Woo, K.Y., Sibbald, R.G., Ayello, E.A. "D-Debridement," *Ostomy Wound Management Supplement*, p. 13-14, April 2009.

37. Sibbald, R.G., Woo, K.Y., Ayello, E.A. "Healing Chronic Wounds: DIM before DIME Can Help," *Ostomy Wound Management Supplement*, p.12, April 2009.

CHAPTER 6

Wound Assessment

Sharon Baranoski, MSN, RN, CWCN, APN-CCNS, DAPWCA, FAAN
Elizabeth A. Ayello, PhD, RN, ACNS-BC, CWON, MAPWCA, FAAN
Diane K. Langemo, PhD, RN, FAAN

Objectives

After completing this chapter, you'll be able to:

- state the reasons for performing a wound assessment
- differentiate between partial- and full-thickness injury
- list the parameters of a complete wound assessment
- describe useful photographic techniques for wound documentation
- discuss wound documentation using an electronic medical record and electronic health record.

THE WOUND

Reliable, consistent, and accurate wound description and documentation are essential components of a wound assessment. Not only does it provide objective data to confirm wound healing, but it can also serve to alert clinicians about wound deterioration.[1] Wound description and documentation also enhances communication among healthcare providers, patients, and care settings.[1,2] Assessment of chronic wounds is important because several clinical characteristics, such as new or increasing pain, new or increasing cellulitis, new or increasing purulent or non-purulent drainage and significant undermining, have been reported to constitute a wound emergency.[2]

The management of acute and chronic wounds has progressed into a highly focused area of practice, with physicians, nurses, therapists, and other professionals expanding their practice in this challenging arena. Care plans, treatment interventions, case management and discharge planning, as well as ongoing patient and wound management, are all based on the initial and subsequent wound assessments. The total patient assessment, inclusive of any comorbid conditions and lifestyle, must also be a part of any comprehensive wound assessment. This chapter addresses the key assessment parameters of a patient with a wound admitted to any healthcare setting, including the importance of a history and physical examination, how to assess a wound, essential practice points, and examples of accurate and thorough documentation tools.

A wound is a disruption of normal anatomic structure and function.[3] Wounds are classified as either acute or chronic. Acute wounds can be result from trauma or surgery. According to Larazus and colleagues,[3] acute wounds proceed through an orderly and timely healing process with the eventual return of anatomic and functional integrity. Chronic wounds, on the other hand, fail to proceed through this process and lose the cascade effect of wound healing and sustained anatomic and functional integrity. Stated simply, wounds may be classified as those that repair themselves or can be repaired in an orderly and timely process (acute wounds) and those that don't (chronic wounds).[3] See chapter 5 for a more detailed description of wound healing.

In the United States, the Centers for Medicare and Medicaid Services (CMS) is considering changing its current definition of a chronic wound. The current CMS definition of a chronic wound includes a time frame of greater than 30 days' duration for complete healing.[4]

The etiology or cause of the wound must be determined before appropriate interventions can be implemented. In the United States, states differ as to which clinicians can legally diagnose and assess the type of wound or the stage/category of a pressure ulcer, so check your specific state practice act for your discipline. Getting the differential diagnosis right is not always easy, but learning the typical characteristics of a wound type can be helpful. Wounds may have a surgical, traumatic, neuropathic, vascular, or pressure-related etiology. For example, an acute wound caused by a bite (animal, insect, spider, or human) needs a different care plan than a wound caused by a burn. A patient who has an animal bite may require additional testing to rule out damage to nerves, tendons, ligaments, or bone, as well as determination of rabies or rabies vaccination status of the animal and the need for tetanus immunization.[5] The pathologic etiology will provide the basis for additional testing and evaluation to start the wound assessment process. (See *Practice Point: The nine C's of wound assessment.*)

INITIAL PATIENT ASSESSMENT

Obtain a thorough history and a complete physical examination on every patient admitted into your care. Obtaining a patient history provides information on relevant disease processes, comorbidities, medications the patient is taking, and family history of conditions that can impact the etiology of the wound. In addition, the patient history may reveal information that explains previous wound healing concerns, infection, and other core information needed to develop the plan of care. A detailed patient medical and social history should direct additional questioning on any abnormal lab findings as well as a history of diabetes, vascular conditions, or an immune-compromised state. Therapies received as part of a prior health condition, such as radiation at the site of a wound, are also important factors that can contribute to impaired healing and delay appropriate management strategies.[1] (See "Radiation wounds" in chapter 23, Palliative wound care.) Use the assessment data to determine whether the wound is healable, non-healable, or palliative.

Family support and patient and family functional abilities should be evaluated as well. Involving other services and/or departments (for example, social work, case management, pastoral care) early in the care planning process is crucial to developing a comprehensive plan for the wound patient. Case managers can be invaluable in determining the continuity of

---

 PRACTICE POINT

The nine C's of wound assessment

Wound assessment is needed for the following nine reasons:

- Cause of the wound
- Clear picture of what the wound looks like
- Comprehensive picture of the patient
- Contributing factors
- Components of the wound care plan
- Communication to other healthcare providers
- Continuity of care
- Centralized location for wound care information
- Complications from the wound.

care across healthcare settings by asking the following questions during the initial assessment:

- Can the patient care for himself or herself?
- Is there a caregiver available to assist with care after discharge?
- Can the patient change his or her own dressings?
- Who will put on and help remove compression stockings?
- Can the patient afford to purchase the necessary wound products/items?
- Does the patient/family know how to care for the stockings or other equipment?

Asking these questions is vital to conducting a comprehensive assessment of the wound patient.

PHYSICAL EXAMINATION

A head-to-toe physical examination should be performed. Evaluation of the skin, including any skin folds, pressure points, old scars or lesions, indications of previous surgeries, and the presence of vascular, neuropathic, or pressure ulcers, should be noted. The appearance of the skin, nails, and hair on the extremities should be assessed. Appraisal of skin color, temperature, capillary refill, pulses, and edema are also important elements of a thorough physical examination.

Different types of wounds require different considerations. Dehisced surgical wounds may have opened due to an infection or may heal poorly due to underlying disease processes, current medications (such as steroids), or malnutrition. Hemosiderin staining (reddish-brown color), caused by the chronic leakage of red blood cells into the soft tissue of the lower leg, is a classic sign of venous insufficiency and often seen in a person with a venous ulcer. If not managed with compression, this leakage often leads to venous ulcers. Arterial ulcers often present with the classic signs of hair loss, weak or absent pulse, and very thin, shiny, taut skin. Neuropathic ulcers require intense evaluation to determine the extent of the neuropathy. Patients with diabetes are prone to callus formations and pressure points even when off-loading interventions are in place.

Both are easily noted on examination. (See color section, Hemosiderin deposit, page C2.)

In persons with darkly pigmented skin, early detection of ulceration that relies only on visual inspection by the clinician to note erythema and color changes (such as a stage/category I pressure ulcer) remains a clinical challenge. The lack of a tool to help clinicians detect erythema in darkly pigmented skin hampers early detection of tissue injury. In a recent study in which 28 of 56 subjects had darkly pigmented skin, the authors showed that use of multispectral images of the ulcers resulted in algorithms that enhanced detection of erythema in darkly pigmented skin.[6]

A comprehensive patient examination will reveal areas of concern for wound development and can pinpoint wound origins as well as why healing is not progressing in some wounds. Based on the comprehensive assessment and the determination as to whether a wound is healable, non-healable, or palliative, appropriate goals and treatment plan can be developed.[7] Developing realistic goals and care plans, performing regular follow-up examinations, and ensuring patient adherence to the plan of care are all key markers for successful outcomes. (See chapters on specific wound types for more details.)

WOUND ASSESSMENT AND CLASSIFICATION

Wound assessment—a written record and picture of the current status and progress of a wound—is a cumulative process of observation, data collection, and evaluation. As such, it's an important component of patient care. A wound assessment includes a record of your initial assessment, ongoing changes in and around the wound, and treatment interventions. The initial assessment serves as the baseline for

PRACTICE POINT

Because a wound can change rapidly, it is important to assess wounds for changes that could signal the need to modify treatment.[8]

future comparisons, with ongoing assessments occurring regularly and when significant changes occur throughout the healing process.

Although the frequency of wound assessment is often determined by individual agency or institutional guidelines, treatment modalities, regulatory guidelines, and wound characteristics also play a role in determining assessment frequency.[9] According to the most recent international guidelines, pressure ulcers should be evaluated at a minimum on admission, weekly, and with any signs of deterioration.[8] Frequency of assessment is also determined by wound severity, the patient's overall condition, the patient's environment, and the goals and plan of care.[9] Acute-care patients often receive wound assessments daily or with each dressing change. In long-term care facilities, wounds must be assessed on admission, with each dressing change, and at least weekly.[10] Home-care assessments are usually based on the frequency of the home visits but often occur weekly and/or with each licensed nurse visit. Regardless of the setting, however, the frequency of assessments should be determined by the wound characteristics observed at the previous dressing change, the

significance of wound changes from one assessment to the next, as well as on the physician's or other practitioner's orders. Patient interventions should be implemented based on the baseline and subsequent wound assessment data. (See *Practice Point: When to reassess a wound*.)

Although wound assessment needs to be in compliance with the regulatory requirements specific to the care setting, no written standard exists outlining the type and amount of information to include in a wound assessment. Likewise, no single documentation chart, tool, or electronic medical record (EMR) has been designated as the most effective. Banfield and Shuttleworth found that wound assessments were documented significantly more frequently when an assessment chart or form is used and that using a chart or form improves the nurses' assessment skills.[11] The best assessment form is one that is used consistently by the facility's staff. Forms that can be completed easily and quickly are more likely to be used on a regular basis. If the staff finds a form too long or difficult, that form is less likely to be used.

A minimal wound assessment should include a thorough assessment of the whole patient, identification of the cause of the wound, and wound characteristics such as type of wound, location, size, depth, exudate and tissue type(s) present, and periwound condition. (See *color section, Geography of chronic wounds*, page C3.)

PRACTICE POINT
When to reassess a wound

Assessment provides indicators of successful treatment interventions and attainment of achievable outcomes and guides decisions about product changes. Reassess the patient's wound:

- before and after any surgical or specialized procedures
- weekly for a pressure ulcer[8]
- if the wound noticeably deteriorates
- if the wound becomes odorous, has new purulent exudate, or becomes more painful
- upon observing any other significant change in the condition of the wound, including at time of transfer or discharge
- after the patient has returned from another facility.

PRACTICE POINT

CMS's suggestion for minimal pressure ulcer assessment for residents in long-term care facilities includes[10]:

- Location and staging
- Size
- Exudate
- Pain
- Color and type of wound bed tissue
- Description of wound edges and surrounding tissue

Wounds can be classified using several different approaches. The partial- versus full-thickness model is used primarily by physicians and clinicians for wounds other than pressure ulcers. Damage to the epidermis and part of the dermis constitutes a partial-thickness wound. Abrasions, skin tears, blisters, and skin-graft donor sites are common examples of partial-thickness wounds. Full-thickness wounds extend through the epidermis and dermis and may extend into the subcutaneous tissue, fascia, and muscle. Partial-thickness wounds heal by resurfacing or reepithelialization. Full-thickness wounds heal by secondary intention through the formation of granulation tissue, contraction and, finally, reepithelialization, which of course requires a longer time period for healing.[4]

Pressure ulcers and neuropathic ulcers have their own staging and classification systems to indicate the depth of injury and healing methods. Use the specific system for the type of wound. (See chapter 13, Pressure ulcers, and chapter 16, Diabetic foot ulcers, for more information.)

Assessing the severity of a burn is a two-part process. Burn injuries are described by the extent of the body burned using one of several methods for estimating burn size, such as the Rule of Nines[12] or the Lund and Browder Chart.[13] (See *The rule of nines*.) The depth of a burn injury is described by clinical observation

The rule of nines

The rule of nines estimates the amount of body surface that has been burned. In adults, the body is divided into sections of 9% or multiples of 9%. The percentages used in the rule of nines differ between adults and children.

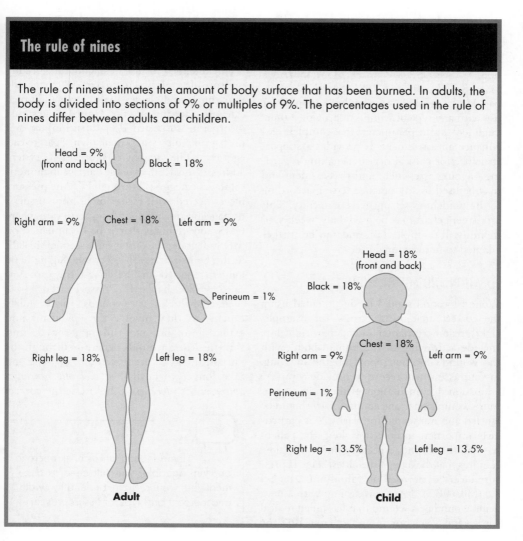

Head = 9%
(front and back)   Black = 18%

Right arm = 9%   Chest = 18%   Left arm = 9%

Perineum = 1%

Right leg = 18%   Left leg = 18%

Adult

Head = 18%
(front and back)

Black = 18%

Right arm = 9%   Chest = 18%   Left arm = 9%

Perineum = 1%

Right leg = 13.5%   Left leg = 13.5%

Child

of the anatomic layer of the skin involved (for example, superficial, partial-thickness, full-thickness, or subdermal burns).

Obviously, there are many parameters to consider when performing a comprehensive wound assessment. Each clinical agency needs to develop a protocol that all clinicians should learn and follow to ensure consistency of assessment. Whether using stage/category, or partial- and full-thickness terminology, the one constant is clinical assessment. Assessment data give the healthcare provider a mechanism by which to communicate, improve continuity among disciplines, and establish and modify appropriate treatment modalities.

Elements of a wound assessment

In 1992, Ayello developed a mnemonic for pressure ulcer assessment and documentation.[14] (See *Pressure ulcer ASSESSMENT chart.* See also *Wound ASSESSMENTS chart,* page 108.) The mnemonic has been adapted for use with any type of wound to provide a thorough look at the parameters that complete and enhance an assessment. It provides a support structure for clinical decision-making regarding ongoing assessment and reassessment and may be used in any practice setting according to the guidelines set up by your facility. This assessment chart may be used daily, weekly, or monthly. It's simple, fast, and can be further adapted to fit individual use.

LOCATION AND AGE OF WOUND

Wound location should be documented using the correct anatomical terms—for example, right greater trochanter rather than right hip. Include a drawing of the human body, with the wound's location noted on the drawing, in your assessment record to provide complete admission documentation. If there are two or more wounds near one another, they should be labeled and numbered for clarity. It is particularly important to note how long the patient has had the wound, especially since CMS now requires that the date of the oldest stage II pressure ulcer be recorded on Minimum Data Set 3.0 (M0300B.3).[15] Are you dealing with a new, acute wound or a wound that has failed to heal for several weeks or months? Time isn't the

sole determinant of acute versus chronic wound status. Although 30 days is often used for designation as chronic status, the more important criterion is whether or not the wound is making progress toward healing.[13,14]

In addition to wound duration, documentation of the etiology of the wound, if known, is important. For example, if a patient reported that she spilled hot coffee on her amputated stump, causing a blister that evolved into a full-thickness wound due to trauma and insufficient arterial supply, it would be incorrect to classify the wound as a pressure ulcer.

WOUND SIZE AND STAGE/CATEGORY

The joint National Pressure Ulcer Advisory Panel (NPUAP)–European Pressure Ulcer Advisory Panel (EPUAP) classification system[8] is only intended for use in staging/categorizing pressure ulcers. It was revised in 2009 to include four numerical stages with two additional categories for use in the United States that incorporate suspected deep tissue injury and unstageable ulcers into their own separate categories.[8] The staging/categorization system addresses the depth of tissue damage in numerical stages/categories I through IV. Any pressure ulcer covered with eschar or necrotic tissue is unstageable, including in long-term care where CMS now requires that it be documented on MDS 3.0 under the unstageable section M0300F in the United States.[15,16] Reverse staging is no longer required in the long-term care setting.[15,16] (See chapter 13, Pressure ulcers.)

Partial-thickness wounds heal fairly quickly as they involve the epidermis and extend into, but not through, the dermis. Full-thickness wounds penetrate through the fat and involve muscle, tendon, or bone and take longer to heal. (See *Necrotic, unstageable pressure ulcer,* page 109.) Use the correct

---

▶ PRACTICE POINT

Even though an ulcer is necrotic and unstageable, you still need to document the wound size for length, width, and percent and type of tissue present.

Pressure ulcer ASSESSMENT chart

PATIENT'S NAME: _____   AGE: _____ ❑ M ❑ F

DATE: _____   TIME: _____   NUMBER OF PRESSURE ULCERS: _____

A Anatomic location of wound
❑ Sacrum
❑ Elbow ❑ R ❑ L
❑ Trochanter ❑ R ❑ L   ❑ Incisional
❑ Ischium ❑ R ❑ L   ❑ Other
❑ Heel ❑ R ❑ L
❑ Lateral malleolus ❑ R ❑ L

Age of wound
_____days or _____months patient has had the pressure ulcer
_____ Date of oldest stage II pressure ulcer (MDS 3.0)

S size
_____cm length _____cm width_____cm depth

Shape
❑ Oval ❑ Round
❑ Other _____

Stage/Grade/Category
Pressure ulcer
❑ I ❑ II ❑ III ❑ IV
❑ sDTI
❑ Unstageable—Unable to determine stage; ulcer is necrotic
Wagner ulcer grade for neurotrophic ulcers:
❑ 0 ❑ 1 ❑ 2 ❑ 3 ❑ 4 ❑ 5

S sinus tract, tunneling, undermining, fistulas
❑ Sinus tract, tunneling (narrow tracts under the skin) at _____ o'clock_____cm

❑ Undermining (bigger area [than tunneling] of tissue destruction—area is more like a cave than a tract)

E exudate
Color
❑ Serous ❑ Serosanguineous
❑ Sanguineous ❑ Green ❑ Brown

Amount
❑ Scant ❑ Moderate ❑ Large

Consistency
❑ Clear ❑ Purulent

S sepsis
❑ Local ❑ Systemic ❑ None

S surrounding skin
❑ Dark ❑ Discolored ❑ Erythematous
❑ Intact ❑ Swollen
❑ Other _____

M margins
❑ Attached (edges are connected to the sides of the wound)
❑ Not attached (edges aren't connected to the sides of the wound)
❑ Rolled (edges appear rounded or rolled over)

Maceration
❑ Present ❑ Not present

E erythema
❑ Present ❑ Not present

Epithelialization
❑ Present ❑ Not present

Eschar (necrotic tissue)
❑ Yellow slough ❑ Black ❑ Soft
❑ Hard ❑ Stringy

Area around eschar is:
❑ Dry ❑ Moist ❑ Reddened

N necrotic tissue
❑ Present ❑ Not present

Nose
❑ Odor present ❑ Odor not present

Neovascularization (blood vessels are visible)
❑ Present ❑ Not present

T tissue bed
❑ Granulation tissue present
❑ Not present

Tenderness to touch
❑ No pain
❑ Pain present
❑ On touch
❑ Anytime
❑ Only when performing ulcer care

Patient getting pain medication:
❑ Yes ❑ No

Tension
❑ Tautness, hardness present
❑ Not present

Temperature
❑ Skin warm to touch
❑ Skin cool to touch
❑ Normal

_____

Wound ASSESSMENTS chart

PATIENT'S NAME:_____

AGE: _____

ASSESSMENT DATE:_____

REASSESSMENT DUE DATE:_____

Wound etiology:
- ❏ Surgical ❏ Arterial ❏ Venous
- ❏ Pressure ulcer ❏ Neurotrophic/DM ulcer
- ❏ Skin tear ❏ Trauma ❏ Other

A anatomic location of wound
- ❏ Upper/lower chest ❏ Abdomen
- ❏ Back ❏ Head ❏ Ear ❏ R ❏ L
- ❏ Sacrum ❏ Coccyx ❏ Ischium ❏ R ❏ L
- ❏ Trochanter ❏ R ❏ L
- ❏ Elbow ❏ R ❏ L ❏ Arm ❏ R ❏ L
- ❏ Leg ❏ R ❏ L ❏ Foot ❏ R ❏ L
- ❏ Heel ❏ R ❏ L
- ❏ Lateral malleolus ❏ R ❏ L
- ❏ Medial malleolus ❏ R ❏ L

Age of wound
- ❏ Acute—Date of onset: _____
- ❏ Chronic—Date of onset: _____

S size, shape, stage
_____cm L_____cm W_____cm Depth

Shape
- ❏ Oval ❏ Round ❏ Irregular
- ❏ Other _____

Stage
Stage of pressure ulcer
❏ I ❏ II ❏ III ❏ IV ❏ unstageable ❏ sDTI
Wagner ulcer classification
❏ 0 ❏ 1 ❏ 2 ❏ 3 ❏ 4 ❏ 5

S sinus tract, tunneling, undermining, fistulas
- ❏ Sinus tract ❏ Tunneling
- ❏ Undermining ❏ Fistula ❏ None
Located _____at _____o'clock, _____cm depth

E exudate
Amount:
- ❏ None ❏ Scant ❏ Moderate
- ❏ Large
Color: ❏ Serous
❏ Serosanguineous ❏ Sanguineous
Consistency: ❏ Clear ❏ Purulent
Odor: ❏ Present

S sepsis
- ❏ Systemic ❏ Local ❏ Both ❏ None

S surrounding skin
- ❏ Intact ❏ Erythematous ❏ Edematous
- ❏ Induration ❏ Warm ❏ Cool
- ❏ Discolored ❏ Dry ❏ Other _____

M Maceration
- ❏ Not present
- ❏ Present: _____cm,
location_____

E edges, epithelialization
- ❏ Edge attached ❏ Edge not attached
- ❏ Edges rolled

_____

- ❏ Surgical incision approximated
- ❏ Surgical incision open
- ❏ Sutures/staples intact
- ❏ Epithelialization present: _____ cm
- ❏ Epithelialization not present

N necrotic tissue
- ❏ Not Present ❏ Present
Type
- ❏ Yellow slough ___% ❏ Black ____%
- ❏ Soft ❏ Hard ❏ Stringy
Percentage of wound (check closest percentage):
- ❏ 100% of wound ❏ <75% ❏ >75%
- ❏ <50% ❏ >50% ❏ <25% ❏ >25%
- ❏ Other: _____ %

T tissue of wound bed
- ❏ Granulation not present
- ❏ Granulation present _____ amount%

Tenderness or pain
(0 being no pain, 10 being intense pain)
Pain scale score
0 1 2 3 4 5 6 7 8 9 10
Circle appropriate number

Pain present:
- ❏ on touch ❏ anytime
- ❏ only when performing wound care
- ❏ during dressing change
- ❏ other (specify) _____
Pain management: Specify method _____
- ❏ Not effective ❏ Effective

S status
Wound status: Initial assessment date _____
- ❏ Improved: date _____
- ❏ Unchanged: date _____
- ❏ Healing: date _____
- ❏ Deteriorating: * date _____
*Notify physician
- ❏ Supportive therapy
  - ❏ compression ❏ off-loading
  - ❏ pressure redistribution devices
  - ❏ other _____
- ❏ Patient's perception on quality of life ____
- ❏ Case management/social services needs
- ❏ Nutrition consultation requested
- ❏ PT/OT
- ❏ Referral to other departments _____
Initial assessment:
Signature _____Title _____
Date _____
Reassessment:
Signature _____Title _____
Date _____

Necrotic, unstageable pressure ulcer

Shown here is a pressure ulcer that's unstageable because its base is covered with eschar. Be sure to measure the pressure ulcer's length, width, and percent and type of necrotic tissue. Document your findings.

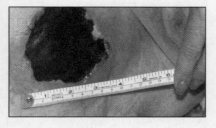

classification/staging system for the specific wound type, for example, Meggitt-Wagner for diabetic ulcers (see chapter 16, Diabetic foot ulcers), CEAP (clinical, etiology, anatomy, pathophysiology) for venous (see chapter 14, Venous disease and lymphedema management), or Payne-Martin for skin tears (see chapter 4, Skin: an essential organ).

WOUND MEASUREMENT

Measurement of a wound is an important component of wound assessment and provides valuable information on wound progression or non-progression as well as assessment of the effectiveness of clinical interventions. Wound measurement is particularly important in determining clinical effectiveness for research purposes. Consistency and accuracy in how the wound is measured are important for determining changes in the wound over time and for comparing the effectiveness of various treatments. Consistency is best assured when the agency develops and disseminates a protocol for wound measurement that staff can follow. It is also important to use consistent patient positioning every time a wound is measured.[8]

Wound measurement methods can be simple or sophisticated, two-dimensional (wound surface area) or three-dimensional (wound volume). A variety of systems are used to measure wounds and assess healing. These include wound tracing, width and length measurements, computerized wound-documenting systems (which can be one-, two-, or three-dimensional), and digital photography.[1,17] A new hand-held portable device that combines a digital camera with a scanner unit that plugs into a standard personal digital assistant has reportedly been useful in the community setting for assessment and documentation of venous and diabetic ulcers.[1]

Changes in wound measurements, such as a decrease in size, are used as an indicator of healing. Surgical incisions can be measured using length (for example, "incision line is 8 cm long"). Wounds should not be measured using objects, such as a dime or half-dollar, but rather should be measured in centimeters or millimeters depending on the size of the wound.

Area

The simplest and most common method of wound measurement is the linear method using a paper or plastic ruler marked in centimeters and millimeters. The NPUAP Position on Wound Area Measurement, outlined in a 2008 study by Langemo and colleagues,[18] is to measure the greatest head-to-toe length and the greatest side-to-side width perpendicular (90-degree angle) to each other.[19] If this method is used consistently, then measurements over time should become more reliable and comparable. (See *Wound measurement,* page 110.) Linear measurement is inexpensive, readily available, causes little to no discomfort, and is used frequently by most clinicians.[18,20] However, use caution with this method, as it assumes that the wound area is a rectangle or square, which is rarely ever the case, and nearly always overestimates the size of the wound.[21] Regardless of which method is used, what's most important is to have an agency protocol that the staff understands and that is being implemented consistently.

Another way to measure area is to multiply length by width in square centimeters (cm^2). This adds a third dimension of depth, which is then added to the linear measurement if desired.[21,22] If the wound is open, depth can be

Wound measurement

Linear measurements of a wound should be taken at the greatest length head-to-toe and the greatest width side-to-side, with measurements taken perpendicular to each other (90-degree angle), as shown below.

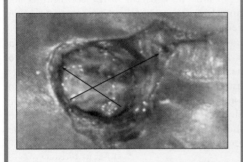

Determining wound depth

The depth of a wound can be measured by placing a clean cotton-tipped applicator, into the wound and comparing the marked area against a centimeter measuring device.

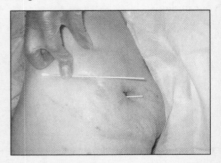

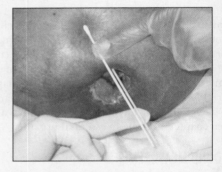

assessed by placing either a clean cotton-tipped applicator or a centimeter measuring device into the deepest part of the wound, marking it, and then measuring it upon removal. (See *Determining wound depth*.)

Planimetry is a method where a wound tracing is made on metric graph paper with a 4-cm or 8-cm grid. The completed squares, within the traced wound edges, are then counted to yield an approximate area in square centimeters.[23] Minimal training is needed to use this method, the acetate tracing medium is inexpensive and disposable, and the wound area can be determined immediately.[21]

The area of a wound area can also be measured non-invasively by stereophotogrammetry (SPG), using a digital camera and computer software. A target plate is placed within the plane of the wound to be photographed. The digital photo is then downloaded to the computer screen where the wound edges are traced, along with the length and width, using a computer-pointing device or mouse. The software automatically calculates the area as well as the length and width.[21] A color picture of the wound along with the measurements taken during each visit can be printed on a chart sheet for the patient record. This method allows for

Evidence-Based Practice

Using SPG to measure wounds is the most accurate and reliable method. Digital planimetry has fairly good reliability.[21, 24]

accurate, reproducible measurements of irregular wounds and is noninvasive.[21, 24]

Volume

As most wounds extend below the skin surface, they are three-divmensional, generally irregular, and, at times, cone-shaped. To that end, volume becomes an important variable and needs to be calculated. The most commonly used technique to assess wound volume is to measure the three dimensions of length, width, and depth and multiply those measurements by one another (L × W × D = volume cm^3).[22] Caution should be used, however, as this equation assumes that the base and surface area are the same size, which is generally not the case. The net effect is overestimation of wound volume.

Other techniques include molds, fluid instillations, the Kundin device, and SPG. Molds and fluid installations are imprecise and time-consuming, uncomfortable for the patient, and can potentially contaminate the wound.[23] The Kundin device is a plastic-coated, disposable, three-dimensional gauge with three arms for measuring length, width, and depth.[25] Wound volume is calculated via a mathematical formula that assumes the shape of the wound lies somewhere between a cylinder and a sphere.[25] Measuring volume using the Kundin device is a convenient, relatively inexpensive, user-friendly technique.[25] As mentioned previously, SPG measures the depth and area of a wound and inputs that information into software that calculates wound volume using the Kundin device formula. In one study, SPG was found to have the greatest reliability and least error of measurement.[22] When the Kundin device and SPG were compared using wound models, SPG was the more accurate method. However, more research is needed.

SINUS TRACTS, UNDERMINING, AND FISTULAS

Sinus tracts/tunnels, undermining, and fistula formation delay the healing cascade. Intervening early with the appropriate medical, surgical, and nursing actions is paramount to healing these complicated wounds.

Sinus tracts

A sinus tract (or tunnel) is a channel that extends from any part of the wound and may pass away from the wound through subcutaneous tissue and muscle. The channel or pathway, together with the wound itself, involves an area larger than the visible surface of the wound. The sinus or tunnel will result in dead space and has a potential for abscess formation, further complicating the healing process. Sinus tracts are common in dehisced surgical wounds and may also be present in neuropathic wounds, arterial wounds, and pressure ulcers. Documenting sinus tracts is an important element in assessment because it enables the clinician to evaluate potential treatment interventions and to identify reasons for non-healing. Treatment interventions involve loosely packing the dead space with an appropriate dressing to stimulate granulation tissue production and the contraction process. Document what goes into the tract to see that it is removed during dressing changes. The goal is to close the sinus tract first, while allowing the outside of the wound to remain open and fully heal.

Measurement of a sinus tract can be made by inserting a clean cotton-tipped applicator, a centimeter measuring device, or a gloved finger into the bottom or end of the tract, marking it, and then measuring it upon removal. This must be done very carefully to avoid injury during measurement. (See *Determining wound depth*.)

Undermining

Undermining is tissue destruction that occurs around the wound perimeter underlying intact skin; in these wounds, the edges have pulled away from the wound's base. (See *Undermining*, page 112.) Pressure ulcers that have been subjected to a shearing force often present with undermining in the area of the greatest shear. Undermining is also seen when the opening of the wound is smaller than the affected tissue below the dermis and in desiccated wound beds.

Documentation of the location and amount of undermining is important. Clinicians can document using the clock figure, with the head as the 12 o'clock position (for example, "undermining from 2 to 6 o'clock, measures 3 cm") or using percentages (for example, "75% of the wound has undermining measuring 2 cm from 12 to 9 o'clock"). Undermining may also be more extensive in one part of a wound than another. This, too, should be documented appropriately. Interventions include loosely packing or tucking all undermined areas to prevent buildup of debris and dead tissue

Undermining

Undermining, shown in the photographs below, is tissue destruction that occurs around the wound perimeter underlying intact skin.

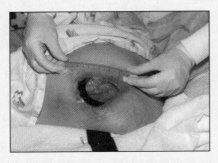

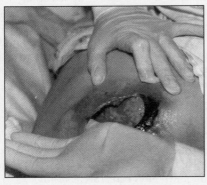

and applying an appropriate dressing, such as hydrogel, gauze, or alginate dressing.

The degree of undermining can be measured using the same method as for sinus tracts.

Fistulas

Fistulas can develop in surgical wounds and in deep, severe pressure ulcers. A fistula connects viscous organs together (for example, a rectovaginal fistula) or connects a viscous organ to the skin (for example, an entero-cutaneous fistula).[23] Fistulas are named by using the point of origin, such as the rectum, and the point of exit, such as the vagina. Management of a patient with a fistula is complex and intense and demands critical thinking and technical skills.[23] Fistulas can take weeks or months to heal. The presence of feces in the area of a fistula is a significant concern. In addition, the patient with a fistula is often malnourished and may require weeks of intense nutritional therapy to improve his or her condition. (See chapter 19 for more on fistulas.)

EXUDATE AND ODOR

Exudate is accumulated fluids in a wound; these fluids may contain serum, cellular debris, bacteria, and leukocytes. Exudate may appear as dry, dehydrated, dead, or nonviable tissue (non-draining) or be moist and draining. Exudate assessment includes noting the amount (small, moderate, large), color, consistency, and odor.[26] Certain microorganisms, such as *Pseudomonas aeruginosa*, have a characteristic odor. (See *Classifying exudate*. See also *LOWE© skin barriers for wound margins: 20-second enablers for practice,* page 114.)

Exudate may be serous (clear or pale yellow), serosanguineous (serous or blood tinged), sanguineous (bloody), or green brown. The consistency may be thick, milky, or purulent.

SEPSIS

Sepsis or bacteremia is caused by anaerobes and gram-negative bacteria and can occur in any susceptible wound. Assessment for the presence of sepsis should include consideration of erythema, warmth, edema, purulent or increased drainage, induration, increased tenderness or pain, and crepitus or fluctuance.[8,27,28] If sepsis is present, it's important to determine whether the infection is local or systemic. Interventions are based on accurate assessment and laboratory support.

The best method to culture a wound to determine the presence of sepsis remains controversial. Typically, tissue biopsy followed by fluid aspiration is the gold standard. These options may not be available in all settings, however, and many clinicians lack the skill necessary to perform them. The swab method, in which the wound must be cleaned and thoroughly dried prior to swabbing for a culture, continues to be used

Classifying exudate

Wound exudate can be classified in two ways—by type or amount.

Type (color and consistency)

Exudate may exist as a single form or in combinations (for example, serosanguineous):

- Serous or clear fluid
- Sanguineous for blood
- Purulent pus made up of inflammatory cells and tissue debris that can result from infection or an inflammatory process

Amount

The amount of exudate may indicate that the cause of the wound has not been treated (for example, edema due to venous insufficiency), that congestive heart failure is present (look for bilateral involvement and extension above the knee), that low albumin levels have occurred (malnutrition, kidney or liver disease), or that infection is present (check for signs or symptoms). Amounts of exudate include:

- none
- small—there's just a detectable discharge when the dressing is removed, less than 33%
- moderate—exudate is covering less than 67% of the dressing surface
- large—exudate is covering more than 67% of the dressing surface.

in many settings. After first cleansing the wound, culture viable tissue in the wound bed to identify the presence and type of microorganisms.[27] Culturing of wounds is important in determining whether infection is present. Malodorous wounds should also be documented. However, make sure the odor is from the wound—not the dressing change, which is a common mistake. The clinician must first cleanse the wound prior to assessing and documenting malodor. Certain organisms—such as *Pseudomonas*—have a distinct odor that is easily recognized by the trained clinician. (See chapter 7, Wound bioburden and infection, for more detailed information on infection and culturing.)

SURROUNDING SKIN/PERIWOUND

The skin surrounding a wound also provides valuable information to the assessing clinician. Erythema and warmth may indicate inflammation, cellulitis, or infection. Interruptions in periwound skin integrity (denudation, erosion, papules, or pustules) may indicate allergic reactions to tape or dressing adhesive.

PRACTICE POINT

Cleanse the wound prior to assessing for malodor. Remember that not all odor indicates infection; certain dressings develop a distinct odor when exudates interact with them (for example, alginates). Odor may also indicate the need to change the dressing more often.

Moisture-associated skin damage caused by wound drainage can lead to maceration of the periwound skin. Maceration or desiccation may be a sign that the dressing is too moist or too dry for the amount or type of exudate. Ensure that the dressing used can adequately absorb the amount of drainage present without having to be changed frequently. Palpation should be done with the fingertips around a wound surface. This may reveal induration (hard to touch) or fluctuance (bubbly, fluid wave), which are abnormal fluid accumulations indicative of further tissue damage or abscess. Although new research provides us with a different understanding of where the wound ends[30] and the surrounding skin begins, assessment of surrounding tissue does provide useful information for the ongoing evaluation and future wound-care interventions.

LOWE© skin barriers for wound margins: 20-second enablers for practice

Exudate may indicate that the cause of the wound has not been treated (for example, edema due to venous insufficiency), congestive heart failure is present (look for bilateral involvement and extension above the knee), low albumin (malnutrition, kidney or liver disease), or infection (check for symptoms or signs).

Periwound skin needs protection from exudate by using absorbent dressings over the wound and protecting the periwound skin. You can choose from four ways to protect the external skin of a wound. Try using this memory jogger to remember them: LOWE© (from Old English, meaning to approve of, prompt, or to humble oneself).

Type	Advantages	Disadvantages
Liquid film Forming acrylate • No sting • Skin preparation etc.	• Transparent surface that resists removal • Low incidence of reactions	• Some skin sealants may evaporate and dry out • Lack of availability on some institutional formularies
Ointments • Petrolatum • Zinc oxide	• Relatively cheap and easy to apply	• Petrolatum liquefies with heat • Zinc oxide ointment does not allow visualization of underlying wound margin • Ointment vehicle may interfere with the action of ionized silver • Reactions to the adhesive can occur

Windowed dressing
• Framing of wound margin with protective adhesive
  – Hydrocolloid
  – Film
  – Acrylate
  – Silicone etc.
	• Provides a good seal around the wound edge
	• Some products facilitate visibility of the wound margins
		• If seal is compromised, moisture may accumulate under the dressing

External collection devices	• External pouching may help in locations where an external seal is difficult (e.g., perirectal area)	• Devices need to be monitored for external seal *Note: These devices do not replace a search for the cause of the excessive exudate and the need to correct the cause.*

Ayello, E.A., and Sibbald, R.G. LOWE© "Skin Barriers for Wound Margins: 20 Second Enablers for Practice." *Advances in Skin & Wound Care* 19(5):237, 2006.

MACERATION

As stated above, moisture-associated skin damage from wound exudate may cause maceration of the periwound skin. Maceration is a softening of the skin surrounding a wound caused by excess drainage or pooling of fluid on intact skin and appears as a white, waterlogged area. It may be caused by inadequate management of exudate or an increase in exudate due to changes in the wound tissue. Maceration may be prevented by using an appropriate barrier cream around the wound, changing the dressing more often, or selecting a more absorbent dressing. (See *color section, Maceration,* page C3.)

EDGES AND EPITHELIALIZATION

Epithelialization is the regeneration of the epidermis across a wound surface.[23] The epithelial wound edge is continuous and often difficult to see. As wound migration proceeds from the edges toward the center, the portion covered with epithelium appears pearly or silver and shiny. Because it is thin and fragile, this area is easily damaged. The edge of a wound may be attached to the wound bed, unattached (undermining), or rolled inward. (See *color section, Wound edges with epithelialization* and *Rolled edges,* page C4.) Wound edges should be assessed as part of a thorough evaluation of the wound.

Examining the wound edges may reveal whether the wound is acute or chronic and can often provide clues as to the wound's etiology. For example, a wound with inflamed edges or violaceous with undermined borders may indicate pyoderma gangrenosum. A wound with edges rolled inward may be too dry, causing the wound edges to seek more moisture from the wound bed. A wound that is covered in necrotic tissue, desiccated, or deprived of oxygenation will exhibit poorly defined wound margins.[23]

Epithelialization can also occur in the middle of a wound bed if hair follicles or new cell growth is present. The appearance of new tissue at the wound edge can be measured in centimeters or by the percentage of wound coverage (for example, "0.3 cm of epithelial tissue surrounds the wound" or "wound is 25% epithelialized"). The degree of epithelialization is often overlooked.

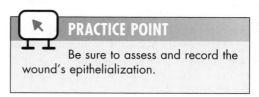

NECROTIC TISSUE

Necrotic tissue is dead, devitalized, avascular tissue that provides an ideal medium for bacterial proliferation and may inhibit healing. It's a well-known theory that wound healing is optimized when all necrotic tissue is removed from the wound bed. Necrotic tissue may present as yellow, gray, brown, or black. As it becomes dry, it presents as thick, hard, leathery black eschar.[23,29] Yellow, stringy necrosed tissue is referred to as slough.[23] Document the type and percent of necrotic tissue in the wound bed. For example, the wound bed may be 100% necrotic or 25% granular with 75% necrotic tissue. (See *color section, Wound terminology,* page C5.)

WOUND BED TISSUE

The wound bed tissue reveals the phase and progress of wound healing through observation of its color, degree of moisture—a moist wound bed facilitates movement of fibroblasts and macrophages, as well as collagenase, and other chemicals, across the wound bed, resulting in healing—and amount of epithelialization.[23,29] The wound bed may be pale pink, pink, red, yellow, or black. Clean, granular wounds are typically described as red, and wounds with devitalized slough are described as yellow. Brown and black wounds are typically those with necrotic tissue or eschar or desiccated tissue; these wounds need to be debrided because this type of tissue slows the healing process.[23]

Is the wound bed moist or dry? The presence of moisture or dry tissue will guide you in selecting the right dressing to create an environment that supports healing. Do you see new tissue growth—epithelialization at the wound edges or within the wound bed? Is granulation tissue present—that is, beefy red tissue with a granular or gritty appearance?

Documentation should be based on your observations.[31] Is the wound 100% granular tissue, or is it 25% filled with slough (yellow tissue) or necrotic (dead) tissue? All three tissue types can be found in the same wound, and assessing the amount of each type of tissue will help you determine the appropriate treatment and document the outcome of care based on improvement or deterioration, as indicated by wound tissue characteristics. Outcomes can then be tracked by percentage of improvement toward a clean granular wound bed (for example, "the wound progressed from 75% necrotic tissue to 100% granular tissue").

Tenderness to touch or the amount of pain the patient reports—both in the wound itself and in the surrounding tissue—are also essential parts of your assessment. Wound pain is one of the secondary signs of infection. It's important to differentiate between constant and episodic pain (such as pain that occurs only with dressing changes). Use a validated pain assessment scale accepted by your facility. (See chapter 7, Wound bioburden and infection, and chapter 12, Pain management and wounds.)

Assessing and measuring healing

Although wound assessment and measurement are important, so is documenting wound healing. There is growing research on the best ways to determine the healing rates of different types of chronic wounds (pressure, venous, and diabetic neuropathic ulcers) as well as expected healing rates at 4 weeks.[32, 33] The NPUAP–EPUAP 2009 clinical practice guidelines state that, for a pressure ulcer, one should "expect some signs of healing in most individuals within two weeks."[8] A variety of tools are available to assess and document healing in clinical practice, including the Pressure Sore Status Tool (PSST),[34,35] the Pressure Ulcer Scale for Healing (PUSH),[36] and the Toronto Symptom Assessment System for Wounds (TSAS-W).[37]

Originally developed for pressure ulcers, the PSST has been revised by the author, Dr. Barbara Bates-Jensen, to be used for all wounds and is now referred to as the Bates-Jensen Wound Assessment Tool (BWAT).[38] The BWAT includes 13 wound factors to be tracked over time, each of which is scored numerically. Wound location and shape are not scored. The total of the 13 factors reflects overall wound status.[38]

The PUSH tool, developed and revised by the NPUAP,[36] has been validated by research. This tool allows for the quick and reliable assessments necessary to monitor pressure ulcer healing over time and should be used at least weekly.[36,39] Three scores are developed: one is for surface area (L × W), one indicates drainage amount, and the third is for tissue type. The total score, which is the sum of these three factors, is plotted on a healing record (or graph) to depict healing over time. Although originally developed by the NPUAP to quantify healing in pressure ulcers, a recent study by Hon and colleagues[40] provides evidence that this tool is valid for monitoring and evaluating the progress of venous and diabetic ulcers.

The TSAS-W, which can be completed by either the patient or caregiver,[37] quantifies 10 wound-related symptoms. The patient or the caregiver ranks each symptom from 0 to 10. In a test on 531 patients, this tool was found to be useful for all wound types.

Another tool is the DESIGN from Japan, which is used to classify severity and monitor healing of pressure ulcers. The tool uses six factors to classify and assess healing: *d*epth, *e*xudate, *s*ize, *i*nfection, *g*ranulation, *n*ecrosis. Reported inter-rater reliability is good with both patients and photos, and there is very good correlation with the BWAT.[41]

WOUND DOCUMENTATION ESSENTIALS

Documentation is an essential component of wound assessment. Every wound assessment should be documented thoroughly, accurately, and legibly, with an accompanying signature as well as the date and time of the assessment. Wounds should be documented on the patient's admission, weekly, with each dressing change, upon any significant change in the wound, and upon discharge.

As mentioned earlier, the initial assessment and documentation become a baseline comparison for all future assessments. It is recommended that each clinical agency have a consistent chart form and format for wound documentation. All facilities should follow the wound assessment policy as determined by their setting-specific regulations. These include the mandated Outcome and Assessment Information Set (OASIS)[42] for home care or the MDS 3.0 for long-term care.[15] (See chapter 2, Regulation and wound care.)

The continuous assessment record and evaluation (CARE) tool[43]

The Deficit Reduction Act of 2005 directed the CMS to develop a Post Acute Care (PAC) Payment Reform demonstration. The CARE Tool Project was initiated in 2008 to standardize patient assessment information and utilize the data to guide Medicare payments. A report on the CARE Tool Project will be submitted to Congress in 2011. Dr. Jean DeLeon has been actively involved with the project and has shared the following information with us.

The CARE Tool is a database designed to measure the health and functional status of patients as they leave one healthcare setting and enter another. This type of information can help assess whether patients with similar diagnoses and severity are being treated in more than one setting and which setting is the most efficacious and cost-effective.

There are three phases to the initiative. Phase I of the project[43] started in the Chicago area in the summer of 2007. The pilot test involved five types of facilities: acute care, long-term acute care, independent rehabilitation, skilled nursing, and home health care. The goal in this phase was to evaluate the tool's application in different care settings and

refine the components. Additionally, a cost and resource use (CRU) tool was piloted in various PAC settings in the Boston area. The CRU tool was used to measure the amount of time various medical staff members spent with particular patients. It did not focus on the specific nature of the intervention received by the patient. The goal in using the CRU tool was to identify fixed and variable costs within each PAC setting. More geographic areas were added in late 2007.

Phase II, which started in March 2008, also included all five healthcare settings. The CARE Tool data were collected on all Medicare beneficiaries upon discharge from the acute setting and on admission and discharge from the PAC settings. The CRU data were collected intermittently from selected sites participating in phase II for 2-week periods throughout the study period. Phase III is an expansion of the project to more geographic areas.

The four major domains included in the tool are medical, functional, cognitive and social/environmental factors. The assessment items are designed to eventually replace existing Medicare assessment forms such as OASIS, the Resident Assessment Instrument MDS, and the Inpatient Rehabilitation Facility–Patient Assessment Instrument (IRF-PAI). The CARE Tool is a Web-based reporting system for the Medicare program and as such allows for incorporating advances in evidence-based medicine.

The CARE Tool questions can be broken down into core items and supplemental items. The core items are asked of every patient in that setting, regardless of condition. The supplemental items, however, are only asked of

---

PRACTICE POINT

It's important to remember that in the United States, the OASIS and MDS are regulatory documentation tools—neither tool is considered a comprehensive wound assessment.

CARE tool: PAC admission

This instrument uses the phrase "2-day assessment period" to refer to the day of admission and the next calendar day (ending at 11:59 PM), or, if the patient is admitted after noon, add an additional calendar day.

I. Skin integrity (complete during the 2-day assessment period)

  a. Presence of pressure ulcers

    i. Is this patient at risk of developing pressure ulcers?

    ii. Does this patient have one or more unhealed pressure ulcer(s) at stage 2 or higher or is the ulcer unstageable?

      1. If No, *Skip to Major Wounds.*

    iii. If the patient has one or more stage 2-4 or unstageable pressure ulcers, indicate the number of unhealed pressure ulcers at each stage.

    iv. Number of unhealed stage 2 ulcers known to be present for more than 1 month.

      1. If the patient has one or more unhealed stage 2 pressure ulcers, record the number present today that were first observed more than 1 month ago, according to the best available records. If the patient has no unhealed stage 2 pressure ulcers, record "0." If the patient has 8 or more unhealed stage 2 pressure ulcers, record "8." If unknown, record "9."

    v. If any unhealed pressure ulcer is stage 3 or 4 (or if eschar is present), record the most recent measurements for the LARGEST ulcer (or eschar).

    vi. Indicate if any unhealed stage 3 or stage 4 pressure ulcer(s) has undermining and/or tunneling (sinus tract) present.

  b. Major wound (excluding pressure ulcers)

    i. Does the patient have one or more major wound(s) that require ongoing care because of draining, infection, or delayed healing?

      1. If No, *Skip to Turning Surfaces Not Intact.*

    ii. Number of major wounds

      1. Delayed healing of surgical wound

      2. Trauma-related wound (e.g., burns)

      3. Diabetic foot ulcers

      4. Vascular ulcer (arterial or venous including diabetic ulcers not located on the foot)

      5. Other (e.g., incontinence associated with dermatitis, normal surgical wound healing). Please specify.

  c. Turning surfaces not intact

    i. Indicate which of the following turning surfaces have either a pressure ulcer or major wound. (*Check all that apply*)

      1. Skin for all turning surfaces is intact

      2. Right hip not intact

      3. Left hip not intact

      4. Back/buttocks not intact

CARE tool: PAC admission. Retrieved May 26, 2010 from www.ascp.com/advocacy/cms/upload/ApndxB-MASTERCARETool103107.pdf.

patients who have a specific condition. These are meant to measure severity or the degree of need for patients with that condition. For example, in the section on skin integrity, the core question asks whether there is a stage II or greater ulcer. Supplemental questions would only apply to those patients who answered yes to that question. (See *CARE Tool: PAC admission.*)

The discharge section for wound care is the same as the admission section. During Phase II of the demonstration project, three additions were made to the skin integrity section. First, wound depth was included in the data collection. Second, instructions specified that pressure ulcers should not be reversed staged. Third, a new item was added to measure complex wound management with positioning and skin traction that required at least two persons or extensive management by one person.

The demonstration project is currently in Phase III. The PAC Payment Reform demonstration is a novel Web-based initiative that strives to consolidate and standardize patient assessment throughout care settings. Combined with the CRU tool, the data may help CMS refine reimbursement and quality measures.

Wound photography

Photographs can provide a visual record of the wound. When done correctly, they can assist the clinician in clinical care decisions and provide documentation support in the case of ligitation.[44] Standardization of when and how to photograph wounds is paramount. Several wound care organizations, including the NPUAP,[45] the Wound Ostomy and Continence Society,[46] and the American Professional Wound Care Association,[47] have position statements regarding wound photography on their websites. It is important to remember, however, that photographs do not replace bedside wound assessments.

When using film photography, it's necessary to permanently mark on the photograph • the date and time it was taken as well as patient identification information. The photo should also include a sample measure in each frame, such as a 10-cm strip of paper tape.[45] For the best clarity when using digital photography, a camera no smaller than 1.5 megapixels is recommended.[45] However, because digital photos can be altered, the identifying data must be encoded permanently. When periodic photos are taken, distortion of the photos can be a problem due to body contour, angle of the body in a bed, angle and distance of the camera from the patient, and lighting. Some photo software packages use a target plate in the photo and the software; once the photo is downloaded, it can automatically calculate wound area and volume as well as length and width.[45]

Wound photographs can quickly and accurately represent a wound's appearance if the proper equipment is used in the correct way.[48,49] Clinicians need appropriate training and must consistently follow a wound photography protocol. The angle at which the camera is held to the wound makes a difference. Using the wrong camera angle can result in an improperly photographed wound that appears larger than it truly is. (See *Proper photo technique,* page 120.) Other strategies to enhance wound photos have been described elsewhere in the literature.[17, 50]

Electronic medical records and electronic health records

The electronic medical record (EMR) is the legal record created in hospitals and healthcare environments that is the source of data for the electronic health record (EHR). The EHR represents the ability to easily share medical information among stakeholders and to have a patient's information follow him or her through the various modalities of care in which he or she engages. EHRs are reliant on EMRs being in place, and EMRs will never reach their full potential without interoperable EHRs in place.[51]

A system of dedicated wound EMRs supports comprehensive and consistent care in patients with wounds. It promotes patient safety, facilitates evidence-based care,[49] and helps eliminate disparities in care regardless of

Proper photo technique

Used correctly, photography can be a great tool in documenting the appearance of a wound. Holding the camera at the appropriate angle is imperative to accurately document wound size.

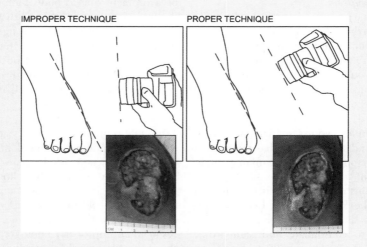

IMPROPER TECHNIQUE   PROPER TECHNIQUE

(Rennert, R., Golinko, M., Kaplan, D., Flattau, A., Brem, H. Standardization of wound photograph using the wound electronic Medical Record. *Advances in Skin & Wound Care* 22[1]:32-38, 2009.)

care setting because the interdisciplinary team has access to objective wound assessment data.[2] In one large urban center, the use of an objective wound EMR decreased chronic wound emergencies.[2]

Telemedicine

Teleassessment and telemanagment are terms used to describe the "assessment and management of a wound at a distance using electronic information and communication technologies."[17] The potential of telemedicine to enhance wound treatment in the home has been described in the literature. In one randomized controlled study of 103 participants with 160 pressure ulcers or non-healing surgical wounds receiving home care in conjunction with telemedicine, the average healing or improvement rate was 51 days for pressure ulcers and 34 days for surgical wounds. The role of telemedicine in wound healing continues to evolve.[52] In another descriptive comparative study of home care nurses with 43 adult patients, the use of digital photography rather than simply reporting resulted in a decreased chance of under- or over-treating the patients' wounds.[53] Use of digital images in telemedicine also resulted in the unexpected finding of more information than just what was revealed by conventional inspection, such as the identification of other factors in the patient's environment beyond the local wound bed that may have inhibited wound healing.[53] These included, for example, the patient's bed, wheelchair, redistribution devices, and shoes.[53] In areas of the country where weather can prohibit travel to a wound care center or the patient is unable to be transported, telemedicine has been an immense facilitator of timely and appropriate wound assessment and treatment. Truly this was an example of the importance of treating the "whole patient and not just the hole in the patient."

SUMMARY

Wound assessment—an appraisal of a patient's condition based on clinical signs and symptoms, laboratory data, and medical history—is an integral part of wound management. Assessment has become a highly specialized area of care, requiring well-developed observational skills and current knowledge. The use of current terminology is vital to accurate assessment and communication. Use of the

Wound ASSESSMENTS[14] chart or WOUND PICTURE[31] mnemonic can provide a fast, ongoing, and accurate assessment for patients with wounds.[33] (See *WOUND PICTURE*.) Other tools that quantify wound characteristics, such as the BWAT,[38] PUSH,[36] TSAS-W,[37] or DESIGN,[41] can help the clinician track wound healing. Proper assessment of wound parameters provides clinicians with the information they need to make the decisions that guide the wound care team to suitable interventions, management, and care strategies. Technology will continue to help clinicians with documentation. Unless standardized techniques and protocols are followed, wound photos can hinder, rather than help with treatment care decisions. EMRs and their important role in EHRs are the wave of the future. These advances, coupled with the use of telemedicine, ensure that the future of wound assessment and documentation looks promising.

WOUND PICTURE

When assessing wounds in your patient, use the mnemonic, **WOUND PICTURE**, for a fast and accurate assessment.

Wound or ulcer location
Odor Assess before and during all dressing changes
Ulcer category, stage (for pressure ulcer) or classification (for diabetic ulcer), and depth (partial-thickness or full-thickness)
Necrotic tissue
Dimension of wound (shape, length, width, depth); drainage color, consistency, and amount (scant, moderate, large)

Pain (When it occurs, what relieves it, patient's description, patient's rating on scale of 0 to 10)
Induration (Surrounding tissue hard or soft)
Color of wound bed (Red-yellow-black or combination)
Tunneling (Record length and direction —toward patient's right, left, head, feet)
Undermining (Record length and direction, using clock references to describe)
Redness or other discoloration in surrounding skin
Edge of skin loose or tightly adhered? Edges flat or rolled under

From *Wound Care Made Incredibly Easy*, 2nd ed. Philadelphia: Lippincott, Williams & Wilkins, 2006.

PATIENT SCENARIO

Clinical Data

Mr. X is a 54-year-old gentleman with a painful stage IV pressure ulcer on the right trochanter. There is large amount of light beige exudate that has some blood in it. There is a small amount of black eschar in the wound bed, while the rest of the wound bed is red and granular.

Case Discussion

After the nurse removes the dressings and cleanses the pressure ulcer, she completes the wound assessment chart documentation. (See Pressure ulcer ASSESSMENT chart, page 107.)

Wound etiology: Pressure ulcer

Anatomic location: right trochanter; date of onset: chronic, 6 weeks ago
Stage/category: IV; size: 7.5 × 6.2 × 2.5 cm (LxWxD); Shape: circular
Sinus tract/tunneling: none present; undermining: 0.75 cm from 1 o'clock to 4 o'clock
Exudate: large amount, thin, tannish/serosanguineous; malodorous drainage
Sepsis: local
Surrounding skin: erythematous, intact, slightly swollen; temperature: skin warm to touch
Maceration: not present
Edges/epithelialization: attached and slightly rolled; epithelialization: small amount present, .05 cm
Necrotic tissue: present; black, <10%
Tissue wound bed: granulation, present 90%; tenderness to touch: pain present; anytime; pain scale 9/10
Status: initial assessment date, 6/23/10; nutritional, PT consult ordered 6/23/10

Signature: A Nurse RN_____

SHOW WHAT YOU KNOW

1. Initial wound assessment involves all of the following <u>except</u>:
    A. observation.
    B. data collection.
    C. evaluation.
    D. surgical debridement

    ANSWER: D. *Wound assessment involves observation, data collection, and an ongoing evaluation process. Surgical debridement is an intervention for the management of wound care.*

2. A wound that has tissue damage through the epidermis and partially into the dermis would be classified as:
    A. superficial.
    B. partial-thickness.
    C. full-thickness.
    D. subdermal.

    ANSWER: B. *A superficial wound involves only the epidermis and the dermis is still intact. A full-thickness wound extends through the dermis. A subdermal wound extends into underlying structures below the skin such as bone, muscle, or tendon.*

3. In assessing a wound, you find an area of tissue destruction under the edge of the patient's wound. This is best described as:
    A. a sinus tract.
    B. maceration.
    C. fistula.
    D. undermining.

    ANSWER: D. *A sinus tract/tunnel is a channel that involves an area larger than the visible surface of the wound. Maceration is the softening of the surrounding skin usually from exposure to or excess wound drainage. A fistula is an opening between two organs or between an organ and the skin.*

4. Which of the following wound photography techniques is <u>incorrect</u>?
    A. Include a measuring device in the photo.
    B. Permanently mark the date and time of the photo in the picture.
    C. Hold the camera at 90-degree angle to the wound.
    D. Digital photos should be at least 1.5 megapixels.

    ANSWER: C. *Holding the camera at a 90-degree angle rather than perpendicular to the wound plane can cause distortion of the wound size in the photo. A, B, and D are correct techniques that should be part of a wound photo protocol.*

5. Which of the following statements about electronic health records is <u>false</u>? They are:
    A. the same as electronic medical records.
    B. reliant on electronic medical records being in place.
    C. an important way of sharing medical information across stakeholders.
    D. a modality of care that holds promise to promote patient safety across care settings.

    ANSWER: A. *electronic health records and electronic medical records are different. The electronic medical record is a legal record within a special institution, such as a hospital, while an electronic health records uses the electronic medical record as a source of information to share patient data across care settings. Options B, C, are D are true.*

REFERENCES

1. Romanelli, M., Dini, V., Rogers, L.C., Hammond, C.E., Nixon, M.A. "Clinical Evaluation of a Wound Measurement and Documentation System," *WOUNDS* 20(9):258-264, 2008.
2. Golinko, M.S., Clark, S., Rennert, R., Flattau, A., Boulton, A.J., Brem, H. "Wound Emergencies: The Importance of Assessment, Documentation and Early Treatment using a Wound Electronic Medical Record," *Ostomy Wound Manage* 55(5):54-61, 2009.
3. Larazus, G.S., et al. "Definitions and Guidelines for Assessment of Wounds and Evaluation of Healing," *Archives of Dermatology* 130(4):489-93, April 1994.
4. Centers for Medicare and Medicaid Services (CMS). "Usual Care of Chronic Wounds Meeting, March 29, 2005." Retrieved June 11, 2006 from *http://www.cms.gov/mcd/viewmcac.asp?from2=viewmcac.asp&where=index&mid=28&*.
5. Bower, M.G. "Evaluating and Managing Bite Wounds," *Advances in Skin & Wound Care* 15(2): 88-90, March-April 2002.
6. Sprigle, S., Zhang, L., Duckworth, M. "Detection of Skin Erythema in Darkly Pigmented Skin using Multispectral Images," *Advances in Skin & Wound Care*, 22(4):172-9, 2009.
7. Okan, D., Woo, K., Ayello, E.A., Sibbald, R.G. "The Role of Moisture Balance in Wound Healing," *Advances in Skin and Wound Care*, 20(1):39-53, 2007.
8. National Pressure Ulcer Advisory Panel (NPUAP) and European Pressure Ulcer Advisory Panel (EPUAP). Prevention and treatment of pressure ulcers: clinical practice guideline. Washington, DC: National Pressure Ulcer Advisory Panel, 2009.
9. Conley, M. "Wound, Ostomy, Continence Nurses Society Pressure Ulcer Evaluation: Best Practice for Clinicans," *WOCN Society*, p. 9, 2008.
10. Centers for Medicare and Medicaid Services (CMS). "Pressure Ulcers. Revised Guidance for Surveyors in Long Term Care." Tag F-314, issued November 12, 2004. Retrieved June 11, 2006 from *http://new.cms.hhs.gov/manuals/downloads/som107ap_pp_guidelines_ltcf.pdf*.

11. Banfield, K.R., and Shuttleworth, E. "A Systematic Approach with Lasting Benefits: Designing and Implementing a Wound Assessment Chart," *Professional Nurse* 8(4):234- 38, January 1993.

12. "Burn Percentage in Adults: Rule of Nines." Retrieved September 30, 2010 from *www.emedicinehealth.com/burn_percentage_in_adults_rule_of_nines/article_em.htm*.

13. The Royal Children's Hospital Melbourne. "Clinical Practice Guidelines: Burns." Retrieved May 26, 2010 from *www.rch.org.au/clinicalguide/cpg.cfm?doc_id=5158*.

14. Ayello, E. "Teaching the Assessment of Patients with Pressure Ulcers," *Decubitus* 5(7):53-4, July 1992.

15. Centers for Medicare and Medicaid Services. "Nursing Home Quality Initiatives: MDS 3.0 Overview." Retrieved May 26, 2010 from *http://www.cms.hhs.gov/NursingHomeQualityInits/01_Overview.asp#TopOfPage*.

16. Levine, J.M. Roberson, S., Ayello, E.A. (2010). "Essentials of MDS 3.0, Section M, Skin Condition," *Advances in Skin & Wound Care* 23(6):273-284; quiz 285-6.

17. Ahn, C., Salcido, R.S. "Advances in Wound Photography and Assessment Methods," *Adv Skin Wound Care.* 2008;21(2):85-93, 2008.

18. Langemo, D., Anderson, J., Hanson, D., Hunter, S., Thompson, P. "Measuring Wound Length, Width and Area: Which Technique?" *Advances in Skin & Wound Care* 21(1):42-5, quiz 46-7, 2008.

19. Cutler, N.R., George, R., Seifert, R.D., et al. "Comparison of Quantitative Methodologies to Define Chronic Pressure Ulcer Measurements," *Decubitus* 6:22-30, 1993.

20. National Pressure Ulcer Advisory Panel and European Pressure Ulcer Advisory Panel. Prevention and Treatment of Pressure Ulcers: Clinical Practice Guideline. Washington DC: National Pressure Ulcer Advisory Panel; 2009

21. Langemo, D.K., Melland, H., Hanson, D., Olson, B., Hunter, S., Henly, S. "Two-dimensional Wound Measurement: Comparison of 4 Techniques," *Advances in Skin & Wound Care* 11(7):337-43, 1998.

22. Langemo, D.K., Melland, H., Olson, B., Hanson, D., Hunter, S., Henly, S. "Comparison of 2 Wound Volume Measurement Methods," *Advances in Skin & Wound Care* 14(4):190-6, 2001.

23. Bryant, R.A. Nix, N.P. *Acute and Chronic Wounds, Current Management Concepts,* 3rd ed. St. Louis: Mosby–Year Book, Inc., 2007.

24. Frantz, R.A., and Johnson, D.A. "Stereophotogrammetry and Computerized Image Analysis: A Three-dimensional Method of Measuring Wound Healing," *Wounds* 4:58-64, 1992.

25. Kundin, J.I. "A New Way to Size Up a Wound," *Am J Nurs* 1:206-207, 1989.

26. Ayello, E.A., and Sibbald, R.G. "LOWE© Skin Barriers for Wound Margins: 20 Second Enablers for Practice," *Advances in Skin & Wound Care* 19(5):237, 2006.

27. Harding, K.A., Carville, K., Cuddigan, J., Fletcher, J., Fuchs, P., et al. "Wound Infection in Clinical Practice: Shaping the Future. An International Consensus Document," *Int Wound J* 5 Suppl 3:1-11, 2008.

28. Mouton, C.P., Bazaldua, O.V., Pierce, B., Espino, D.V. "Common infections in Older Adults," *Am Fam Physician* 63(2):257-268, 2001.

29. Maklebust, J., and Sieggreen, M. *Pressure Ulcers: Guidelines for Prevention and Management,* 3rd ed. Springhouse, Pa.: Springhouse Corp., 2000.

30. Stojadinovic, O., et al. "Role of B-Catenin and C-myc in the Inhibition of Epithelialization and Wound Healing," *American Journal of Pathology* 167(1):59-69, 2005.

31. *Wound Care Made Incredibly Easy,* 2nd ed. Philadelphia: Lippincott, Williams & Wilkins, 2006.

32. Jessup, R.L. "What Is the Best Method for Assessing the Rate of Wound Healing? A Comparison of 3 Mathematical Formulas," *Advances in Skin & Wound Care* 19(3):138,140-42, 145-46, 2006.

33. Van Rijswijk, L. "Full-thickness Pressure Ulcers: Patient and Wound Healing Characteristics," *Decubitus* 6(1):16-21, 1993.

34. Bates-Jensen, B. "The Pressure Sore Status Tool a Few Thousand Assessments Later," *Advances in Wound Care* 10(5):65-73, 1997.

35. Bates-Jensen, B.M. "A Quantitative Analysis of Wound Characteristics as Early Predictors of Healing in Pressure Sores" [Abstract]. Dissertation Abstracts International, 59:11. Los Angeles, CA: University of California, Los Angeles; 1999.

36. National Pressure Ulcer Advisory Panel. "PUSH Tool." Retrieved April 15, 2010 from *http://www.npuap.org/PDF/push3.pdf*.

37. Maida, V., Ennis, M., Kuziemsky, C. "The Toronto Symptom Assessment System for Wounds: A New Clinical and Research Tool," *Advances in Skin and Wound Care* 22(10):468-74, 2009.

38. Harris, C. Bates-Jensen, B, Parslow, N., et al. Bates-Jensen Wound Assessment Tool, "Pictorial Guide Validation Project," *JWOCN* 37(3)253-59, May/June 2010.

39. Stotts, N.A., et al. "Testing the Pressure Ulcer Scale for Healing (PUSH) and Variations of the PUSH," Paper presented at the 11th Annual Symposium on Advanced Wound Care, April 18-22, 1998, Miami Beach, Fla.

40. Hon, J., Lagden, K., McLAren, A., O'Sullivan, D., Orr, L., Houghton, P.E., Woodbury, M.G. "A Prospective, Multicenter Study to Validate use of the Pressure Ulcer Scale for Healing (PUSH©) in

Patients with Diabetic, Venous and Pressure Ulcers," *Ostomy Wound Management* 56(2):26-36, 2010.

41. Sanada, H., Moriguchi, T., Miyachi, Y., Ohura, T., Nakajo, T., Tokunaga, K., et al. "Reliability and Validity of DESIGN, a Tool that Classifies Pressure Ulcer Severity and Monitors Healing," *J Wound Care* 13(1):13-18, 2004.

42. Centers for Medicare and Medicaid Services. "Home Health Quality Initiatives: OASIS C." Retrieved September 20, 2010 from *www1.cms.gov/HomeHealthQualityInits/06_OASISC.asp*.

43. CARE tool: PAC admission. Retrieved May 26, 2010 from www.ascp.com/advocacy/cms/upload/ApndxB-MASTERCARETool103107.pdf.

44. International Expert Wound Care Advisory Panel, Ayello, E.A., Capitulo, K.L., Fife, C.E., Fowler, E., Krasner, D.L., Mulder, G., Sibbald, R.G., Yankowsky, K.W. "Legal Issues in the Care of Pressure Ulcer Patients: Key Concepts for the Healthcare Providers: A Consensus Paper from the International Expert Wound Care Advisory Panel," *WCET Journal* 29(1):8-22, 2009.

45. National Pressure Ulcer Advisory Panel. "FAQ: Photography for Pressure Ulcer Documentation." Retrieved September 30, 2010 from *http://www.npuap.org/DOCS/PhotographyFaq.doc*.

46. WOCN Society. "Photography in Wound Documentation." Retrieved September 30, 2010 *from http://www.wocn.org/pdfs/WOCN_Library/Position_Statements/photoposition.pdf*.

47. American Professional Wound Care Association. "Proposed APWCA Photographic Guidelines for Wounds." Retrieved October 11, 2010 from *http://www.apwca.org/guidelines/photographic.cfm*.

48. Sullivan, V. "In Focus: The Photography Forecast," *Today's Wound Clinic* 2(2):30-31,33, 2008.

49. Rennert, R., Golinko, M., Kaplan, D., Flattau, A., Brem, H. "Standardization of Wound Photograph using the Wound Electronic Medical Record," *Advances in Skin & Wound Care* 22(1):32-38, 2009.

50. Rennert, R., Golinko, M., Yan, A., Flattau, A., Tomic-Canic, M., Brem, H. "Developing and Evaluating Outcomes of an Evidence-based Protocol for the Treatment of Osteomyelitis in Stage IV Pressure Ulcers: A Literature and Wound Electronic Medical Record Database Review," *Ostomy Wound Manage* 55(3):42-53, 2009.

51. Garets, D., David, M. "Electronic Medical Records vs. Electronic Health Records: Yes, there is a difference. A HIMSS Analytics™ White Paper." Updated January 26, 2006. Retrieved May 26, 2010 from www.himssanalytics.org.

52. Terry, M., Halstead, L.S., O'Hare, P., Gaskill, C., Ho, P.S., Obecny, J., James, C., Lauderdale, M.E. "Feasibility Study of Home Care Wound Management using Telemedicine," *Advances in Skin & Wound Care* 22(8):358-64, 2009.

53. Buckley, K.M., Adelson, L.K., Agazio, J.G. "Reducing the Risks of Wound Consultation: Adding Digital Images to Verbal Reports," *JWOCN* 36(2)163-170, 2009.

CHAPTER 7

Wound Bioburden and Infection

Sue E. Gardner, PhD, RN
Rita A. Frantz, PhD, RN, FAAN

Objectives

After completing this chapter, you'll be able to:
- distinguish between colonization, critical colonization, and infection in a chronic wound
- identify the most valid method of determining a wound infection
- explain the effects of antiseptics on chronic wound tissue
- identify conditions in which antimicrobial therapy is indicated for treatment of a chronic wound.

BIOBURDEN IN WOUNDS

The human body is in constant contact with multiple microorganisms originating from both endogenous and exogenous sources.[1] These microorganisms are usually present without any evidence of infection because a balance exists between host resistance and microbial growth. Infection occurs when this equilibrium is upset, either because of lowered host defenses or increased microorganism quantity or virulence. Infection is directly related to the number and virulence of the organisms, which overcome host resistance.[2]

The skin provides a physical and chemical barrier to microorganisms. Many microorganisms are able to survive on the skin and are known as skin colonizers, or normal flora. Normal flora may actually inhibit the growth of more virulent microorganisms and, therefore, serve a protective function. This mutually beneficial relationship between host and microorganism is referred to as a *commensal relationship*. Some normal florae are transient colonizers; they merely survive, don't multiply, and can easily be removed. Resident florae, on the other hand, multiply and are permanent.

Breaks in the skin, including wounds, allow microorganisms to access deeper tissue and structures where they can more readily adhere and multiply.[2] Host response to microorganisms in the wound is multifaceted. Nonspecific host responses occur regardless of microbial species; whereas specific host responses are triggered by specific microorganisms and involve the immune system. Regardless, nonspecific and specific responses are essential for preventing invasion of wound microorganisms into vital tissue and organs.

Nonspecific responses include phagocytosis by polymorphonuclear leukocytes (PMNs) and macrophages and inflammation. Although the mechanism of inflammation evolved to protect humans from microorganisms in particular,[3] the inflammatory response can be elicited from any type of tissue injury. Thus, the first phase of wound healing is referred to as the *inflammatory phase* (see chapter 5, Acute and chronic wound healing); the cascade of events that occur during this phase is essential to activating the healing process.

INFLAMMATION

Inflammation is integral to microbial resistance. It's triggered by endogenous (host sources) and exogenous (microbial) mediators.

Endogenous mediators, such as cytokines and growth factors, arise from mast cells, PMNs, macrophages, the complement system, and immune cells. These cells release mediators in response to contact with microorganisms or microbial products. Endogenous mediators are also released in response to tissue injury unrelated to microorganisms, such as injury caused by surgical procedures or trauma.

Exogenous mediators are produced by microorganisms. Most notable is endotoxin, which is produced by gram-negative bacteria. If released into the blood, endotoxin activates all inflammatory mechanisms at once, resulting in septic shock. Exotoxins are inflammatory mediators released by bacteria. Many bacterial exotoxins are extremely chemotactic; that is, they attract leukocytes. However, many bacterial toxins don't elicit inflammation directly. They indirectly elicit inflammation by activating mast cells and macrophages or by evoking an adaptive immune response, which then produces inflammatory mediators.[3,4]

The release of inflammatory mediators results in localized vasodilation and increased blood flow to the area of injury. The accompanying increase in vascular permeability promotes a rapid influx of phagocytic cells, complement, and antibody to the wound site. Collectively, these events remove microorganisms and debris as well as bacterial toxins and enzymes. These physiological responses to injury are expressed by the signs of inflammation, including erythema, heat, edema, and pain.[3,5,6]

Inflammation is characterized as being either acute or chronic.[3,7] Acute inflammation is the initial response to tissue invasion or injury and includes pronounced vascular changes and the predominance of PMNs at the site of injury.[7] Again, this type of inflammation can result from microorganisms or any type of tissue injury. Chronic inflammation occurs if the invasion or injury of tissue isn't resolved and persists over a long period

of time. The vascular response becomes less pronounced during chronic inflammation and the predominant leukocyte at the site of injury shifts to macrophages.[3,7] Chronic inflammation is also characterized by the proliferation of fibroblasts and scar tissue.[6,7]

INFECTION

When host resistance fails to control the growth of microorganisms, localized wound infection results. Uncontrolled localized infection of a wound can lead to deep, more severe infections such as extensive cellulitis, osteomyelitis, bacteremia, and sepsis. More subtly, localized wound infection impairs healing and is thought to be an important cause of wound chronicity.[8] This more subtle level of wound bioburden is often referred to as "critical colonization."[9]

The persistent presence of microorganisms leads to the influx of phagocytes, which release proteolytic enzymes, inflammatory mediators, and free radicals. The cumulative effect of these substances in the wound is additional tissue injury and wound deterioration.[10] Moreover, inflammatory mediators produce localized thrombosis and vasoconstriction, resulting in a hypoxic wound environment that in turn promotes further bacterial proliferation, thus establishing a destructive, prolonged inflammatory cycle.[11] The immune response (that is, specific host responses) may be down-regulated in an attempt to limit self-destruction.

The proliferative phase of wound healing is also affected by wound infection. Bacteria and bacterial toxins stimulate macrophages to produce an excessive angiogenic response. The resultant granulation tissue is edematous, somewhat hemorrhagic, and more fragile.[12] Although the collagen content of infected wounds is higher than the collagen content of noninfected wounds, collagenolytic activity is also higher, resulting in wound breakdown.[13,14] Migration of epithelial tissue is inhibited by bacteria and bacterial toxins, and new epithelium is prone to lysis and desiccation by neutrophil proteases.[15,16] Finally, wound contraction is inhibited in the presence of large numbers of bacteria.[17]

> ▶ **PRACTICE POINT**
>
> Wound infection prolongs the inflammatory phase and disrupts the proliferative phase of wound healing.

Defining infection

"Wound infection is a serious problem that can lead to delay in discharge as well as adverse patient complication such as sepsis, amputation and even death."[18] Wound infection has been defined as the invasion and multiplication of microorganisms in wound tissue resulting in pathophysiologic effects or tissue injury.[19] Of particular importance in this definition is the fact that invasion and multiplication of microorganisms occurs in the *wound tissue*. (See *Key elements of wound infection*.) Thus, wound infection can be differentiated from wound contamination and colonization. (See *color section*, *Progression of bacterial balance to bacterial damage in a chronic wound*, page C6.)

Wound contamination is the presence of bacteria on wound surfaces with no multiplication of bacteria.[20-22] Other organisms are permanent colonizers and replicate, or multiply, on the wound surface. Wound colonization is characterized by the replication of microorganisms on the wound surface without invasion of wound tissue and no host immune response.[2] Some of these colonizers may be involved in a mutually beneficial relationship with the host preventing the adherence of more virulent organisms in the wound bed. These organisms include *Corynebacterium* species, coagulase-negative staphylococci, and viridans streptococci.[11]

The mere presence or multiplication of microorganisms on the wound surface doesn't necessarily constitute wound infection. Contamination and colonization with wound microorganisms is a condition common to all wounds healing by secondary intention and, in fact, is a prerequisite to the formation of granulation tissue.[1,9,23] In contrast, wound infection is the invasion and multiplication of microorganisms in the wound tissue beneath the wound surface. Thus, for an infection to be present, the microorganisms must be present in viable tissue.

> **Key elements of wound infection**
>
> - Wound infection occurs in wound tissue, not on the surface of the wound bed.
> - Wound infection occurs in viable wound tissue; it isn't a phenomenon of necrotic tissue, eschar, or other debris contained in the wound bed.
> - Wound infection is caused by invasion and multiplication of microbes in the wound.
> - Wound infection is manifested by a host reaction or tissue injury.

> ▶ **PRACTICE POINT**
>
> Contamination and colonization of a wound with microorganisms doesn't constitute infection.

The presence of microorganisms in wound pus, necrotic tissue, or slough isn't evidence of tissue invasion. These nonviable substances are known to support bacterial growth,[24] and debridement of this tissue is essential to prevent infection. However, the presence of microorganisms in necrotic tissue that hasn't invaded viable tissue doesn't constitute wound infection.

Multiplication of microorganisms is another key element of the definition; that is, microorganisms must replicate and produce large enough numbers to cause injury or impair healing.

Another key element in the definition is that the invading organisms must produce host responses or tissue injury. The concepts of host response and pathophysiologic tissue injury are interrelated; that is, they both present clinical signs and symptoms. As previously described, host response produces the signs and symptoms associated with inflammation. Tissue injury produces other signs and symptoms.

Identifying infection

Despite the known deleterious effect of infection on healing,[25,26] the identification and diagnosis of localized wound infection and/or critical colonization is fraught with ambiguity in clinical practice. This is especially true for chronic wounds, which heal by secondary intention. (See chapter 5, Acute and chronic wound healing.)

▶ PRACTICE POINT

The first sign of critical colonization may be delayed wound healing as evidenced by no change in wound size (L × W) or increasing exudate.[9]

Conversely, the identification and diagnosis of localized infection of acute wounds—such as surgical incisions—is less equivocal because most of these wounds display a clinically apparent, robust inflammatory response. The normal time frame for inflammation associated with the wounding event (for example, a surgical procedure) is 3 to 5 days.[19] Inflammation that persists past 3 to 5 days is considered indicative of wound infection.[27]

Like acute wound infections, the identification of deep, more severe infections is often easier due to the development of overt systemic signs and symptoms. For example, extensive erythema, elevated body temperature, elevated white blood cell count, and elevated blood sugar in people with diabetes are readily apparent. Similarly, osteomyelitis should always be considered if a wound probes to bone because exposed bone is usually indicative of osteomyelitis, especially in diabetic foot ulcers.[28]

Evidence-Based Practice

A wound that has exposed bone or that can be probed to the bone with a sterile instrument should be evaluated for osteomyelitis.[29]

However, identifying milder, localized infection or critical colonization in chronic wounds is much more problematic for a variety of reasons. First, chronic wounds by definition are slow to heal or don't heal at all. Although many factors may account for impaired healing, wound bioburden has always been suspected as a major deterrent to healing and an important cause of wound chronicity. Second, the manifestation of inflammation may be altered in chronic wounds because of population-specific factors. For example, the inflammatory response to bacteria may be influenced by age,[30] presence of diabetes, tissue perfusion and oxygenation, other aspects of immunocompetence, and anti-inflammatory drug use.

Finally, considerable disagreement exists regarding what constitutes wound infection in the chronic wound.[31] In addition to this lack of consensus, the value of wound cultures in identifying infection is a source of confusion for clinicians and a source of debate among experts. However, despite the confusion surrounding identification of localized chronic wound infection, an operative definition of wound infection can provide a foundation from which clinicians can approach identification and diagnosis in a rational, consistent manner.

Methods to identify wound infection

In practice, wound infection is identified and diagnosed based on clinical signs and symptoms of infection or on the findings from wound cultures. The advantages and disadvantages of using these methods can be evaluated in light of the key elements contained in the definition of wound infection.

CLINICAL SIGNS AND SYMPTOMS

The most common and clinically practical method for identifying wound infection is to monitor for clinical signs and symptoms of infection. Clinical signs and symptoms of wound infection reflect host response to invasion or tissue injury. They can be detected by direct observation of the wound and periwound area or be reported by the patient. The clinical signs and symptoms of wound infection can be divided into those that comprise the classic signs of infection and those that are specific to secondary wounds (that is, tissue injury).

The classic signs and symptoms of infection are pain, erythema, edema, heat, and purulent exudate.[3,5,6,18] As indicators of infection, they're a reflection of the host's response to invading organisms. The first four of these signs are also known as the signs of inflammation, which can be elicited by tissue damage unrelated to infection.[3] Purulent exudate is the result of bacterial exotoxins recruiting white blood cells to the wound. However, it's the host reaction, expressed by the classic signs and symptoms of infection, that distinguishes an infected wound from one that's merely colonized or contaminated according to some authors.[23] For example, the American Diabetes Association (ADA) Consensus Conference on diabetic foot wound care (1999) defined localized infection in diabetic foot ulcers as purulence or two or more signs of inflammation.[32]

PRACTICE POINT

The classic signs of infection are pain, erythema, edema, heat, and purulent exudate.

The classic signs and symptoms of infection are believed to be reliable indicators of infection in acute wounds such as surgical incisions. In surgical wounds, inflammation occurs after wounding but should subside within 5 days.[33] The Centers for Disease Control and Prevention's (CDC) definition of a surgical site infection (SSI) reflects the confidence placed in clinical signs and symptoms to identify SSIs.[34]

CDC criteria for surgical site infection

The Centers for Disease Control and Prevention (CDC) has established the following criteria to define surgical site infection (SSI).

Superficial incisional SSI	Deep incisional SSI	Organ/space SSI

Involves only skin or subcutaneous tissue of the incision and at least one of the following:
• purulent drainage from the superficial incision
• organisms isolated from aseptically obtained culture of fluid or tissue from the incision
• at least one of the following, unless negative culture:
  – pain or tenderness
  – localized swelling
  – redness or heat
  – incision opened by surgeon
• diagnosis of SSI by the surgeon or attending physician.
	Involves deep soft tissues (such as fascia and muscle layers) of the incision and at least one of the following:
	• purulent drainage from the deep incision but not organ/space
	• deep incision spontaneously dehisces or is deliberately opened by surgeon with one of the following symptoms, unless negative culture:
	  – fever greater than 100.4° F (38° C)
	  – localized pain
	• an abscess
	• diagnosis of deep SSI by surgeon or attending physician.
		Involves any part of the anatomy (other than the incision) opened or manipulated during operation and at least one of the following:
		• purulent drainage from a drain placed in organ/space
		• organisms isolated from aseptically obtained culture of fluid or tissue in organ/space
		• an abscess or other evidence of infection
		• diagnosis of an organ/space SSI by a surgeon or attending physician.

Source: Horan, T.C., et al. "CDC Definitions of Nosocomial Surgical Site Infections, 1992; A modification of CDC Definitions of Surgical Wound Infections," *American Journal of Infection Control* 20(5):271-74, October 1992.

(See *CDC criteria for surgical site infection.*) SSIs are defined as infections occurring within 30 days of the operative procedure and are categorized as superficial incisional, deep incisional, or organ/space. The presence of purulent drainage is sufficient criteria as are signs of inflammation accompanied by a positive culture.

Unlike acute wounds, the classic signs and symptoms are not always present in chronic wounds[35] or diabetic foot ulcers[36] with high wound bioburden. This may be due to diminished systemic or local inflammatory responses among populations with a high prevalence of chronic wounds, such as patients with diabetes and those with peripheral vascular disease or autoimmune disorders. Similarly, immunosuppressed patients with acute wounds may not express classic signs of infection despite high wound bioburden. The only exception is the symptom of pain, which may occur in people with compromised immune function and be the only apparent symptom of infection.[37]

Evidence-Based Practice

The classic signs and symptoms of infection may not be present in chronic wounds or in patients who are immunosuppressed.

Evidence-Based Practice

Pain may be the only classic sign of wound infection present in immune-compromised patients.

Additional signs and symptoms specific to secondary wounds have been proposed as indicators of infection.[38] These signs and symptoms include:

- serous drainage with concurrent inflammation
- delayed healing
- discoloration of granulation tissue
- friable granulation tissue
- pocketing at the base of the wound
- foul odor
- wound breakdown.

PRACTICE POINT

Granulation tissue bleeds easily due to bacterial stimulation of vascular endothelial growth factors (VEGF).[9]

All of these signs and symptoms, with the exception of pocketing, were found to be valid indicators of localized infection in a sample of chronic wounds.[35] Among a sample of diabetic foot ulcers, all were found to be valid with the exception of pocketing, friable granulation tissue, and wound breakdown.[36] Moreover, delayed healing may be the only apparent sign. According to the clinical practice guideline published by the Agency for Health Care Policy and Research (now the Agency for Healthcare Research and Quality), "a clean pressure ulcer should show some evidence of healing within 2 to 4 weeks."[39] Although many factors have been associated with delayed healing, wound infection, or critical colonization, may be a primary contributor.[8] When it's the only sign readily apparent, delayed healing should stimulate further assessment of wound bioburden by clinicians.[39]

PRACTICE POINT

Delayed healing may be the only sign of infection in some wounds.

Although using clinical signs and symptoms of infection to monitor wounds for infection is congruent with the definition of infection, the assessment of these parameters is quite subjective.[40] Therefore, the clinical signs and symptoms checklist[41] (CSSC) was developed to assess for the presence of such signs and symptoms of infection in chronic wounds. (See *Clinical signs and symptoms checklist*, pages 132–133.) The CSSC provides a precise description for each of the clinical signs and symptoms. Although more research regarding the validity and reliability of this checklist is needed, preliminary findings indicate that the reliability of the items

Clinical signs and symptoms checklist

Signs and symptoms	**check (+) if present**

Increasing pain in the ulcer area

The patient reports increased level of peri-ulcer pain since the ulcer developed. Ask him to select the most appropriate statement for current level of ulcer pain from the following choices:
1. I can't detect pain in ulcer area.
2. I have less ulcer pain now than I had in the past.
3. The intensity of the ulcer pain has remained the same since the ulcer developed.
4. I have more ulcer pain now than I had in the past.

If the patient selects number 4, his pain is increasing. Write n/a if the patient can't respond to the question.

Erythema

The presence of bright or dark red skin or darkening of normal ethnic skin color immediately adjacent to the ulcer opening indicates erythema.

Edema

The presence of shiny, taut skin or pitting impressions in the skin adjacent to the ulcer but within 4 cm from the ulcer margin indicates edema. Assess pitting edema by firmly pressing the skin within 4 cm of ulcer margin with a finger, release and waiting 5 seconds to observe indentation.

Heat

A detectable increase in temperature of the skin adjacent to the ulcer but within 4 cm of the ulcer margin as compared with the skin 10 cm proximal to the wound indicates heat. Assess differences in skin temperature using the back of your hand or your wrist.

Purulent exudate

Tan, creamy, yellow, or green thick fluid that's present on a dry gauze dressing removed from the ulcer 1 hour after the wound was cleaned and dressed indicates purulent exudate.

Sanguinous exudate

Bloody fluid that's present on a dry gauze dressing removed from the ulcer 1 hour after the wound was cleaned and dressed indicates sanguinous exudate.

Serous exudate

Thin, watery fluid that's present on a dry gauze dressing removed from the ulcer 1 hour after the wound was cleaned and dressed indicates serous exudate.

Delayed healing of the ulcer

The patient reporting no change, or an increase in the volume or surface area of the ulcer, over the preceding 4 weeks indicates delayed healing. Ask the patient if the ulcer has filled with tissue or is smaller around than it was 4 weeks ago.

Discoloration of granulation tissue

Granulation tissue that is pale, dusky, or dull in color compared with surrounding, healthy tissue. Note variations of normal, beefy-red appearance of granulation tissue.

Clinical signs and symptoms checklist (continued)

Signs and symptoms	check (+) if present
Friable granulation tissue Bleeding of granulation tissue when gently manipulated with a sterile cotton-tipped applicator indicates friable tissue.	☐
Pocketing at base of wound The presence of smooth, nongranulating pockets of ulcer tissue surrounded by beefy red granulation tissue indicates pocketing.	☐
Foul odor The ulcer may have a putrid or distinctively unpleasant smell.	☐
Wound breakdown Small open areas in newly formed epithelial tissue not caused by reinjury or trauma indicate wound breakdown.	☐

Adapted with permission of HMP Communications from Gardner, S.E., et al. "A Tool to Assess Clinical Signs and Symptoms of Localized Chronic Wound Infection: Development and Reliability," *Ostomy/ Wound Management* 47(1):40-47, January 2001.

on the CSSC is acceptable.[41,42] Moreover, the CSSC provides clinicians with information on assessing the lesser-known signs and symptoms specific to secondary wounds.

Compounding the subjective limitations of using signs and symptoms to identify wound infection is the lack of clear guidelines regarding the number of signs and symptoms that need to be present to constitute infection. Increasing pain and wound breakdown were found to be sufficient signs of infection in a small study ($n = 36$) of chronic wounds, but none were necessary.[35] Further, it's unclear how assessment of clinical signs and symptoms leads to decisions regarding wound infection status.[40] As mentioned previously, the ADA suggests that purulent exudate or the presence of two signs of inflammation be used to define infection in diabetic foot ulcers.[32] In practice, the presence of frankly obvious signs and symptoms of infection often triggers treatment or wound cultures to guide selection of antimicrobials.

A practical clinical approach using the mnemonics NERDS and STONES[9] can help identify superficial and deep infection. (See *NERDS©* and *STONES©*, page 134. See also *color section*,

NERDS, page C7, and *STONES*, pages C8–C9.) Based on a cross-sectional validation study, Woo and colleagues (2009)[42a] found that the presence of any three NERDS signs had a sensitivity of 73% and a specificity of 81% when compared with semi-quantitative swab cultures with scan or light growth. They also found that any three STONES signs had a sensitivity of 90% and a specificity of 69% when compared with semi-quantitative swab cultures with moderate to heavy growth. Early recognition of infection is crucial so that appropriate systemic treatment can be started and further damage can be prevented.[9]

Evidence-Based Practice

Increasing pain and wound breakdown are sufficient signs of wound infection. Any three NERDS signs are indicative of critical colonization, while any three STONES signs are indicative of deep infection.

NERDS© and STONES©

Superficial infection
- **N**on-healing wounds
- **E**xudate wounds
- **R**ed and bleeding wound surface granulation tissue
- **D**ebris (yellow or black necrotic tissue) on the wound surface
- **S**mell or unpleasant odor from the wound

Deep infection
- **S**ize bigger
- **T**emperature increased
- **O**s (prone to or exposed bone)
- **N**ew or satellite areas of breakdown
- **E**xudate, erythema, edema
- **S**mell

Source: Sibbald, R. G., et al. "Increased Bacterial Burden and Infection: The story of Nerds and Stones," *Advances in skin & wound care* 19(8):447-61, October 2006.

PRACTICE POINTS

Wound cultures are used to diagnose wound infection when it isn't clinically obvious.

The ADA suggests that purulent exudate or the presence of two or more signs of inflammation are indicative of infection in diabetic foot ulcers.

Using a Delphi process of international interdisciplinary wound experts, Cutting and colleagues tried to determine which clinical signs and symptoms of infection are present in all wounds as well as any that are specific to a particular wound.[43] They determined that cellulitis, malodor, pain, delayed healing, wound deterioration or breakdown, and an increased amount of exudate are common to all wounds (except for acute wounds healing by primary intention and full-thickness burns). Symptoms or criteria that had the highest score for infection in a particular wound are as follows: crepitus for pressure ulcers; phlegmon for neuropathic/diabetic ulcers; increase in local skin temperature for venous ulcers; and dry necrosis, which may turn moist and boggy at the edges of the necrotic tissue, for arterial disease–associated tissue breakdown.[43] (See *Ranking of clinical infection indicators by wound type.*)

Patient Teaching
Observing for signs of infection

Infection from a sore can develop in the tissue surrounding the sore or it can spread throughout the body. Signs of an infection in the surrounding tissue include redness, warmth, or swelling around the sore; increased pain; foul odor; drainage that thickens and assumes a more intense tan, creamy, yellow, or green color; red wound tissue that bleeds easily; and new areas of skin breakdown in proximity to the sore. Signs that the infection may be spreading throughout the body include increased temperature, fever or chills, weakness, confusion or difficulty concentrating, and rapid heartbeat. These signs should be observed for on a daily basis and reported to a healthcare provider if they occur.

WOUND CULTURES AND SPECIMENS

Like clinical signs and symptoms, the identification of wound infection based on culture findings may be inconclusive. Nonetheless, numerous methods are available for clinical and research purposes. The methods presented

Ranking of clinical infection indicators by wound type

Acute wounds: Primary
Cellulitis
Pus/abscess
Delayed healing
Erythema ± induration
Hemopurulent exudate
Malodor
Seropurulent exudate
Wound breakdown/enlargement
Increase in local skin temperature
Edema
Serous exudates with erythema
Swelling with increase in exudate volume
Unexpected pain/tenderness

Acute wounds: Secondary
Cellulitis
Pus/abscess
Delayed healing
Erythema 6 induration
Hemopurulent exudate
Increase in exudate volume
Malodor
Pocketing
Seropurulent exudates
Wound breakdown/ enlargement
Discoloration
Friable granulation tissue that bleeds easily
Increase in local skin temperature
Edema
Unexpected pain/tenderness

Diabetic foot ulcers
Cellulitis
Lymphangitis
Phlegmon
Purulent exudate
Pus/abscess
Crepitus in the joint
Erythema
Fluctuation
Increase in exudate volume
Induration
Localized pain in a normally asensate foot

Malodor
Probes to bone
Unexpected pain/tenderness
Blue-black discoloration and hemorrhage (halo)
Bone or tendon becomes exposed at base of ulcer
Delayed/arrested wound healing despite offloading and debridement
Deterioration of the wound
Friable granulation tissue that bleeds easily
Local edema
Sinuses develop in an ulcer
Spreading necrosis/ gangrene
Ulcer base changes from healthy pink to yellow or grey

Arterial leg ulcers
Cellulitis
Pus/abscess
Change in color/viscosity of exudates
Change in wound bed color*
Crepitus
Deterioration of wound
Dry necrosis turning wet
Increase in local skin temperature
Lymphangitis
Malodor
Necrosis—new or spreading
Erythema
Erythema in peri-ulcer tissue — persists with leg elevation
Fluctuation
Increase in exudate volume
Increase in size in a previously healing ulcer
Increased pain
Ulcer breakdown

Venous leg ulcers
Cellulitis
Delayed healing despite appropriate compression therapy
Increase in local skin temperature

Increase in ulcer pain/change in nature of pain
Newly formed ulcers within inflamed margins of pre-existing ulcers
Wound bed extension within inflamed margins
Discoloration, e.g., dull, dark brick red
Friable granulation tissue that bleeds easily
Increase in exudate viscosity
Increase in exudate volume
Malodor
New onset dusky wound hue
Sudden appearance/increase in amount of slough
Sudden appearance of necrotic black spots
Ulcer enlargement

Pressure ulcers
Cellulitis
Change in nature of pain
Crepitus
Increase in exudate volume
Pus
Serous exudate with inflammation
Spreading erythema
Viable tissues become sloughy
Warmth in surrounding tissues
Wound stops healing despite relevant measures
Enlarging wound despite pressure relief
Erythema
Friable granulation tissue that bleeds easily
Malodor
Edema

Burns: Partial-thickness
Cellulitis
Ecthyma gangrenosum
Black/dark brown focal areas of discoloration in burn
Erythema
Hemorrhagic lesions in subcutaneous tissue of burn wound or surrounding skin
Malodor

(continued)

Ranking of clinical infection indicators by wound type *(continued)*

Spreading peri-burn erythema (purplish discoloration or edema)
Unexpected increase in wound breadth
Unexpected increase in wound depth
Discoloration
Friable granulation tissue that bleeds easily
Sub-eschar pus/abscess formation
Increased fragility of skin graft
Increase in exudate volume
Increase in local skin temperature
Loss of graft
Edema
Onset of pain in previously pain-free burn
Opaque exudates

Rejection/loosening of temporary skin substitutes
Secondary loss of keratinized areas

Burns: Full-thickness
Black/dark brown focal areas of discoloration in burn
Cellulitis
Ecthyma gangrenosum
Erythema
Hemorrhagic lesions in subcutaneous tissue of burn wound or surrounding skin
Increased fragility of skin graft
Loss of graft
Onset of pain in previously pain-free burn
Spreading peri-burn erythema (purplish discoloration or edema)

Sub-eschar pus/abscess formation
Unexpected increase in wound breadth
Discoloration
Friable granulation tissue that bleeds easily
Malodor
Edema
Opaque exudate
Rapid eschar separation
Rejection/loosening of temporary skin substitutes
Secondary loss of keratinized areas

Key:

HIGH	Mean score 8 or 9
MEDIUM	Mean score 6 or 7
LOW	Mean score 4 or 5

---

*black for aerobes, bright red for *Streptococcus,* green for *Pseudomonas*

Results of the Delphi process identifying criteria in six different wound types
Used with permission: Medical Education Partnership LTD, 2005.

Source: Cutting, K. F., et al. "Clinical Identification of Wound Infection: A Delphi Approach," in *EWMA Position Document—Identifying Criteria for Wound Infection.* London, MEP Ltd., pp 6-9, 2005.

here are limited to those most commonly used in practice.

Wound cultures require two steps. The first step is the acquisition of a specimen from the wound. The second step includes the laboratory procedures used to grow, identify, and quantify the microorganisms. Clinicians are directly responsible for the first part and must be aware of laboratory processes included in the second to acquire an appropriate wound specimen and effectively transport the specimen to the laboratory.

The three most common types of wound specimens are:

• wound tissue
• needle-aspirated wound fluid
• swabs.

The tissue biopsy method consists of aseptically removing a piece of viable wound tissue with a scalpel or punch biopsy instrument. Wound tissue specimens are the most congruent with the first two elements that define wound infection if the specimens are samples from viable tissue rather than necrotic tissue. Among a sample of 41 wounds of mixed etiology, the quantitative tissue biopsy method had a sensitivity of 100%, a specificity of 93.5%, and an accuracy of 95.1% in predicting the success of delayed closure.[44] Based on these and other data, the tissue biopsy became the gold standard specimen for wound cultures.[45] Unfortunately, tissue biopsy cultures are invasive, skill-intensive (both from clinician and laboratory perspectives), and unavailable in many settings. Therefore, they aren't commonly used in practice but are often used in research of wound microbiology.

The needle-aspiration technique obtains fluid through multiple insertions of a 22-gauge needle into the tissue surrounding the wound. The needle is attached to a 10-cc syringe.[46] Although studies have compared needle aspiration technique with both quantitative tissue biopsy and swab cultures, the sensitivity, specificity, and accuracy of quantitative needle aspiration remains unclear due to methodological limitations.[45-47] However, this may be the best technique for specimen collection when focal collections of tissue fluid or abscess formations exist close to the wound.[48]

The most practical and widely available method for obtaining wound specimens is the swab culture. However, the usefulness of this method is extremely contentious. Since this method samples only wound surface organisms (as opposed to organisms within the tissue), many believe it's ineffectual as a measure of infection.[39] In addition, it may be difficult to recover anaerobic organisms from swab specimens.[27] However, others defend the role of swab cultures in monitoring infection, emphasizing its entrenchment in clinical practice.[49]

The swab techniques most commonly used or advocated in the literature are swabs of wound exudate, swabs taken using a broad Z-stroke over the entire wound bed, and swabs using the technique described by Levine and colleagues.[27,48,50-55]

Wound cleaning is advocated prior to obtaining swabs using either Z-stroke or Levine's technique in order for the culture to isolate wound tissue microorganisms as opposed to microorganisms associated with wound exudate, topical therapies, or nonviable tissue.[27,54] Moistening the swab with normal saline or transport medium is also recommended prior to specimen collection.[47,54] Moistening the swab is believed to provide more precise data than a dry swab.[56] Swabs using the broad Z-stroke entail rotating the swab between the fingers as the wound is swabbed from margin to margin in a 10-point zigzag fashion.[48] Because a large portion of the wound surface is sampled, the specimen collected may reflect surface contamination rather than tissue bioburden.[27]

The Levine technique consists of rotating a swab over a 1-cm^2 area with sufficient pressure to express fluid from within the wound tissue (see photo).[50] This technique is believed to be more reflective of "tissue" bioburden than swabs of exudate or swabs taken with a Z-stroke.[27] Theoretically, the Levine technique is the best technique for wound swabbing provided the wound is cleaned first and the area sampled is over viable tissue, not necrotic tissue or eschar.[27]

Although the accuracy of swab cultures as compared with biopsy cultures had been studied, the findings from these studies provided little information from which to base clinical practice.[47,49,50,57-60] The most serious methodological problem presented by these studies is that the specific swabbing techniques employed were not described. Swabbing techniques vary greatly according to wound preparation, area of the wound sampled, duration of sampling, and even the type of swab employed (for example, alginate).[45] To address

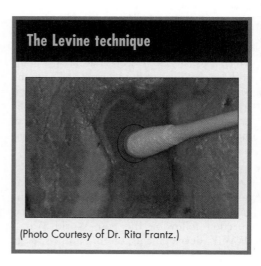

The Levine technique

(Photo Courtesy of Dr. Rita Frantz.)

this problem, we compared culture findings from swab specimens obtained using wound exudate, the Z-stroke technique, and Levine's technique with culture findings from viable wound specimens.[61] We found that culture findings based on swab specimens obtained using Levine's technique were more accurate and concordant with culture findings based on tissue specimens than swabs taken with either wound exudate or the Z-stroke technique. In her systematic review of the literature and clinical guideline, Bonham also concluded that Levine's technique was the most appropriate for obtaining swab specimens of the wound.[62]

PRACTICE POINT

Levine's technique provides culture findings most comparable to tissue specimens because this technique attempts to sample microorganisms from within the wound tissue, not just from the wound surface.

Analyzing cultures and specimens

Laboratory procedures for the microbiological analysis of wound specimens include isolation and identification of the microorganisms alone or in combination with quantification of the microorganisms isolated. When done alone, isolation and identification is referred to as qualitative culture; when done in conjunction with quantification, it's referred to as quantitative culture. Quantitative cultures provide information regarding the type of organisms present in addition to the number of organisms present, which is usually expressed as number per gram of tissue, milliliter of fluid, or swab. The number of organisms present provides information regarding the rate of microorganism multiplication; therefore, quantitative cultures reflect the third key element of wound infection more completely than qualitative cultures.

Qualitative cultures. The recovery, isolation, and identification of microorganisms gained importance in identifying wound infection following the post–World War I (WWI) development of organism-specific

antimicrobials.[63] According to the CDC, one sufficient criteria of SSI is an "organism isolated from an aseptically obtained culture of fluid or tissue."[34] By this definition, an organism present in the tissue of the wound indicates infection. It's important to note that this CDC criterion implies that isolation of organisms must be from within the tissue or tissue fluid, not isolation of organisms from the wound surface. The CDC defines pressure ulcer infection as the presence of two of the following clinical findings: (1) redness, tenderness, or swelling of wound edges and (2) organisms isolated from a needle aspiration, tissue biopsy, or blood culture.[64] Clinical signs and symptoms of infection must be present along with isolation of an organism known to cause disease.

Acute wounds often contain skin flora, such as staphylococci and diphtheroids.[2] Chronic wounds, with their distinctive environment, often contain larger numbers and types of microorganisms than acute wounds. These wounds have large amounts of exudate, necrotic tissue and eschar, large surface areas, and deep cracks and crevices suitable for a variety of microbial species. Chronic wounds have been associated with anaerobes and multiple types of organisms.[65-67] Common organisms isolated from chronic wounds are *Proteus mirabilis, Escherichia coli,* and *Streptococcus, Staphylococcus, Pseudomonas, Corynebacterium,* and *Bacteroides* species.[18,65,66,68-70] Limited data indicate that the presence of *P. mirabilis, Pseudomonas aeruginosa,* and *Bacteroides,* an anaerobe, deter healing of chronic wounds.[71,72] Non-healing chronic wounds were also associated with the presence of *E. coli,* group D *Streptococcus,* and other anaerobic cocci.[58] Although the presence of methicillin-resistant *Staphylococcus aureus* (MRSA) in chronic wounds presents a problem for infection control in healthcare settings, the association between colonization with MRSA and subsequent infection or bacteremia is unclear.[73] Only the presence of beta-hemolytic *Streptococcus* is considered to be a notable threat in the chronic wound at levels less than 105 organisms per gram of tissue.[48,63,74] Nonetheless, qualitative cultures have a role in the monitoring of wounds and in guiding antibiotic selection for infected wounds. Qualitative cultures are accomplished by plating wound specimens on solid media, identifying isolates using standard microbiological procedures, and testing for antibiotic sensitivity. Qualitative cultures from swab specimens obtained using Levine's technique were found to be highly concordant with qualitative cultures from tissue specimens.[61] In terms of recovering any and all organisms, swab specimens obtained using Levine's technique were 78% concordant with tissue specimens. Concordance with respect to recovering the specific organisms *S. aureus, P. aeruginosa,* and beta-hemolytic *Streptococcus* was 96%, 96%, and 99%, respectively.

PRACTICE POINT

Beta-hemolytic *Streptococcus* is considered a notable threat in wounds regardless of the number of these microorganisms present.

PRACTICE POINT

Gram-positive organisms are the first to invade wounds with decreased host resistance followed by gram-negative then anaerobic organisms.[9]

Quantitative cultures. Although Pasteur suggested that the invasion of microorganisms in the body was related to quantity of inoculation, French WWI surgeons were the first to base wound management on the number of organisms present.[75-77] The relationship between bacterial quantity, wound infection, and sepsis was given attention in the 1960s. Krizek and Davis[78] found that fatal sepsis was associated with visceral or blood cultures greater than 10^6 or 10^7 organisms per gram of tissue or milliliter of blood. These researchers also demonstrated that fatal wound sepsis was related to the number of bacteria in the wound.[79] In addition, Noyes and colleagues[80] found that wound exudates with greater than 10^6 bacteria per milliliter were associated with invasive infection. The U.S. Army Surgical Research Unit provided a series of studies that found burn wound

sepsis was associated with bacterial levels exceeding 10^5 organisms per gram of tissue.[81-83] Quantity of bacteria was also inversely linked to chronic wound healing.[25,44,71,72] These studies, along with earlier findings that clean wounds harbor microorganisms, provided the foundation from which quantitative culturing was added as a method of diagnosing infection.[44] The Agency for Health Care Policy and Research clinical practice guideline, Treatment of Pressure Ulcers, embraced quantitative culture as the gold standard to diagnose pressure ulcer infection.[39,84] More than 10^5 organisms per gram of tissue, milliliter of fluid, or swab has been adopted by many as the critical value for diagnosing wound infection.[23,25,30,39,63,85] Although references to greater than 10^5 have been interpreted as $100,000^1$ or $1,000,000^{86}$ organisms per gram of tissue, greater than 1,000,000 organisms per gram of tissue is the preferred critical value.[87]

Swab specimens can be quantitatively or semi-quantitatively processed. Wound tissue specimens must be of sufficient weight to ensure validity of findings—around 0.25 g of tissue.[86] Quantitative swab cultures are placed in 1 ml of dilutant and vortexed to release microorganisms from the swab. This fluid is then serially diluted, plated, and incubated, usually in aerobic conditions only. However, the recovery of anaerobes from swab specimens has been described through the use of an anaerobic transport container.[88] Plates are read for type and quantity of organisms and quantification is expressed as number or organisms per swab or gram of tissue. Similarly, wound aspirate is diluted, plated, and incubated. Quantification is expressed as the number of organisms per ml of fluid.[46]

We compared the quantitative culture findings from swab specimens obtained using Levine's technique with quantitative culture findings from tissue specimens in a sample of chronic wounds.[61] A critical threshold of 37,000 organisms per swab had a sensitivity of 90% and specificity of 57% when the true infection status of the wound was defined as 1,000,000 or more organisms per gram of tissue. Although this was the first study to examine different critical thresholds for swab specimens, further study is needed to identify the optimal critical threshold for practice.

Semi-quantitative swabs are inoculated onto solid media and streaked on four quadrants. The number of colony-forming units is counted in each quadrant and results are reported from 1 to 4+. Dow and colleagues[48] suggest that 4+ should be used as the cut-off for diagnosing infection.

In summary, the identification of wound infection remains ambiguous and uncertain. Monitoring wounds for the clinical signs and symptoms of infection is an important component of wound assessment. Indicators of inflammation are especially important markers in acute wounds, such as SSIs. However, the signs and symptoms associated with inflammation may not be present in some patients with acute wounds or in patients with chronic wounds. The signs specific to secondary wounds may be useful in these cases and should be incorporated into clinical assessment. Wounds suspected of infection, especially those with delayed healing, are often cultured to confirm the diagnosis. While qualitative cultures provide useful information in wounds that are demonstrating obvious clinical signs of infection, they may not be as useful in diagnosing infection in the absence of signs and symptoms unless certain pathogens are isolated. In the absence of clinical signs and symptoms, quantitative cultures are the gold standard method for diagnosing localized wound infection.

MANAGING WOUND BIOBURDEN

Controlling wound bioburden requires a multifaceted approach consisting of one or more of the following:

- correction of the host factors that contributed to the infection
- removal of devitalized tissue and foreign debris
- initiation of antimicrobial therapy.

Although not all of these interventions will be indicated in every case of wound infection, they each have a role to play in either reducing the number of microorganisms or enhancing host resistance.

The presence of host factors that reduce resistance to infection are often overlooked in management of wound bioburden. Judicious attention to restoration of adequate blood supply and tissue oxygen, provision of nutritional support, maintenance of glycemic control, reduction of edema, and protection from mechanical forces on the wounded tissue will aid in restoring the balance between host resistance and microorganisms. Failure to address these host factors may contribute to continued proliferation of microorganisms despite initiation of other treatment modalities.

Because necrotic tissue provides an excellent medium for growth of microorganisms, removal of devitalized tissue and debris is an essential step in treating wound infection. When devitalized tissue is adherent to the wound bed, wound debridement is indicated.

Debridement may also be indicated when a chronic wound persists without adequate management of wound bacteria, allowing organisms to invade the deeper tissue. Methods of wound debridement are addressed in chapter 8, Wound debridement.

Wound cleaning

Host factors such as foreign debris and contaminants on the surface of the wound can harbor microorganisms or provide nutrients for their growth. Wound cleaning is a process that removes these less adherent inflammatory contaminants from the wound surface and renders the wound less conducive to microbial growth. However, the process of wound cleaning can also create tissue trauma. Effective wound cleaning requires selection of methods that minimize chemical and mechanical trauma to wound tissue while removing surface debris and contaminants. Although definitive research is lacking to guide selection of wound cleaning methods, the available practice evidence suggests using a nontoxic cleaning solution in combination with a delivery device that will create sufficient mechanical forces to remove the surface debris while limiting tissue injury.

CLEANING AGENTS

The usefulness of specific agents to correct host factors depends on a balance between their antibacterial properties and their cytotoxicity to wound healing cells, such as white blood cells (WBCs) and fibroblasts.[89] For the majority of wounds, isotonic saline is adequate to clean the wound surface. A *Cochrane* review concluded that water, although not isotonic, is a suitable alternative, as long as it's free of any potential contaminants.[90] Because the fluid has only brief contact with the wound surface, it isn't crucial that the solution be isotonic (0.9% sodium chloride). If you choose to use an isotonic solution, however, an inexpensive saline solution can be prepared by combining one teaspoon of noniodized salt in one quart of water. (See *Patient Teaching: Preparing saline solution at home,* page 142.)

If the wound surface is heavily laden with surface debris, a commercial wound cleaner may be used. These agents contain surface-active agents or surfactants that by the nature of their chemical polarity break the bonds that attach wound contaminants. The intensity of their chemical reactivity is directly related to their cleaning capacity and cytotoxicity. Thus, selection of a wound cleaner needs to weigh cleaning capacity against potential toxicity to cells in the wound.

Evidence regarding the safety of wound cleaners is difficult to interpret due to the lack of standardized methods for testing these agents. At present, the majority of available evidence comes from in vitro studies comparing wound cleaners under experimentally controlled conditions. The earliest such study evaluated the relative toxicity of various commercial wound and skin cleaners according to their effect on the viability of PMNs.[91] PMNs were exposed to increasing 1:10 dilutions of test cleaners for 30 minutes and analyzed for viability and phagocytic function. The toxicity index was defined as the amount of dilution required to achieve PMN viability and phagocytic function compared with that obtained by cells exposed to a balanced salt solution. Generally, toxicity levels of wound cleaners ranged from 10 to 1,000 while skin cleaners were 10,000. A second study of wound cleaner cytotoxicity evaluated the effects of five wound cleaning products on the viability of human fibroblasts, red blood cells, and WBCs in culture.[92] Although the results were similar, the findings related to specific agents varied somewhat from those reported by Foresman et al.[91] One cleaner was found to be considerably more toxic in this study, a result of the sample tested failing to meet the manufacturer's specification for pH. A more recent study evaluated the toxicity index of several current formulations of skin and wound cleansers using both fibroblasts and keratinocytes.[93] Collectively, these studies confirm that skin cleaners, which are formulated to break the chemical bonds that bind fecal matter to the skin, are stronger and more toxic than wound cleaners.

Evidence-Based Practice

Skin cleaners should never be used for wound cleaning due to their toxicity.

Patient Teaching
Preparing saline solution at home

To prepare saline solution at home, tell the patient to combine 1 teaspoon of noniodized salt with 1 quart of distilled water, stirring until the salt is completely dissolved. The solution can be stored for up to 1 week, at room temperature, in a tightly covered glass or plastic container.

Evidence-Based Practice

Use of wound cleansers on wounds heavily laden with debris must be balanced against the potential toxicity to wound healing cells.

Antiseptic agents have historically been used to control bacterial levels in chronic wounds. (See *Antiseptic agents historically used to treat chronic wounds.*) This practice was based on the well-documented finding that bacteria suspended in a test tube of fluid medium are rapidly killed when exposed to an antiseptic. However, in order for an agent to be effective in the environment of a chronic wound, an agent must be able to penetrate into contaminated tissue in an active form and in sufficient concentration to achieve bactericidal activity. Because antiseptics bind chemically to multiple organic substrates that are normally present in chronic wounds, they may fail to reach bacteria in the wound tissue when used in standard clinical concentrations.[94-96] Thus, they're unable to create an effective antibacterial effect. Furthermore, antiseptics are toxic to all cells with which they come into contact, including WBCs and fibroblasts.

The cytotoxic properties of antiseptics have been well documented in vitro and in vivo.[89,97-104] Furthermore, the addition of an antiseptic to wound cleaners has been shown to increase the toxicity index of the agent to 10,000 on average.[105] Although multiple clinical studies are cited to support the benefits of using antiseptic agents in healing chronic wounds, they fail to distinguish the antimicrobial effect of the antiseptic from other bacteria-reducing treatments that are being simultaneously administered, such as debridement or absorption of wound exudate, including bacteria and their toxins.[106-109] Although some clinicians have reported using antiseptics for specific clinical indications, such as to demarcate a gangrenous wound and limit bacterial invasion of surrounding tissue, to date, no scientifically valid clinical studies have documented the antibacterial benefits of using antiseptic agents in chronic wounds.[110-112]

 PRACTICE POINT

Antiseptics shouldn't be used as a cleaning agent for wounds.

Antiseptic agents historically used to treat chronic wounds

Acetic acid

Aluminum salts

Boric acid

Chlorhexidine

Gentian violet

Hexachlorophene

Hydrogen peroxide

Hypochlorite (Dakin's solution)

Iodine, povidone-iodine

Merthiolate

Silver nitrate

CLEANING DEVICES

The effectiveness of wound cleaning is influenced by the type of cleaning device used to deliver the solution to the wound surface. It's essential that the method used provide sufficient force to remove surface contaminants and debris while minimizing trauma to the wound. A variety of scrubbing cloths, sponges, and brushes are available for wound cleaning. Although evidence related to their efficacy is limited, it has been demonstrated that wounds cleaned with coarse sponges were significantly more susceptible to infection than those scrubbed with smoother sponges.[113] Furthermore, when compared with saline, wound cleaners containing surfactant were found to decrease the coefficient of friction between the scrubbing device and wound tissue.

Wound irrigation, as opposed to a cleaning device, promotes wound cleaning by creating hydraulic forces generated by the fluid stream. In order for the irrigation to be effective in cleaning the wound, the force of the irrigation stream must be greater than the adhesion forces that hold the debris to the surface of the wound. Multiple studies have substantiated that increasing pressure of a fluid stream improves removal of bacteria and debris from the wound.[114,115] Wound irrigation pressures of 10 lb per square inch (psi) and 15 psi are more effective than pressures of 1 and 5 psi in removing debris and bacteria from the wound surface; however, increasing the irrigation pressure to 20 psi or greater doesn't significantly improve the efficacy of cleaning.

When irrigation is delivered with a mechanical irrigation device, such as those used for dental hygiene, greater pressures are attainable than with other methods. Although clinical studies of mechanical irrigation devices used on crushing trauma wounds have confirmed that cleaning with a pressure of 70 psi produces significantly more effective removal of bacteria and debris than cleaning with 25 or 50 psi,[116-118] lower pressures are generally desirable in chronic wounds. However, even with pressures as low as 10 psi, bacteria and debris removal with mechanical irrigation devices was significantly more effective than results obtained from irrigation with a bulb syringe.

Although high pressure optimizes wound cleaning, the risk of dispersing fluid into adjacent wound tissue or along tissue planes is increased when higher pressures are used for irrigation.[119-121] The magnitude of this dispersion is related to the amount of fluid stream pressure. Research on the animal model established that irrigation at 70 psi produced greater dispersion of fluid into the tissue than irrigation with a 35-ml syringe and a 19-gauge needle (8 psi).[121] Moreover, when a single orifice tip was used to irrigate experimental wounds, extensive fluid penetration occurred at pressures greater than 30 psi.[120] This dispersion of fluid did not occur when a multi-jet tip was used to deliver the irrigation stream. Collectively, this evidence supports avoiding irrigation pressures of greater than 15 psi for wound cleaning.

While high pressures should be avoided in performing wound irrigation, it's also necessary to create sufficient hydraulic forces with the fluid stream to overcome the adhesion forces holding debris to the wound surface. Research on experimental wounds in the animal model found that irrigation pressures of 1 and 5 psi removed significantly less wound debris than did pressures of 10 and 15 psi.[115] The use of a needle and syringe to deliver fluid to wound tissue is generally regarded as a convenient method of providing effective irrigation pressure. A 35-ml syringe and a 19-gauge needle or angiocatheter has been shown to deliver an irrigation stream at 8 psi.[122] This study also demonstrated that irrigation with a 19-gauge needle and a 35-ml syringe was significantly more effective than bulb syringe irrigation in removing wound bacteria and preventing the development of infection in experimental wounds.[122] Additional evidence of the effectiveness of a needle and syringe method of irrigation over the bulb syringe was established in a clinical experimental study of trauma wounds treated within 24 hours of injury with either a standard bulb syringe (0.05 psi) or a 12-ml syringe and 22-gauge needle (13 psi).[123] A significant decrease was observed in both wound inflammation and wound infection in those wounds cleaned with the syringe and needle compared with the bulb syringe. The collective evidence regarding the effect of fluid stream pressure on removal of wound debris and bacteria supports using an irrigation pressure of 5 to 15 psi for wound cleaning.

A variety of needle and syringe combinations can be used to achieve the desired range of irrigation pressure. The size of the syringe and the needle gauge determine the amount of pressure of the fluid stream. Since the force depressing the plunger is distributed over a larger surface area, the larger the syringe, the less the force. With a 19-gauge needle, 6-, 12-, and 35-ml syringes will produce pressures of 30, 20, and 8 psi, respectively. The opposite effect occurs by increasing the size of the needle. Since the larger the lumen of the needle, the greater will be the flow of fluid, needles of 25-, 21-, and 19-gauge will create pressures of 4, 6, and 8 psi, respectively, when used with a 35-ml syringe.

A number of devices capable of delivering saline under pressure have been made available commercially. Although the claim is made that these devices produce a 19-gauge stream at 8 psi, no evidence exists to support this assertion. In a preliminary report of the pressure dynamics of one of these devices, measurement of pressure was limited to the pressure within the pressurized canister system, not the actual force of the fluid stream against the wound surface.[124]

PRACTICE POINT

Wound irrigation can be accomplished with a variety of medical tools and specially made devices.

Evidence-Based Practice

Research indicates that the optimum pressure for wound cleaning is between 5 and 15 psi.

In addition to varying the amount of pressure used for wound irrigation, the fluid stream can be delivered in either a pulsatile or continuous flow pattern. The benefit of delivering wound irrigation with a pulsatile as compared with a continuous fluid stream hasn't been substantiated in experimental studies.[114,117,118] Although several commercially available battery-powered, disposable irrigation systems (Davol, Inc., Cranston, RI; Stryker Instruments, Kalamazo, MI; Zimmer, Inc., Dover, OH) deliver pulsatile fluid streams with different spray patterns and remove the fluid and wound debris with suction, their wound healing efficacy in comparison with other irrigation methods remains to be established.[31,125-127] However, a recent animal study comparing pulsed lavage and bulb syringe irrigation showed reduced bacterial levels with pulse lavage irrigation.[128] At the present time, their primary benefit appears to be their portability and capability to serve as an alternative to whirlpool therapy for patients with chronic wounds, which aren't amenable to whirlpool, or for patients when whirlpool therapy isn't accessible.

PRACTICE POINT

Pulsatile irrigation devices don't appear to be better than nonpulsatile devices, but they may be useful for patients who don't have access to a whirlpool.

An alternate approach to wound irrigation is the whirlpool bath. It cleans the wound by exposing the entire wound bed and surrounding skin to agitating water generated by jets in the sides of the whirlpool tub. Only two studies have investigated the cleaning effectiveness of whirlpool and these are methodologically confounded with wound irrigation, which was provided at the end of the whirlpool therapy.[129,130] The benefit of the whirlpool bath is thought to be derived from the prolonged exposure of the wound to water, which softens wound debris and makes it more amenable to removal. For this reason, the whirlpool is best suited for use with chronic wounds containing thick slough or necrotic tissue. Since it isn't possible to control the amount of pressure being exerted on the wound surface in a whirlpool bath, once the devitalized tissue has been cleared from the wound, the whirlpool should be discontinued to avoid disrupting new granulation tissue forming in the wound. Extreme caution must also be taken to ensure that the wound doesn't come in close contact with the water jets, since the high pressure they generate could cause further tissue injury.

A more recently developed technology that assists with removing fluids from a wound is negative-pressure wound therapy (NPWT). Fluid removal is accomplished by placing foam or gauze dressing into the wound, sealing it with a semi-occlusive covering, and applying subatmospheric pressure through an evacuation tube coupled to a computer-modulated pump. The suction action created by the subatmospheric pressure facilitates removal of stagnant fluid from a wound. Although removal of stagnant wound fluid with NPWT is thought to decrease wound bioburden, research findings have been mixed. In a randomized trial comparing NPWT and conventional moist gauze therapy, quantitative bacterial load, as measured by tissue biopsy, did not change significantly in either treatment group.[131] However, the NPWT wounds showed a significant decrease in nonfermentative gram-negative bacilli and an increase in *S. aureus*. Similarly, in a study of 65 patients with acute or chronic wounds who were randomized to initial treatment with vacuum-assisted closure or a "modern" dressing, there was no significant reduction in bacterial clearance.[132] In contrast, others have reported a trend toward reduction in bacterial load using semi-quantitative superficial swabs.[133,134] Additionally, Morykwas and colleagues found a 1,000-fold decrease in the number of bacteria in experimentally inoculated wounds of pigs that had been treated with NPWT for 4 days.[135] Variation in sampling techniques and methods of analyses of wound specimens have contributed to these discrepant findings.

Evidence for use of NPWT with antimicrobial solution instillation has been reported in the literature.[136] Case studies of infected acute wounds using this new treatment modality are being evaluated. Continued research will help us determine the effectiveness of this new treatment strategy.

ANTIMICROBIAL THERAPY

When removal of necrotic tissue doesn't reduce bacterial burden to a level compatible with healing, additional interventions to reduce the number of organisms on the wound surface are indicated. These antimicrobial therapies consist of elemental topical antimicrobials and antibiotics, both topical and systemic. These agents act directly on the microorganisms, destroying the bacteria and preventing development of new colonies.

The clinical use of antimicrobials to control bacterial burden in chronic wounds has been characterized by misconceptions and controversy. As a result, they have frequently been used too extensively or for too long a time. The lack of valid indicators of chronic wound infection has further complicated the selection and use of antimicrobial therapy. Research evidence has documented that systemic antibiotics are of no value in reducing bacterial counts in chronic, granulating wounds.[137] Furthermore, the presence of purulent exudate, a recognized sign of infection in an acute wound, isn't a sufficient indicator of the need to initiate antimicrobial therapy to treat a chronic wound. Given the current state of ambiguity regarding valid clinical signs and symptoms of chronic wound infection, the decision to initiate antimicrobial therapy is best guided by the failure of a wound to make progress toward healing despite the absence of devitalized tissue. The main indications for topical antibiotic use revolve around superficial wound infection, or critical colonization, in which there is impaired wound healing, pale fragile granulation tissue, or suspected or confirmed high microbial burden, without periwound cellulitis. Applying the NERDS and STONES mnemonics reveals that these indicators are consistent with critical colonization but not deep infection. Topical elemental antimicrobials are formulated from elements such as silver, copper, gold, or zinc. (See *Topical antibiotics traditionally used to control bioburden in chronic wounds*, page 146.) The specific formulation of the antimicrobial agent is crucial to its effectiveness in reducing bacterial burden without destroying cells essential to healing. Iodine is an example of an agent that, in its elemental form, is toxic to cells that promote healing. However, when formulated as *cadexomer iodine* gel, it slowly releases iodine from its microspheres while absorbing bacteria.[138,139] An in vitro study of varying concentrations of cadexomer iodine demonstrated that it is nontoxic to human fibroblasts in culture in concentrations of up to 0.45%; the study also showed that chronic wounds treated with cadexomer iodine revealed reepithelialization on biopsy.

Topical agents formulated with silver have long been a part of the antibacterial armamentarium. Using the ionized form of silver (Ag+), these agents exert bacteriostatic properties through the action of the silver cation on proteins. The Ag+ binds to proteins in the bacterial cell wall, disrupting its integrity and resulting in death of the cell. Silver-containing wound care products include pure silver, creams, and sustained-release dressings. Research evidence regarding the efficacy of these agents is most substantial for the cream formulations (silver sulfadiazine 2% or 7%). Topical cream formulations have been shown to reduce bacterial density, vascular margination, and migration of inflammatory cells in chronic leg ulcers.[140] The efficacy of silver sulfadiazine cream in reducing bacterial burden in chronic wounds was substantiated in a randomized trial of 45 patients with a single infected pressure ulcer who were randomly assigned to receive silver sulfadiazine cream, povidone-iodine solution, or saline gauze dressings.[106] Standard care consisting of debridement, pressure reduction, and nutritional support was provided to all subjects. In 100% of the ulcers treated with silver sulfadiazine cream, the bacterial levels were reduced to 10^5 or less per gram of tissue during the 3-week study period, while only 78.6% of the povidone-iodine solution–treated ulcers and 63.6% of the saline gauze–treated ulcers achieved these reductions in bacterial levels. Overall, ulcers treated with silver sulfadiazine responded more rapidly, with one-third

Topical antibiotics traditionally used to control bioburden in chronic wounds
Mafenide acetate (Sulfamylon)
Metronidazole (Flagyl®, Metizol, MetroGel)
Mupirocin (Bactroban)
Nitrofurazone (Furacin)
Polysporin
Silver sulfadiazine (Silvadene)

achieving bacterial levels of less than 10^5 within 3 days and half of the ulcers reaching this level within 1 week. These data support limiting treatment with silver-based creams to no more than 2 weeks. Limiting the use of effective topical antibiotics to short durations with high doses can minimize the potential for selection or development of more resistant bacteria. If clinical evidence of improvement has not occurred with 2 weeks of treatment, other host factors that may be contributing to decreased bacterial resistance should be explored.

Evidence-Based Practice

Research suggests that topical elemental antimicrobial therapy with silver-based creams be limited to 2 weeks.

A more recently developed topical delivery system, the silver-impregnated dressing, has been shown to have antimicrobial effects on a broad spectrum of organisms.[141] However, many questions remain regarding the dosage of silver released into the wound and the potential for delays in healing if the silver cation binds to fibroblasts and epithelial cells. Reports of industry-conducted in vitro studies demonstrate that different silver-containing dressings release different amounts of silver over time.[137a] There are preliminary indications that the toxic dosage of silver differs depending on whether the fibroblasts and epithelial cells are in a mono-layer or in a three-dimensional matrix.[142] The potential adverse consequences in epithelializing wounds was demonstrated in a controlled study of matched pair skin graft donor sites treated with a non-antimicrobial foam dressing or a nanocrystalline silver dressing. Although there were no differences in bacterial counts between the two treatment groups, reepithelialization was significantly slower in the wounds treated with the silver dressing.[143] At the present, in vivo evidence to establish the safety and efficacy of silver-containing dressings is lacking. Recent reviews of the research literature confirm that clinical evidence of benefit for silver-containing dressings is lacking.[144-146] An evaluation of multiple elements of dressing performance, including silver content, rate of silver release, and antibacterial activity, concluded that the dressing should be selected based on standard clinical parameters rather than on a dressing's silver content or release activity.[147] Therefore, given the ambiguity in the evidence surrounding silver-containing dressings, discretion should be exercised in using them as a method of reducing microorganisms on wound surfaces, and treatment periods should be limited to 4 weeks in duration. Their use should be discontinued when reepithelialization is observed in the wound.

Topical antibiotics exert their antimicrobial effects through selective binding to chemical targets on the bacterial cell wall. Since human cell membranes lack these chemical targets, topical antibiotics have negligible effect on cells that promote wound healing. Although numerous antibiotics are available for topical application, research confirming the potential utility of topical antibiotics in reducing bacterial burden in chronic wounds is limited to two randomized controlled trials. In one study, 31 patients with pressure ulcers were treated with topical gentamicin cream and standard treatment consisting of debridement, cleaning, pressure reduction, and nutritional support (experimental group). These patients demonstrated significant improvement, while only three of the nine given standard treatment alone improved.[71] Serial bacteriological and pathological observations made over a 1- to 4-week treatment period showed a rapid reduction in bacterial counts to levels less than 10^6/ml in all ulcers treated with gentamicin. Furthermore, analysis of quantitative bacterial counts in relation to clinical outcome revealed an absolute correlation between significant clinical improvement and a fall in the bacterial count to less than 10^6/ml and between no clinical improvement and the persistence of counts greater than 10^6/ml. The efficacy of silver sulfadiazine in reducing bacterial counts was also demonstrated in the previously noted randomized trial of 45 patients with pressure ulcers.[106] In this study, all of the ulcers treated with topical silver sulfadiazine achieved bacterial levels of 10^5 or less per gram of tissue following 3 weeks of treatment.

Although clinical studies provide evidence supporting the utility of topical antibiotics in reducing bacterial burden in chronic wounds, these agents can cause adverse reactions in some patients. Reports of permanent hearing loss with topical 1% neomycin solution and acute anaphylactic reactions with topically applied bacitracin suggest that careful monitoring is indicated when using these agents.[148,149] Additionally, since there's a risk of selecting out resistant strains of bacteria, antibiotics that are used to treat infections systemically shouldn't be used in a topical form on chronic wounds. For this reason, despite the reported effectiveness of gentamicin in reducing bacterial levels in pressure ulcers, alternative topical antibiotics are indicated that won't produce resistant bacterial strains to systemic forms of the antimicrobial agent. Furthermore, since topical antibiotics are limited in the range of species they are effective against, it is important to judiciously select the specific antibiotic based on the organism present in the wound.

While topical antibiotics have demonstrated effectiveness in reducing bacterial burden when the area of involvement is localized, they're generally regarded as inadequate to control more extensive tissue involvement, such as advancing cellulitis. In these instances, systemic antibiotic therapy is indicated. Since the type of organisms and degree of invasiveness will vary, the choice of antimicrobial therapy will need to be individualized. Unfortunately, little research evidence exists to guide selection of antibiotics to treat chronic wound infections. Generally, chronic wound infections are treated empirically with antibiotics that have a narrow but sufficient spectrum of coverage. Care should be taken to avoid routine or extended periods of treatment. Less acute forms of chronic wound infection are treated with oral antibiotics. However, parenteral therapy may be indicated when the infection involves deeper tissue and is accompanied by systemic signs, such as fever, chills, and elevated WBC count. Regardless of the route, the effectiveness of any systemic antibiotic in reducing bacterial burden will be dependent on the adequacy of the patient's peripheral circulation. In those instances where peripheral vascular disease compromises blood flow to the infected tissue, systemic antimicrobial therapy may produce no clinical improvement in the wound.

> **PRACTICE POINT**
>
> The effectiveness of systemic antibiotics is dependent on an adequate blood supply to the wound.

Several adjuvant therapies have shown potential as interventions for reducing bacterial burden in chronic wounds. Hyperbaric oxygen therapy, administered by intermittent inhalation of pure oxygen at a pressure greater than 1 atmosphere, has been shown to promote PMN microbicidal efficacy in diabetic foot ulcers.[150] Ultraviolet (UV) light has long been recognized for its bactericidal effects derived from in vitro studies. The effect of UV light has been demonstrated in a clinical study of 22 patients with chronic wounds containing high bacteria levels as determined by quantitative swab culture.[151] Following one 180-second

UV-C treatment session, cultures showed a statistically significant reduction in predominant bacteria ($P = .001$) and significant reductions in MRSA ($P < .05$) and *S. aureus* ($P < .01$).[152]

Additionally, exposure of wound tissue to electrical current using an electrical stimulation device has been shown in animal studies to exert bacteriostatic and bactericidal effects on microorganisms known to infect chronic wounds. In a study of 20 patients with burn wounds that had been unresponsive to conventional therapy for 3 months to 2 years, application of direct current stimulation for 10 minutes twice weekly produced a quantitatively lower level of microorganisms.[152] However, the antibacterial effect of pulsed current, the more commonly used electrical stimulation modality in current practice, remains unclear. There is evidence that the voltage that would be required to produce an antibacterial effect would create profound muscle contractions, making it not applicable in clinical practice.[153-155]

SUMMARY

Most of our understanding of wound infection has been derived from the study of acute wounds. As wound healing science has evolved, it has become clear that chronic wounds are distinctly different environments where host resistance has been overwhelmed by bacterial burden. The classic signs and symptoms of infection are well recognized. However, they're based on assessments made of acute wounds and aren't valid in the chronic wound. While indicators of chronic wound infection remain ambiguous, substantial evidence shows that necrotic tissue harbors microorganisms. Therefore, debridement of necrotic tissue in the wound bed is an essential first step to reducing bacterial burden. Regular wound cleaning with a noncytotoxic solution, using sufficient force to remove surface contaminants and debris while minimizing trauma, is an important adjunct to reduce surface contaminants. In those instances where these measures aren't sufficient to restore a balance between host resistance and bacterial burden, antimicrobials that act directly on the bacteria are indicated.

PATIENT SCENARIO

Clinical Data

Mr. L is a well-nourished 70-year-old who lives independently with his wife. His past medical history is negative for diabetes, pulmonary disease, and cardiac disease. His hypertension is well controlled with hydrochlorothiazide. He presents to the wound clinic for the first time for an open wound on the medial aspect of his lower left leg (Fig. 7-1A). He sustained a crushing injury to his left lower leg 20 years ago and has had a wound on the medial aspect since that time. Multiple skin grafts have failed. On clinical examination, erythema is noted around the periwound area. There is no increase in skin temperature and no apparent edema. He denies increasing pain in the wound area and reports that the wound has not increased in size. The wound measures 3.9 × 2.5 cm. The wound bed contains some granulation tissue and a small amount of yellow surface debris. There is a distinctive foul odor with a small amount of yellow-tinged exudate. The mnemonic NERDS® produces four NERDS signs. A quantitative tissue culture reveals the presence of S. aureus, diphtheroids, and *P. aeruginosa*. The microbial load of the organisms present is less than 10^6 per gram of tissue. Doppler waveform studies and pulse volume recordings reveal normal triphasic vessels.

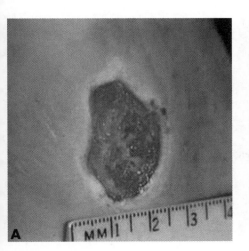 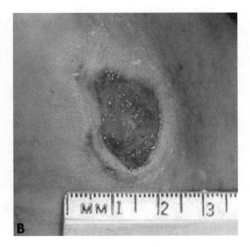

Figure 7-1. (**A**) Baseline photo. (**B**) The appearance of the wound after 2 weeks of topical antibiotic therapy. (Photo courtesy of S. Gardner. See also *color section*, *Patient Scenarios*, page C42, for the color versions of these images.)

Case Discussion

Based on the signs and symptoms, the enabler NERDS, and the wound culture data, it was determined that Mr. L's wound was critically colonized or superficially infected. Having confirmed the presence of adequate circulation and a normal nutritional state, local treatment consisted of twice-daily cleansing with normal saline using a 35-ml syringe and 19-gauge Angiocath followed by topical application of silver sulfadiazine (Silvadene) and covering with a foam dressing. Following 2 weeks of treatment, the wound bed was free of debris and healthy granulation tissue filled the wound space (Fig. 7-1B). The periwound erythema and foul odor had resolved. The wound had decreased in size to 2.7 × 1.6 cm.

1. Which of the following distinguishes a wound colonized with bacteria from one that's infected?
   A. An infected wound will have purulent exudate; a colonized wound won't.
   B. An infected wound will have organisms present in viable tissue; a colonized wound won't.
   C. An infected wound will always have necrotic tissue; a colonized wound won't.
   D. An infected wound will have a positive swab culture; a colonized wound won't.

   ANSWER: B. *For a wound to be infected, organisms must be present in viable tissue and not limited to the wound surface. Purulent exudate may be observed in a colonized wound as well as one that's infected. While necrotic tissue does contain organisms, a wound can be infected without the presence of necrotic tissue. Both an infected wound and a colonized wound will produce a positive swab culture. For the wound to be infected, the organisms must be present in the tissue and not limited to the surface of the wound that has contact with the culture swab.*

2. Which of the following is the most valid indicator of a wound infection?
   A. A swab culture showing large amounts of Staphylococcus
   B. The presence of erythema in the periwound area
   C. Quantitative culture of tissue showing 1,000,000 organisms/g of tissue
   D. Large amounts of serosanguineous exudate on dressings

   ANSWER: C. *Quantitative cultures provide a count of the actual number of organisms present in a standard gram of tissue taken from beneath the wound surface in the wound tissue. Although quantitative swab cultures are fairly comparable to quantitative tissue cultures, tissue cultures remain the gold standard. Erythema is one of the classic signs of inflammation and may arise in response to any type of tissue injury, including, but not limited to, infection. Serosanguinous exudate contains serum and a small number of red blood cells and may be indicative, but not conclusive, of infection.*

3. Antiseptics are a deterrent to healing of clean, granulating wounds because they:
   A. interfere with absorption of nutrients.
   B. discolor the wound tissue.
   C. irritate surrounding skin.
   D. are harmful to fibroblasts and other cells.

   ANSWER: D. *Antiseptics have been documented as toxic to fibroblasts. Although some antiseptics can bleach out the color of wound tissue, this isn't what causes them to disrupt the repair process. While many antiseptics can cause skin irritation if allowed to come in contact with the periwound surface, this isn't the mechanism that interferes with wound repair.*

4. Topical antibiotics for treatment of chronic wounds should be:
   A. used routinely to reduce high bacterial levels.
   B. used routinely to prevent infection.
   C. avoided unless necrotic tissue is present.
   D. avoided in absence of signs of infection.

   ANSWER: D. *Treatment with topical antibiotics is indicated only when signs of infection are present. However, it's important to recognize that a chronic wound may not present with the same signs of infection as an acute wound. Treatment with topical antibiotics isn't indicated unless the wound is infected. Routine use of topical antibiotics for prevention of infection is unnecessary and can lead to development of resistant organisms. Using topical antibiotics in the presence of necrotic tissue isn't effective.*

(continued)

5. Which of the following correctly describes the Levine technique for wound culturing?
A. Obtain a tissue specimen using a sterile scalpel.
B. Aspirate wound fluid using a 21-gauge needle and 10-ml syringe.
C. Swab necrotic tissue prior to cleaning the wound.
D. Rotate swab over a 1-cm-square area with sufficient pressure to express fluid from within the wound tissue.

ANSWER: D. *Rotating a swab over a 1-cm-square area to express fluid from within the wound describes the Levine technique. Using a sterile scalpel and aspirating wound tissue with a needle and syringe are alternate methods of obtaining a wound specimen for culture. C is incorrect. You should never culture necrotic tissue.*

REFERENCES

1. Robson, M.C. "Wound Infection: A Failure of Wound Healing Caused by an Imbalance of Bacteria," *Surgical Clinics of North America* 77(3):637-50, June 1997.
2. Bowler, P.G. "Wound Pathophysiology, Infection, and Therapeutic Options," *Annals of Medicine* 34:419-27, September 2002.
3. Majno, G. *Cells, Tissues, and Disease: Principles of General Pathology.* New York: Oxford University Press, 2004.
4. Abraham, S.N. "Discovering the Benign Traits of the Mast Cell," *Science and Medicine* 3(5):46-55, September-October 1997.
5. McGeer, A., et al. "Definitions of Infection for Surveillance in Long-term-care Facilities," *American Journal of Infection Control* 19(1):1-7, February 1991.
6. Thomson, P.D., and Taddonio, T.E. "Wound Infection," in Krasner, D., and Kane, D., eds., *Chronic Wound Care,* 2nd ed. Wayne, PA: HMP Communications, 1997.
7. Larocco, M. "Inflammation and Immunity," in Porth, C.M., ed., *Pathophysiology: Concepts of Altered Health States,* 4th ed. Philadelphia: Lippincott Williams & Wilkins, 1994.
8. Tarnuzzer, R.W., and Schultz, G.S. "Biochemical Analysis of Acute and Chronic Wound Environments," *Wound Repair and Regeneration* 4(3):321-26, July-September 1996.
9. Sibbald R.G., et al. "Increased Bacterial Burden and Infection: The Story of Nerds and Stones," *Advances in Skin & Wound Care* 19(8):447-61, October 2006.
10. Heggers, J.P., and Robson, M.C. "Prostaglandins and Thromboxanes," in Ninneman, J., ed., *Traumatic Injury-infection and Other Immunological Sequelae.* Baltimore, MD: University Park Press, 1983.
11. Dow, G. "Infection in Chronic Wounds," in *Chronic Wound Care: A Clinical Source Book for Healthcare Professionals,* 3rd ed. Wayne, PA: HMP Communications, 2001.
12. Hunt, T.K., et al. "A New Model for the Study of Wound Infection," *Journal of Trauma* 7(2):298-306, March 1967.
13. Bucknall, T.E. "The Effect of Local Infection upon Wound Healing: An Experimental Study," *British Journal of Surgery* 67(12):851-55, December 1980.
14. Dunphy, J.E. "The Cut Gut," *American Journal of Surgery* 119(1):1-8, January 1970.
15. Lawrence, J.C. "Bacteriology and Wound Healing," in Fox, J.A., and Fischer, J., eds., *Cadexomer Iodine.* Stuttgart: Schattauer Verlag, 1983.
16. Orgill, D., and Demling, R.H. "Current Concepts and Approaches to Wound Healing," *Critical Care Medicine* 16(9):899-908, September 1988.
17. Stenberg, B.D., et al. "Effect of bFGF on the Inhibition of Contraction Caused by Bacteria," *Journal of Surgical Research* 50(1):47-50, January 1991.
18. Renyi, R. "The International Wound Infection Institute: A Global Platform for the Clinical Management of Infected Wounds," *World Council of Enterostomal Therapists Journal* 29(2):27-33, 2009.
19. American College of Surgeons: Committee on the Control of Surgical Infections. *Manual on Control of Infection in Surgical Patients.* Philadelphia: Lippincott Williams & Wilkins, 1976.
20. Baxter, C., and Mertz, P.M. "Local Factors that Affect Wound Healing," *Nursing RSA Verpleging* 7(2):16-23, February 1992.
21. Gilchrist, B. "Treating Bacterial Wound Infection," *Nursing Times* 90(50):55-58, December 1994.
22. Hutchinson, J.J., and McGuckin, M. "Occlusive Dressings: A Microbiologic and Clinical Review," *American Journal of Infection Control* 18(4):256-68, August 1990.

23. Stotts, N.A., and Hunt, T.K. "Pressure Ulcers: Managing Bacterial Colonization and Infection," *Clinics in Geriatric Medicine* 13(3):565-73, August 1997.

24. Barnett, A., et al. "A Concentration Gradient of Bacteria within Wound Tissue and Scab," *Journal of Surgical Research* 41(3):326-32, September 1986.

25. Lookingbill,D.P.,etal. "BacteriologyofChronicLeg Ulcers," *Archives of Dermatology* 114(12):1765-68, December 1978.

26. Robson, M.C., et al. "Wound Healing Alterations Caused by Infection," *Clinics in Plastic Surgery* 17(3):485-92, July 1990.

27. Stotts, N.A., and Whitney, J.D. "Identifying and Evaluating Wound Infection," *Home Healthcare Nurse* 17(3):159-65, March 1999.

28. Kravitz, S. "Infection: Are we defining it accurately?" *Advances in Skin & Wound Care* 19(4):176, May 2006.

29 Grayson, M.L., et al. "Probing to Bone in Infected Pedal Ulcers: A Clinical Sign of Underlying Osteomyelitis in Diabetic Patients," *Journal of the American Medical Association* 273(9):721-23, March 1995.

30. Gilchrist, B. "Infection and Culturing," in Krasner, D., and Kane, D., eds., *Chronic Wound Care,* 2nd ed. Wayne, PA: HMP Communications, 1997.

31. Cicione, J. "Making Waves," *Case Review* 26-29, July-August 1998.

32. American Diabetes Association. "Consensus Conference on Diabetic Foot Wound Care," *Diabetes Care*, 22(8):1354-60, August, 1999.

33. Stotts, N.A. "Promoting Wound Healing," in Kinney, M.R., et al., eds., *AACN's Clinical Reference for Critical Care Nursing*, 4th ed. St. Louis: Mosby–Year Book, Inc., 1998.

34. Horan, T.C., et al. "CDC Definitions of Nosocomial Surgical Site Infections, 1992: A Modification of CDC Definitions of Surgical Wound Infections," *American Journal of Infection Control* 20(5):271-74, October 1992.

35. Gardner, S.E., et al. "The Validity of the Clinical Signs and Symptoms Used to Identify Localized Chronic Wound Infection," *Wound Repair and Regeneration* 9(3):178-86, May-June 2001.

36. Gardner, S.E. et al. "Clinical Signs of Infection in Diabetic Foot Ulcers with High Microbial Loads," *Biological Research for Nursing* 11(2):119-28. October 2009.

37. Steed, D.L. "Diabetic Wounds: Assessment, Classification, and Management," in Krasner, D., and Kane, D., eds., *Chronic Wound Care,* 2nd ed. Wayne, PA: HMP Communications, 1997.

38. Cutting, K.F., and Harding, K.G. "Criteria for Identifying Wound Infection," *Journal of Wound Care* 3(4):198-201, June 1994.

39. Bergstrom, N., et al. *Treatment of Pressure Ulcers. Clinical Practice Guideline, Number 15. AHCPR Publication No. 95-0652.* Rockville, Md.: Agency for Health Care Policy and Research, Public Health Service, U.S. Department of Health and Human Services, December 1994.

40. Cutting, K.F. "Identification of Infection in Granulating Wounds by Registered Nurses," *Journal of Clinical Nursing* 7(6):539-46, November 1998.

41. Gardner, S.E., et al. "A Tool to Assess Clinical Signs and Symptoms of Localized Chronic Wound Infection: Development and Reliability," *Ostomy Wound Management* 47(1):40-47, January 2001.

42. Gardner, S.E. et al. "The Reliability of the Clinical Signs and Symptoms Checklist in Diabetic Foot Ulcers," *Ostomy Wound Management* (in press).

42a. Woo, K.Y., & Sibbald, R.G. "A Cross-sectional Validation Study of Using NERDS and STONES to Assess Bacterial burden," *Ostomy Wound Management* 55(8):40-48, August 2009.

43. Cutting, K.F., et al. "Clinical Identification of Wound Infection: A Delphi Approach," in *EWMA Position Document—Identifying Criteria for Wound Infection.* London: MEP Ltd, pp 6-9, 2005.

44. Robson, M.C., and Heggers, J.P. "Bacterial Quantification of Open Wounds," *Military Medicine* 134(1):19-24, January 1969.

45. Stotts, N.A. "Determination of Bacterial Burden in Wounds," *Advances in Wound Care* 8(4):46-52, July-August 1995.

46. Lee, P., et al. "Fine-needle Aspiration Biopsy in Diagnosis of Soft Tissue Infections," *Journal of Clinical Microbiology* 22(1):80-83, July 1985.

47. Rudensky, B., et al. "Infected Pressure Sores: Comparison of Methods for Bacterial Identification," *Southern Medical Journal* 85(9): 901-903, September 1992.

48. Dow, G., et al. "Infection in Chronic Wounds: Controversies and Treatment," *Ostomy Wound Management* 45(8):23-40, August 1999.

49. Donovan, S. "Wound Infection and Wound Swabbing," *Professional Nurse* 13(11): 757-59, August 1998.

50. Levine, N.S., et al. "The Quantitative Swab Culture and Smear: A Quick, Simple Method for Determining the Number of Viable Aerobic Bacteria on Open Wounds," *Journal of Trauma* 16(2):89-94, February 1976.

51. Morison, M.J. *A Colour Guide to the Nursing Management of Wounds.* Oxford: Blackwell Scientific, November-December 1992.

52. Pagana, K., and Pagana, T.J. *Mosby's Diagnostic and Laboratory Test Reference.* St. Louis: Mosby–Year Book, Inc., 1992.

53. Alvarez, O., et al. "Moist Environment for Healing: Matching the Dressing to the Wound," *Ostomy Wound Management* 21:64-83, Winter 1988.

54. Cooper, R., and Lawrence, J.C. "The Isolation and Identification of Bacteria from Wounds," *Journal of Wound Care* 5(7):335-40, July 1996.

55. Cuzzell, J.Z. "The Right Way to Culture a Wound," *American Journal of Nursing* 93(5):48-50, May 1993.

56. Georgiade, N.G., et al. "A Comparison of Methods for the Quantitation of Bacteria in Burn Wounds I: Experimental Evaluation," *American Journal of Clinical Pathology* 53(1):35-39, January 1970.

57. Bill, T.J., et al. "Quantitative Swab Culture versus Tissue Biopsy: A Comparison in Chronic Wounds," *Ostomy Wound Management* 47(1): 34-37, January 2001.

58. Sapico, F.L., et al. "Quantitative Microbiology of Pressure Sores in Different Stages of Healing," *Diagnostic Microbiology of Infectious Diseases* 5(1):31-38, May 1986.

59. Basak, S., et al. "Bacteriology of Wound Infection: Evaluation by Surface Swab and Quantitative Full Thickness Wound Biopsy Culture," *Journal of the Indian Medical Association* 90(2):33-34, February 1992.

60. Herruzo-Cabrera, R., et al. "Diagnosis of Local Infection of a Burn by Semiquantitative Culture of the Eschar Surface," *Journal of Burn Care & Rehabilitation* 13(6):639-41, November-December 1992.

61. Gardner, S.E. et al. "Diagnostic Validity of Three Swab Techniques for Identifying Chronic Wound Infections," *Wound Repair and Regeneration* (in press).

62. Bonham, P.A. "Swab Cultures for Diagnosing Wound Infections: A Literature Review and Clinical Guideline," *Journal of Wound, Ostomy & Continence Nursing* 36(4):389-95, Jul-Aug 2009.

63. Robson, M.C., and Heggers, J.P. "Quantitative Bacteriology and Inflammatory Mediators in Soft Tissue," in Hunt, T.K., et al., eds., *Biological and Clinical Aspects of Soft and Hard Tissue Repair.* New York: Praeger Pubs., 1984.

64. Garner, J.S., et al. "CDC Definitions for Nosocomial Infections, 1988," *American Journal of Infection Control* 16(3):128-40, June 1988.

65. Peromet, M., et al. "Anaerobic Bacteria Isolated from Decubitus Ulcers," *Infection* 1(4):205-207, December 1973.

66. Chow, A.W., et al. "Clindamycin for Treatment of Sepsis by Decubitus Ulcers," *Journal of Infectious Disease* 135(suppl):S65-S68, March 1977.

67. Vaziri, N.D., et al. "Bacterial Infections in Patients with Chronic Renal Failure: Occurrence with Spinal Cord Injury," *Archives of Internal Medicine* 142(7):1273-76, July 1982.

68. Bryan, C.S., et al. "Bacteremia Associated with Decubitus Ulcers," *Archives of Internal Medicine* 143(11):2093-95, November 1983.

69. Gilchrist, B., and Reed, C. "The Bacteriology of Chronic Venous Ulcers Treated with Occlusive Hydrocolloid Dressings," *British Journal of Dermatology* 121(3):337-44, September 1989.

70 Trengove, N.J., et al. "Qualitative Bacteriology and Leg Ulcer Healing," *Journal of Wound Care* 5(6):277-80, June 1996.

71. Bendy, R.H., et al. "Relationship of Quantitative Wound Bacterial Counts to Healing of Decubiti: Effect of Topical Gentamicin," *Antimicrobial Agents and Chemotherapy* 4:147-55, 1964.

72. Daltrey, D.C., et al. "Investigation into the Microbial Flora of Healing and Non-healing Decubitus Ulcers," *Journal of Clinical Pathology* 34(7):701-705, July 1981.

73 Roghmann, M.C., et al. "MRSA Colonization and the Risk of MRSA Bacteraemia in Hospitalized Patients with Chronic Ulcers," *Journal of Hospital Infection* 47(2):98-103, February 2001.

74. Leaper, D.J. "Defining Infection," *Journal of Wound Care* 7(8):373, September 1998.

75. Absolon, K.B., et al. "From Antisepsis to Asepsis: Louis Pasteur's Publication on 'The Germ Theory and its Application to Medicine and Surgery,'" *Review of Surgery* 27(4):245-58, July-August 1970.

76. Elek, S.D. "Experimental Staphylococcal Infections in the Skin of Man," *Annals of the New York Academy of Science* 65:85, 1956.

77. Hepburn, H.H. "Delayed Primary Suture of Wounds," *British Medical Journal* 1:181-83, 1919.

78. Krizek, T.J., and Davis, J.H. "Endogenous Wound Infection," *Journal of Trauma* 6(2):239-48, March 1966.

79. Krizek, T.J., and Davis, J.H. "Experimental Pseudomonas Burn Sepsis: Evaluation of Topical Therapy," *Journal of Trauma* 7(3):433-42, May 1967.

80. Noyes, H.E., et al. "Delayed Topical Antimicrobials as Adjuncts to Systemic Antibiotic Therapy of War Wounds: Bacteriologic Studies," *Military Medicine* 132(6):461-68, June 1967.

81. Lindberg, R.B., et al. "The Successful Control of Burn Wound Sepsis," *Journal of Trauma* 5(5):601-16, September 1965.

82. Shuck, J.M., and Moncrief, J.A. "The Management of Burns: Part I. General Considerations and the Sulfamylon Method," *Current Problems in Surgery* 352, February 1969.

83. Teplitz, C., et al. "Pseudomonas Burn Wound Sepsis. I. Pathogens of Experimental Burn Wound Sepsis," *Journal of Surgical Research* 4:200-16, May 1964.

84. Rodeheaver, G.T., and Frantz, R.A. "14. Guideline: Bacterial Control," in Bergstrom, N., and Cuddigan, J., eds., *Treating Pressure Ulcers.*

Guideline Technical Report, Number 15, Volume 1. Rockville, Md.: U. S. Department of Health and Human Services, Public Health Service, Agency for Health Care Policy and Research, AHCPR Publication No. 96-N014, 1994.

85. Krizek, T.J., and Robson, M.C. "Evolution of Quantitative Bacteriology in Wound Management," *American Journal of Surgery* 130(5):579-84, November 1975.

86. Heggers, J.P. "Variations on a Theme," in Heggers, J.P., and Robson, M.C., eds. *Quantitative Bacteriology: Its Role in the Armamentarium of the Surgeon.* Boca Raton, FL: CRC Press, 1991.

87. Robson, M.C. Personal communication, May 29, 2002.

88. Johnson, S. et al. "Use of an Anaerobic Collection and Transport Swab Device to Recover Anaerobic Bacteria From Infected Foot Ulcers in Diabetics," *Clinical Infectious Diseases* 20(Suppl 2):S289-S290, June 1995.

89. Lineaweaver, W., et al. "Topical Antimicrobial Toxicity," *Archives of Surgery* 120(3):267-70, March 1985.

90. Fernandez R.S., et al. "Water for Wound Cleansing (Review)," *The Cochrane Database of Systemic Reviews Issue 4*, Hoboken, NJ: John Wiley & Sons, Ltd., 2006.

91. Foresman, P.A., et al. "A Relative Toxicity Index for Wound Cleansers," *Wounds* 5(5):226-31, September-October 1993.

92. Wright, R.W., and Orr, R. "Fibroblast Cytotoxicity and Blood Cell Integrity Following Exposure to Dermal Wound Cleansers," *Ostomy Wound Management* 39(7):33-36, 38, 40, September 1993.

93. Wilson, J.R., et al. "A Toxicity Index of Skin and Wound Cleansers Used on *in Vitro* Fibroblasts and Keratinocytes," *Advances in Sin & Wound Care* 18(7):373-378, July 2005.

94. Zamora, J.L., et al. "Inhibition of Povidone-iodine's Bactericidal Activity by Common Organic Substances: An Experimental Study," *Surgery* 98(1):25-29, July 1985.

95. Fleming, A. "The Action of Chemical and Physiological Antiseptics in a Septic Wound," *British Journal of Surgery* 7:99-129, February 1919.

96. Lacey, R.W. "Antibacterial Activity of Povidone Towards Non-sporing Bacteria," *The Journal of Applied Bacteriology* 46(3):443-49, June 1979.

97. Cooper, M.L., et al. "The Cytotoxic Effects of Commonly Used Topical Antimicrobial Agents on Human Fibroblasts and Keratinocytes," *Journal of Trauma* 31(6):775-84, June 1991.

98. Teepe, R.G., et al. "Cytotoxic Effects of Topical Antimicrobial and Antiseptic Agents on Human Keratinocytes In Vitro," *Journal of Trauma* 35(1):8-19, July1993.

99. Branemark, P.I., and Ekholm, R. "Tissue Injury Caused by Wound Disinfectants," *Journal of Bone and Joint Surgery American* 49(1):48-62, January 1967.

100. Brennan, S.S., et al. "The Effect of Antiseptics on the Healing Wound: A Study Using the Ear Chamber," *British Journal of Surgery* 72(10):780-82, October 1985.

101. Cotter, J.L., et al. "Chemical Parameters, Antimicrobial Activities, and Tissue Toxicity of 0.1% and 0.5% Sodium Hypochlorite Solutions," *Antimicrobial Agents Chemotherapeutics* 9(1):118-22, July 1985.

102. Brennan, S.S., et al. "Antiseptic Toxicity in Wounds Healing by Secondary Intention," *Journal of Hospital Infection* 8(3):263-67, November 1986.

103. Becker, G.D. "Identification and Management of the Patient at High Risk for Wound Infection," *Head and Neck Surgery* 8:205-10, January-February 1986.

104. Viljanto, J. "Disinfection of Surgical Wounds without Inhibition of Normal Wound Healing," *Archives of Surgery* 115:253-56, March 1980.

105. Hellewell, T.B., et al. "A Cytotoxicity Evaluation of Antimicrobial and Non-antimicrobial Wound Cleansers," *Wounds* 9(1):15-20, January 1997.

106. Kucan, J.O., et al. "Comparison of Silver Sulfadiazine, Povidone-iodine and Physiologic Saline in the Treatment of Chronic Pressure Ulcers," *Journal of the American Geriatric Society* 29(5):232-35, May 1981.

107. Carrel, A., and Dehelly, G. *The Treatment of Infected Wounds.* New York: Hoeber, 1917.

108. American Medical Association. *AMA Drug Evaluation,* 10th ed. Chicago: American Medical Association, 1994.

109. Sundberg, J., and Meller, R. "A Retrospective Review of the Use of Cadexomer Iodine in the Treatment of Chronic Wounds," *Wounds* 9(3): 68-86, May-June 1997.

110. Sibbald, R.G. "Topical Antimicrobials," *Ostomy Wound Management* 49(5A Suppl):14-18, May 2003.

111. Edwards, R., & Harding, K.G. "Bacteria and Wound Healing," *Current Opinion in Infectious Diseases* 17(2):91-96, April 2004.

112. Falanga, V. "The Chronic wound: Impaired Healing and Solutions in the Contest of Wound Bed Preparation," *Blood Cells and Molecular Disease* 31(1):88-94, January-February 2004.

113. Rodeheaver, G.T., et al. "Mechanical Cleaning of Contaminated Wounds with a Surfactant," *American Journal of Surgery* 129(3):241-45, March 1975.

114. Madden, J., et al. "Application of Principles of Fluid Dynamics to Surgical Wound Irrigation," *Current Topics in Surgical Research* 3:85-93, 1971.

115. Rodeheaver, G.T., et al. "Wound Cleaning by High Pressure Irrigation," *Surgical Gynecology and Obstetrics* 141(3):357-62, September 1975.

116. Grower, M.F., et al. "Effect of Water Lavage on Removal of Tissue Fragments from Crush Wounds," *Oral Surgery Oral Medicine Oral Pathology* 33(6):1031-36, June 1972.

117. Green, V.A., et al. "A Comparison of the Efficacy of Pulsed Mechanical Lavage with That of Rubber-bulb Syringe Irrigation in Removal of Debris from Avulsive Wounds," *Oral Surgery Oral Medicine Oral Pathology* 32(1):158-64, July 1971.

118. Stewart, J.L., et al. "The Bacteria-removal Efficiency of Mechanical Lavage and Rubber-bulb Syringe Irrigation in Contaminated Avulsive Wounds," *Oral Surgery Oral Medicine Oral Pathology* 31(6):842-48, June 1971.

119. Bhaskar, S.N., et al. "Effect of Water Lavage on Infected Wounds in the Rat," *Journal of Periodontology* 40(11):671-72, November 1969.

120. Carlson, H.C., et al. "Effect of Pressure and Tip Modification on the Dispersion of Fluid Throughout Cells and Tissues During the Irrigation of Experimental Wounds," *Oral Surgery Oral Medicine Oral Pathology* 32(2):347-55, August 1971.

121. Wheeler, C.B., et al. "Side Effects of High Pressure Irrigation," *Surgical Gynecology and Obstetrics* 143(5):775-78, November 1976.

122. Stevenson, T.R., et al. "Cleansing the Traumatic Wound by High Pressure Syringe Irrigation," *Journal of the American College of Emergency Physicians* 5(1):1721, January 1976.

123. Longmire, A.W., et al. "Wound Infection Following High-pressure Syringe and Needle Irrigation" [Letter to the editor], *American Journal of Emergency Medicine* 5(2):179-818, March 1987.

124. Singer, A.J., et al. "Pressure Dynamics of Various Irrigation Techniques Commonly Used in the Emergency Department," *Annals of Emergency Medicine* 24(1):36-40, July 1994.

125. Loehne, H. "Pulsatile Lavage with Concurrent Suction," in Sussman, C., and Bates-Jensen, B.M., eds., *Wound Care: A Collaborative Practice Manual for Physical Therapists and Nurses,* 1st ed. Gaithersburg, MD: Aspen Pubs., 1998.

126. Ho, C., et al. "Healing with Hydrotherapy," *Advances for Directors in Rehabilitation* 7(5):45-49, 1998.

127. Morgan, D., and Hoelscher, J. "Pulsed Lavage: Promoting Comfort and Healing in Home Care," *Ostomy Wound Management* 46(4):44-49, April 2000.

128. Haynes, L.J., et al., "Comparison of Pulsavac and Sterile Whirlpool Regarding the Promotion of Tissue Granulation," *Physical Therapy* 74(5 Suppl):S4, May 1994.

129. Bohannon, R.W. "Whirlpool Versus Whirlpool Rinse for Removal of Bacteria from a Venous Stasis Ulcer," *Physical Therapy* 62(3):304-308, March 1982.

130. Neiderhuber, S., et al. "Reduction of Skin Bacterial Load with Use of Therapeutic Whirlpool," *Physical Therapy* 55(5):482-86, May 1975.

131. Moues, C.M., et al. "Bacterial Load in Relation to Vacuum-assisted Closure Wound Therapy: A Prospective Randomized Trial," *Wound Repair and Regeneration* 12(1):11-17, January-February 2004.

132. Braakenburg, A. et al. "The Clinical Efficacy and Cost Effectiveness of the Vacuum-assisted Closure Technique in the Management of Acute and Chronic Wounds: A Randomized Controlled Trial," *Plastic and Reconstructive Surgery* 118(2):3907, August, 2006.

133. Deva, A.K., et al. "Topical Negative Pressure in Wound Management," *Medical Journal of Australia* 173(3):128-31, August 2000.

134. Pinocy, J., et al. "Treatment of Periprosthetic Soft Tissue Infection of the Groin Following Vascular Surgical Procedures by Means of a Polyvinyl Alcohol-vacuum Sponge System," *Wound Repair Regeneration* 11(2):104-9, March-April 2003.

135. Morykwas, M.J., et al. "Vacuum-assisted Closure: A New Method for Wound Control and Treatment: Animal Studies and Basic Foundation," *Annals of Plastic Surgery* 38(6):553-62, June 1997.

136. Gabriel, A., Shores, J., Bernstein, B., et al. "A Clinical Review of Infected Wound Treatment with Vacuum-assisted Closure (V.A.C.) Therapy: Experience and Case Series." *International Wound Journal* 6(suppl 2):1-25, October 2009.

137. Robson, M.C., et al. "The Efficacy of Systemic Antibiotics in the Treatment of Granulating Wounds," *Journal of Surgical Research* 16(4):299-306, April 1974.

137a. Ovington, L.G. "The Truth About Silver," *Ostomy Wound Management* 50(9A Suppl):1S-10S, September, 2004.

138. Stadelmann, W.K., et al. "Impediments to Wound Healing," *American Journal of Surgery* 176(Suppl 2A):39S-47S, August 1998.

139. Zhou, L.H., et al. "Slow Release Iodine Preparation and Wound Healing: *In Vitro* Effects Consistent with Lack of *In Vivo* Toxicity in Human Chronic Wounds," *British Journal of Dermatology* 146(3):365-74, March 2002.

140. Fumal, I., et al. "The Beneficial Toxicity Paradox of Antimicrobials in Leg Ulcer Healing Impaired by a Polymicrobial Flora: A Proof-of-Concept Study," *Dermatology* 70(Suppl 1):70-74, 2002.

141. Bowler, P.G., et al. "Microbicidal Properties of a Silver-containing Hydrofiber Dressing Against a Variety of Burn Wound Pathogens," *Journal of Burn Care Rehabilitation* 25(2):192-96, March-April 2004.

142. Poon, V.K.M., et al. "*In vitro* Cytotoxicity of Silver: Implications for Clinical Wound Care," *Burns* 30(2):140-47, March 2004.

143. Innes, M.E., et al. "The Use of Silver Coated Dressings on Donor Site Wounds: a Prospective, Controlled Matched Pair Study," *Burns* 27(6): 621-27, September 2001.

144. Bolton, L. "Are Silver Products Safe and Effective for Chronic Wound Management?" *Journal of Wound, Ostomy & Continence Nursing* 33(5):469-477, September/October, 2006.

145. Tomaselli, N. "The Role of Topical Silver Preparation in Wound Healing." *Journal of Wound, Ostomy & Continence Nursing* 33(4):367-380, July/August, 2006.

146. Bergin, S.M., and Wraight, P. "Silver Based Wound Dressings and Topical Agents for Treating Diabetic Foot Ulcers," *The Cochrane Collaboration*, Issue 5, 2010.

147. Parsons, D. et al. "Silver Antimicrobial Dressings in Wound Management: A Comparison of Antibacterial, Physical, and Chemical Characteristics," *Wounds* 17(8):22-232, August 2005.

148. Johnson, C.A. "Hearing Loss Following the Application of Topical Neomycin," *Journal of Burn Care and Rehabilitation* 9(2):162-64, March-April 1988.

149. Schechter, J.F., et al. "Anaphylaxis Following the Use of Bacitracin Ointment. Report of a Case and Review of the Literature," *Archives of Dermatology* 120(7):909-11, July 1984.

150. Zamboni, W.A., et al. "Evaluation of Hyperbaric Oxygen for Diabetic Wounds: A Prospective Study," *Undersea Hyperbaric Medicine* 24(3):175-79, September 1997.

151. Thai, T.P., et al. "Effect of Ultraviolet Light C on Bacterial Colonization in Chronic Wounds," *Ostomy Wound Management* 51(10):32-45, October 2005.

152. Fakhri, O., et al. "The Effect of Low-Voltage Electric Therapy on the Healing of Resistant Skin Burns," *Journal of Burn Care Research* 8(1):15-18, January-February 1987.

153. Guffey, J.S., et al. "*In Vitro* Bactericidal Effects of High Voltage Pulsed Current Versus Direct Current Against *Staphylococcus aureus*," *Journal of Clinical Electrophysiology* 1(1):5-9, January 1989.

154. Kincaid, C., et al. "Inhibition of Bacterial Growth *In Vitro* Following Stimulation with High Voltage, Monophasic, Pulsed Current," *Physical Therapy* 69(8):651-55, August 1989.

155. Szuminsky, N.J., et al. "Effect of Narrow, Pulsed High Voltages on Bacterial Viability," *Physical Therapy* 74(7):660-67, July 1994.

CHAPTER 8

Wound Debridement

Elizabeth A. Ayello, PhD, RN, ACNS-BC, CWON, MAPWCA, FAAN
Sharon Baranoski, MSN, RN, CWCN, APN-CCNS, DAPWCA, FAAN
R. Gary Sibbald, BSc, MD, MEd, FRCPC (Med)(Derm), MACP, FAAD, HAPWCA
Janet E. Cuddigan, PhD, RN, CWCN

Objectives

After completing this chapter, you'll be able to:

- state the purpose of debriding a wound
- list criteria for *not* debriding a necrotic wound
- describe types of debridement, including sharp/surgical, mechanical, maggot, enzymatic, and autolytic
- compare the advantages and disadvantages of each type of debridement
- select the most appropriate method of debridement depending on patient preference, clinician expertise, and healthcare system resources.

SPEEDING THE HEALING PROCESS

Debridement is an important component of the wound bed preparation (WBP) management model.[1] After considering the cause of the wound and patient-centered concerns, debridement is a necessary step in local wound care.[1,2] Debridement is the removal of necrotic tissue, exudate, bacteria, and metabolic waste from a wound in order to improve or facilitate the healing process.[3] Accumulation of necrotic tissue usually results from poor blood supply, a prolonged inflammatory process, bacterial damage, or an untreated cause of the wound (for example, increased interstitial pressure or other mechanical, chemical, or traumatic injury). In otherwise healthy people, natural debridement keeps pace with the accumulation of dying tissue in a wound. If the host resistance is impaired by poor nutrition, continued pressure damage, or other comorbidities such as diabetes, medical intervention is required to facilitate wound healing.

The primary purpose of debridement is to reduce or remove dead and necrotic tissue in a healable wound because this tissue is a proinflammatory stimulus and a culture medium for bacterial growth.[1,3] The removal of dead and necrotic tissue is necessary to reduce the biological burden of the wound in order to control and prevent wound infection, especially in deteriorating wounds.[4] Debridement allows the practitioner to visualize the sides and base of a wound more accurately to determine whether viable tissue is present. (Keep in mind that a pressure ulcer that is covered with necrotic tissue cannot be numerically staged until debridement is completed.). Necrotic tissue that is not removed not only impedes wound healing but also can result in spread of bacterial damage to deeper tissue, causing surrounding cellulitis, osteomyelitis, and the possibility of septicemia, limb amputation, or death. By removing necrotic tissue, debridement creates an acute wound within a chronic wound, restoring circulation and allowing adequate oxygen delivery to the wound site.[5]

For a wound to heal, it must have a microenvironment free from the nonviable tissue that serves as a bacterial culture medium to increase organism proliferation.[6] Oxygen is a primary requirement for this energy-dependent metabolic process to occur. The production of free radicals kills bacteria, facilitating the proliferation of fibroblasts and epithelial cells, which are crucial for wound healing. However, bacteria that are present in hypoxic conditions compete with healing tissue for nutrients and produce exotoxins and endotoxins that damage newly generated, mature cells. This setting of hypoxia and bacteria interrupts the fundamental wound healing process of fibroblast migration into the extracellular matrix. Fibroblasts, which produce the fibrils of collagen, help lay the foundation for new cell growth. This process allows a chronic wound stuck in the inflammatory stage to move to the proliferative stage, promoting new tissue formation and laying the foundation for healing with the necessary recruitment of fibroblasts to deposit collagen.[6]

Leukocytes—primarily polymorphonuclear leukocytes—are the primary cells of the inflammatory process of wound healing. They enter the wound and remove devitalized tissue and foreign material. Collaboration of local enzymes (proteolytic, fibrinolytic, or collagenolytic) also helps to dissolve and remove devitalized tissue. Because collagen comprises approximately 75% of the skin's dry weight, the overall endogenous collagenase is considered to be one of the main regulators of tissue remodeling in the process of wound healing. Remodeling is part of the healing process in which the wound restructures into its final functional image.

After a wound is cleaned, macrophages are recruited; they, in turn, recruit fibroblasts, which deposit collagen and fill the wound with scar tissue. An acute wound with a good blood supply and essential nutrients generally "heals" within 14 days—but this doesn't represent the total healing process. Remodeling, or maturation, typically takes another 4 weeks, making the total healing process about 6 weeks. Other factors may be involved in the healing process as well. For example, a wound that appears in an area of rich blood supply such as the scalp will heal faster than a wound in an area with a lesser blood supply. Collagen breakdown and collagen buildup occur in equal degrees, resulting in an appropriate-appearing scar. However, excess collagen can form a keloid or hypertrophic scar. A hypertrophic scar represents disordered collagen within the scar tissue of a healed wound. A keloid extends beyond the wound margin with a greater disorganization of collagen fibers.

Identifying necrotic tissue

Dead or necrotic tissue may be loose and moist, or dry and firm. This tissue is identified by its moist, yellow, green, or gray appearance and may become thick and leathery with a dry black eschar. (See *color section*, *Eschar*, page C10.) Oxygen and nutrients can't penetrate a wound that is impaired by necrotic tissue. Dead tissue is the breeding ground for bacteria, and the eschar may mask an underlying abscess.[7] Necrotic tissue that is soft, moist, stringy, and yellow is referred to as slough (devitalized/avascular) tissue).[8-10] While some clinical experts have questioned whether slough is in fact tissue or an inflammatory by-product,[11] the National Pressure Ulcer Advisory Panel (NPUAP)/European Pressure Ulcer Advisory Panel (EPUAP) clinical practice guideline, entitled "Prevention and Treatment of Pressure Ulcers," did define slough as "soft, moist, devitalized (avascular) tissue. It may be white, yellow, tan, or green and it may be loose or firmly adherent."[12] (See *color section*, *Slough*, page C10.) Regardless of whether slough is or is not tissue, clinicians agree that it must be removed in acute and chronic wounds in order for the wounds to heal.[9-13]

In general, removing necrotic tissue restores the local vascular supply to the wound and improves healing. However, debriding too much viable tissue can destroy the collagen structural framework for healing. Some wounds shouldn't be debrided at all. Exercise caution, for example, in dealing with necrotic ulcers on ischemic limbs, which may have poor perfusion.[1,12] Debriding heel ulcers remains controversial because of problems with perfusion and the small amount of tissue that covers the calcaneus bone.[9,12] There is consensus that an adequate vascular supply is necessary prior to debridement of ulcers in the lower extremities.[1,9,12] The controversy revolves around whether to debride stable, adherent eschar with no exudate or signs of infection; some clinicians believe that although caution is indicated, all necrotic heels should be debrided.[1,8-10,12,13] Wounds become larger with debridement, something that should be discussed with the patient/family.

Pyoderma gangrenosum is one example of a wound that should not be debrided. Debridement will exacerbate the active lesions and increase the size of the raised active border.[2] A raised active border indicates an acute inflammatory reaction, and debridement would stimulate the infiltrate even more through a process called *pathergy*.[2] Septicemia is another condition that requires serious caution before initiating debridement. The wounds of patients with septicemia should not be debrided unless the patient is receiving systemic antibacterial coverage.[2]

PRACTICE POINT

Monitor stable necrotic heels for odor and signs of edema, erythema, fluid wave, or drainage, which may signal the need for debridement.[12]

PRACTICE POINT

It's often important to watch the line of demarcation between viable and necrotic tissue for signs of further tissue breakdown or softening eschar.

Chronic wound care begins with treating the cause and patient-centered concerns, including pain and activities of daily living. Assess individual patients to determine whether the wound is healable, maintenance, or non-healable. To assess healability, an adequate blood supply needs to be present.[1,12] Palpable pulses in the foot indicate a pressure in excess of 80 mm Hg and enough blood supply for healing to occur. This finding could equate to an ankle-brachial pressure index of 0.6 or higher. If there is a sufficient blood supply and the cause has been corrected (compression for venous ulcers and pressure offloading for diabetic neurotrophic foot ulcers), the ulcer is healable. For pressure ulcers, the source of tissue damage needs to be corrected, including high blood pressure, poor nutrition, friction and shear, decreased mobility, or excess local moisture. Active debridement can be coupled with moisture and bacterial-balanced dressings.

A maintenance wound is one that has a sufficient blood supply for healing but is unable to heal due to patient or health delivery system factors. Debridement and local wound care should then be conservative for maintenance wounds. A non-healable or palliative wound does not have enough blood supply to heal; therefore, debridement should be conservative and limited to soft slough with a local antimicrobial (such as povidone-iodine or chlorhexidine) and moisture reduction to reduce local bacteria.

Although it is acknowledged that debridement is a critical first step in preparing the wound bed for healing, all of the recommendations on debridement from the international NPUAP/EPUAP clinical practice guideline are at the C level of knowledge.[12] (See *Debridement Recommendations: NPUAP/EPUAP Clinical Practice Guideline,* page 160.)

Wound bed preparation (WBP) is the management of a wound to accelerate endogenous healing or to facilitate the effectiveness of other therapeutic measures.[1,3,13] The original TIME model—**T**issue nonviable or deficient, **I**nfection or inflammation, **M**oisture imbalance, **E**pidermal margin non-advancing or undermining[3]—has been reconceptualized to the **DIME**© model.[1,12,13] (See *TIME is now DIME: Wound bed preparation DIME© model,* page 161.)[13] As mentioned, you should first identify and treat the cause of the wound, address patient-centered concerns, and provide local wound care. (See *Best practices for preparing the wound bed,* page 162.)[13]

Debridement recommendations: NPUAP/EPUAP Clinical Practice Guideline

1. Debride devitalized tissue within the wound bed or edge of pressure ulcers when appropriate to the individual's condition and consistent with overall goals of care. (Strength of Evidence = C)

2. Select the debridement method(s) most appropriate to: the individual's condition; goals of care; ulcer/periulcer status; type, quantity, and location of necrotic tissue; care setting; and professional accessibility/capability. (Strength of Evidence = C)

3. Use mechanical, autolytic, enzymatic, and/or biosurgical methods of debridement when there is no urgent clinical need for drainage or removal of necrotic tissue. (Strength of Evidence = C)

4. Perform surgical debridement in the presence of advancing cellulitis, crepitus, fluctuance, and/or sepsis secondary to ulcer-related infection. (Strength of Evidence = C)

5. Sharp/surgical debridement must be performed by specially trained, competent, qualified and licensed healthcare professionals consistent with local legal and regulatory statutes. (Strength of Evidence = C)

6. Use sterile instrument to sharply/surgically debride. (Strength of Evidence = C)

7. Use sharp debridement with caution in the presence of: immune incompetence, compromised vascular supply to the limb, lack of antibacterial coverage in systemic sepsis. Relative contraindications include anticoagulant therapy and bleeding disorders. (Strength of Evidence = C)

8. Refer individuals with Category/Stage III or IV pressure ulcers with undermining, tunneling, sinus tracts, and/or extensive necrotic tissue that cannot be easily removed by the other debridement methods for surgical evaluation as is appropriate with the individual's condition and goals of care. (Strength of Evidence = C)

9. Manage pain associated with debridement. (Strength of Evidence = C)

10. Perform a through vascular assessment prior to debridement of lower extremity pressure ulcers (e.g., rule out arterial insufficiency). (Strength of Evidence = C)

11. Do not debride stable, hard dry eschar in ischemic limbs(Strength of Evidence = C)

   11.1 Assess the wound daily for signs of erythema, tenderness, edema, purulence, fluctuance, crepitance, and/or malodor (i.e., signs of infection). (Strength of Evidence = C)

   11.2 Consult a vascular surgeon urgently in the presence of the above symptoms. (Strength of Evidence = C) (Strength of Evidence = C)

   11.3 Debride urgently in the presence of the above symptoms if consistent with the individual's wishes and overall goals of care (Strength of Evidence = C)

12. Perform maintenance debridement on a chronic pressure ulcer until the wound bed is covered with granulation tissue and free of necrotic tissue. (Strength of Evidence = C)

National Pressure Ulcer Advisory Panel and European Pressure Ulcer Advisory Panel. *Prevention and Treatment of Pressure Ulcers: Clinical Practice Guideline.* Washington, DC: National Pressure Ulcer Advisory Panel, 2009, pp 77-80.

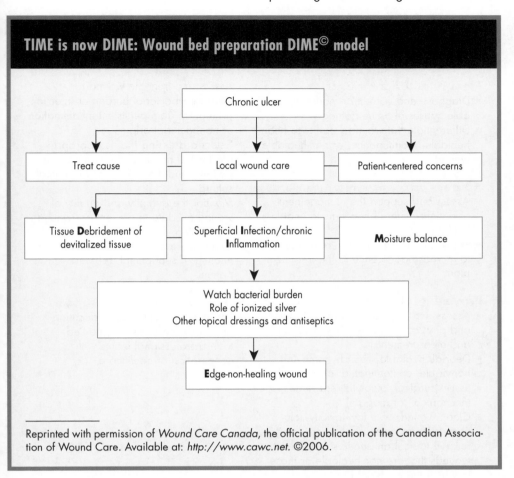

TIME is now DIME: Wound bed preparation DIME© model

Chronic ulcer

Treat cause — Local wound care — Patient-centered concerns

Tissue **D**ebridement of devitalized tissue — Superficial **I**nfection/chronic **I**nflammation — **M**oisture balance

Watch bacterial burden
Role of ionized silver
Other topical dressings and antiseptics

Edge-non-healing wound

Reprinted with permission of *Wound Care Canada*, the official publication of the Canadian Association of Wound Care. Available at: *http://www.cawc.net.* ©2006.

PRACTICE POINT

Save time and use the DIME[1,3,13] acronym in preparing the wound bed for healing.

- **D**ebridement
- **I**nfection or inflammation
- **M**oisture imbalance
- **E**dge-non-healing

Predebridement teaching

Patient-centered care should include teaching about the purpose and usual expecta-

tions of the debriding process. This process needs to be explained and understood by the patient and family *before* initiating treatment. Include in your teaching the debridement method that will be used and the desired outcome. It is vital that the patient and family understand why the necrotic tissue is being removed. Some laypersons mistakenly believe that necrotic tissue is a "scab" (eschar) and is a sign of healing. They need to know that epithelium needs a firm granulation base to migrate optimally toward the center of a wound. Delayed healing will result if epithelial margins need to migrate down valleys under eschar or over hypertrophic or unhealthy granulation tissue. Similarly, patients and families need to know that the

Best practices for preparing the wound bed

Identify and treat the cause
- Diagnose and correct or modify treatable causes of tissue damage
- Differentiate the wound's ability to heal: healable, maintenance, or non-healable wound

Address patient-centered concerns
- Assess and support the management of patient-centered concerns to enable healing
- Provide patient education and support to increase adherence to the treatment plan

Provide local wound care
- Assess and monitor the wound history and physical characteristics (location and measurements)
- Debride healable wounds, removing nonviable, contaminated, or infected tissue (surgical, autolytic, enzymatic, mechanical, or maggot)
- Clean wounds with low-toxicity solutions (such as normal saline or water); reserve topical antiseptic solutions for wounds that are non-healable or those in which the bacterial burden is of greater concern than the stimulation of healing

- Assess and treat the wound for increased bacterial burden or infection; distinguish from persistent inflammation of nonbacterial origin
- Select a dressing that is appropriate for the needs of the wound, the patient, and the caregiver or clinical setting
- Monitor the quantity and quality of wound exudate to prevent periwound maceration
- Evaluate expected rate of wound healing; if suboptimal, reassess patient

Provide organizational support
- For improved outcomes, education and evidence base must be tied to interprofessional teams with cooperation of healthcare systems

Reprinted with permission *Wound Care Canada*, the official publication of the Canadian Association of Wound Care. Available at: http://www.cawc.net ©2006. All Rights Reserved. Secondary source: Sibbald, R.G., et al. "Best Practice Recommendations for Preparing the Wound Bed: Update 2006," *Wound Care Canada* 4(1):15-29, 2006.

wound will change during the debridement process because an acute wound is created within a chronic wound to stimulate the healing process. For example, tell them to expect a wound to become larger in size.

DEBRIDEMENT METHODS

Mechanical, sharp/surgical, enzymatic, and autolytic are the common methods of debridement.[1,2,9,12-17] However, a resurgence in

Overview of debridement methods

Method	Considerations	Contraindications
Surgical/sharp		
Necrotic tissue is removed using a scalpel, scissors, forceps, or curette	• Urgent need for debridement • Highly selective • Rapid results • Pain unless the patient has neuropathy; analgesia often needed • Risk of hemorrhage/complications • Cost; use of special equipment • Requires patient consent • Requires special training and expert confidence level (including anatomic knowledge) • Must distinguish between necrotic and healthy tissues • Can be done at bedside • May require an operating room and systemic anesthetics for extensive procedures • Anticoagulant therapy	• Malignant wounds • Patients with clotting/bleeding abnormalities • Ischemic tissue • Unstable • Underlying dialysis fistula, prosthesis, or arterial bypass graft • Caution with wounds involving hands and face • Caution with immunocompromised patients
Autolyic		
Endogenous enzymes present in wound fluid interact with moist dressing to soften and remove necrotic tissue	• Need for minor or moderate debridement • Patient has a decreased or minimal risk of wound infection • Performed in any setting • Can be used with other methods • Selective • Safe, easy to use • Painless and soothing when dressing in place • Slow • Risk of maceration to surrounding skin • Removal of some dressings may be painful • Odor • Secondary dressing needed for some types of primary dressings • Absorptive dressing can dehydrate the wound bed	• Some dressings cannot be used with infected wounds • Exposed tendon/bone • Friable skin • Deep extensive wounds • Severe neutropenia • Immunocompromised patients

(continued)

Overview of debridement methods (continued)

Method	Considerations	Contraindications
Mechanical		
Wet-to-dry: moist dressing is applied to wound, allowed to dry, and removed with force	• Larger wounds • Nonsurgical candidates • Nonselective • Painful • Frequent dressing changes required, may need to be done 2 to 3 times a day; not cost-effective • May macerate surrounding skin • Bleeding • Dressing fibers stick to wound and can cause a foreign body reaction • May disperse bacteria when removed • Traditional more than a modern accepted practice	• Clean wounds
Hydrotherapy: moving water dislodges loose debris	• Increases circulation to wound bed • May macerate periwound skin • Time-consuming • May cause trauma to wound bed and lead to bacterial contamination of wound and environment • Labor-intensive • Theoretical risk of fluid embolism or promotion of infection with irrigation • Healthcare professional needs personal protective equipment due to aerosolization • Can impede venous blood flow in legs	• Clean wounds • Presence of diabetic neuropathy
Pulsed lavage: irrigation combined with suction	• Bed-bound patients • Wound with large amount of necrotic tissue	• Clean wounds

(continued)

Overview of debridement methods (continued)

Method	Considerations	Contraindications
Maggot larvae (*Lucillia sericata*—green bottle fly)		
Break down necrotic tissue and digest bacteria	• Psychological distress to patients or clinicians • Allergic reaction • Potential for increased pain in ischemic wounds • Time-consuming • Selective debridement • Rapid • Costly • May be painless • Decrease bacterial load • Bedside use • Can be used for various wound types, including infected wounds	• Allergies to adhesives, fly larvae, eggs, soybeans • Patients with bleeding abnormalities • Deep, tunneled wounds
Enzymatic		
Enzymes degrade and remove necrotic tissue	• Patient on anticoagulants • Can be used on infected wounds • Cost-effective • Bedside use • Selective debridement • Decreased wound trauma • Cost varies • Usually daily application in United States • Sting/inflammation around wound with some enzymes • Not used with heavy metal salts (silver and mercury) • May need cross-hatching of eschar • Clinicians need to document in patient's medication record because enzymes are prescribed drugs	• Clean wounds • Allergy to component of the enzyme preparation

Source: Kirshen, C., et al. "Debridement: A Vital Component of Wound Bed Preparation," *Advances in Skin & Wound Care* 19(9):506-17, quiz 518-519, November-December, 2006.

the use of older methods, such as maggots (biological or larval therapy), has become accepted practice in some wound care centers.[2,15] (See *Overview of debridement methods*, pages 163–165.)[2]

Mechanical debridement

Methods of mechanical debridement include wet-to-dry dressings, hydrotherapy (whirlpool), and wound irrigation (pulsed lavage).[10,12-14] Mechanical debridement may be more painful than other debridement methods, and the healthcare provider should consider premedicating the patient for pain. Both whirlpool and pulsed lavage (see chapter 9, Wound treatment options) require special equipment and skill. All of the mechanical methods are considered nonselective debridement; that is, they don't always discriminate between viable and nonviable tissue. Mechanical methods may be harmful to healthy granulation tissue on the surface of the wound and lead to bleeding, trauma, and disruption of the collagen matrix along with the necrotic tissue.

> **▶ PRACTICE POINT**
>
> Mechanical debridement may be painful; consider premedicating the patient for pain.

WET-TO-DRY DRESSINGS

Despite the drawbacks, such as pain and the necessary application up to three times per day, the use of wet-to-dry dressings to debride a wound unfortunately remains a common treatment in all healthcare settings. This method involves placing a moist saline gauze dressing on the wound surface and removing it when it's dry. The removal of the dried gauze dressing facilitates removal of devitalized tissue and debris from the wound bed. However, newly formed granulation tissue and new cell growth are also removed. To prevent pain and to help remove the dry gauze, clinicians often wet the dressing before removal. However, this defeats the purpose of aggressively removing dead tissue. This type of debridement requires significant nursing time and although the materials may be relatively inexpensive, the overall cost can often be greater than other techniques.

A wet-to-dry dressing can be used when a moderate to large amount of necrotic tissue is present and surgical intervention is not an immediate option. Because of pain and the removal of viable tissue, the Centers for Medicare and Medicaid Services (CMS) has stated in its revised surveyors guidance on pressure ulcers that use of wet-to-dry dressings should be limited.[18] CMS also states that wet-to-dry dressings should not be used in a clean, granulating wound. Instead, they recommend use of moist wound therapy dressings, which are discussed in chapter 9, Wound treatment options.

HYDROTHERAPY

Hydrotherapy (or whirlpool) debridement may be indicated for patients with large wounds that need aggressive cleaning or softening of necrotic tissue. It is contraindicated in granulating wounds because it can macerate and injure the wound bed. Hydrotherapy should be discontinued after necrotic tissue has been removed from the wound bed.

Hydrotherapy is performed by putting the patient's wound in a whirlpool bath and letting the swirling waters soften and loosen dead tissue. This procedure is usually performed in the physical therapy department, with an average treatment duration of 10 to 20 minutes up to twice per day. Operators should carefully monitor the water temperature to prevent burns. The water should be tepid (80° to 92° F [26.7° to 33.3° C]) or close to body temperature (92° to 96° F [33.3° to 35.5° C]).

This type of debridement may cause periwound maceration, traumatize the wound bed, and put the patient at risk for waterborne infections such as *Pseudomonas aeruginosa*. The potential for cross-contamination between patients is also a concern. Both patients and healthcare workers may be exposed to health risks associated with aerosolization. To minimize infection risks, the whirlpool tank must be cleaned thoroughly with an appropriate disinfectant after each use.

PULSED LAVAGE

Pulsed lavage debridement is often indicated for patients with large amounts of necrotic tissue and for those in whom other debridement methods are not an option. It is accomplished by using specialized equipment that combines a pulsating irrigation fluid with suction.[19] With pulsed lavage, you can clean and debride a wound at variable irrigation pressures (measured in pounds per square inch [psi]). The pulsatile action and effective wound bed debridement may improve granulation tissue growth. This treatment takes 15 to 30 minutes and should be done twice daily if more than half of the wound contains necrotic tissue.

Patients may need to be premedicated for comfort before beginning the procedure. Safe and effective ulcer irrigation pressures ranges from 4 to 15 psi.[8] Controlling the amount of water pressure is critical during this procedure. Because fluid is being forced at the wound directly, the risk of driving organisms deep into the wound tissue is a concern. In addition, inhalation of contaminated water droplets or mist is possible for the clinician and the patient.

> ### PRACTICE POINT
>
> Always use appropriate equipment to prevent excess lavage pressure. Wear personal protective equipment to prevent splash injury, including eye and face protectors as well as an impervious gown. Remember to administer pain medication to the patient before the procedure.

Sharp/surgical debridement

Sharp/surgical debridement includes the use of a scalpel, forceps, scissors, hydrosurgery devices, or lasers to remove dead tissue.[16,17,20,21] Sharp debridement is considered by many clinicians to be the gold standard of debridement.[21] It can cause pain, so a topical anesthetic, such as lidocaine cream or gels, may be required.[22] Patients may also need follow-up appointments for serial debridement.

Because viable tissue may also be removed inadvertently with this method, excellent judgment must be used when performing sharp debridement.[16,17,21-23] The clinician must be able to differentiate where and what to cut, identifying, for example, a tendon versus slough because both are yellow in color.[16,17,21-23] (See *color section, Differentiating tendon from Slough*, page C10.) Clinicians need guidance in discerning the line of demarcation between viable and nonviable keratinocytes at the wound edge. As shown in *Margin of debridement* (page 168), most clinicians can identify the stalled edge of a chronic wound (location A), where the keratinocytes, which are the cells that close the surface of the wound, cannot migrate across the wound bed. Research suggests that the wound edge really extends to location B[24,25] and that debriding only to this boundary may be inadequate as it leaves behind impaired cells.[24,25] Therefore, adequate debridement of a chronic wound needs to extend beyond the point at which the keratinocytes have lost the ability to move (edge of the callus tissue at location B) to where the cells can move to heal the wound (location C). Clinicians may need to rethink the distance from the wound edge (location A) that they need to debride. Research focuses on an easy way for clinicians to identify how far from the wound edge to perform debridement, based on the pathology of the abnormal keratinocytes at the wound edge.[24,25] (Also see *color section, The wound "bar code,"* page C11.)

Nonviable surgical debridement must be distinguished from sharp/surgical debridement, which may remove viable tissue on the wound surface to a bleeding base and thus create an acute wound within a chronic wound.[1-3,13,21] This procedure is usually done by experienced physicians or surgeons. In the United States, only physicians can perform surgical debridement in the operating room with hydrosurgery devices. Individual states

Margin of debridement

The *solid black line* (A) indicates a non-healing edge. The *outer gray and white broken lines* (B and C) indicate two possible margins of debridement. Location B is the edge of the wound, whereas location C is the presumed location of the healing edge of the wound where keratinocytes have the ability to migrate and participate in the wound healing process. Therefore, debride to Location C.

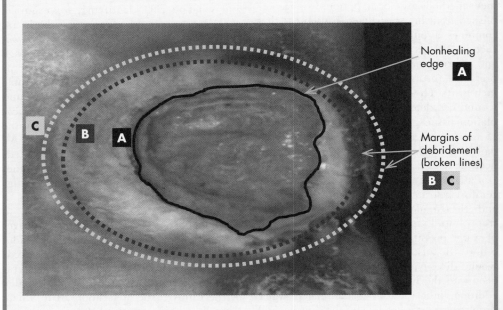

(Adapted from Tomic-Canic, M., Ayello, E.A., Stojadinovic, O, Golinko, M.S., Brem, H. "Using Gene Transcription Patterns [Bar Coding Scans] to Guide Wound Debridement and Healing [Figure 4, Biologically based margins of debridement]," *Advances in Skin & Wound Care* 21[10]: 487-92, 2008.)

may allow nurses, physical therapists, and physician assistants with appropriate licensing and training to perform some sharp debridement procedures with a scalpel, forceps, or scissors.

The use of sharp debridement is based on expert opinion and clinical data. Steed et al.[26] reanalyzed data from multisite clinical trials that tested the use of recombinant human platelet-derived growth factor (rhPDGF) in neuropathic diabetic foot ulcers. These authors found significantly higher healing rates in treatment facilities in which more frequent and complete surgical debridement to bleeding tissue was performed rather than simply removal of the pericallus. The removal of loose bright friable granulation tissue from the surface of an ulcer removes senescent fibroblasts as well as bacteria that may be arranged in biofilms, leading to damage to the underlying tissue. Surgical debridement is used for adherent eschar and devitalized or dead slough on the wound surface. This method can be used in infected wounds and should be the first choice for wounds demonstrating signs of advancing cellulitis or sepsis. Small wounds may be debrided at the bedside, but extensive wounds— for example, a stage IV pressure ulcer— may require debridement in the operating room. Physicians have reported that the use of hydrosurgery devices has decreased the number of times that debridement was needed.[20] (See *Hydrosurgery device*.) Surgical/ sharp debridement must be performed with extreme caution in patients taking anticoagulant medications. The medication may need to be held for a short period of time prior to the procedure. Patients with prolonged bleeding may be best treated with other methods of debridement. (See *color section, Surgical wound debridement case series*, page C12. See also *Sharp debridement at the bedside*, page C13.)

> **PRACTICE POINT**
>
> Exercise caution when performing surgical/sharp debridement on any patient who has been on a prolonged course of anticoagulant therapy.

Enzymatic debridement

Enzymatic debridement is considered safe, effective, and easy to perform. Enzymes are effective wound surface cleaning agents that accelerate eschar degradation and debridement. The removal of debris helps a chronic wound move from the inflammatory stage to the proliferative stage, resulting in enhanced wound healing.[27] Enzymatic agents are an ideal option for patients who are not candidates for surgery, for patients receiving care in a long-term facility or at home where other debridement methods may

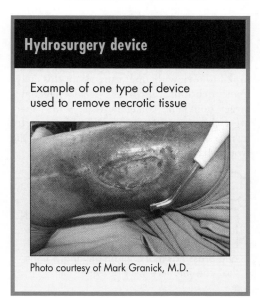

Hydrosurgery device

Example of one type of device used to remove necrotic tissue

Photo courtesy of Mark Granick, M.D.

not be available, and for patients receiving maintenance debridement.[28] Enzymatic debridement is accomplished by applying topical enzymatic agents to devitalized tissue. These agents will digest and dissolve necrotic tissue in the wound bed by breaking down collagen, elastin, and other parts of the abnormal devitalized wound matrix.[2,5,13] Before applying the topical enzymatic agent, crosshatching or scoring can be performed to enhance local penetration of the agent.[29]

If infection has spread beyond the ulcer (as in advancing cellulitis), immediate removal of necrotic tissue is usually recommended. Surgical debridement and then nonenzymatic debridement should be considered. Enzymes often can be used alone, to break down the eschar before sharp debridement, or in conjunction with mechanical debridement.[28] Some topical antibiotics are compatible with enzymatic debriding agents and may be used in conjunction with the treatment.[16,17,30]

Enzymes that act on necrotic tissue are categorized as proteolytics, fibrinolytics, and collagenases, depending on the tissue component they target. Because papain urea enzymatic debriding agents target eschar, they are often used on necrotic wounds. However, the Food and Drug Administration removed papain ureas from use in the United States as of 2008.[31] Those practicing outside the United States, where papain urea is available, are urged to review the literature about this enzymatic debriding agent.[27,29,32-34] Collagenases target nonviable collagen tissue while sparing viable tissue, thereby making them useful in necrotic wounds with slough tissue at the wound base.[30]

PRACTICE POINT

Silver and other metals, including zinc oxide, can inactivate enzymes; be careful when selecting cleaning agents and dressings that contain any ingredients that can interfere with enzyme action.[30]

Enzymes are a prescription drug and require a physician's or prescriber's order. Collagenase is usually applied once per day. Before reapplying any enzymatic agent, thoroughly clean the wound with normal saline or a wound cleanser to remove any residual enzymatic ointment and loose wound debris.[29] Avoid solutions with metal ions, such as mercury or silver, when using collagenase, as they may inactivate the enzyme.[30]

If it is within your state's scope of practice and permitted by your facility, crosshatching or scoring the eschar with a scalpel (#11 or #15 blade), without cutting deep enough to cause bleeding, is recommended prior to applying the enzyme to let the debriding agent penetrate into the eschar. After scoring is complete, apply a thin layer (about the thickness of a nickel) of enzymatic ointment onto the necrotic tissue. Cover the wound with an appropriate dressing to keep it moist and let the debriding agent work.[29,30,35]

Various types of dressings can be used with enzymatic debriders. Avoid covering the wound with a dressing that contains any component that could interfere with the effectiveness of the enzyme. For example, because heavy metals are known to interfere with collagenase enzymatic debriders, do not use them in combination with a silver antimi-

crobial dressing.[29,30,35] (For more information on dressing types, see chapter 9, Wound treatment options.) Follow the specific manufacturer's directions for the particular enzyme you're using. Because these are prescribed drugs, also be sure to record the application of the enzyme in the patient's medication record.

Collagenase is derived from *Clostridium histolyticum*. It may be more effective than papain urea at degrading collagen and elastin and is thought to work from the bottom of the wound up.[33] Research supports collagenase as a more selective enzyme that may be more effective in controlling or reducing pain when compared with other debridements.[29,36] Collagenase up-regulates the migration of keratinocytes over the wound bed and stimulates granulation.[37,38] Muller and colleagues found debridement with collagenase to be quicker and more cost-effective than autolytic debridement with a hydrocolloid dressing in 24 patients with pressure ulcers.[39] Research by Riley and Herman[40] has shed new light on the role keratinocytes play in wound healing and how wound healing is influenced by different substances, including enzymes. This research found that collagenase doubled keratinocyte growth and migration; the increase was fivefold when heparin-binding epidermal-like growth factor was added.[40] In an in vitro study, Mekkes and colleagues found increased healing rates with collagenase and ineffective debridement with fibrinolysin (desoxyribonuclease).[41] Collagenase has also been shown to reduce scarring in partial-thickness burn wounds, which has crucial implications for a patient's quality of life.[42]

The optimal method for enzymatic debriding agents has been the subject of much controversy. Research has also shown some differences between papain urea and collagenase use. While overall healing rates for papain urea and collagenase were not significantly different in one study, papain urea did debride eschar at a faster rate.[43] However, another study found that papain-urea decreased keratinocyte migration by 50%.[40]

The search for new enzymes continues. Mekkes et al. have reported on Antarctic krill as an effective debriding agent,[44] while a systematic review by Bradley and colleagues failed to provide evidence to support the use of enzymatic agents over other methods.[45]

Autolytic debridement

Autolytic debridement uses the body's endogenous enzymes to slowly remove necrotic tissue from the wound bed. In a moist wound, phagocytic cells and proteolytic enzymatic enzymes can soften and liquefy the necrotic tissue that is then digested by macrophages. Autolytic debridement can be facilitated with appropriate dressings in the superficial wound that contains little necrotic tissue or a larger, deeper pressure ulcer.[1,2,13,16,17,19] Underlying these concepts is the requirement of adequate circulation and nutrition.[2] Autolytic debridement may take longer than other methods; however, it represents a less stressful method to the patient and wound than mechanical debridement. This method of debridement is contraindicated in infected wounds.

Autolytic debridement is easy to perform and involves applying a moisture-retentive topical dressing, such as a semi-occlusive or occlusive dressings; types include transparent films, hydrocolloids, hydrogels, and calcium alginate dressings.[2] (See chapter 9, Wound treatment options.) Wound fluid accumulates under the dressing, aiding in the lysis of necrotic tissue. This method is pain-free in patients with adequate tissue perfusion.

Studies have compared the efficacy of hydrogel dressings and mechanical debridement with wet-to-dry dressings.[46-48] Several researchers[46-48] have concluded that autolytic debridement with a hydrogel is more time- and cost-effective, resulting in faster healing when compared with wet-to-dry dressings. One case report found that use of a clear acrylic dressing promoted autolytic debridement and had the added advantage of being able to view the wound without removing the dressing.[49] Schimmelpfenning & Mollenhauer[49] and Konig et al.[50] found that autolytic debridement with moist interactive dressings was equal in efficacy to enzymatic methods using collagenase. Smith's *Cochrane* review on debridement

in diabetic ulcers concluded that hydrogels were more effective than gauze.[51]

PRACTICE POINT

Be sure to tell the patient and family that fluid accumulating under the dressing is a normal part of the debridement process. Discolored wound fluid may not signal a wound infection.

Monitor the wound for signs of infection, such as odor, increasing exudate or wound size, periwound erythema, edema, warmth, or increased pain, and discontinue autolytic debridement if these symptoms occur. Immunocompromised patients should be assessed frequently for any indication of infection. Autolytic debridement isn't the treatment of choice in severely infected wounds; in fact, it may lead to more severe infection and is therefore contraindicated in these situations. Surgical consult is warranted with appropriate medical management of the infection.

Maggot therapy (biological or larval therapy)

Maggot therapy was widely used in the early part of the 20th century. It fell out of favor due in part to the "disgust factor" and the use of newer modalities such as antimicrobial agents in wound treatments. With Europe leading the way, there has been a resurgence in the use of larval therapy in the United States.[52,53] In this type of debridement, several applications of sterilized medicinal *Lucilia sericata* (greenbottle fly) maggots are placed in the wound bed every 2 to 3 days.[54] (See *Maggots in heel wound*, page 172.) (Also see *color section*, *Maggot therapy*, pages C14–C15.) The specific application technique for how the maggots are actually put in the wound varies. Some place the maggots directly into the wound so they can roam around (free-range), and others place the maggots contained in a device such as a pouch or tea bag–like sack.[55] Early evidence

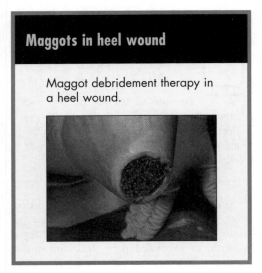

Maggots in heel wound

Maggot debridement therapy in a heel wound.

supports that free-range maggot therapy maximizes debridement benefits compared with maggots that are contained in pouches or sacks and then placed in the wound.[55]

Just how do these larvae accomplish debridement? The mechanism by which maggot therapy works is believed to be by the enzymes the maggots secrete. These substances are proteinases that degrade the necrotic tissue.[56] The maggots also digest bacteria, making them effective in wounds with resistant bacteria strains.[57,58] A recent prospective randomized study provided evidence that complete lysis of methicillin-resistant *Staphylococcus aureus* (MRSA) and *Candida albicans* occurred within 24 hours when maggots were applied to 48 culture plates.[59] This effect continued to be observed for 5 days.[59] Maggots also encourage healing by stimulating granulation tissue.

Prospective trials on the efficacy of maggot therapy have reported debridement and evidence of decrease in wound size.[60,61] Some case studies have reported the efficacy and selectivity of maggot debridement therapy.[62,63] Mumcuoglu[64] has reported significant debridement (80% to 85%) with clinical application of maggots as well as

the prevention of amputation and bacterial spread.

Maggots can be used in almost all wounds. Richardson[65] and Thomas[66] reviewed current best practices. However, some contraindications for their use include a life- or limb-threatening wound, psychological distress or the "ick factor," bleeding abnormalities, and deep-tracking wounds.[52] The literature is unclear about some aspects of maggot use. Sherman[67] says that maggots should not be used in the presence of osteomyelitis or critical ischemia associated with arterial insufficiency, but Claxton et al. disagree.[52] Maggots are cost-effective when used properly and have the potential to help in situations where other resources are not available.[68] Despite the potential for psychological distress, most patients, as well as healthcare professionals, were satisfied with the treatment in one study.[62]

Something else to consider with maggot therapy is the level of pain it causes. There are conflicting reports about the level of expected pain with maggot debridement therapy. Sometimes, pain is minimal or absent.[69] In one report, however, 25% of patients with superficial painful wounds complained of increased pain during treatment with maggots.[56] These patients need analgesics for pain management. The type of wound might make a difference as to whether the patient has pain during therapy. In a retrospective study, Steenvorde et al.[70] found that diabetic patients, the majority of whom had neuropathy (n = 21), did not experience increased pain, while 40% (n = 8) of nondiabetic patients experienced pain when being treated with maggots.

Choosing a debridement method

Does it matter which type of debridement you use on a wound? "No one method of debridement has been proven optimal for pressure ulcers," according to the Wound, Ostomy and Continence Nurses Society (WOCN).[9]

Given the various and conflicting evidence about the different debridement options, choosing the right way to debride wounds can be challenging. Answering the following questions can help guide you in choosing the best debridement method for your patient.[1,2,12,13,16,17,71] Remember, your choice may be limited by the availability of the various debridement methods in your facility or healthcare system.

HOW MUCH TIME DO YOU HAVE TO DEBRIDE?

Infected wounds require immediate attention and may require surgical debridement after systemic antimicrobial therapy has been initiated. The patient's clinical condition and the amount of time that you can devote to a treatment may influence your choice.

WHAT ARE THE WOUND CHARACTERISTICS?

Consider the size, depth, location, amount of drainage (and whether it is increasing), presence (and extent) or absence of infection, and etiology of the wound.

HOW SELECTIVE A METHOD IS NEEDED?

Determine the risk for damage to healthy tissue when necrotic tissue is removed.

WHAT METHODS ARE PERMITTED?

Check that the intended debridement method is allowed by your state's practice act and by your facility. For example, using a scalpel to crosshatch eschar requires specialized training and licensure.

WHAT'S THE CARE SETTING?

Some resources available in a hospital aren't practical in the home and may not even be available in a long-term care facility.

HOW MUCH DEBRIDEMENT IS ENOUGH?

How do you know when you've debrided enough? Assess the tissue in the wound bed: When most of the wound surface is covered with granulation tissue and the necrotic tissue is gone, you've debrided enough.

Saap and Falanga[72] developed a method to assess adequacy of wound debridement. Their Debridement Performance Index may make more effective comparisons between different debridement methods and facilitate more predictive prognostic information.[72]

Falanga[73] has proposed that chronic wounds need constant debridement because maintenance debridement is an important part of the WBP in these wounds. In the past, debridement was regarded as a singular event based on the visible assessment of the wound. Now, however, it's thought that frequent, limited, maintenance debridement will keep the biological burden low and stimulate growth factors.[13,74-76] Maintenance debridement may prove challenging in the future due to proposed reimbursement changes in the United States based on the place in which debridement can be done as well as the frequency of the procedure.

SUMMARY

Debridement is an essential step in the WBP management process. Although surgical debridement is the fastest way of removing necrotic tissue from a wound, it may not be appropriate for all patients in all healthcare settings. The selection of the correct method of debridement should be based on the individual patient and the degree of necrosis present. By knowing the options for debridement, you can help prepare the wound bed and assist your patient on the road to healing.

PATIENT SCENARIO

Clinical Data

Mrs. AA is 55-year-old female patient who presented with a painful left large toe. She has type 2, adult-onset, non–insulin-dependent diabetes mellitus with neuropathy. There is a palpable dorsalis pedis pulse, and her pain is aggravated by wearing shoes.

The best approach to this patient includes all the components in the WBP paradigm of treating the cause and patient-centered concerns before addressing the components of local wound care (**DIME: D**ebridement, **I**nfection/persistent inflammation, **M**oisture balance, and then the **E**dge effect for advanced therapies if wounds are not healing at the expected rate when all the components of WBP have been corrected).

For patient-centered concerns, the pain that has developed in a neuropathic foot with loss of protective sensation should alert the clinician to the disruption of deeper structures with infection (e.g., osteomyelitis) or a Charcot joint (acute inflamed bony structure due to multiple small pathological fractures).

Case Discussion

In this case, physical examination revealed a keratotic cap on the left second toe that required debridement (Figure 8-1A). Vascular supply was assessed prior to surgical debridement. The palpable pulse indicated a local pressure of 80 mm Hg or higher, which was deemed adequate for healing. As is often seen in patients with neuropathy, removal of the surface of the callus revealed encasement of the toenail that had rotated under the tip of the toe with the claw deformity. When the nail and callus were removed, there was a small ulcer that probed to bone (Figure 8-1B). This indicates a high probability of osteomyelitis, which was confirmed with an X-ray showing erosion of the phalangeal bone. Following debridement, a calcium alginate dressing was applied for hemostasis (Figure 8-1C). With this type of dressing, the calcium donated from the dressing assists in local hemostasis while the sodium exchanged for the calcium creates a sodium alginate hydrogel for moist interactive healing, avoiding a pro-inflammatory hemorrhagic crust formation.

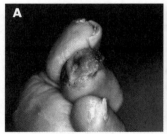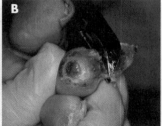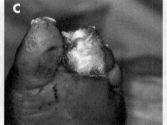

Figure 8-1. **(A)** Keratotic cap on the left second toe. **(B)** A small ulcer probing to bone was revealed when the nail and callus were removed. **(C)** Calcium alginate dressing applied for hemostasis after debridement. (See also *color section*, *Patient scenarios*, page C43.)

The treatment principles employed in this case can be remembered with the mnemonic **VIPS**:

- **V**ascular supply with a palpable pulse was adequate for healing (if the pulse is not palpable, an ankle-brachial pressure index, toe pressures, or transcutaneous oxygen determination can be obtained to assess healability).

- **I**nfection: The osteomyelitis was treated with 3 months of oral clindamycin (good bone penetration with gram-positive and anaerobe coverage) combined with ciprofloxacin (gram-negative coverage including *Pseudomonas*), with resolution of the pain and osteomyelitis.

- **P**ressure: The callus was due to pressure in the toe-box of the patient's shoes. This was corrected with the ordering of deep-toed shoes and orthotics to remove local pressure.

- **S**harp surgical debridement was performed, including removal of the nail to reveal the osteomyelitis sinus. Maintenance debridement may also be necessary when callus periodically re-forms.

This case illustrates the need for holistic patient care with treatment of cause (VIPS), pain control (acetaminophen with codeine), and then local wound care with debridement and the use of calcium alginate followed by a silver alginate dressing.

SHOW WHAT YOU KNOW

1. Which statement about the purpose of debridement is correct? Debridement:
   A. is not essential for wound healing.
   B. removes debris so cell movement is enhanced.
   C. removes necrotic tissue in order to enhance the wound's biologic burden.
   D. reduces the need for moist wound healing.

   ANSWER: B. *Debridement is the removal of debris so that cell movement can be enhanced. A is incorrect because most wounds need debridement to heal; C is incorrect because necrotic tissue increases the wound's biologic burden; and D is incorrect because wounds need moist healing.*

2. Which sign in a stable necrotic heel would signal a need for debridement?
   A. exudate
   B. presence of thick, leathery eschar
   C. an impending inspection by a regulator
   D. yellow slough

   ANSWER: A. *Exudate is a sign of infection, which signals the need for debridement. Other signs are erythema and fluid wave. The other options are incorrect.*

3. Which method is an example of mechanical debridement?
   A. Collagenases
   B. Maggots
   C. Film dressings
   D. Pulsed lavage

   ANSWER: D. *Pulsed lavage is a method of mechanical debridement. Collagenases are enzymes, maggots secrete natural collagenase, and film dressings are a method of autolytic debridement.*

(continued)

4. A resident in a long-term care facility is on Coumadin and needs debridement for a necrotic ulcer on his sacrum. Which of the following methods of debridement would be <u>least</u> indicated?
   A. Surgical
   B. Enzymatic
   C. Mechanical
   D. Autolytic

   ANSWER: A. *Because the resident is on Coumadin and bleeding can occur, surgical debridement would be least indicated. Also, the appropriate personnel and equipment may not be available in the patient's long-term care facility. The other options are correct.*

5. Which method of debridement would be best to use initially for a hospitalized client with an infected large sacral pressure ulcer?
   A. Surgical
   B. Enzymatic
   C. Mechanical
   D. Autolytic

   ANSWER: A. *Time is of the essence, and surgical debridement is the quickest method that can be used with infected wounds. Because the client is hospitalized, the appropriate personnel and equipment to perform this method of debridement are available. The other options are incorrect.*

REFERENCES

1. Sibbald, R.G, Orsted, H.L., Coutts, P.M., Keast, D.H. "Best Clinical Practices for Preparing the Wound Bed: Update 2006," in MacDonald, J.M., Geyer, M.J. (eds.), *Wound Management and Lymphedema.* Geneva: World Health Organization, 2010, pp. 35-61.
2. Kirshen, C., et al. "Debridement: A Vital Component of Wound Bed Preparation," *Advances in Skin & Wound Care* 19(9):506-17, quiz 518-19, November-December, 2006.
3. Schultz, G.S., et al. "Wound Bed Preparation: A Systematic Approach to Wound Management," *Wound Repair and Regeneration* 11(suppl 1): S1-S28, March 2003.
4. Ramasastry, S.S. "Chronic Problem Wounds," *Clinical Plastic Surgery* 25(3):367-96, July 1998.
5. Ayello, E.A., et al. "Skip the Knife: Debriding Wounds Without Surgery," *Nursing 2002* 32(9): 58-63, September 2002.
6. Wysocki, B. "Wound Fluids and the Pathogenesis of Chronic Wounds," *Journal of Wound, Ostomy and Continence Nursing* 23(6):283-90, November 1996.
7. Edlich, R.F., et al. "The Biology of Infections: Sutures, Tapes, and Bacteria," in Hunt, T.K. (ed.), *Wound Healing and Wound Infection: Theory and Surgical Practice.* New York: Appleton-Century-Crofts, 1980.
8. Bergstrom, N., Bennett, M.A., Carlson, C.E., et al. *Treatment of Pressure Ulcers. Clinical Practice Guideline, No. 15,* AHCPR Publication No. 95-0652. Rockville, MD: Agency for Health Care Policy and Research, December 1994.
9. Wound, Ostomy and Continence Nurses Society. *Guideline for Prevention and Management of Pressure Ulcers #2: WOCN Clinical Practice Guideline Series,* Mount Laurel, NJ, June 2010.
10. Brem, H., et al. "Protocol for Treatment of Diabetic Foot Ulcers," *American Journal of Surgery* 187(suppl 1):1S-10S, 2004.
11. Black, J., Baharestani, M., Black, S., et al. "An Overview of Tissue Types in Pressure Ulcers: A Consensus Panel Recommendation." *Ostomy Wound Management* 56(4)28-44, 2010.
12. National Pressure Ulcer Advisory Panel and European Pressure Ulcer Advisory Panel. *Prevention and Treatment of Pressure Ulcers. Clinical Practice Guideline.* Washington, DC: National Pressure Ulcer Advisory Panel, 2009.
13. Sibbald, R.G., et al. "Best Practice Recommendations for Preparing the Wound Bed: Update 2006," *Wound Care Canada* 4(1):15-29, 2006.

14. Keast, D.H., Parslow, N., Houghton, P.E., Norton, L., Fraser, C. *Best Practice Recommendations for the Prevention and Treatment of Pressure Ulcers: Update 2006*. Canadian Association of Wound Care. Available at *http://www.cawc.net/images/uploads/wcc/4-1-vol4no1-BP-PU.pdf*. Accessed January 20, 2010.

15. Beitz, J.M. "Wound Debridement: Therapeutic Options and Care Considerations," *Nursing Clinics of North America* 40(2):233-49, 2005.

16. Ayello, E.A, Cuddigan, J.E. "Debridement: Controlling the Necrotic/Cellular Burden," *Advances in Skin & Wound Care* 17(2):66-75; quiz 76-78, March 2004.

17. Ayello, E.A., Cuddigan, J.E. "Conquer Chronic Wounds with Wound Bed Preparation," *Nurse Practitioner* 29(3):8-25; quiz 26-27, 2004.

18. Centers for Medicare and Medicaid Services (CMS). "Tag F-314: Pressure Ulcers. Revised Guidance for Surveyors in Long Term Care." Issued Nov 12, 2004. Available at *http//cms.gov/transmittals/Downloads/R4SOM.pdf*. Accessed October 10, 2010.

19. Scott, R., and Loehne, H. "Five Questions and Answers About Pulsed Lavage," *Advances in Skin & Wound Care* 13(3, part I):133-34, May-June 2000.

20. Mosti, G., and Mattaliano, V. "The Debridement of Chronic Leg Ulcers by Means of a New, Fluidjet-based Device," *Wounds* 18(8):227-37, August 2006.

21. Leaper, D. Sharp techniques for wound debridement. World Wide Wounds. Available at *http://www.worldwidewounds.com/2002/december/Leaper/Sharp-Debridement.html*. Accessed July 17, 2006.

22. Williams, D., Enoch, S., Miller, D., et al. "Effect of Sharp Debridement Using Curette on Recalcitrant Nonhealing Venous Leg Ulcers: A Concurrently Controlled, Prospective Cohort Study," *Wound Repair and Regeneration* 13:131-37, March-April 2005.

23. Ashworth, J., and Chivers, M. "Conservative Sharp Debridement: The Professional and Legal Issues," *Professional Nurse* 17(10):585-88, June 2002.

24. Brem, H., et al. "Molecular Markers in Patients with Chronic Wounds to Guide Surgical Debridement," *Molecular Medicine* 13(1-2):30-39, 2007.

25. Tomic-Canic, M., Ayello, E.A., Stojadinovic, O, Golinko, M.S., Brem, H. "Using Gene Transcription Patterns (Bar Coding Scans) to Guide Wound Debridement and Healing," *Advances in Skin & Wound Care* 21(10):487-92, 2008.

26. Steed, D.L., et al. "Effect of Extensive Debridement and Treatment on the Healing of Diabetic Foot Ulcers. Diabetic Ulcer Study Group," *Journal of the American College of Surgeons* 183(1):61-64, July 1996.

27. Wright, J.B., and Shi, L. "Accuzyme Papain-Urea Debriding Ointment: A Historical Review," *Wounds* 15(4):2S-12S, April 2003.

28. Falanga, V., Brem, H. Ennis, W.J. et al., "Maintenance Debridement in the Treatment of Difficult-to-Heal Chronic Wounds. Recommendations of an Expert Panel." *Ostomy Wound Management* Supplement:2-15, June 2008.

29. Ramundo, J., Gray, M. "Collagenase for Enzymatic Debridement. A Systematic Review." *Journal of Wound, Ostomy & Continence Nursing* 36(6S):S4-S11, 2009.

30. Shi, L., Carson, D. "Collagenase Santyl Ointment. A Selective Agent for Wound Debridement." *Journal of Wound Ostomy & Continence Nursing* 36(6S):S12-S16, 2009.

31. Smith, R.G. "Enzymatic Debriding Agents: An Evaluation of the Medical Literature," *Ostomy Wound Management* 54(8):16-34, 2008.

32. Hebda, P.A., and Lo, C. "Biochemistry of Wound Healing: The Effects of Active Ingredients of Standard Debriding Agents—Papain and Collagenase—on Digestion of Native and Denatured Collagenous Substrates, Fibrin and Elastin," *Wounds* 13(5):190-94, 2001.

33. Hebda, P.A., et al. "Evaluation of Efficacy of Enzymatic Debriding Agents for Removal of Necrotic Tissue and Promotion of Healing in Porcine Skin Wounds," *Wounds* 10(3):83-96, 1998.

34. Falanga, V. "Wound Bed Preparation and the Role of Enzymes: A Case for Multiple Actions of Therapeutic Agents," *Wounds* 14(2):47-57, February 2002.

35. McCallon, S.K., Hurlow, J. "Clinical Applications for the Use of Enzymatic Debriding Ointment and Broad-spectrum Bacteriostatic Foam Dressing." *Journal of Wound, Ostomy & Continence Nursing* 36(6S):S17-S24, 2009.

36. Hansbrough, J.F., et al. "Wound Healing in Partial-Thickness Burn Wounds Treated with Collagenase Ointment versus Silver Sulfadiazine Cream," *Journal of Burn Care and Rehabilitation* 16(Pt 1):241-47, 1995.

37. Pilcher, B.K., Dumin, J.A., Sudbeck, B.D., et al. "The Activity of Collagenase-1 Is Required for Keratinocyte Migration on a Type I Collagen Matrix," *Journal of Cell Biology* 137:1445-57, 1997.

38. Burgos, A., Gimenez, J., Moreno, E., et al. "Collagenase Ointment Application at 24- versus 48-hour Intervals in the Treatment of Pressure Ulcers. A Randomized Multicentre Study," *Clinical Drug Investigation* 19:399-407, 2000.

39. Muller, E., van Leen, M.W., Bergmann, R. "Economic Evaluation of Collagenase-containing

Ointment and Hydrocolloid Dressings in the Treatment of Pressure Ulcers," *Pharmacoeconomics* 19:1209-16, 2001.

40. Riley, K.N., and Herman, I.M. "Collagenase Promotes the Cellular Responses to Injury and Wound Healing In Vivo," *Journal of Burns and Wounds* 4:112-24, July 2005.

41. Mekkes, J.R., et al. "Quantitative and Objective Evaluation of Wound Debriding Properties of Collagenase and Fibrinolysin/Desoxyribonuclease in a Necrotic Ulcer Animal Model," *Archives of Dermatological Research* 290:152-57, 1998.

42. Frye, K.E., Luterman, A. "Decreased Incidence of Hypertrophic Burn Scar Formation with the Use of Collagenase, An Enzymatic Debriding Agent," *Wounds* 17(12):32-36, December 2005.

43. Alvarez, O.M., et al. "A Prospective, Randomized, Comparative Study of Collagenase and Papain-urea for Pressure Ulcer Debridement," *Wounds* 14:293-301, 2002.

44. Mekkes, J.R., et al. "Efficient Debridement of Necrotic Wounds Using Proteolytic Enzymes Derived from Antarctic Krill: A Double-blind, Placebo-controlled Study in a Standardized Animal Wound Model," *Wound Repair & Regeneration* 6(1):50-57, January 1998.

45. Bradley, M., et al. "The Debridement of Chronic Wounds: A Systematic Review," *Health Technology Assessment* 3(17 Pt 1):iii-iv, 1-78, 1999.

46. Mulder, G.D. "Cost-effective Managed Care: Gel versus Wet-to-dry for Debridement," *Ostomy Wound Management* 41(2):68-70, 72, 74 passim, March 1995.

47. Thomas, S., et al. "Clinical Experience with a New Hydrogel Dressing," *Journal of Wound Care* 5:132-33, 1996.

48. Trudgian, J. "Investigating the Use of Aquaform Hydrogel in Wound Management," *British Journal of Nursing* 9:943-48, 2000.

49. Schimmelpfenning, D., and Mollenhauer, S. "Use of a Clear Absorbent Acrylic Dressing for Debridement," *Journal of Wound Ostomy & Continence Nursing* 33(6):639-42, November/December 2006.

50. Konig, M., Vanscheidt, W., Augustin, M., Kapp, H. "Enzymatic versus Autolytic Debridement of Chronic Leg Ulcers: A Prospective Randomised Trial," *Journal of Wound Care* 14:320-23, July 2005.

51. Smith, J. "Debridement of Diabetic Foot Ulcers," *Cochrane Database of Systematic Reviews* (4):CD003556, 2002.

52. Claxton, M.J., et al. "5 Questions—and Answers—About Maggot Debridement Therapy," *Advances in Skin & Wound Care* 16:99-102, 2003.

53. Bolton, L.L. "Evidence Corner, Maggot Therapy," *Wounds* 18(9):A19-A22, September 2006.

54. Courtenay, M., et al. "Larva Therapy in Wound Management," *Journal of the Royal Society of Medicine* 93(2):72-74, 2000.

55. Steenvorde, P., et al. "Maggot Debridement Therapy: Free-range or Contained? An In Vivo Study," *Advances in Skin & Wound Care* 18:430-35, October 2005.

56. Chambers, L., et al. "Degradation of Extracellular Matrix Components by Defined Proteinases from the Greenbottle Larva *Lucilia sericata* Used for the Clinical Debridement of Non-healing Wounds," *British Journal of Dermatology* 148:14-23, 2003.

57. Wollina, U., et al. "Biosurgery in Wound Healing: The Renaissance of Maggot Therapy," *Journal of the European Academy of Dermatology and Venereology* 14:285-89, 2000.

58. Rayner, K. "Larval Therapy in Wound Debridement," *Professional Nurse* 14:329-33, February 1999.

59. Margolin, L., Gialanella, P. "Assessment of the Antimicrobial Properties of Maggots." *International Wound Journal* 7:202-4, 2010.

60. Sherman, R.A. "Maggot versus Conservative Debridement Therapy for the Treatment of Pressure Ulcers," *Wound Repair & Regeneration* 10:208-14, 2002.

61. Sherman, R.A. "Maggot Debridement Therapy for Treating Non-healing Wounds," *Wound Repair & Regeneration* 8:327, 2000.

62. Sherman, R.A., et al. "Maggot Debridement Therapy in Outpatients," *Archives of Physical Medicine and Rehabilitation* 82:1226-29, 2001.

63. Tanyuksel, M., et al. "Maggot Debridement Therapy in the Treatment of Chronic Wounds in a Military Hospital Setup in Turkey," *Dermatology* 10:115-18, 2005.

64. Mumcuoglu, K.Y. "Clinical Applications for Maggots in Wound Care," *American Journal of Clinical Dermatology* 2:219-27, 2001.

65. Richardson, M. "The Benefits of Larval Therapy in Wound Care," *Nursing Standard* 19(7):70, 72, 74 passim, 2004.

66. Thomas, S., Andrews, A., Jones, M. "The Use of Larval Therapy in Wound Management," *Journal of Wound Care* 7:521-24, 1998.

67. Sherman, R.A. "Maggot Therapy for Foot and Leg Wounds," *International Journal of Lower Extremity Wounds* 1:135-142, June 2002.

68. Wayman, J., et al. "The Cost Effectiveness of Larval Therapy in Venous Ulcers," *Journal of Tissue Viability* 10(3):91-94, 2000.

69. Kitching, M. "Patients' Perceptions and Experiences of Larval Therapy," *Journal of Wound Care* 13(1):25-29, 2004.

70. Steenvoorde, P., et al. "Determining Pain Levels in Patients Treated with Maggot Debridement Therapy," *Journal of Wound Care* 14:485-88, November 2005.

71. Mosher, B.A., et al. "Outcomes of Four Methods of Debridement Using a Decision Analysis Methodology," *Advances in Wound Care* 12(2):81-88, March 1999.

72. Saap, L.J., and Falanga, V. "Debridement Performance Index and Its Correlation with Complete Closure of Diabetic Foot Ulcers," *Wound Repair & Regeneration* 10:354-59, 2002.

73. Falanga, V. "Wound Bed Preparation and the Role of Enzymes: A Case for Multiple Actions of Therapeutic Agents," *Wounds* 14(2):47-57, March 2002.

74. Steed, D.L. "Debridement," *American Journal of Surgery* 187(5A):71S-74S Review, May 2004.

75. Vowden, K.R., and Vowden, P. "Wound Debridement, Part 1: Non-sharp Techniques," *Journal of Wound Care* 8:237-40, 1999.

76. Vowden, K.R., and Vowden, P. "Wound Debridement, Part 2: Sharp Techniques," *Journal of Wound Care* 8:291-94, June 1999.

CHAPTER 9

Wound Treatment Options

Sharon Baranoski, MSN, RN, CWCN, APN-CCRN, DAPWCA, FAAN
Elizabeth A. Ayello, PhD, RN, ACNS-BC, CWON, MAPWCA, FAAN
Andrea McIntosh, RN, BSN, CWOCN, APN
Linda Montoya, RN, BSN, CWOCN, APN
Pamela Scarborough, DPT, MS, CDE, CWS

Objectives

After completing this chapter, you'll be able to:
- explain moist wound therapy
- select dressings based on assessment of wound characteristics
- list indications for use of dressings by categories
- state the advantages and disadvantages for each dressing category
- use the principles of care in dressing selection
- discuss the use of advanced therapies.

A CHALLENGE FOR CLINICIANS

This is an exciting and challenging time for wound care clinicians as a new understanding of the biology of healing wounds has given rise to many new wound care treatments and therapies. Although we are gaining new knowledge as to the biology of wound healing, "we can no longer care only for the wound itself; we must step back and look at the entire human being who happens to have a wound that needs healing."[1] Being able to differentiate among the various treatment options, when and how to apply them, in what combinations, and when to change them has indeed become both an art and a science. "With the emergence of more complex products, we will be increasingly required to use these products appropriately to maximize their impact. As a better understanding of the wound environment becomes available, our ability to tailor our approach and better treat the patient as a whole increases."[2]

Providing quality care for your wound patients starts with an analysis of the patient's individualized wound assessment and continues with developing a plan of care, selecting the proper product, and reevaluating the plan of care as appropriate. Wound dressings can present a challenging decision for clinicians. Moist wound healing, moisture-balanced dressings, and certainly the principles of optimal wound interventions are key concepts needed to support the healing process. As clinicians try to heal wounds faster, the marketplace continues to provide many more treatment choices. Currently there are reported to be more than 500 different types of dressings available to manage patients with wounds.[3] Keeping abreast of wound dressing choices and various application techniques, as well as which product to use and when, is an ambitious task for all clinicians.

MOIST WOUND HEALING

Wound healing in the 21st century has certainly changed. There have been more advances in wound care over the past four decades than during the previous 2,000 years. This wound care revolution has been due in part to Dr. Winter's discovery (in the 1960s) of the importance of moist wound healing in experimental animals.[4] Hinman and Maibach[5] paralleled these findings of faster resurfacing in partial-thickness wounds in humans. Their research efforts laid the foundation for understanding the importance of moisture and moisture loss in wound healing. The concept of moist wound healing and moisture-balanced dressings is now commonly accepted by most clinicians throughout the world as best practice.

We now understand that wound healing must take place in a moist environment. Epithelial cells require moisture to migrate from the wound edges to reepithelialize or resurface the wound. This process is likened to "leap-frogging" of the cells. In a dry wound, these cells have to burrow down underneath the wound bed to find a moist area upon which to "march" or move forward. (See *Epithelial cell migration in an open wound*.)

The concept of moist wound healing based on wound physiology and characteristics required

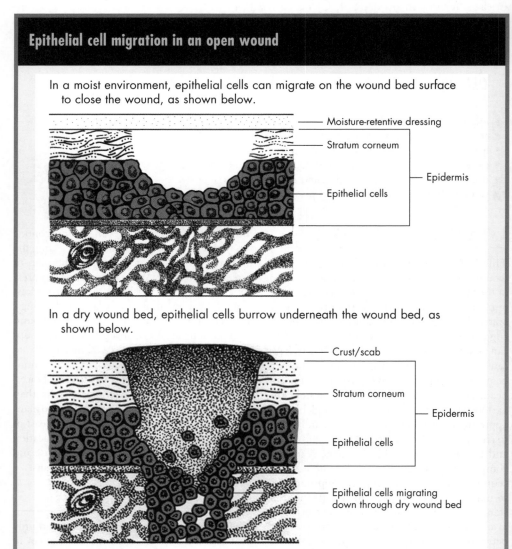

Epithelial cell migration in an open wound

In a moist environment, epithelial cells can migrate on the wound bed surface to close the wound, as shown below.

- Moisture-retentive dressing
- Stratum corneum
- Epithelial cells
- Epidermis

In a dry wound bed, epithelial cells burrow underneath the wound bed, as shown below.

- Crust/scab
- Stratum corneum
- Epidermis
- Epithelial cells
- Epithelial cells migrating down through dry wound bed

that new dressing materials be developed to replace the passive coverings that had been used in the past, which evolved from such "natural" coverings as feathers, lint, grease, milk, wine, mud, leaves, and other concoctions. Today's wound dressings are actively involved in stimulating cell proliferation and encouraging epithelial cells to migrate. Moisture-balanced or moisture-retentive dressings also act as a barrier against bacteria and absorb excess wound fluid, creating opportune conditions for healing.[5-8] Formerly, wound dressings were used primarily to protect the wound from secondary infection by forming a barrier against bacteria and absorbing wound fluid. The greatest advantage of contemporary dressings is the maintenance of moist wound conditions, which is in contrast to the "classical gauze techniques" that led to the formation of a dry, firmly adhering scab.[9] Today's dressings promote rapid healing, act as a barrier, decrease or eliminate pain, require fewer changes, provide autolytic debridement, and can be cost-effective if used appropriately.

Despite the benefits of newer dressing products, wet-to-dry gauze is still popular with many physicians, especially surgeons who have not been influenced by the development of modern wound dressings.[10] In a study by Pieper and colleagues[11] of 1,638 wounds treated in the home setting, the most commonly used dressing for all types of wounds ($n = 406$) was dry gauze. No dressing (that is, an uncovered wound) was the second most common treatment ($n = 252$), and saline-moistened gauze ($n = 145$) was third. Advanced moisture-retentive dressings comprised less than 25% of all dressings used. So despite four decades of information on the benefits of moist wound therapy, some physicians may still revert back to the "old methods."

Research by Kim et al.[12] suggests that a saline gauze dressing acts as an osmotic dressing. As water evaporates from the saline dressing, it becomes hypertonic. Because the body wants to maintain homeostasis by reestablishing isotonicity, wound fluid is drawn into the gauze dressing. In addition to water, wound fluid includes blood and proteins. These substances form an impermeable layer on the dressing that prevents wound fluid from "wetting" the dressing; the net result is

that the dressing dries out. The removal of a wet-to-moist dressing that has dried may then cause reinjury of the wound, resulting in pain and delayed wound healing.[10]

Pain at dressing removal is a frequent complaint heard by patients whose gauze dressings have dried into their wound. In "Principles of Best Practice: "Minimising Pain at Wound Dressing-related Procedures. A Consensus Document,"[13] the World Union of Wound Healing Societies recommends that clinicians use dressings that minimize pain and trauma during application and removal.[13]

Gauze dressings don't present a barrier to bacteria. Lawrence[14] demonstrated in an in vitro study that bacteria can pass through up to 64 layers of dry gauze. Once the gauze is moistened, it's even less effective as a barrier against bacteria. Infection rates are higher in wounds in which gauze is used as compared with wounds that are covered with transparent films or hydrocolloids.[15,16]

Successful wound healing depends on maintaining a moist environment. A balanced moist wound environment facilitates cellular growth and collagen proliferation within a healthy noncellular matrix.[17] The right balance of moisture is critical to wound healing. Too much moisture in the wound bed can impair the healing process, damage surrounding skin, and cause periwound maceration. Excess moisture must be managed with an appropriate wound dressing, thereby preventing further tissue destruction and deterioration of the wound bed.[17]

Film and hydrocolloid were among the first dressing materials that could maintain a moist wound-healing environment. New application techniques had to be learned and, more importantly, the clinical significance of wound fluid findings understood. The accumulation of light greenish–yellow fluid seen collecting under film dressings has caused us to relearn what is a normal expectation in a healing wound. Even the different nuance of wound odors has been cause for new learning. For example, different odors occur as wound fluid interacts with different dressing materials. A wound being treated with alginate dressings, which are made from seaweed, may smell like "low tide."

The new generation of moisture-balanced dressings can maintain the right environment conducive to wound healing. These dressing may have occlusive, semi-occlusive, absorptive, hydrating, autolytic, debriding, or hemostatic characteristics. Various wound dressing types will be discussed later in the chapter.

TREATMENT DECISIONS

The myriad of products available for wound care have enhanced the overall management of patients, but they have also created confusion about selecting the appropriate product. Optimal wound interventions should be dependent on the basic principles of wound care, attentive wound assessment, and expected outcomes. A complete wound assessment should be the driving element in all treatment decisions. (See chapter 6, Wound assessment.) Wound assessment should be based on the principles of wound care. (See *Principles of care: The MEASURES acronym.*)

Wound treatment decisions must be patient centered. What are the patient's goals and preferences? Local wound care starts with a thorough assessment of the wound and a comprehensive collection of data about the patient's overall status. Wound assessment parameters can assist with treatment choices and decisions for appropriate dressing selection.[18] (See *Wound care decision algorithm.*)

Once a thorough, individualized wound assessment is complete, choosing dressings and treatments becomes a clinical decision that is mutually arrived at with the patient based on data collected during the assessment and the overall expected outcome.

PRACTICE POINT

Dressing choices = Wound assessment + Principles of wound care

---

Treatment goals may aim to achieve a clean wound, heal the wound, maintain a clean wound bed, or place the patient in another setting to continue care. Clinicians should match the wound assessment characteristics with the dressing characteristics or function. The goal of care then becomes *using the right product on the right wound at the right time.* For example, a granular, nondraining moist or wet wound needs to maintain a moisture balance that is conducive to healing. The primary dressing choice would be a product that maintains a moist environment but doesn't cause maceration or desiccation of the wound bed. In another example, the goal of dressing selection for a necrotic draining wound is to loosen or soften the eschar for surgical debridement or to assist in autolytic debridement of the wound (see chapter 8, Wound debridement), absorb the excess exudate, and prevent trauma to surrounding tissue.

Principles of care: The MEASURES acronym

Minimize trauma to wound bed
Eliminate dead space (tunnels, tracts, undermining)
Assess and manage the amount of exudates
Support the body's tissue defense system
Use nontoxic wound cleansers
Remove infection, debris, and necrotic tissue
Environment maintenance, including thermal insulation and a moist wound bed
Surrounding tissue, protect from injury and bacterial invasion

© Sharon Baranoski

PRACTICE POINT

If the wound is dry, add moisture. If the wound has drainage, absorb it. If the wound has necrotic tissue, debride it.

Wound care decision algorithm

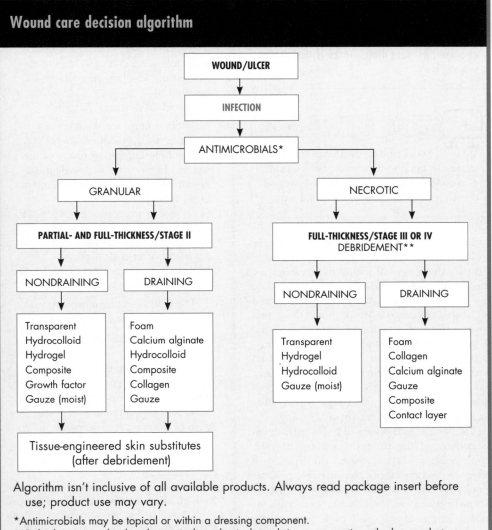

```
                    WOUND/ULCER
                         │
                      INFECTION
                         │
                   ANTIMICROBIALS*
          ┌──────────────┴──────────────┐
       GRANULAR                       NECROTIC
```

| PARTIAL- AND FULL-THICKNESS/STAGE II | FULL-THICKNESS/STAGE III OR IV DEBRIDEMENT** |

NONDRAINING	DRAINING	NONDRAINING	DRAINING
Transparent Hydrocolloid Hydrogel Composite Growth factor Gauze (moist)	Foam Calcium alginate Hydrocolloid Composite Collagen Gauze	Transparent Hydrogel Hydrocolloid Gauze (moist)	Foam Collagen Calcium alginate Gauze Composite Contact layer

Tissue-engineered skin substitutes
(after debridement)

Algorithm isn't inclusive of all available products. Always read package insert before use; product use may vary.

*Antimicrobials may be topical or within a dressing component.
**Debridement may be done by surgical, mechanical, autolytic, or enzymatic methods— products vary.

Adapted with permission from Baranoski, S. McIntosh, A. and Galvan, L. Wound Care Essentials: Practice Principles Lecture, Clinical Symposium on Advances in Skin & Wound Care. San Antonio, TX. October 2009.

Clinicians need to reassess the wound status when completing dressing changes so that appropriate treatment interventions can be implemented. It's important to also understand that once the characteristics of the wound assessment change, so may the dressing choice. All wound products come with product information and instructions to guide the user in appropriate use of that product. The most appropriate dressing should be selected based on consideration of the patient, the wound, and the site.[19] (See *Characteristics of an ideal dressing,* page 186, and *NICE© for dressing decision making,* pages 187–188. See also *Wound dressings categories,* pages 222–239.)

PRACTICE POINT

Wound dressings should be changed to meet the characteristics of the wound bed.

PRACTICE POINT

Read and understand the information in the package insert before using a wound care product. Not all wound dressings will function in the same way.

Dressings that come in contact with the wound bed are considered primary dressings. Primary dressings fall within three categories: those that maintain adequate moisture, those that absorb excess moisture, and those that add moisture.[9] Secondary dressings are those that cover a primary dressing or secure a dressing in place. Clinicians should know which dressings are safe to be put into the wound itself and which are used as securement products. Several dressings on the market act as both primary and secondary dressings. Again, what wound characteristics are you addressing?

Dressing selections should also include an assessment of the patient's outcome of care. High-priced, inappropriate dressings are often used when a more cost-effective product would suffice. Outcome is commonly driven by institutional setting. Acute care patients whose length of stay is 4 to 5 days usually won't achieve healing as their outcome, but they will achieve a moist, clean wound bed that supports the healing environment. Home care and long-term care settings may have a goal of healing or maintaining the current status of the wound based on the overall health status of the patient. Wound outcomes need to be patient-focused and realistic with regard to the length of time a patient is cared for.

The clinician also needs to keep in mind that one of the primary goals of care is the prevention of wound related-infection. Infection is a common complication of all open wounds. Open wounds are colonized with bacteria, which means that low numbers of bacteria are always

Characteristics of an ideal dressing

Use the following characteristics to determine the ideal dressing for your patient.
The ideal dressing should:
• maintain a moist environment
• facilitate autolytic debridement
• be conformable for the range of use needed (such as to fill tunneling, undermining, or sinus tracts to eliminate dead space)
• come in numerous shapes and sizes
• be absorbent
• provide thermal insulation
• act as a bacterial barrier
• reduce or eliminate pain at the wound site; Pain-free removal.

The following considerations can be used to evaluate the dressing:
• number of days the dressing can remain in place
• reason for change or removal
• appearance of dressing (soiled or intact)
• ease of dressing application
• ease of dressing removal
• ease of dressing maintenance
• ease of teaching about dressing to caregiver.

Adapted with permission from Seaman, S. "Dressing Selection in Chronic Wound Management," *Journal of the American Podiatric Medical Association* 92(1):24-33, January 2002.

present on the wound surface.[20] Wounds that are critically colonized can be managed with antimicrobial or antiseptic dressings that provide sustained release of various agents, such as silver or cadexomer iodine.[21] If a wound fails to respond, the clinician should consider switching to a product with a different mechanism of action.[20] Reviewing the NICE model for dressing selection can help streamline your decision process.[17] (See Chapter 7, Wound bioburden, for more information regarding wound infection and bioburden.)

NICE© for dressing decision making

There are thousands of dressings available and the clinician needs to decide which dressing to select for a particular wound. Ask yourself the following questions about the wound to help determine the dressing that is NICE© to use:

- Is there any **N**ecrotic tissue that needs to be debrided? (Make sure the wound has the ability to heal; if not, however, moist interactive dressings and active surgical debridement to bleeding tissue are contraindicated.)
- Is the wound **I**nfected or inflamed? (Clinicians often look for more than one sign or symptom before diagnosing infection.)
- Do the specific wound **C**haracteristics, such as location, need to be considered? (If the wound is around the anus, a waterproof adhesive dressing may be preferred.) Is pain an issue?
- Is there any **E**xudate; if so, why, how much, and what are the color and consistency?

Exudate may indicate that the cause of the wound has not been treated (for example, edema due to venous insufficiency); that congestive heart failure is present (look for bilateral involvement and extension above the knee); that albumin levels are low (malnutrition, kidney, or liver disease); or that infection is present. Periwound skin needs protection from exudate by using absorbent dressings and protecting the periwound skin. Select a dressing by answering the four questions. Remember, it's NICE© to pick the right dressing.

Letter	Key information to know	Caution
Necrotic tissue Slough, eschar	• Wet-to-dry dressings are a non-selective method of mechanical debridement. • Autolytic debridement of tissue is best accomplished with hydrogels, hydrocolloids, and alginate dressings. • With dressing-stimulated autolytic debridement, watch for secondary infection and remove unwanted slough with dressing change.	• Dressings are a slower method of debridement compared with sharp/surgical methods. • There is limited use of wet-to-dry dressings as a debridement method. • Some dressings cannot be used or caution is urged in necrotic wounds; check with the manufacturer for any contraindications for use. • Removal of non-viable tissue is a critical step in preparing the wound bed for healing.
Infection/inflammation	• Consider using antimicrobial dressings (for example, silver or iodine). • Infected wounds may require more frequent dressing changes.	• Not all dressings can be used in infected wounds; check with the manufacturer for the specific brand indicated for use.

(continued)

NICE© for dressing decision making (continued)

Letter	Key information to know	Caution
Characteristics	• Select and reassess a dressing based on location of the wound, such as the use of conformable dressings for hard-to-fit areas. • Waterproof dressings may be used if incontinence is an issue. • Consider the patient's pain and select dressings that may promote comfort and pain reduction.	• Change dressings when they become soiled from feces or urine. • Different dressings can remain in place for different lengths of time; check with the manufacturer for recommended frequency for dressing changes. • Avoid dressings that may increase or contribute to wound pain and consider systemic pain management strategies.
Exudate	• Match the absorbency of the dressing (none, low, moderate, heavy) to the amount of exudate from the wound. • Assess surrounding skin to evaluate for macerations.	• Surrounding skin needs to be protected from wound drainage; refer to the enabler LOWE©. Search for the cause of the excessive exudate and the need to correct the cause. Exudate may be an indicator of infection.

© E.A. Ayello and R.G. Sibbald.

The practice of using the same wound dressing during the entire healing period is no longer valid. *All* wounds under the care of clinicians should be assessed a minimum of once a week and more often if notable changes occur. The type of wound, status of the wound, clinical setting, and regulatory compliance may dictate a different interval of assessment, however. Be aware of practice regulations for your facility or institution. (See chapter 6, Wound assessment.)

Wound assessment is the cumulative process of observing the wound itself as well as observing the patient and collecting and evaluating data. For many patients, weekly reassessment will provide the indices of successful treatment and guide decisions that suggest product changes. As the wound characteristics change, so too should the choice of the wound dressing.

Indeed, several different types of products may be needed as the wound progresses through the stages of healing.

Dressings should be matched carefully to the wound, the patient, and the setting. For example, a deep wound with a large amount of drainage will require a highly absorbent dressing such as alginate or foam. As the depth and amount of drainage decrease, a dressing such as a hydrogel, hydrocolloid, or film might be used.

PRACTICE POINT

Don't use film dressings with higher moisture vapor rates developed for use over IV line sites on open wounds.

Economic considerations for nurses

- Clean, rather than sterile, dressings and gloves can usually be used in the home for chronic wounds (refer to your agency's policy).
- Saline solution can be made at home by adding 1 teaspoon of salt to 1 quart of boiling water.[21]
- Dressings shouldn't be left open or at the patient's bedside.
- Cost of product selected and resources available for financial assistance should be considered.
- Frequency of dressing changes and cost-effective use of materials should be considered.
- Fistula management may use pouching versus dressing.
- Nursing time per dressing change should be considered.
- The overall effectiveness of the treatment should be an economic consideration.

Adapted with permission from Baranoski, S. "Wound Dressings: A Myriad of Challenging Decisions," *Home Healthcare Nurse* 23(5):307-17, May 2005.[6]

Over the course of healing, the treatment plan will change as the wound is filled with granulation tissue and epithelialization occurs. Economic factors should also be considered when selecting dressings. The overall cost and effectiveness of treatment, cost of materials, nursing time, and frequency of dressing changes over time all impact the economic burden of care.[22,23] (See *Economic considerations for nurses*.)

The notion that all wounds are alike has also changed. An understanding of the etiology of the wound is essential for appropriate care.[21] Local wound care products as well as supportive care must be individualized for the particular wound. For example, a venous stasis ulcer might require a highly absorptive dressing as well as the necessary compression

therapy. A variety of two- to four-layered compression bandages beyond the classic "Unna boot" are now available. Further, checking for ankle-brachial index and/or toe pressures using a Doppler is part of the total care of a patient with a peripheral vascular ulcer or history of diabetic neuropathies.[17]

USING WOUND HEALING BIOLOGY TO SELECT TREATMENT

An example of increased understanding of the "cellular biology" of wound healing and technology is the use of growth factors in wound care. All growth factors are proteins that are secreted by cells and have the ability to stimulate cell division, a positive action during the wound healing process.[24] Growth factors are now available either derived from a patient's own platelets or in a drug form dispensed in a tube to apply to certain wounds. Research continues as to what combination, what quantity, and when growth factors will best enhance wound healing

Yet another way technology is providing new options for wound management is in the use of tissue-engineered skin equivalents or substitutes for healing chronic wounds.

What the future holds for the use of gene therapy in wound healing is yet to be seen. The use of gene delivery or microencapsulation in advanced wound therapy is being investigated.[24]

Moist wound therapy and dressing options

The essential function of a wound dressing is to provide the right environment to enhance and promote wound healing. Research over the past 50 years has led to the generally accepted phenomenon that moist wound dressings create an optimal environment for wounds to heal faster and with less scar formation. The work of Orland[25] and Winter[4] led to the development of moist wound dressings as a clinical intervention to treat wounds.

George Winter is often cited as the father of moist wound healing. His laboratory work comparing the effect of air drying versus occlusive dressings on epithelialization in the animal model is generally considered a landmark study.[4,26] Fear of increasing infection with occlusive therapy slowed the development of moist wound therapy dressings, however, and 16 years passed between Winter's study and the development of what is considered the first moist wound therapy dressing, OpSite. Continued research, clinician experiments, and interest in wound healing in general have led many companies to develop an assortment of moist wound treatment dressings. However, this has created a challenge for healthcare providers, who struggle to keep up with the ever-increasing number of new products and new technologies.

The following synopsis reviews the major dressing categories and provides helpful practice points on what, when, and how to use these dressings.

TRANSPARENT FILM DRESSINGS

Transparent film dressings, so named for their "see-through" properties, are thin polyurethane membranes. They are coated with an adhesive that allows them to adhere to the wound margins without sticking to the actual wound (Fig. 9-1).

Transparent films have no absorptive capacity but do transmit moisture vapor and are semipermeable to gases. These dressings imitate the outer skin layer to provide a moist environment, similar to a blister. This covering allows epithelial cells to migrate over the surface of the wound. Fluid may accumulate under these dressings. This fluid is sometimes mistaken for pus, a sign of infection. The fluid is a useful adjunct to create an autolytic environment, thereby inducing a cleaner wound surface. When excess fluid accumulates or leaks out from the sides of the dressing, the dressing needs to be changed. Maceration of periwound skin can occur if these dressings are not changed in a timely manner.

Transparent film dressings provide a valuable protective barrier against outside contaminants, fluid, and bacteria. Transparent films also add a layer of protection to the wound bed to minimize further damaging trauma.[17] They provide protection from friction and aid in autolytic debridement and pain control. Film makes an excellent secondary dressing as well. Most films can be left on for up to 7 days. These dressings are indicated for wounds with absent or low levels of exudate.[7,8,17] Transparent films can be used on a variety of wound types, such as stage I and II pressure ulcers, superficial wounds, minor burns, or lacerations; over sutures, catheter sites, donor sites, and superficial dermal ulcers; and for protection of the skin against friction. Transparent dressings can be used on central lines, peripherally inserted central catheter lines, and infected wounds.

In addition, some of the newer transparent films currently on the market also contain ionic silver.

Practice Essentials

- Apply transparent film dressings to healthy skin; use with caution on aging and fragile skin.
- These dressings aren't recommended for use on infants or small children.
- These dressings may be used on dry to minimally moist wounds.
- Don't use transparent film dressings on exudating wounds.
- Transparent film dressings make excellent secondary dressings.
- Not all film dressings can be used on infected wounds.
- Change the dressing when fluid reaches the edge of the dressing, when the seal is broken, or when the adhesive bond is compromised.
- When removing the dressing, lift the corner and pull the film toward the outside of the wound to break the adhesive barrier.
- Avoid roughness when removing the film; gently stretch the corner of the dressing and support the skin as you remove the dressing.
- Skin protective wipes and sprays can be used on the periwound area before applying the dressing. Skin wipes also provide an

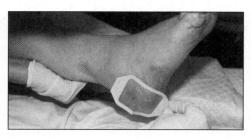

Figure 9-1. Transparent film dressing.

additional seal to prevent the dressing edges from rolling.
- Always read the package insert before applying the dressing because product usage may vary.
- Numerous sizes and shapes are available.

> **PRACTICE POINT**
>
> Transparent film and hydrocolloid dressings are known for their ability to maintain existing moisture levels in the wound.

HYDROCOLLOID DRESSINGS

Hydrocolloid dressings were introduced in the 1980s and were the mainstay for wound management for many years. Hydrocolloids are impermeable to gases and water vapor.[27] These wafer-shaped dressings (Fig. 9-2) are composed of opaque mixtures of adhesive, absorbent polymers, pectin gelling agents, and sodium carboxymethylcellulose. Hydrophilic particles within the dressing react with the wound fluid to form a soft gel over the wound bed. According to Choucair and Phillips,[27] some hydrocolloid dressings provide an acidic environment and some act as a bacterial or viral barrier. Their translucent appearance allows for viewing of the amount of exudate absorbed and fluid accumulated under the dressing.

Hydrocolloid dressings may have a noticeable odor during dressing changes. This is normal in the absence of clinical signs of infection. Some hydrocolloids may also leave residue in the wound bed.

Hydrocolloid dressings have evolved into a shape that fits most wounds and locations. They're sold in wafer, sheet, paste, and powder forms and are available in many sizes. Adhesive properties and ability to absorb exudate vary by product. Because most of these dressings are adhesive, care must be taken when using on fragile skin. Correct application requires the dressing to be bigger than the actual wound size. For optimal dressing adherence, the dressing must extend at least 1″ (2.5 cm) onto the healthy skin surrounding the wound. The dressing should be changed as recommended by the manufacturer. This could be from 3 to 7 days and often depends on the amount of exudate. Many of the newer hydrocolloids have other absorptive ingredients added, such as alginate, collagen, and sustained-released silver ions.

Hydrocolloids are indicated for minimally to moderately heavy exudating wounds, abrasions, skin tears, lacerations, pressure ulcers, dermal wounds, granular wounds, or necrotic wounds as well as under compression wraps. Some of the second-generation hydrocolloids are more absorptive and can be used in heavily exudating wounds. Hydrocolloids do not absorb fluids rapidly, which is valuable when wound exudate levels are in transition from higher to lower quanitites.[9] Hydrocolloids also provide a moist environment that is conducive to autolytic debridement. Excessive granulation (hyper-granulation tissue) and maceration can occur if the dressing isn't changed appropriately. Hydrocolloids are often used as a preventive dressing on high-risk areas (sacrum, heels) and around surgical wounds to protect the skin from frequent tape removal.

Practice Essentials
- Change the dressing every 3 to 7 days, or before it reaches its maximal absorption or when fluid reaches within 1″ of the edge.
- Not all hydrocolloid dressings can be used on infected wounds. Check product insert.
- These dressings aren't recommended for undermining, tunnels, or sinus tracts.
- Hydrocolloid dressings may be cut to fit the wound area, such as on an elbow or heel.
- These dressings may be used as primary or secondary dressings or over other wound filler products.

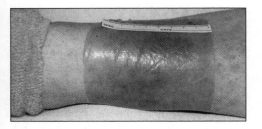

Figure 9-2. Hydrocolloid dressing.

- Remove the dressing by starting at a corner and gently rolling it off the wound; don't pull to remove.
- Flush out any residue with saline or wound cleanser.
- Skin protective wipes or sprays may be used on the periwound area to enhance adherence.
- Picture-framing with paper tape may prevent the dressing edges from rolling.

HYDROGEL DRESSINGS

Hydrogel dressings have provided clinicians with a viable means to hydrate or, stated differently, donate moisture to dry wound beds.

Hydrogel dressings are marketed in multiple formats containing varying amounts of water in various polymer matrices. Hydrogels are available as amorphous gels, three-dimensional sheets, or amorphous gels impregnated into other mesh-type dressings (Fig. 9-3). Their unique cross-linked polymer structure entraps water and reduces the temperature of the wound bed by up to 5° C.[27] This moist environment facilitates autolysis and removal of devitalized tissue.

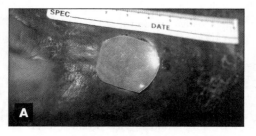

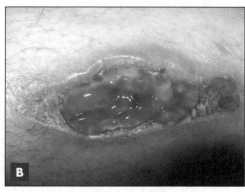

Figure 9-3. (A) Hydrogel dressing. (B) Amorphous hydrogel dressing.

The main application for hydrogels is hydrating dry wound beds and softening and loosening slough and necrotic wound debris. Hydrogels have a limited absorptive capacity due to their high water concentration. Some hydrogels have other ingredients, such as alginates, collagen, or starch, to enhance their absorptive capacity and will absorb low to moderate amounts of exudate. Absorptive capability varies by product and type of gel. They can be used for many types of wounds, including pressure ulcers, partial- and full-thickness wounds, and vascular ulcers. Their soothing and cooling properties also make them excellent choices for use in skin tears, dermabrasion, dermal wounds, donor sites, and radiation burns.

Maceration can be a concern for clinicians. Periwound skin areas need to be protected from excess hydration; therefore, protective barriers are often recommended. One of the benefits of a hydrogel is that it can be used with topical medications or antibacterial agents. Hydrogels are packaged as sheets, tube gels, sprays, and impregnated gauze pads or strips for packing tunneling and undermined areas within the wound bed. Some require a secondary dressing to secure the hydrogel; new versions have adhesive borders. Some newer versions also contain ionic silver and can be left on for several days. Hydrogels with silver should not be used in combination with enzymatic debriding agents because the silver can inactivate the enzymatic.

Practice Essentials
- Don't use hydrogels with heavily draining wounds or on intact skin.
- Daily dressing changes may be necessary due to evaporation of the hydrogel. Some sheet hydrogels may last for several days. Check daily to maintain a moist environment.
- Protect the surrounding skin with a skin barrier ointment, wipe, or spray.
- Watch for areas of maceration on surrounding skin.

FOAM DRESSINGS

Foam dressings are highly absorbent and are usually made from a polyurethane base with a heat- and pressure-modified wound contact layer (Fig. 9-4).[28] Foam dressings are permeable to both gases and water vapor, and their hydrophilic properties allow for absorption of exudate into the layers of the foam.

Foam dressings are some of the most adaptable dressings for wound care. They are indicated for wounds with moderate to heavy exudate, prophylactic protection over bony prominences or friction areas, partial- and full-thickness wounds, granular or necrotic wound beds, skin tears, donor sites, under compression wraps, surgical or dermal wounds, in combination with other primary dressings, and wounds of any etiology. They can also be used on infected wounds, if changed daily.[19] The second generation of foams is also available with controlled-released ionic silver. These dressings must have exudates for the silver ion to be released.

Foams shouldn't be used on dry eschar wound beds because they could cause further desiccation of the wound site. Foams may be used in combination with topical treatments and/or enzymatic debriders. Foams are available in many sizes and shapes, including cavity (pillow type) dressings. Not all foam dressings have an adhesive border, so they'll need to be secured with tape. However, new foam products have emerged with adhesive borders. Caution with fragile skin may be warranted.

Practice Essentials
- Not all foams have FDA approval for use on infected wounds—be sure to check the package insert.

- Foam dressings can be left in place for up to 3 to 7 days, depending on the amount of exudate absorption.
- Removal of these dressings is usually trauma-free.
- Foam dressings can be cut to fit the size of the wound.
- Skin wipes or sprays can be used to protect the periwound area from maceration.
- Non-adhesive border dressings will require taping or wraps to secure.
- Make sure you put the *correct* side of the foam dressing in contact with the wound bed.

CALCIUM ALGINATE DRESSINGS

Calcium alginate dressings provide yet another choice for clinicians to use in managing highly exudative wounds (Fig. 9-5). Alginate dressings are absorbent, non-adherent, biodegradable, nonwoven fibers derived from brown seaweed, composed of calcium salts of alginic acid and mannuronic and galuronic acids.[27,28]

When alginate dressings come in contact with sodium-rich solutions such as wound drainage, the calcium ions undergo an exchange for the sodium ions, forming a soluble sodium alginate gel. This gel maintains a moist wound bed and supports a therapeutic healing environment. Alginates can absorb 20 times their weight; this may vary based on the particular product. They are extremely beneficial in managing large draining cavity wounds, pressure ulcers, vascular ulcers, surgical incisions, wound dehiscence, tunnels, sinus tracts, skin graft donor sites, exposed

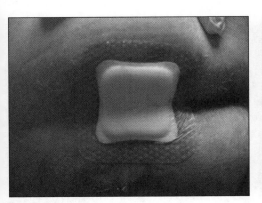

Figure 9-4. Foam dressing.

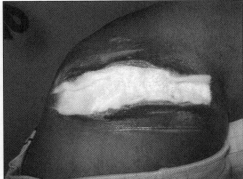

Figure 9-5. Calcium alginate dressing.

tendons, and infected wounds. Additionally, their hemostatic and absorptive properties make them useful on minor-bleeding wounds. Alginates are contraindicated for dry wounds, eschar-covered wounds, surgical implantation, or third-degree burns.

Alginates are available in sheet, pad, and rope forms and in numerous sizes. Some newer calcium alginate dressings also contain controlled-release ionic silver; these calcium alginate–silver dressings should not be used in combination with enzymatic debriding agents. Alginate dressings are usually changed daily or as indicated by the amount of drainage. One drawback is that these dressings can dry out and adhere to the wound bed. Using appropriate secondary dressings that help to maintain a gelling state is recommended.[9] Early wound care interventions may warrant more frequent dressing changes due to high volume of drainage. As fluid management is attained, the frequency of dressing changes can be decreased.

Practice Essentials
- Calcium alginate dressings provide easy application and trauma-free removal.
- These dressings are a good choice for undermined or tunneled draining wounds.
- Calcium alginate dressings require a secondary dressing.
- These dressings may leave fiber residue, which can be removed by flushing with saline.
- Calcium alginate dressings facilitate autolytic debridement.
- These dressings can be used on infected wounds, with or without ionic silver.
- These dressings are cost-effective if used appropriately.

PRACTICE POINT

In order to release the silver ion, moisture/exudate must be present when controlled-release ionic silver is used in combination with other types of dressings (hydrogels, hydrocolloids, foams, etc.).

COMPOSITE DRESSINGS

A combination of materials makes up a single-layered composite dressing. These dressings have multiple functions, such as a bacterial barrier, absorptive layer, foam, hydrocolloid, or hydrogel.[28] Additionally, they must have an adhesive border and semi-adherent or non-adherent properties. These dressings are conformable and are available in numerous sizes and shapes.

However, not all composite dressings provide a moist environment; many are used or created by using a secondary dressing. They are also referred to as *island dressings*.

Practice Essentials
- Use composite dressings with caution when treating a patient with fragile skin.
- Composite dressings are easy to apply.
- These dressings may be used on infected wounds and with topical products.
- They may facilitate autolytic or mechanical debridement.
- Frequency of dressing change depends on the wound type and the manufacturers' recommendations.
- These dressings may adhere to wound bed; use caution when removing them.

COLLAGEN DRESSINGS

Collagen is a major protein of the body and is necessary for wound healing and repair. Collagen dressings are derived from bovine hide (cowhide). Collagen dressings are either 100% collagen or may be combined with alginates or other products. They are a highly absorptive, hydrophilic, moist wound dressing (Fig. 9-6).

Seaman[19] suggests that collagen powders, particles, and pads are useful in treating highly exudative wounds. If the wound has low to

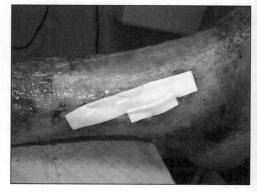

Figure 9-6. Collagen dressing.

moderate exudate, sheets should be used. If the wound is dry, gels should be used. Collagen dressings can be used on granulating or necrotic wounds and on partial- or full-thickness wounds.[19] They may be used with other topical agents.

A collagen dressing should be changed every 3 to 7 days. If wound infection is present, then daily dressing change is recommended. Collagen dressings require a secondary dressing for securement.

Practice Essentials
- Use collagen dressings with caution when treating patients with fragile skin if adhesive secondary dressings are also being used.
- These dressings are contraindicated for patients who are sensitive to bovine products.
- Don't use these dressings on dry wounds or third-degree burns.
- Collagen dressings are easy to remove.
- Their gel properties prevent these dressings from adhering to the wound bed.
- Collagen dressings facilitate a moist wound environment and may be used with other topical products.
- Change collagen dressings daily if used on infected wounds.

CONTACT LAYER DRESSINGS

Contact layer dressings are a single layer of a woven net that acts as a low adherence material when applied to wound surfaces.[28] A contact layer dressing is applied directly to the wound and acts as a protective interface between the wound and the secondary dressings. Their main purpose is to allow exudate to pass through the contact layer and into the secondary dressing. They are often used with ointments, creams, or other topical products such as growth factors or tissue-engineered skin substitutes. Contact layer dressings aren't recommended for dry wounds or third-degree burns. Check the package insert for clarification as to which wounds the product can be used on. Various sizes and shapes are available. Frequency of dressing changes is dependent on the etiology of the wound and the amount of exudate.

Practice Essentials
- Contact layer dressings aren't recommended for dry wounds or third-degree burns.

- Contact layer dressings are easy to apply and are secured with a secondary dressing.
- They protect the wound bed during dressing changes.

ANTIMICROBIAL DRESSINGS

Antimicrobial dressings have added a new dimension to the wound dressing arena. Clinicians now have several choices of dressings when dealing with wound infections. These new dressings are different than topical antibiotic therapy. They provide the benefit of an antimicrobial effect against bacteria and a moist environment for healing. The active ingredient may be silver ions, cadexomer iodine, or polyhexamethylene biguanide (Fig. 9-7). Antimicrobial dressings do not replace the need for systemic antibiotic therapy; rather, they serve as an adjunct in treating wound infections As research continues and new products become available, this classification of wound dressing will expand. Antimicrobial dressings are available in a variety of forms: transparent dressings, gauze, island dressings, foams, and absorptive fillers to name a few. Some of these dressings can remain in place for 7 days.

Practice Essentials
- Antimicrobial dressings are an adjunct in treating wound infections.
- Frequency of dressing change varies among antimicrobials.
- Antimicrobial dressings are used in wounds with high bacterial bioburden or in wounds

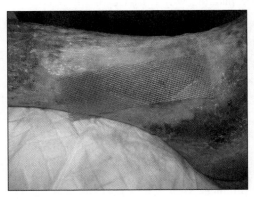

Figure 9-7. Silver dressing.

that are critically colonized to prevent wound infection.

• Antimicrobial dressings may be used under compression wraps to prevent infection in wounds with a high bacterial bioburden.

Advanced therapies
TISSUE-ENGINEERED SKIN SUBSTITUTES

Technology has spawned a new generation of skin substitute materials to advance wound healing and provide all the characteristics of natural skin. Skin substitutes were originally were designed to replace autografts, which are the harvesting of a patient's own skin to apply to a burn or wound.[9] Tissue engineering is the development of materials that combine novel substances with living cells to yield functional tissue equivalents, such as skin substitutes.[19] Current skin substitutes may be comprised of epidermal cells, dermal cells, or both supported by a biodegradable matrix.[9] Products containing both epidermal and dermal cells are referred to as bilayered.[9]

Two tissue-engineered products containing living cells are approved for use in the United States. Apligraf® and Dermagraft® both contain living cells derived from neonatal foreskin. A single foreskin can produce over 200,000 units of the product.[26] Apligraf is a bilayered skin product consisting of a dermal equivalent composed of type I bovine collagen that contains living human dermal fibroblasts as an overlying cornified epidermal layer of living human keratinocytes. Apligraf doesn't contain Langerhans' cells, melanocytes, or endothelial cells, perhaps explaining why it isn't clinically rejected. It contains only human fibroblasts and is tested extensively for infectious agents. Dermagraft is a cryopreserved human fibroblast-derived dermal skin substitute indicated for use in the treatment of full-thickness diabetic foot ulcers.[29, 30] When the Dermagraft is placed on an ulcer, the mesh material is gradually absorbed and the human cells grow into place, replacing the damaged skin.[30] Dermagraft is not recommended for use on infected wounds or wounds with sinus tracts. It should not be used in patients who are sensitive to bovine products.[30]

Different tissue-engineered skin products are approved for various applications such as use on venous ulcers, diabetic ulcers, and burns. Additional applications will most likely be available in the future. Skin substitutes are surgically applied by a physician; however, several applications may be needed before healing is attained. Prior to application, the wound bed preparation process needs to be strictly followed. Wounds are debrided, moisture balance maintained, and infection monitored.

The wound may be cultured prior to the procedure and appropriate oral antibiotic therapy used, as well as an antimicrobial wound dressing, to prevent "losing" the graft. If infection does occur, it can be successfully handled with various topical medications. The graft site must be protected from injury; the secondary dressing is changed without disturbing the graft site. Tissue-engineered skin holds a promising future for wound care patients.

Practice Essentials
• Skin substitutes will only adhere to a clean wound bed.
• Watch for signs and symptoms of infection.
• Don't debride the yellow caramelized crust at the edges or in the wound; this is the growth factor and you may be removing the tissue-engineered skin substitute. This is important to teach physicians and staff who are changing the wound dressings.
• Don't allow the graft site to adhere to a secondary dressing.

▶ PRACTICE POINT

To date, no skin substitute is able to completely replicate normal, uninjured skin.[9]

Biophysical technologies

Unlike acute wounds, chronic wounds do not heal spontaneously and within the expected time frame. The application of exogenous energies has been shown to enhance cellular

Categories and types of biophysical agents

Category	Biophysical agents
Mechanical/kinetic	• Subatmospheric/negative pressure • Atmospheric (hyperbaric and topical oxygen) • Kinetic (whirlpool, pulsatile lavage)
Electrical/electromagnetic	• Electrical stimulation • Electromagnetic fields • Phototherapy: infrared, ultraviolet, coherent (laser), monochromatic (light-emitting diode)
Acoustic	• High-frequency ultrasound • Low-frequency ultrasound

Adapted from Biophysical Agents in Pressure Ulcer Management, National Pressure Ulcer Advisory Panel and European Pressure Ulcer Advisory Panel. *Prevention and Treatment of Pressure Ulcers: Clinical Practice Guideline.* Washington, DC: National Pressure Ulcer Advisory Panel, pp 90-95, 2009.

and tissue responses. This section discusses some of these energies and devices.

There is a plethora of current research supporting the use of exogenous energies to improve healing in chronic wounds. The newer terminology for these devices is biophysical technologies or energies. Biophysical technologies include physical modalities that create tissue changes at the tissue/cellular level. These agents include electrical, light, sound, and mechanical energies, all of which have been used to promote soft tissue regeneration in both acute and chronic wounds.[31] Biophysical agents are divided into three primary categories: mechanical or kinetic, electrical/electromagnetic, and acoustic. (See *Categories and types of biophysical agents*.)

When deciding which biophysical agent to choose, it is important that the clinician consider the evidence that supports the use of these interventions. In addition, the clinician must not only know how to use the equipment correctly and safely but also be able to identify where in the wound healing sequelae of events these devices should be used to best augment the desired tissue response. The

delivery of these energies should be under the direction and supervision of a licensed healthcare professional who has been educated and trained and is considered competent in the use, safety, selection, application, and monitoring of biophysical agents.[31] It is of critical importance to know and understand not only the indications for these devices but also the contraindications and precautions associated with these energies.

NEGATIVE-PRESSURE WOUND THERAPY

Negative-pressure wound therapy (NPWT) was developed in the early 1990s in Europe and launched in the United States in 1997. This biophysical agent is indicated for a variety of wound types. (See *Indications and contraindications for NPWT,* page 198.) In general, NPWT is indicated for full-thickness wounds such as stage III and IV pressure ulcers and other deep wounds that require assistance with contraction and granulation tissue formation. Some NPWT systems are appropriate for tunnels, tracts, and undermining.

Indications and contraindications for NPWT

Indications	Contraindications
• Diabetic foot ulcers • Pressure ulcers (stage III & IV) • Venous insufficiency ulcers • Arterial insufficiency ulcers • Full-thickness burns • Surgical wounds (especially infected sternal wounds) • Postoperative and dehisced surgical wounds • Traumatic wounds • Explored fistulas • Skin grafts and flaps	• Exposed vital organs (treatment may continue after the organ has been covered by Vicryl absorbable mesh) • Inadequately debrided wounds; granulation tissue that will not form over necrotic tissue • Untreated osteomyelitis or sepsis within the vicinity of the wound • Presence of untreated coagulopathy • Necrotic tissue with eschar • Malignancy in the wound (negative-pressure therapy may lead to cellular proliferation) • Allergy to any component required for the procedure

NOTE: Indications and contraindications vary slightly by manufacturer. Please refer to manufacturer's recommendations for the particular unit to be used.

Adapted from Agency for Healthcare Research and Quality. "Negative Pressure Wound Therapy Devices," Available at: http://www.ahrq.gov/clinic/ta/negpresswtd/npwtd02.htm. Accessed September 2, 2010.

NPWT applies subatmospheric pressure, or suction, to the wound bed by way of a mechanical unit that is attached to a dressing through a plastic tube (Fig. 9-8). Several types of dressings are used with these devices, including foam, moistened cotton gauze, and nonwoven polyester layers joined by a silicone elastomer.[32,33] The dressings are covered with a transparent film that seals the wound and dressing to maintain the vacuum effect. Foam or gauze containing silver or other antibiotics is available from some manufacturers. When using gauze, a non-adherent dressing should be placed next to the wound bed and then the moistened gauze applied on top to fill the wound. Manufacturers recommend initially changing the dressing 48 hours after beginning treatment, then two to three times per week as indicated by the wound's response to the NPWT intervention.[32-38]

Once the dressing is applied, an evacuation tube runs from the wound through the dressing, drawing excess exudate away from the wound and into a canister attached to the other end of the tubing. The canister is attached to a vacuum pump that provides either continuous or intermittent negative pressure, adjusted for the type of wound being treated. Negative pressure created by the pump is in the range of 0 to 200 mm Hg depending on the system used.[34-36]

The application and type of dressing vary by the specific manufacturer and the goals for use of the device. NPWT reportedly facilitates wound closure and healing through several mechanisms of action, including[31]:

• removing third space edema, which improves nutrient and oxygen delivery
• removing wound exudate, which is a medium for bacterial colonization

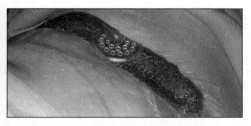

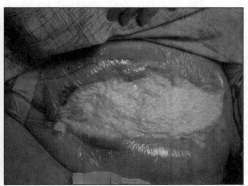

Figure 9-8. Negative-pressure wound therapy.

- decreasing harmful levels of pro-inflammatory agents, such as matrix met-alloproteases (MMPs), found in chronic wounds
- facilitating wound retraction or contraction
- promoting angiogenesis.

One theory as to how NPWT enhances wound closure is that the externally applied stress creates macro-strain and micro-strain in the wound bed and in individual cells.[39-42] Macro-strain is the physical response that can be seen immediately as the negative pressure contracts the wound.[39] In addition, this mechanical stress creates changes at the cells' surface (also known as micro-deformations), causing growth factors and cytokines to "up-regulate" fibroblastic activity, increasing production of the extracellular matrix and cell proliferation within the wound and ultimately creating new granulation tissue.[39-42] This increase in the rate of granulation tissue formation has been noted in several studies using NPWT.[39-42]

According to the National Pressure Ulcer Advisory Panel (NPUAP),[31] wound volume was significant reduced and healing was more rapid in pressure ulcers treated with NPWT compared with other traditional wound treatments.

It has been suggested that NPWT assists in preparing the wound bed for closure once granulation tissue has been well established.[42] When a wound is filled with newly synthesized granulation tissue, resurfacing by epithelial cells can take place more readily.[42]

It is important that the wound be debrided of as much necrotic tissue as possible before using the NPWT device. The exact percentage of necrotic tissue that can be present in the wound bed varies according to manufacturer as well as facility and clinician protocols. In general, it is best to have the wound bed *free* of necrotic tissue prior to application of the NPWT device.

Safety must be taken into consideration when using these devices. In November 2009, the FDA released a Preliminary Public Health Notification Safety Alert[43] describing deaths and serious complications associated with the use of NPWT systems. The FDA had received reports of six deaths and 77 injuries associated with NPWT systems over a 2-year period in relation to bleeding, primarily in conjunction with anticoagulation therapy.

PRACTICE POINT

NPWT should be used cautiously when there is active bleeding, when the patient is on anticoagulants, when there is difficult wound hemostasis, or when placing the dressing in proximity to blood vessels.

Practice Essentials
- Dressing changes should be performed according to the specific manufacturer's directions.
- Be sure to apply skin sealant to the entire periwound area under the drape to assist in preventing blistering and excoriation when removing the adhesive drape.
- Check the manufacturer's directions to see how long the suction unit can be off until the dressing must be changed

ELECTRICAL SIMULATION

In the 18th and 19th centuries, when Galvani[44,45] and Matteucci[46] made preparations of cut sciatic nerve and muscle tissue from an excised frog leg, they found that small electrical currents were generated at the cut points. The electric potentials associated with these cut points are now referred to as injury potentials. In 1860, German physiologist Emil Du Bois Reymond[47] measured a direct current flow out of a cut in his finger and observed the disappearance of these currents when the wounds healed.

Electrical stimulation (ES) has been used for more than three decades to accelerate the rate of chronic wound healing. This energy has been given strength of evidence of A by the NPUAP[31] as an adjunctive therapy for treatment of recalcitrant stage III and IV pressure ulcers. Healthcare professionals who have used ES consider it to be one of the most cost-effective, therapeutically efficacious tissue repair and wound healing accelerators in our wound care tool kit. Unfortunately, ES is often passed over due to lack of knowledge, education, and training among clinicians in the application of this energy.[48] Based on the research in this field of study, the strength-of-evidence rating for this modality was increased from level B to level A in 1999.[49] In 2000, the Paralyzed Veterans of America published a Clinical Practice Guideline titled "Pressure Ulcer Prevention and Treatment Following Spinal Cord Injury,"[50] which stated that ES qualified as a stand-alone intervention and should no longer be classified as an adjunctive therapy. The reported effects of ES in relation to chronic wound healing and tissue repair include increased blood flow,[51] increased tissue oxygenation,[52,53] increased fibroblast proliferation and collagen deposition,[47] increased angiogenesis,[54] decreased wound pain,[55] increased wound tensile strength,[56,57] and decreased diabetic peripheral neuropathic pain.[58]

ES energy may be considered for treatment of lower limbs with severely compromised arterial blood flow. ES energy delivered as high-voltage pulsed current (HVPC) applied to ischemic lower extremities has been shown to increase transcutaneous pulse oximetry and perfusion, with subsequent healing of these legs and feet in patients who were at high risk for amputation.[47]

The application of ES in wound healing includes therapeutic exogenous (externally applied) electrical currents. These currents are delivered to the wound tissues by placing at least two electrodes directly into or around the wound (periwound tissue) (Fig. 9-9B-D) or by applying a stocking or glove electrode garment to the affected limb (Fig. 9-9A.)

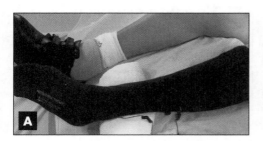
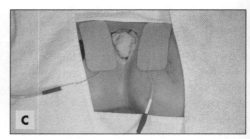
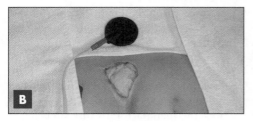
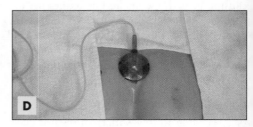

Figure 9-9. Electrical stimulation used to accelerate wound healing via placement of electrodes (B,C,D) and with the use of a stocking electrode garment (A).

ES uses an electrical current to transfer energy to the tissue. This energy produces a number of cellular processes and physiological responses that are important to wound healing, including:

- stimulation of fibroblasts to enhance collagen and DNA synthesis
- increased number of receptor sites for growth factors
- alteration in the direction of fibroblast migration, activation of cells in the wound site, improved tissue perfusion, and decreased edema.[59]

The electrical current may be delivered as low-intensity direct current, HVPC, transcutaneous electrical nerve stimulation, or pulsed electromagnetic energy. However, HVPC has become the current used most often for ES wound treatments in the past decade.

ES is performed by physical therapists or other licensed healthcare professionals who are educated and trained in identifying how and when to apply and change the ES treatment parameters (for example, ES dosage, polarity, electrode placement) according to the wound characteristics. According to Myer,[60] HVPC has a waveform of paired short-duration pulses with a long interpulse interval. It's a pulsed or interrupted monophasic waveform. The duration of treatment is usually 45 to 60 minutes, delivered five to seven times per week. ES is indicated for all types of wounds regardless of the etiology. It is contraindicated for basal or squamous cell carcinoma in the wound or periwound tissue, for osteomyelitis (if the patient is not responding to systemic treatment with antibiotics), for ion residues of iodine or silver in the wound, and over electronic implants or directly over the carotid arteries or heart.[48]

The decision-making process for how to use ES in a specific wound depends on the phase of wound healing and what the clinician is attempting to accomplish. ES delivers a summation of either a positive charge or a negative charge to the tissues. Therefore, it is important to consider what specific outcome the clinician is attempting to create. For instance, if treating an infection is important, the current selected would be a summation of a positive charge to attract the negatively charged neutrophils;

whereas if the goal is to facilitate the proliferative phase for angiogenesis and granulation tissue formation, one would want a summation of the negative current to attract the positively charged fibroblast.

PRACTICE POINT

- Don't place ES electrodes over the carotid sinus, close to the heart, or near the laryngeal musculature. The exception to this rule is when the speech-language pathologist is using the VitalStim stimulator for treating patients with dysphagia.
- ES can be a first line of treatment and should be used in combination with other moist wound therapy interventions.
- When using silver products, ensure that the residue has been well irrigated from the wound prior to using ES.

LIGHT THERAPIES

Light is a form of electromagnetic radiation (EMR) that is very familiar to us. Light comes in different colors, spread across the rainbow of hues known as the visible spectrum. Each color in this spectrum corresponds to a different wavelength. The visible light spectrum ranges from short wavelengths of the violet or purple color to long wavelengths, which are red. Photons of light from the violet end of the spectrum have the highest energies and the highest frequencies, while red photons have lower energies and lower frequencies. Beyond the range of our human vision are the longer wavelengths of the infrared and the shorter wavelengths of the ultraviolet regions of the electromagnetic spectrum (EMS). (See *color section, Electromagnetic spectrum*, page C16.)

Sunlight has been known for many centuries to have beneficial effect on humans. The Egyptians, Greeks, and Chinese all have writings referring to the use of sunlight to treat different conditions and illnesses. Sunlight is still prescribed for certain illnesses today.

Most of the time, however, light therapy, or phototherapy as it is known in the health-care field, involves the application of specific wavelengths to patients using various medical devices.[61]

Phototherapy devices

When discussing phototherapy in wound care today, one is usually referring to a low-level or cold laser, which is used for tissue regeneration, as opposed to coherent laser beams of high-intensity light, which is used for surgical incisions.

Low-level laser therapy in wound healing

Used in Europe and Russia for more than 30 years as an adjunctive modality for wound healing, laser therapy for tissue regeneration is still in its infancy in the United States. "Laser" is an acronym for light amplification by stimulating emissions of radiation. Low-level laser therapy (LLLT) or low-intensity laser therapy (LILT) is also known as *cold laser therapy, photobiomodulation*, or *monochromatic infrared light therapy*. Laser light is always one single color (therefore monochromatic) and is in the infrared (nonvisible) area of the light spectrum. Several studies have demonstrated a positive effect of LLLT on the three overlapping phases of wound healing: inflammation, proliferation, and remodeling. The proposed outcome of LLLT is more rapid wound healing. Dyson and colleagues[62-69] have suggested that this modality can reduce the inflammatory phase, cause earlier initiation of the proliferative phase, and augment the rate of contraction as angiogenesis increases.

More than 2,000 scientific, peer-reviewed studies on the uses of LLLT have been published worldwide. Specific topics have included chronic wound healing, acute soft tissue injuries, shingles, regeneration for both nerve injuries and diabetic peripheral neuropathy, and reducing postoperative pain. There are also a significant number of research articles describing the effects of LLLT on keratinocytes, mast cells, and macrophages and fibroblasts, all of which are critical to the wound healing processes.

Light is applied by a multi-cluster diode probe (Fig. 9-10), a single diode probe, or a

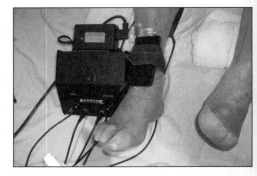

Figure 9-10. Multi-cluster diode probe for use in low-level laser therapy for wound healing.

multi-cluster diode pad. The literature and anecdotal reports indicate that most chronic wounds, including diabetic neuropathic foot ulcers, venous insufficiency, arterial insufficiency, and pressure ulcers, respond well to this treatment intervention.[70-80]

> ### ▶ PRACTICE POINT
>
> When treating with LLLT directly over or in an open wound, apply a thin plastic transparent barrier, such as Saran Wrap™, over the wound or place the pad(s) or probe in a plastic bag to keep them free of contaminants.

Ultraviolet light

Ultraviolet light (UV) has been used for centuries to treat a myriad of health and skin problems in the form of natural sunlight and more recently by artificial UV-generated sources. Ultraviolet light A (UVA) and ultraviolet light B (UVB) are responsible for the pigmentation and erythema (and sometimes blistering) often seen in light-skinned individuals after significant sun exposure. UVB light assists in wound healing by inducing an inflammatory reaction, stimulating the growth of granulation tissue, and promoting breakdown and elimination of dead tissue from the wound.[81]

Ultraviolet light C (UVC) (wavelength 200 to 290 nm) is the form of UV light most often used in the treatment of chronic wounds specifically for its bactericidal effects (Fig. 9-11).

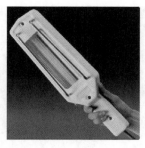

Figure 9-11. Dermawand used in ultraviolet light therapy.

Recent research demonstrated that UVC is capable of killing strains of bacteria in laboratory cultures, in animal tissue, and in patients with chronic ulcers infected with methicillin-resistant *Staphylococcus aureus*.[82,83] In patients with chronic wounds, UVC treatment also reduced the wound bioburden and facilitated wound healing.[84] In addition, in vitro studies have shown that UVC therapy destroyed 100% of antibiotic-resistant bacteria.[85]

The suggested application of UVC is as follows: remove the dressing, debride the wound if not contraindicated, protect the periwound area with petroleum jelly, hold the light perpendicular to wound bed at a distance of 1", and apply UV light.

PRACTICE POINT

Contemporary UV light equipment is usually equipped with distance guards, which ensure correct distance and reproducibility of UV treatments.

Compression therapy

Compression therapy is the foundation for successful management in patients with edematous wounds caused by venous insufficiency and/or lymphedema. Compression therapy wraps are used to manage fluid accumulation and promote sufficient return of venous blood back to the central system and lymph back into the bloodstream. The substances transported by the lymphatic system are called *lymphatic loads* and consist of protein, water, cellular debris, and fat from the digestive system.

These loads are filtered by the regional and central lymph nodes prior to re-entry into the venous system.[86]

It is worth noting that the edema associated with venous insufficiency is different in consistency from the edema or fluid accumulation that is seen in lymphedema. Protein-rich lymphedema fluid appears to be more "viscous" or thicker than the edema associated with venous insufficiency and requires different treatment interventions, including higher compression forces when using wraps or garments. (See chapter 14, Venous disease and lymphedema management.)

Several types of compression wraps are available, and instructions on their application techniques vary. Some have layers that are applied in a spiral fashion, while others are wrapped in a figure-eight configuration, and still others use a combination of the two wrapping techniques. Bandages are also classified by their elasticity. Short-stretch bandages have a smaller degree of stretch than do long-stretch bandages. Short-stretch or rigid compression systems are particularly suited to managing the fluid accumulation of lymphedema and are also indicated for patients with a combination of venous insufficiency and lymphedema in the same leg.[87] An Unna boot is a "short-stretch" system that includes a moist layer impregnated with several substances, including zinc oxide, calamine, and gelatin. This layer molds to the extremity, becoming semirigid when dried and creating high working pressures during ambulation; this improves the calf pump function to facilitate fluid return to the central system and decrease edema in the afflicted extremity.

PRACTICE POINT

When using an Unna's boot, apply a non-adherent dressing over the open wound first so as to avoid damage to the healing tissue when removing the compression dressing.

Long-stretch bandages are so called due to their large amount of extensibility and elastic recoil back to near-original configuration.

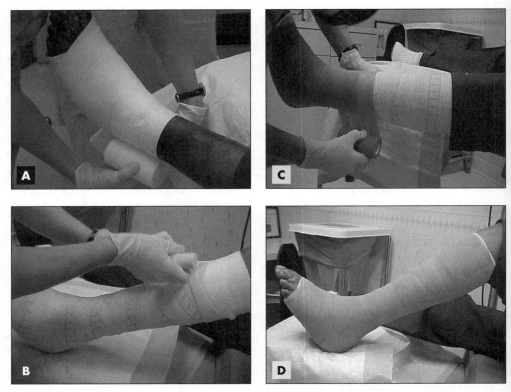

Figure 9-12. Application of a multi-layer compression system. (A) Absorbent padding applied to leg. (B) Application of a light conformable dressing applied in a spiral manner. (C) Flexible cohesive bandage applied over the two other layers, also in a spiral manner. (D) Completed compression wrap.

While short-stretch bandages require the patient to be ambulatory or able to engage the calf muscles effectively (ideally by walking), long-stretch bandages have been shown to be suitable for individuals who are not active or who are non-ambulatory.[87] Clinicians need to be trained and skilled to proficiently and safely apply these compression wraps, keeping in mind that they should be applied according to the manufacturer's detailed directions (Fig. 9-12).

Other compression systems

Some compression systems do not fall into the wrap or bandage category. These include garments that are usually short-stretch systems consisting of material that does not give way during ambulation; these systems often include Velcro straps to help conform the garment to the extremity contours (Fig. 9-13). Application techniques vary according to product; it is important that the clinician read the package insert before applying the compression system.

INTERMITTENT COMPRESSION THERAPY

External pneumatic compression therapy or intermittent compression therapy (ICT) contributes to the healing of venous insufficiency ulcers by collapsing the superficial venous system and forcing blood into the deep system, thus increasing subcutaneous pressure. ICT prevents the leakage of blood, fibrin, and protein from the skin capillaries. In addition to the hemodynamic effect of

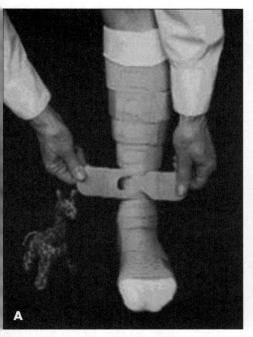
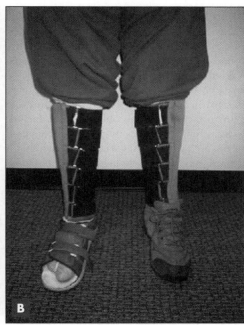

Figure 9-13. Short-stretch bandages, such as the CircAid® (A) and LegAssist® (B), do not give way when the calf muscle pump is exercised. The force of the muscle is directed back into the leg and promotes venous return.

ICT, enhancement of fibrinolysis has been an important outcome of this intervention.[88-90] ICT results in improved circulation with an increase in oxygenated blood flow and the removal of potentially harmful toxic waste from the wound and periwound area.[90]

There is some controversy regarding the use of ICT in patients with lymphedema due to concerns for damaging the superficially located lymphatic anatomical structures.

Application of ICT to the lower extremity is best accomplished with the patient positioned supine and the extremity elevated above the heart. Treatment time varies but usually lasts from 45 to 60 minutes.

ICT is contraindicated for patients with acute deep vein thrombosis or severe peripheral vascular disease. Although not an absolute contraindication, vigilant observation and communication with the patient who has a history of congestive heart failure must be practiced when using any type of compression system. This is important in order to ensure that the heart is not overloaded with

the increased fluid return back to the central system.[90]

▶ PRACTICE POINT

- Compression therapy should be applied cautiously and at lower levels of compression (20 mm Hg) when there is evidence of mild to moderate peripheral arterial disease.
- If a patient presents with mixed etiology of venous and arterial insufficiency, he or she should be monitored diligently to ensure that arterial compromise is not occurring.

Vascular assessment and an ankle-brachial index Doppler study are critically important prior to the use of compression therapy dressings or devices.

(See chapter 14, Venous disease and lymphedema management.)

Growth factors

Growth factors are proteins (polypeptides) that occur naturally in the body. They are found primarily in platelets and macrophages. Various types of growth factors are being researched: epidermal growth factors, platelet-derived growth factor (PDGF), transforming growth factors, and fibroblast growth factors, to list a few. The types of growth factors used in research can be categorized into two major groups: single growth factors manufactured through recombinant DNA technology and multiple growth factors secured from human platelet releasate.[24]

PDGF is the most widely recognized growth factor today. It has been found to be efficacious in the management of diabetic ulcers and in granulating wounds. Becaplermin gel is a PDGF that is available by prescription for use in diabetic wounds.

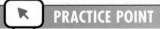

PRACTICE POINT

Becaplermin gel (Regranex) must be kept refrigerated.

Another approach to healing chronic wounds, especially diabetic ulcers, is the exogenous application of autologous platelet-derived concentrate, such as platelet-rich plasma. Platelet-rich plasma contains multiple growth factors. Unlike becaplermin, which is produced by the manufacturer and comes ready to use, platelet-rich plasma is prepared at the point of care for the patient. Blood taken from the patient is mixed with a small amount of anticoagulant citrate dextrose and the solution is then centrifuged to separate the platelets and serum.[91,92] The concentrated platelets are then placed into the specially provided syringe that mixes the concentrate as it is applied to the prepared wound bed as a gel.[91,92]

Although growth factor research is still in its infancy, it holds a promising future for wound care patients.

Hyperbaric oxygen therapy

Most chronic wounds are hypoxic, which means they require an increase in oxygen for adequate wound healing to take place. Hyperbaric oxygen therapy (HBOT) is the delivery of oxygen at pressures greater than normal atmospheric (sea level) pressure or more pressure than one atmosphere absolute (ata). This requires that the entire body be placed in a pressure chamber while 100% oxygen is circulated for the patient to breathe. The barometric pressure can be increased up to three times normal atmospheric pressure (3ata). The physiological effects of systemic oxygen on the human body are more similar to a drug than a physical modality and, like any drug, there is the chance of overdose (oxygen toxicity) and side effects.[7, 93–95]

The Undersea and Hyperbaric Medical Society endorses HBOT and determines treatment protocols and practice standards[93] for the following conditions and type of wounds: air or gas embolism, carbon monoxide poisoning, clostridial myositis and myonecrosis (gas gangrene), crush injury, compartment syndrome and other acute traumatic ischemias, decompression sickness, enhancement of healing in selected problem wounds, exceptional blood loss (anemia), intracranial abscess, necrotizing soft-tissue infections, refractory osteomyelitis, delayed radiation injury (soft tissue and bony necrosis), and compromised skin grafts and flaps.[94] The treatment is delivered by the patient breathing 100% oxygen either in a monoplace chamber, where the entire chamber is pressurized with 100% oxygen, or in a multiplace chamber, which accommodates two or more people and is usually pressurized with air while the patients breathe 100% oxygen via a mask or hood (Fig. 9-14).

Studies have demonstrated that the oxygenation of hypoxic tissue is one of the key mechanisms by which HBOT accelerates wound healing.[95] When patients breathe oxygen at two to three times atmospheric pressure the amount of dissolved oxygen in the blood significantly increases. The subsequent effect is that more oxygen is delivered to the afflicted area by the circulating blood *plasma,* thereby alleviating the wound hypoxia. Although the actual HBOT treatment is only 1 to 2 hours in length, the systemic and local effects are prolonged. The following is a partial list of the principal methods by which HBOT is capable of affecting wound healing.

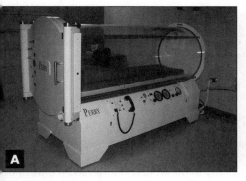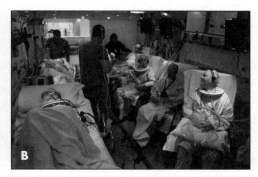

Figure 9-14. Hyperbaric oxygen therapy. (A) Monoplace chamber. (B) Multiplace chamber. (View B courtesy of Jeff Niezgoda, M.D.)

- *Vasoconstrictive effects of oxygen:* Vasoconstriction takes place in both arterial and venous vessels, which reduces edema and congestion while the amount of oxygen supplied by the plasma is increased.[96]
- *Hyperoxygenation of ischemic tissue:* Chronic wounds are frequently hypoxic. HBOT increases tissue partial pressure of oxygen (pO_2), correcting wound hypoxia intermittently[95]. It then allows for acceleration of the wound healing process through a series of actions that continue long after the HBOT session has ended and tissue oxygen levels have returned to pretreatment values.[95, 97, 98]
- *Improved wound metabolism:* The elevation in pO_2 promotes wound healing by directly enhancing fibroblast replication, collagen synthesis, and the processes of neovascularization and epithelialization.[95, 99]
- *Up-regulation of growth factors:* HBOT causes the up-regulation of cytokines, including PDGF, which may be one of the mechanisms by which HBOT enhances angiogenesis.[100, 101]
- *Antibacterial effects:* The increase in available oxygen enhances the leukocyte bactericidal effect, including the killing of aerobic gram-positive (*S. aureus*) and gram-negative organisms in addition to being cytotoxic to anaerobes. Neutrophils or polymorphonuclear cells (PMNs) require oxygen for phagocytosis and killing of bacteria to take place. Should the oxygen tension fall below 30 mm Hg, the efficiency of bactericidal action of PMNs decreases dramatically, leaving the patient at higher risk for infection.[101]

HBOT must be supervised by a hyperbaric-certified physician with expertise and training in this highly specialized treatment modality. HBOT has been shown to improve and accelerate wound healing in all types of chronic wounds, including venous and arterial insufficiency ulcers, burns (thermal), crush injuries, compartment syndrome, refractory osteomyelitis, clostridial myositis and myonecrosis (gas gangrene), delayed radiation injury (soft tissue and bony necrosis), and compromised skin grafts and flaps.[93] Transcutaneous oximetry can be used to predict the effectiveness of hyperbaric therapy. Levels greater than 200 mm Hg measured in a hyperbaric chamber correlate with a high likelihood of benefit from HBOT.

Practice Essentials

- Patients should undergo revascularization when possible. HBOT is used when tissue hypoxia persists after adequate revascularization or if revascularization is not possible but some flow remains.
- HBOT is an adjunctive therapy accompanying good wound care practices.
- Before HBOT is initiated, it is important to consider the patient's compliance and commitment to the time involved. Daily treatments are required, typically 20 to 40 in all, with each treatment lasting 90 minutes.[93] Treatment cost and insurance approval should be considered before initiating HBOT.

ULTRASOUND ENERGY IN WOUND CARE AND HEALING

Therapeutic ultrasound delivers energy through mechanical vibrations in the form of sound waves at frequencies above detection by the human ear (>20 kHz). High-frequency ultrasound is currently used in the range of 1 to 10 MHz for fetal imaging and duplex scanning and has been used in the 1- to 3-MHz range for over six decades to promote soft-tissue injury healing. In addition, high-frequency ultrasound has been implemented to facilitate wound healing. High-frequency ultrasound devices create their effect by running electricity through a crystal in the sound head, causing the crystal to "vibrate." The vibrations are then passed through the sound head via an ultrasound coupling medium into the tissues, causing them to vibrate and creating a local thermal effect.

Ultrasound affects tissue through thermal and nonthermal mechanisms. The thermal effects with greater tissue absorption increase with higher frequencies, whereas nonthermal effects are predominant with lower frequencies and when ultrasound is pulsed.[102]

Recently, low-frequency ultrasound (LFU) has been added to the arsenal of tools available for wound care. Delivery of LFU to wounds has been shown to effectively debride necrotic tissue, eradicate some strains of bacteria from the wound, and facilitate the wound healing process.[103]

LFU therapy is believed to promote wound healing through the processes of cavitation (production and vibration of micron-sized bubbles within the coupling medium and fluids within the tissues) and acoustic streaming (movement of fluids along acoustic boundaries).

The combination of cavitation and acoustic streaming, both of which occur more frequently with kilohertz than megahertz ultrasound, provides a mechanical energy capable of altering cell membrane activity and, therefore, cellular activity.

The LFU effects of microstreaming, and possibly to some degree cavitation, create micro-deformations or shear forces that aid in tissue repair by "up-regulating" the fibroblasts, causing them to proliferate and migrate more readily to the wound site and to become more active, creating a collagen-rich connective tissue matrix. The fibroblasts then differentiate into myofibroblasts to facilitate the contraction process of wound repair.

The mechanical energy from an ultrasound wave is absorbed by an individual protein molecule, theoretically inducing a conformational change. Signal transduction pathways can also be stimulated from ultrasound-generated mechanical energy. This may result in a broad range of cellular effects that impact wound healing, including leukocyte adhesion, growth factor and collagen production, increased angiogenesis, increased macrophage responsiveness, increased fibrinolysis, and increased nitric oxide levels.

There are currently two delivery mechanisms (contact and non-contact) for LFU energy to wounds. The SonicOne (Misonix, Farmingdale, NY) and the Sonoca-180 (Söring, Inc., North Richland Hills, TX) machines deliver ultrasound energy as contact devices, in which the ultrasound probe is in direct contact with the wound surface. The SonicOne operates at a frequency of 22.5 kHz in the continuous or pulsed mode. This allows for deep tissue penetration and causes cell destruction within the wound bed through combined vibrational and cavitational effects. Continuous irrigation provides a medium for cavitation and flushes the wound of fibrin deposits and bacterial growth while preserving the granulation tissue. The Sonoca-180 operates at a frequency of 25 kHz in the continuous mode. This allows the energy to gently loosen necrotic tissue and fibrin layers. An irrigation solution (0.9 % NaCl or Ringer's solution) is used to transmit the ultrasound energy as well as for wound irrigation. Granulation tissue is not negatively affected since these cells react more flexibly to the pressure changes. The cavitation process destroys bacteria.

The MIST Therapy® System (Celleration Inc., Eden Prairie, MN) operates at a frequency of 40 kHz in the continuous mode and is a non-contact LFU device that promotes healing by actively stimulating cells, reducing the bioburden, increasing blood flow to the immediate treatment area, and providing cleansing and gentle debridement.[104]

The Qoustic Wound Therapy System™ (Arobella Medical, LLC, Minneapolis, MN) is a contact/noncontact system operating at a frequency of 35 kHz in either continuous or pulsed mode. It provides selective, precise, and gentle fragmentation of soft and hard tissues, with preservation of healthy tissue through ultrasonic separation of damaged tissue.[105] This cleanses the wound area with less pressure and pain and also improves granulation formation of treated tissue. (See *Low-frequency ultrasound summary and comparison of specifications,* page 210.)

Various clinical studies have evaluated the safety and efficacy of LFU therapy in patients with a variety of wounds, including recalcitrant pressure ulcers, chronic lower-extremity leg and foot ulcers, and diabetic foot ulcers.

> ## PRACTICE POINT
>
> *Ultrasound* cannot be used near parts of the body containing electronic implants/prostheses, on areas of malignancy, or over the lower back or abdomen during pregnancy.

SCAR MANAGEMENT

Patients, clinicians, and researchers are all concerned about scar appearance. Progress has been made in our understanding of the mechanisms involved in producing an exaggerated scar. The scientific principles for scar management and minimization—support, controlled inflammation, adequate hydration, and remodeling/maturation of collagen[106,107]—form the basis of product selection for scar control strategies. (See *SCAR acronym for the practical application of principles for scar management,* pages 212–214.)

Scar control does not rely on a single modality but rather on a number of proven factors whose combination results in a good outcome.

Controlling scar formation is an important part of wound management practice. Widgerow and colleagues[106–108] have described a patented process of applying a cream/gel that contains anti-scar active agents (*Centella asiatica*, oleuropein, dimethicone, *Bulbine frutescens*) to the surface of microporous tape. This process has been used successfully for scar management. Within 2 minutes, the active agents in the gel are absorbed through the tape and on to the scar tissue. The saturated tape continues to work as an occlusive scar dressing. The tape remains in place during patient bathing and is only replaced when it separates from the skin (usually in 3 to 5 days). Gel is reapplied to the tape surface twice a day until scar maturation (white color) begins to occur. Once the scar is maturing well (usually 6 weeks), use of the tape can be stopped and the gel applied directly to the scar.[108] In a comprehensive trial,[107] 170 scars were assessed based on the SCAR acronym (Fig. 9-15; see *color section*, *Scar management*, page C17, for color versions of these images). Hypertrophy was prevented in more than 80% of cases. Hypertrophy and scar exaggeration are seen in 60% to 80% of cases when there is no scar management.[109]

Although often confused as the same, keloid scars are different from hypertrophic scars. Keloid scarring usually has a genetic component, where collagen type 1 is produced in a tumor-like fashion with uncontrolled growth of scar tissue. (See *color section*, *Scar management*, page C17.) The typical wound history includes a well-managed non-infected wound that progressively increases in size and extends over the wound boundary. These scars may be painful, sensitive, and extremely uncomfortable. Treatment (often radiotherapy) is unpredictable and unsatisfactory. The SCAR principles are not applicable to keloid scarring. The different mechanisms between hypertrophic and keloid scars require different product approaches.

SUMMARY

The selection of appropriate wound treatment options must be patient centered and driven by the specific goals of care. A succinct overview of the important characteristics and use of wound dressing products is provided following the References at the end of this chapter. (See *Wound dressing categories,* pages 222–239.)

Low-frequency ultrasound summary and comparison of specifications

Features	SonicOne™	Sonoca-180™	MIST Therapy® System	Qoustic Wound Therapy System™
Frequency	22.5 kHz	20-80 kHz	40 kHz	35 kHz
Intensity	Variable: auto gain control	Variable: 40%-100%	Preset: based on wound size	Variable: 10%-100%
Mode	Continuous or pulsed	Continuous	Continuous	Continuous or pulsed
Coupling	Sterile saline vapor	Sterile saline vapor	Sterile saline vapor	Sterile saline vapor
Controls	Foot pedal	Foot pedal	Button on hand piece	
Treatment time	Usually 2-5 min	Usually 2-5 min	Depends on wound size (3-20 cm)	Usually 2-5 min
Wound contact with applicator	Yes; autoclavable metal probes	Yes; autoclavable metal probes	No; 0.5-1.5 cm disposable applicator	Yes; autoclavable curette shaped
Indications and Clinical Features				
Selective debridement	Yes	Yes	No	Yes
Fibrinolysis	Yes	Yes	Yes	Yes
Antibacterial	Yes	Yes	Yes	Yes
Associated pain	Yes	Yes	No	No
Aerosolization	Yes	Yes	Yes	Yes

Adapted and used with permission from Luther Kloth, PT, MS, FAPTA, CWS, FCCWS.

Selecting from the abundant number of wound dressings that are available today can pose a challenge. Tools such as wound product charts and enablers such as MEASURES© or NICE© give clinicians a model by which to enhance their clinical decision making.

The concepts of moist wound healing and the significance of clinical treatment decisions regarding wound care dressing options described herein are essential elements of your wound care arsenal. Other therapies, such as ES, HBOT, ultrasound, and growth factors, to name a few, are also important wound healing options available for consideration. By using helpful practice points, tables, figures, and product algorithms, the clinician is guided through the milieu of product alternatives. Improving technology and evolving research into wound care dressings and modalities will continue to create new and challenging opportunities for all of us.

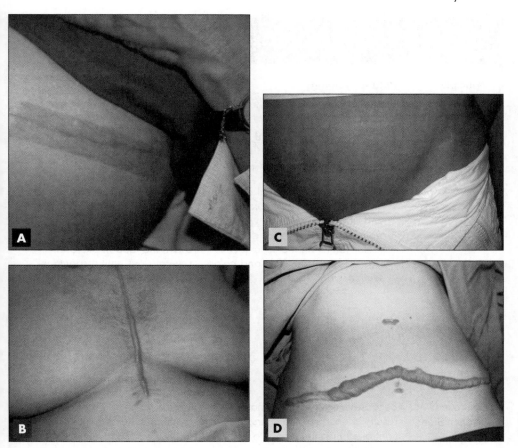

Figure 9-15. (A) Tape applied longitudinally along the direction of the scar. White or flesh-tone tape may be used, with the same effect. (B) Untreated hypertrophic scar in the presternal area; multiple vector forces are working against this scar. (C) The mature treated abdominal scar is flat, white, and non-reactive (note that it is normal for most scars to become hypopigmented to some extent). Compare this scar with the untreated scar. (D) Keloid scarring, which grows like a tumor and flows over the scar boundary, occurs wherever the skin is breached. Its pathogenesis and treatment are different from those of hypertrophic scars. (See also *color section, Scar management*, page C17, for the color versions of these images.) From Widgerow, A. D. "Scar Management: The Principles and Their Practical Application," *World Council of Enterostomal Therapists Journal* 31(1): 18–21, 2011. Used with permission.

SCAR acronym for the practical application of principles for scar management

Principle	Pathophysiology	Proven agents (examples)
Support	• Vector forces increase the production of collagen. • All scars, especially long scars, need support in areas where vector forces continually pull on the scar.[106,107,110,111] For example, in a presternal chest area wound, neck, shoulder, and arm movements as well as weight from the breasts generate vector forces on the scar. (See Fig. 9-15B, page 211, and *color section*, page C17.)	• Microporous tape is the best form of scar support.[107,112,113] • To ensure that there is consistent support for the scar, the tape must be applied longitudinally along the scar path and not at right angles. (See Fig. 9-15A, page 211, and *color section*, page C17.) • Leave the tape in place for several days until it spontaneously separates from the skin. • Premature removal of the tape results in skin stripping, which sets up inflammation with negative consequences on the scar. • Small scars in some areas (face) may not need support.
Controlled inflammation	Because excessive inflammation results in exaggerated scars, controlled inflammation is a sought-after principle in scar management.	• Topical application of olive oil compounds (phenol compounds such as oleuropein in newly pressed olive oils) have anti-inflammatory activity and antimicrobial effects.[114-116] • Oleuropein stimulates proteasome function and fibroblast formation of new collagen.[116] Proteasomes prevent collagen from clumping as they up fragmented protein particles, including fragmented collagen, a process critical to the prevention of clumped collagen. Thus stimulation of proteasomes and inhibition of inflammation are extremely advantageous to the process of scar maturation.

SCAR acronym for the practical application of principles for scar management (continued)

Principle	Pathophysiology	Proven agents (examples)
Adequate hydration	• Hydration of the scar surface is the basis of action of 90% of scar management systems on the market. • Most oils (tissue oils), lotions, and creams have beneficial effects on scars purely on the basis of their hydrative capacities.[117-119] Although this is obviously beneficial, it is limited in terms of the outcome it can produce and affects only one area of scar control. • Normal skin has a mature stratum corneum characterized by minimal transepidermal water loss (TEWL). • Dehydration of the stratum corneum initiates signaling to keratinocytes. These keratinocytes are stimulated to produce cytokines, which activate dermal fibroblasts to synthesize and release collagen. Excessive collagen production leads to abnormal scarring.[120]	• The most effective barrier to TEWL and stratum corneum breach is silicone, in the form of either sheeting or gels (dimethicone).[120-122] • In addition, gel derived from the plant *Bulbine frutescens* has been found to be effective as a hydrating agent; the glycoproteins of this plant extract are large and remain on the surface of the skin long enough to produce effective hydration of the skin.[107,110]

(continued)

SCAR acronym for the practical application of principles for scar management (continued)

Principle	Pathophysiology	Proven agents (examples)
Remodelling/ maturation of collagen	• The quicker the scar matures, the less chance there is of hypertrophy. • Collagen maturation goes through phases, with collagen type III being present in greater levels in the early scarring phase. • As the scar matures, the ratio of type III to type I collagen returns to normal levels.[123] Thus any agent that encourages a return to stable ratios is advantageous to scar outcome. • Transforming growth factor (TGF)-β is the prototype of a protein superfamily that has been recognized as the major fibroproliferative and collagen-stimulating agent involved in excess scarring (particularly TGF-β₁). Many isoforms of the protein exist, most of which share the same fibroproliferative properties. One isoform (TGF-β₃), however, appears to have a protective effect against excess collagen formation counteracting the TGF-β₁ effects.[124]	• Extracts of the *Centella asiatica* plant increase levels of mature collagen and encourage normalization of collagen ratios.[123-125] • Purified extracts (triterpenic fractions, including asiaticoside) isolated from *C. asiatica* have been shown to induce type I collagen synthesis in human dermal fibroblast cells.[123-125] • Asiaticoside down-regulates TGF-β₁ expression and up-regulates TGF-β₃ expression and is also capable of decomposing the products of type I collagen, contributing to the reduction of hypertrophic scar formation.[124] • Laboratory evidence of asiaticoside efficacy was demonstrated in the rabbit ear model, one of the only consistent animal models producing hypertrophic scarring.[126,127]

Adapted with permission from Widegerow, A.D. "Scar Management: The Principles and Their Practical Application," *World Council of Enterostomal Therapists Journal* 31(1):18–21, 2011.

1. Wound dressings have evolved into a new concept of:
   A. dry gauze.
   B. moist wound therapy.
   C. open to air.
   D. wet to dry.
   ANSWER: B. *A, C, and D are all old concepts of wound management.*

2. Which of the following is <u>not</u> a category of moist wound care dressings?
   A. hydrogel dressing
   B. calcium alginate dressing
   C. roller gauze dressing
   D. foam dressing
   ANSWER: C. *Gauze is a form of dry dressing therapy. A, B, and D are moist wound therapy dressings.*

3. Wound dressing selection should be based on the characteristics of the wound. All of the following should be considered when selecting dressings <u>except</u>:
   A. size of dressing.
   B. nurse preference.
   C. moist or dry wound bed.
   D. drainage.
   ANSWER: B. *Nurse preference shouldn't be a parameter of dressing selection. A, C, and D are appropriate dressing parameters.*

4. A disadvantage of transparent film is that it:
   A. is nonabsorptive.
   B. is conformable.
   C. allows wound inspection.
   D. is impermeable to bacteria.
   ANSWER: A. *Transparent film doesn't absorb fluid. B, C, and D are all advantages of transparent film use.*

5. The acronym "MEASURES" is a useful tool for remembering the principles of wound care.
   A. True
   B. False
   ANSWER: A

6. Which one of the following is a dermal skin substitute?
   A. OpSite
   B. Tegaderm
   C. Allevyn
   D. Apligraf
   ANSWER: D. *Apligraf is a bilayered skin substitute. A, B, and C are all moist wound therapy choices.*

(continued)

7. Which one of the following treatment options would <u>not</u> be an appropriate treatment option for a heavily draining wound?
   A. Negative-pressure therapy
   B. Foam dressing
   C. Calcium alginate dressing
   D. Hydrogel amorphous gel

   ANSWER: D. *Hydrogel amorphous gel has minimal ability to absorb drainage, so it is not indicated for use in heavily draining wounds. A, B, and C are all specifically used for heavily draining wounds.*

8. Prior to the application of tissue-engineered skin substitute, the clinician needs to evaluate:
   A. whether the wound bed is free of necrotic tissue.
   B. the patient's immune system status.
   C. that anti-rejection drugs have been administered.
   D. the patient's weight.

   ANSWER: A. *Tissue-engineered skin substitutes must be applied to a wound bed that is free of necrotic tissue and infection. B and C are incorrect as rejection of these products is not an issue. Although the patient's weight may be part of the total care plan, it is not essential to evaluate for use of this product.*

9. All of the following are therapeutic effects of electrical stimulation <u>except</u>:
   A. increased blood flow.
   B. decreased tissue oxygenation.
   C. increased angiogenesis.
   D. decreased wound pain.

   ANSWER: B. *Tissue oxygenation is increased with the use of electrical stimulation. A, C, and D are all correct.*

10. Which one of the following is <u>not</u> a method by which hyperbaric oxygen therapy affects wound healing:
    A. Increased fibroblast replication
    B. Up-regulation of growth factors
    C. Vasodilation effects of oxygen on the blood vessels
    D. Enhanced leukocyte bactericidal effects

    ANSWER: C. *Hyperbaric oxygen therapy causes vasoconstriction not vasodilation in both arterial and venous vessels. A, B, and D are all ways in which hyperbaric oxygen therapy enhances wound healing.*

REFERENCES

1. Ayello, E.A. "20 Years of Wound Care: Where We Have Been, Where We Are Going," *Advances in Skin & Wound Care* 19(1):28-33, January-February 2006.
2. Queen, D. "A Personal Perspective," *International Wound Journal* (1):1, March 2006.
3. Krasner, D., Ed. *WoundSource 2010/11: The Kestrel Wound Product Sourcebook*, 13th ed. Hinesburg, VT: Kestrel Health Information; 2010/11.
4. Winter, G.D. "Formation of the Scab and the Rate of Epithelialization of Superficial Wounds in the Skin of Young Domestic Pigs," *Nature* 193:293-94, 1962.
5. Hinman, C.D., and Maibach, H.I. "Effect of Air Exposure and Occlusion on Experimental Human Skin Wounds," *Nature* 200:377, 1963.

6. Baranoski, S. "Wound Dressings: A Myriad of Challenging Decisions," *Home Healthcare Nurse* 23(5):307-17, May 2005.

7. Baranoski, S. "Wound & Skin Care: Choosing a wound dressing, Part 1," *Nursing 2008* 60-61, January 2008.

8. Baranoski, S. "Wound & Skin Care: Choosing a wound dressing, Part 2," *Nursing 2008* 14-15, February 2008.

9. Ovington, L. "Dressings and Skin Substitutes," in *Wound Healing Evidence-Based Management*, 4th ed. J. McCulloch, and L. Kloth, eds. Philadelphia: FA Davis, 183-86, 2010.

10. Armstrong, M.H., Price, P. "Wet to Dry Dressings: Fact and Fiction." Available at: *www.woundsresearch.com/article/2284*. Accessed August 17, 2010.

11 Pieper, B., et al. "Wound Prevalence, Types, and Treatments in Home Care," *Advances in Skin & Wound Care* 12(3):117-26, May-June 1999.

12. Kim, J.K., et al. "Normal Saline Wound Dressing—Is It Really Normal?" *British Journal of Plastic Surgery* 53(1):42-45, January 2000.

13. "Principles of Best Practice: Minimising Pain at Wound-Dressing-Related Procedures. A Consensus Document." Toronto, ON, Canada: WoundPedia, Inc., 2007.

14. Lawrence, J.C. "Dressings and Wound Infection," *American Journal of Surgery* 167(suppl 1A):1S-24S, January 1994.

15. Hutchinson, J.J. "Prevalence of Wound Infection under Occlusive Dressings: A Collective Survey of Reported Research," *Wounds* (1):123-33, 1989.

16. Hutchinson, J.J. "A Prospective Clinical Trial of Wound Dressings to Investigate the Rate of Infection under Occlusion," in Harding, K (ed.). *Proceedings of the First European Conference on Advances in Wound Management*. London: Macmillan, 1993.

17. Okan, D., Woo, K., Ayello, EA., Sibbald, RG. "The Role of Moisture Balance in Wound Healing," *Advances in Skin & Wound Care* 20:39-53, 2007.

18. Baranoski, S., McIntosh, A., Galvan, L. "Wound Care Essential: Practice Principles Lecture," Clinical Symposium on Advances in Skin & Wound Care, San Antonio, TX.; October 2009.

19. Seaman, S. "Dressing Selection in Chronic Wound Management," *Journal of the American Podiatric Medical Association* 92(1):24-33, January 2002.

20. Doughty, D.B. "Wound Care in Long Term Care: Focus on Infectious Complications," *Safe Practices in Patient Care*, 4(3):1,5-7, 2010.

21. Rodeheaver, G. "Wound Cleansing, Wound Irrigation, Wound Disinfection," in Krasner, D., Rodeheaver, G., Sibbals, RG., eds., *Chronic Wound Care*, 4th ed. Malvern, PA: HMP Communications, 2007.

22. San Miguel, L., Torra I Bou, JE., et.al. "Economics of Pressure Ulcer Care: Review of the Literature on Modern Versus Traditional Dressings," *Journal of Wound Care* 16(1):5-9, January 2007.

23. Payne, W.G., Posnett, J., et al. "A Prospective, Randomized Clinical Trial to Assess the Cost-Effectiveness of a Modern Foam Dressing versus a Traditional Saline Gauze Dressing in the Treatment of Stage II Pressure Ulcers," *Ostomy Wound Management* 55(2):50-55, February 2009.

24. Davidson, J. "Growth Factors and Extracellular Matrix in Wound Repair," in J, Mculloch, L. Kloth, eds., *Wound Healing Evidence-Based Management*, 4th ed. Philadelphia: FA Davis, pp 35-43, 2010.

25. Orland, G. "The Fine Structure of the Interrelationship of Cells in the Human Epidermis," *Journal of Biophysical and Biochemical Cytology* 4:529-35, 1958.

26. Eaglstein, W.H. "From Occlusive to Living Membranes," *Journal of Dermatology* 25(12):766-74, December 1998.

27. Choucair, M., and Phillips. "Wound Dressings," in Fitzpatrick, ed., *Dermatology in General Medicine*. New York: McGraw-Hill Book Co., pp 2954-58, 2000.

28. Hess, C.T. *Clinical Guide: Wound Care,* 6th ed. Philadelphia: Lippincott Williams & Wilkins, 2008.

29. Hess, C.T. (ed.). "Advanced BioHealing Will Offer Dermagraft, TransCyte," *Advances in Skin and Wound Care* 19(7):348, September 2006.

30. Dermagraft®. Available at *www.fda.gov/MedicalDevices/ProductsandMedicalProcedures/DeviceApprovalsandClearances/Recently-ApprovedDevices/ucm085085.htm*. Accessed January 3, 2011.

31. National Pressure Ulcer Advisory Panel and European Pressure Ulcer Advisory Panel. *Prevention and Treatment of Pressure Ulcers: Clinical Practice Guideline*. Washington, DC: National Pressure Ulcer Advisory Panel, Biophysical Agents in Pressure Ulcer Management, pp 90-95, 2009.

32. Agency for Healthcare Research and Quality. "Negative Pressure Wound Therapy Devices." Available at: *http://www.ahrq.gov/clinic/ta/negpresswtd/npwtd02.htm*. Accessed September 2, 2010.

33. Paul, J.C. "Vacuum Assisted Closure Therapy: A Must in Plastic Surgery," *Plastic Surgery Nursing* 25(2):61-5, April-June 2005.

34. Kilpadi, D.V., Stechmiller, J.K., Childress, B., et al. "Composition of Wound Fluid from Pressure Ulcers Treated with Negative Pressure Wound

Therapy Using V.A.C.® Therapy in Home Health," *Wounds* 18(5), 2006.

35. Willy, C., ed. *The Theory and Practice of Vacuum Therapy. Scientific Basis, Indications for Use, Case Reports, Practical Advice.* Ulm, Germany: Lindqvist Book Publishing; 2006, p 405.

36. Borgquist, O., Ingemansson, R., Malmsjo, M. "Negative Pressure Wound Therapy Using Gauze and Foam: An In-detail Study of the Effects on the Wound Bed Including Macro and Microdeformation, Tissue Ingrowth and Wound Bed Histology." Department of Ophthalmology and Department of Cardiothoracic Surgery, Lund University Hospital, Lund, Sweden. Presented at the 24th Annual Clinical Symposium on Advances in Skin & Wound Care in San Antonio, TX, October 22–25, 2009.

37. Weed, T., Ratliff, C., Drake, D.B. "Quantifying Bacterial Bioburden During Negative Pressure Wound Therapy: Does the Wound VAC Enhance Bacterial Clearance?" *Annals of Plastic Surgery* 52(3):276-9, discussion 279-80, March 2004.

38. Moues, C.M., Vos, M.C., van den Bemd, G.J., Stijnen, T., Hovius, S.E. "Bacterial Load in Relation to Vacuum-assisted Closure Wound Therapy: A Prospective Randomized Trial," *Wound Repair and Regeneration* 12(1):11-7, Jan-Feb 2004.

39. Saxena, V., Hwang, C.W., Huang, S., Eichbaum, Q., Ingber, D., Orgill, D.P. "Vacuum-assisted Closure: Microdeformations of Wounds and Cell Proliferation," *Plastic and Reconstructive Surgery* 114(5):1086-96, discussion 1097, October 2004.

40. Scherer, S.S., Pietramaggiori, G., Mathews, J.C., Prsa, M.J., Huang, S., Orgill, D.P. "The Mechanism of Action of the Vacuum-assisted Closure Device," *Plastic and Reconstructive Surgery* 122(3):786-97, September 2008.

41. Malmsjo M., Ingemansson R. Martin R. Huddleston E. "Negative-pressure Wound Therapy using Gauze or Open Cell Polyurethane Foam: Similar Early Effects on Pressure Transduction and Tissue Contraction in an Experimental Porcine Wound Model," *Wound Repair and Regeneration* 17(2):200-205, Mar-Apr. 2009.

42. Morykwas, M.J., Faler, B.J., Pearce, D.J., Argenta, L.C. "Effects of Varying Levels of Subatmospheric Pressure on the Rate of Granulation Tissue Formation in Experimental Wounds in Swine," *Annals of Plastic Surgery* 47(5):547-51, November 2001.

43. U.S. Food and Drug Administration. "Negative Pressure Wound Therapy (NPWT) Systems: Preliminary Public Health Notification." Available at *http://www.fda.gov/Safety/MedWatch/SafetyInformation/SafetyAlertsforHumanMedicalProducts/ucm190704.htm*. Accessed December 28, 2010.

44. Piccolino, M. "Animal Electricity and the Birth of Electrophysiology. The Legacy of Luigi Galvani," *Brain Research Bulletin* 46:381-407, 1998

45. Piccolino, M. "Luigi Galvani's Path to Animal Electricity," *CR Biology* 329:303-318, 2006.

46. Moruzzi, G. "The Electrophysiological Work of Carlo Matteucci," *Brain Research Bulletin* 40:69-91, 1996.

47. Kloth, L., Zhao, M. "Endogenous and Exogenous Electrical Fields for Wound Healing," in McCulloch, J., and Kloth, L., eds., *Wound Healing Evidence-Based Management*, 4th ed. Philadelphia: FA Davis, 2010, pp 450-513.

48. Kloth, L.C. "5 Questions and Answers about Electrical Stimulation," *Advances in Skin & Wound Care* 14(3):156-58, May-June, 2001.

49. Ovington, L.G. "Dressing and Adjunctive Therapies: AHCPR Guidelines Revisited," *Ostomy Wound Management* 45(suppl 1a):94S-106S, 1999.

50. Garber, S.L., et al. "Pressure Ulcer Prevention and Treatment Following Spinal Cord Injury: A Clinical Practice Guideline for Health Care Professionals," *Consortium for Spinal Cord Medicine Clinical Practice Guidelines.* Washington DC: Paralyzed Veterans of America, 2000.

51. Junger, M., et al. "Treatment of Venous Ulcers with Low Frequency Pulsed Current (Dermapulse): Effects on Cutaneous Microcirculation," *Der Hautartz* 18:879-903, 1997.

52. Gagnier, K.A., et al. "The Effects of Electrical Stimulation on Cutaneous Oxygen Supply in Paraplegics," *Physical Therapy* 68:835, 1988,

53. Dodgen, P.W., et al. "The Effects of Electrical Stimulation on Cutaneous Oxygen Supply in Paraplegics," *Physical Therapy* 67:793, 1987.

54. Greenberg, J., et al. "The Effect of Electrical Stimulation (RPES) on Wound Healing and Angiogenesis in Second-degree Burns," Abstract # 44 in *Program and Abstracts of the 13th Annual Symposium on Advanced Wound Care,* Dallas, TX, April 1–4, 2000.

55. Kloth, L.C., McCulloch, J.M. *Wound Healing Alternatives in Management,* 3rd ed. Philadelphia: FA Davis, 2002, pp 271-315.

56. Brown, M., et al. "Electrical Stimulation Effects on Cutaneous Wound Healing in Rabbits," *Physical Therapy* 68:955, 1988,

57. Demir, H., et al. "A Comparative Study of the Effects of Electrical Stimulation and Laser Treatment on Experimental Wound Healing in Rats," *Journal of Rehabilitation Research & Development* 41(2):147-54, March 2004.

58. Kumar, D., and Marshall, H.J. "Diabetic Peripheral Neuropathy: Amelioration of Pain with Transcutaneous Electrostimulation," *Diabetes Care* 20:1702, 1997.

59. Houghton, P.E., and Campbell, K.E. "Therapeutic Modalities in the Treatment of Chronic Recalcitrant Wounds," In Krasner, D., et al., eds., *Chronic Wound Care: A Clinical Source Book for Healthcare Professionals,* 3rd ed. Wayne, PA: Health Management Publications, Inc., 2001, pp 455-468.

60. Myer, A. "The Role of Physical Therapy in Chronic Wound Care," in Krasner, D., et al., eds., *Chronic Wound Care: A Clinical Source Book for Healthcare Professionals,* 3rd ed. Wayne, PA: Health Management Publications, Inc., 2001.

61. Conner-Kerr, T. "Light Therapies," in McCulloch, J., and Kloth, L., eds., *Wound Healing Evidence-Based Management,* 4th ed. Philadelphia: FA Davis, 2010, pp 576-593.

62. Steinlechner, C., Dyson, M. "The Effect of Low Level Laser Therapy on the Proliferation of Keratinocytes," *Laser Therapy* 5(2):65, 1993.

63. Dyson, M., and Young, S. "Effect of Laser Therapy on Wound Contraction and Cellularity in Mice," *Lasers in Medical Science* 1:125, 1986.

64. Dyson, M. "Cellular and Subcellular Aspects of Low Level Laser Therapy," In Ohshiro, T., and Calderhead, R.G., eds., *Progress in Laser Therapy.* London: John Wiley & Sons, 1991, p. 221.

65. Bolton, P.A., et al. "Macrophage Responsiveness to Light Therapy. A Dose Response Study," *Laser Therapy* 2:101-106, 1990.

66. Bolton, P.A., et al. "The Effect of Polarised Light on the Release of Growth Factors from the U-937 Macrophage-like Cell Line," *Laser Therapy* 4: 33-42, 1992.

67. Cheetham, M.J., et al. "Histological Effects of 820 nm Laser Irradiation on the Healthy Growth Plate of the Rat," *Laser Therapy* 2:59, 1992.

68. Bolton, P.A., et al. "The Direct Effect of 860 nm Light on Cell Proliferation and on Succinic Dehydrogenase Activity of Human Fibroblasts in Vitro," *Laser Therapy* 7:55-60, 1995.

69. el Sayed, S.O., Dyson, M. "Effect of Laser Pulse Repetition Rate and Pulse Duration on Mast Cell Number and Degranulation," *Laser in Surgery and Medicine* 19(4):433-3, 1997.

70. Nicolopoulos, N., et al. "The Use of Laser Surgery in the Subtotal Meniscectomy and the Effect of Low-level Laser Therapy on the Healing Potential of Rabbit Meniscus: An Experimental Study," *Lasers in Medical Science* 1(2):109-15, 1996.

71. Crous, L.C., and Malherbe, C.P. "Laser and Ultraviolet Light Irradiation in the Treatment of Chronic Ulcers," *South African Journal of Physiotherapy* 44(3):73-77, 1988.

72. Franek, A., et al. "Does Low Output Laser Stimulation Enhance the Healing of Crural Ulceration? Some Critical Remarks," *Medical Engineering and Physics* 24(9):607-15, 2002.

73. Iusim, M., et al. "Evaluation of the Degree of Effectiveness of Biobeam Low Level Narrow Band Light on the Treatment of Skin Ulcers and Delayed Postoperative Wound Healing," *Orthopedics* 15(9):1023-26, 1992.

74. Lagan, K.M., et al. "Low-intensity Laser Therapy/Combined Phototherapy in the Management of Chronic Venous Ulceration: A Placebo-controlled Study," *Journal of Clinical Laser Medicine and Surgery* 20(3):109-16, 2002.

75. Lucas, C., et al. "The Effect of Low Level Laser Therapy (LLLT) on Stage III Decubitus Ulcers (pressure sores); A Prospective Randomised Single Blind, Multicentre Pilot Study," *Lasers in Medical Science* 15(2):94-100, 2000.

76. Lucas, C., et al. "Efficacy of Low-level Laser Therapy in the Management of Stage III Decubitus Ulcers: A Prospective, Observer-blinded Multicentre Randomised Clinical Trial," *Lasers in Medical Science* 18(2):72-77, 2003.

77. Lundeberg, T., and Malm, M. "Low-power HeNe Laser Treatment of Venous Leg Ulcers," *Annals of Plastic Surgery* 27(6):537-39, 1991.

78. Malm, M., and Lundeberg, T. "Effect of Low Power Gallium Arsenide Laser on Healing of Venous Ulcers," *Scandinavian Journal of Plastic Reconstructive Surgery and Hand Surgery* 25(3):249-51, 1991.

79. Nussbaum, E.L., et al. "Comparison of Ultrasound/Ultraviolet-C and Laser for Treatment of Pressure Ulcers in Patients with Spinal Cord Injury," *Physical Therapy* 74(9):812-23, 1994.

80. Kloth, L.C., and McCulloch, J.M. *Wound Healing Alternatives in Management,* 3rd ed. Philadelphia: FA Davis, 2002, pp. 326-339.

81. Conner-Kerr, T., et al: "UVC Reduces Antibiotic-resistant Bacteria in Vitro," *Ostomy Wound Management* 45:84, 1999.

82. Thai, T., et al. "Effect of Ultraviolet Light C on Bacterial Colonization in Chronic Wounds," *Ostomy Wound Management* 51(10):32-45, 2005.

83. Thai, T., et al. "Ultraviolet Light C in the Treatment of Chronic Wounds with MRSA: A Case Study," *Ostomy Wound Management* 48(11):52-60, 2002.

84. Conner-Kerr, T., et al. "The Effects of Ultraviolet Irradiation on Antibiotic-resistant Bacteria in Vitro," *Ostomy Wound Management* 44:508-11, 1998.

85. Kloth, L.C., and McCulloch, J.M. *Wound Healing Alternatives in Management,* 3rd ed. Philadelphia: FA Davis, 2002, p 335.

86. Hettrick, H. "Lymphedema Complicating Healing," in McCulloch, J.M. and Kloth, L.C., eds., *Wound Healing: Evidence-Based Management,* 4th Ed. Philadelphia: FA Davis, 2010, pp 279-91.

87. McCulloch, J.M. "Compression Therapy," in McCulloch, J.M. and Kloth, L.C., eds., *Wound Healing: Evidence-Based Management*, 4th Ed. Philadelphia: FA Davis, 594-601, 2010.

88. Dai, G.M.S., et al. "An In Vitro Cell Culture System to Study the Influence of External Pneumatic Compression on Endothelial Function," *Journal of Vascular Surgery* 32:977-87, 2000.

89. Kessler, C.M., et al. "Intermittent Pneumatic Compression in Chronic Venous Insufficiency Favorably Affects Fibrinolytic Potential and Platelet Activation," *Blood Coagulation and Fibrinolysis* 7:437, 1996.

90. Alpagut, U., Dayioglu, E. "Importance and Advantages of Intermittent External Pneumatic Compression Therapy in Venous Stasis Ulceration," *Angiology* 56(1), 2005.

91. Frykberg, R., Driver, V.R., et al. "Chronic Wounds Treated with a Physiologically Relevant Concentration of Platelet-rich Plasma Gel: A Prospective Case Series," *Ostomy Wound Management* 56(6):36-44, 2010.

92. McAleer, J.P., et al. "Use of Autologous Platelet Concentrate in a Nonhealing Lower Extremity Wound," *Advances in Skin & Wound Care* 19(7):354-62, September 2006.

93. Gray, M., Ratliff, C.R. "Is Hyperbaric Oxygen Therapy Effective for the Management of Chronic Wounds?" *Journal of Wound, Ostomy and Continence Nursing* 33:21-25, 2006.

94. Gottrup, F., et al. "The Dynamic Properties of Tissue Oxygen in Healing Flaps," *Surgery* 95(5):527-36, 1984.

95. Fife, C. "Hyperbaric Oxygen Therapy Applications in Wound Care," In Sheffield, P., et al., eds., *Wound Care Practice*. Flagstaff, AZ: Best Publishing, 2004, p 664.

96. Wright, J. "Hyperbaric Oxygen Therapy for Wound Healing," *World Wide Wounds,* May 2001.

97. http://www.worldwidewounds.com/2001/april/Wright/HyperbaricOxygen.html.

98. Knighton, D., et al. "Regulation of Wound Healing Angiogenesis-effect of Oxygen Gradients and Inspired Oxygen Concentration," *Surgery* 90:262-70, 1981.

99. Bonomo, S.R., et al. "Hyperbaric Oxygen as a Signal Transducer: Upregulation of Platelet Derived Growth Factor-beta Receptor in the Presence of HBO2 and PDGF," *Undersea Hyperbaric Medicine* 25(4):211-16, 1998.

100. Wu, L., et al. "Effects of Oxygen on Wound Responses to Growth Factors: Kaposi's FGF, But not Basic FGF Stimulates Repair in Ischemic Wounds," *Growth Factors* 12(1):29-35, 1995.

101. Knighton, D.R., et al. "Oxygen as an Antibiotic. The Effect of Inspired Oxygen on Infection," *Archives in Surgery* 119(2):199-204, 1984.

102. Ennis, W.J., et al. "Ultrasound Therapy for Recalcitrant Diabetic Foot Ulcers: Results of a Randomized, Double-blind, Controlled, Multicenter Study," *Ostomy Wound Management* 51(8):24-26, 28-29, 32-39, August 2005

103. Stanisic, M.M., et al. "Wound Debridement with 25 kHz Ultrasound," *Advances in Skin & Wound Care* 18(9):484-90, November-December 2005.

104. Ennis, W.J., et al. "Evaluation of Clinical Effectiveness of MIST Ultrasound Therapy for the Healing of Chronic Wounds," *Advances in Skin & Wound Care* 19(8):437-46, October 2006.

105. Kloth, L.C., Niezgoda, J.A. "Ultrasound for Wound Debridement and Healing," in McCulloch, J.M. and Kloth, L.C., eds., *Wound Healing: Evidence-Based Management*, 4th Ed. Philadelphia: FA Davis, 2010, pp 545-75.

106. Widgerow, A.D., Chait, L.A., Stahls, R., Stahls, P. "New Innovations in Scar Management," *Aesthetic Plastic Surgery* 24:227-34, 2000.

107. Widgerow, A.D., Chait, L.A.C., Stahls, R., Stals, P., Candy, G. "Multimodality Scar Management Program," *Aesthetic Plastic Surgery* 33(4):533, 2009.

108. Widgerow, A.D. "Scar Management: The Principles and Their Practical Application," *World Council of Enterostomal Therapists Journal* 31(1):18-21, 2011.

109. Chan, K.Y., et al. "Silicone Gel in Prevention of Hypertrophic Scar Development in Median Sternotomy Wound," *Plastic and Reconstructive Surgery* 116:1013-20. 2005.

110. Elliot, D., Cory-Pearce, R., Rees, G.M. "The Behaviour of Presternal Scars in a Fair-skinned Population," *Annals of the Royal College of Surgery of England* 67:238, 1985.

111. Meyer, M., McGrouther, D.A. "A Study Relating Wound Tension to Scar Morphology in the Presternal Scar Using Langers Technique," *British Journal Plastic Surgery* 44:291, 1991.

112. Reiffel, R.S. "Prevention of Hypertrophic Scars by Long-term Paper Tape Application," *Plastic and Reconstructive Surgery* 96:1715, 1995.

113. Atkinson, J.A., et al. "A Randomized Controlled Trial to Determine the Efficacy of Paper Tape in Preventing Hypertrophic Scar Formation in Surgical Excisions That Travers Langers Skin Tension Lines," *Plastic & Reconstructive Surgery* 116(6):1648-54. November 2005.

114. Beauchamp, K., et al. "Phytochemistry: Ibuprofen-like Activity in Extra-virgin Olive Oil," *Nature* 437:45-46, September 2005.

115. de la Puerta, R., Martinez-Dominguez, E., et al. "Effect of Minor Components of Virgin Olive Oil on Topical Anti-inflammatory Assays," *Verlag der Zeitschrift für Naturforschung* 55(9-10):814, September-October, 2000.

116. Katsiki, M., Chondrogianni, N., Chinou, I., et al. "The Olive Constituent Oleuropein Exhibits Proteasome Stimulatory Properties In Vitro and Confers Life Span Extension of Human Embryonic Fibroblasts," *Rejuvenation Research* 10(2):157-72, 2007.

117. Sawada, Y., Sone, K. "Hydration and Occlusion Treatment for Hypertrophic Scars and Keloids," *British Journal of Plastic Surgery* 45:599, 1992.

118. Mustoe, T.A , et al. "International Clinical Recommendations on Scar Management" [Review]. *Plastic & Reconstructive Surgery* 110(2):560-71, August 2002.

119. Sawada, Y., Urushidate, S., Nihei, Y. "Hydration and Occlusive Treatment of a Sutured Wound," *Annals of Plastic Surgery* 41:508, 1998.

120. Niessen, F., et al. "The Use of Silicone Occlusive Sheet (Sil-K) and Silicone Occlusive Gel (Epiderm) in the Prevention of Hypertrophic Scar Formation," *Plastic & Reconstructive Surgery* 102(6):1962-72, 1998.

121. Mustoe, T.A. "Evolution of Silicone Therapy and Mechanism of Action in Scar Management," *Aesthetic Plastic Surgery* 32(3):82-92, March 2008.

122. Mustoe, T.A. "The Role of the Epidermis in the Control of Scarring: Evidence for Mechanism of Action for Silicone Gel," *Journal of Plastic, Reconstructive & Aesthetic Surgery* 61(10):1219-25, October 2008.

123. Maquart, F.X., Bellon, G., Gillery, P., Wegrowski, Y., Borel, J.P. "Stimulation of Collagen Synthesis in Fibroblast Cultures by a Triterpene Extracted from *Centella asiatica,*" *Connective Tissue Research* 24(2):107-20, 1990.

124. Zhang T., Tian-zeng, L., Ying Bin, X. "Asiaticoside on Hypertrophic Scars of Transforming Growth Factor-β mRNA and Matrix Metalloproteinase Expression," *Journal of Southern Medical University* 26(1), January, 2006.

125. Bonte, F., Dumas, M., Chaudagne, C., Meybeck, A. "Influence of Asiatic Acid, Madecassic Acid, and Asiaticoside on Human Collagen I Synthesis," *Planta Medica* 60(2):133, April 1994.

126. Ju-Lin, X., Shao-Hai, Q., Tian-Zeng, L., Bin, H., Jing-Ming, T., Ying-Bin, X., Xu-Sheng, L., Bin, S., Hui-Zhen, L.,Yong, H. "Effect of Asiaticoside on Hypertrophic Scar in the Rabbit Ear Model," *Journal of Cutaneous Pathology* 36(2):234-9, February 2009.

127. Saulis, A.S., Mogford, J.H., Mustoe, T.A. "Effect of Mederma on Hypertrophic Scarring in the Rabbit Ear Model," *Plastic and Reconstructive Surgery* 110(1):177-83, July 2002.

Wound dressing categories

Key—Exudate amount: ◊ Dry ♦ Light ♦♦ Moderate ♦♦♦ Heavy

Generic category	Description/ composition	Trade names	
Transparent film ◊	Polyurethane or polymer membrane with porous adhesive layer that varies in thickness and allows oxygen to pass through and moisture vapor to escape	3M Tegaderm 3M Tegaderm HP Bioclusive BlisterFilm CarraSmart Film ClearSite Comfeel Film Dermatell	
Transparent film with silver ◊	Ionic silver from a controlled-release barrier film	Arglaes	
Hydrocolloid ♦ ♦♦	Occlusive or semi-occlusive dressing that consists of gelatin, pectin, and car-boxymethylcellulose Impermeable to bacteria and other contaminants	3M Tegasorb 3M Tegasorb Thin Comfeel Plus Cutinova Hydro DermaFilm DuoDERM CGF DuoDERM Extra Thin & Paste DuoDERM Signal Exuderm LP Exuderm Odor Shield Exuderm Satin	Hydrocol MPM Excel Nu-DERM ProCol RepliCare RepliCare Thin Restore Restore CX Restore Plus SignaDRESS Sorbex Ultec Ultec Pro
Hydrocolloid with silver ♦ ♦♦	Sustained release of silver ions	Contreet	

Indications	Advantages and benefits	Disadvantages
Donor sites Primary and secondary dressings Partial thickness wounds Pressure ulcers, Stages I and II Superficial burns Secondary dressing Peripheral IVs Abrasions	Wound inspection Impermeable to external fluids and bacteria Conformable Promote autolytic debridement Prevention/reduces friction Change every 5 to 7 days or prn if leakage noted Numerous sizes available Waterproof	Nonabsorptive May adhere to fragile skin Not for draining wounds Fluid retention may lead to maceration of peri-wound area Third-degree burns
Post op incisions Central lines, CVPs, and PICC lines Infected wounds Highly colonized wounds	Antimicrobial Same advantages as transparent films	Sensitivity to silver Will inactivate enzymatic debriding agents Same disadvantages as transparent films
Pressure ulcers, Stages II & III Partial and full thickness wounds Under compression wraps/stockings Preventive dressing for high-risk friction areas Secondary dressing or under taping procedures First- and second-degree burns	Facilitates autolytic debridement Self-adherent Impermeable to fluids/bacteria Conformable Reduces wound pain Thermal insulation Long wear time—3 to 7 days, depending on exudate	Contraindicated with muscle, bone, or tendon Not recommended for heavily draining wounds, sinus tracts, or fragile skin May be difficult to remove Contraindicated for third-degree burns
Infected wounds Highly colonized wounds	Antimicrobial Can be left on up to 7 days Same advantages as hydrocolloid dressings	Sensitivity to silver Must have exudate for ionic silver to be released Will inactivate enzymatic debriding agents Same disadvantages as hydrocolloid dressings

(continued)

Wound dressing categories (continued)

Generic category	Description/ composition	Trade names	
Hydrogel ◊ ♦	Water or glycerin based, non-adherent; contains 80% to 99% water; numerous sizes and forms (gels, sheets, strips, and gauze available)	3M Tegaderm Hydrogel Amerigel Aqua Flo AquaSite Aquasorb Biolex CarraDres Hypergel Iamin Hydrating Gel IntraSite Gel Normlgel Purilon Gel Restore Gel SAF-Gel	CarraSmart Carrasyn Gel Curafil Gel Curagel Curasol Gel DermaGauze Elastro-Gel, Plus Elta FlexiGel Skintegrity SoloSite TenderWet Transigel Vigilon Woun'Dres Hydrogel Xcell
Hydrogel with silver ◊ ♦	Controlled-release ionic silver	SilvaSorb Gel	
Foam ♦♦ ♦♦♦	Hydrophilic polyurethane or gel film–coated foam, non-adherent layer absorptive wound dressing	3M Foam Allevyn Allevyn Cavity Biatain CarraSmart COPA COPA Island COPA Plus DermaFoam DermaLevin Flexzan Gentleheal LoProfile Foam	Lyofoam Mepilex Mitraflex Optifoam Polyderm Polymem PolyWic Quadrifoam Sof-Foam Tielle Tielle Plus VigiFoam

Indications	Advantages and benefits	Disadvantages
Pressure ulcers, Stages II to IV Partial and full thickness wounds Dermabrasion Painful wounds Dermal ulcers Radiation tissue damage First- and second-degree burns Skin tears Donor sites Necrotic wounds	Non-adherent Trauma-free removal/soothing to patient Rehydrates the wound bed Reduces wound pain Can be used with topical medications Can be used in cavities or tunnels Softens and loosens necrosis and slough 24 to 72 hour dressing change, depending on the form of gel	Some require secondary dressing to secure May macerate periwound skin Not recommended for heavily draining wounds Contraindicated for third-degree burns
Infected wounds Highly colonized wounds	Antimicrobial Can be left on up to 3 days Non-adherent Rehydrates the wound bed	Sensitivity to silver Not recommended for use in conjunction with topical medications Will inactivate enzymatic debriding agents Same disadvantages as hydrogel dressings
Partial and full thickness wounds Pressure ulcers, Stages II to IV Surgical wounds Dermal ulcers Under compression wraps/stocking Tunneling and cavity wounds (varies; check package insert)	Non-adherent Trauma-free removal Conformable, easy to apply and remove Frequency of dressing change depends on amount of drainage 3 to 5 day dressing change Available with adhesive and nonadhesive border in various shapes and forms	Not recommended for nondraining wounds Not recommended for dry eschar May require secondary dressing May macerate periwound area if not changed appropriately Contraindicated for third-degree burns

(continued)

Wound dressing categories (continued)

Generic category	Description/composition	Trade names	
Foam with silver ♦♦ ♦♦♦	Controlled-release ionic silver	Contreet Foam Polymem Silver Optifoam AG	
Calcium alginate ♦♦ ♦♦♦	Nonwoven composite of fibers from calcium-sodium alginate, a cellulose-like polysaccharide, manufactured from brown seaweed; forms a soft gel when in contact with wound exudate	3M Tegagen HI & HG Alginate Algicell Algiderm AlgiSite CarraGinate Carrasorb H Curasorb Dermaginate Kalginate Kaltostat Kaltostat Fortex	Maxorb Extra CMC Alginate Melgisobr NU-DERM Alginate Polymem Alginate Restore CalciCare SeaSorb Sorbsan
Calcium alginate with silver ♦♦ ♦♦♦	Controlled-release ionic silver	Algidex Ag Alginate	Maxorb Ag (Alginate & Hydrofiber) Silvercel
Composites ♦ ♦♦ ♦♦♦	Combination of two or more physically distinct products manufactured as a single dressing that provides multiple functions; may include a bacterial barrier, absorptive layer, foam, hydrocolloid, or hydrogel; semi-adherent or non-adherent	3M Tegaderm Absorbent Pad Alldress CombiDERM CombiDERM ACD Comfortell CompDress Island	Covaderm Plus Covrsite DermaDress Epigard Stratasorb Telfa Island Viasorb

Indications	Advantages and benefits	Disadvantages
Infected wounds Highly colonized wounds	Antimicrobial Some can be left on up to 7 days Same advantages as foam dressings	Sensitivity to silver Must have exudate for silver to be released Will inactivate enzymatic debriding agents Same disadvantages as foam
Partial and full thickness wounds Pressure ulcers, Stages III and IV Dermal ulcers/dehisced wounds Post-op wounds for hemostasis Sinus tracts, tunnels, or cavities Donor sites	Trauma-free removal Can be used with tunneling and undermining Hemostatic properties for minor bleeding Change every day to every other day Available in sheets, ropes, and within other composite type dressings	Contraindicated for dry eschar, third-degree burns, surgical implantation, and heavy bleeding May require secondary dressing Gel may have odor during dressing change.
Infected wounds Highly colonized wounds	Antimicrobial Change every 3 days or prn Same advantages and benefits as calcium alginate dressings	Sensitivity to silver Must have exudate for silver to be released Will inactivate enzymatic debriding agents Same disadvantages as calcium alginate dressings
Primary and secondary dressings for partial and full thickness wounds Pressure ulcers, Stages I to IV Dermal ulcers Surgical incisions	Conformable Multiple sizes and shapes available Easy to apply and remove Most include adhesive border Frequency of dressing change dependent on wound type (check package insert)	Adhesive borders may limit use on fragile skin. Some contraindicated for Stage IV ulcers (check package insert) May not provide moist wound environment

(continued)

Wound dressing categories (continued)

Generic category	Description/ composition	Trade names
Composites with silver ◆ ◆◆ ◆◆◆	Transparent film with an alginate pad	Arglaes Island
Enzymatic debriders ◊ ◆ ◆◆ ◆◆◆	Prescriptive collagenase ointment that digests collagen	Collagenase/ Santyl Iruxol Mono Novuxol
Collagen ◆ ◆◆ ◆◆◆	Major protein of the body; dressing stimulates cellular migration and contributes to new tissue development derived from bovine, porcine, or avian sources	Cellerate Rx Gel Cellerate Rx Powder ColActive Fibracol Kollagen-Medifil Particles/Gel/Pads Kollagen-SkinTemp Promogran Matrix Stimulen
Collagen with silver ◆ ◆◆ ◆◆◆	Releases silver ions that are antimicrobial while collagen binds with MMP (matrix metalloproteases) in chronic wound exudate	ColActive Ag Prisma Matrix

Antimicrobial therapies

Non-adherent antimicrobial dressings that protect against bacteria and/or decrease bacterial load

◆ ◆◆	Cadexomer iodine– impregnated: Immediate and controlled-release of cadexomer iodine	Iodoflex Pad Iodosorb Gel

Indications	Advantages and benefits	Disadvantages
Infected wounds Highly colonized wounds	Antimicrobial Can be left in place up to 5 days Advantages and benefits same as composite dressings	Sensitivity to silver Must have exudate for silver to be released Will inactivate enzymatic debriding agents Same disadvantages as composite dressings
To debride necrotic wounds, pressure ulcers, dermal ulcers, post-op wounds	Collagen in healthy tissue is not attacked. Nonsurgical method of debridement Requires daily dressing changes	Adversely affected by certain detergents, acidic solutions, and heavy metal ions such as mercury and silver
Chronic non-healing wounds Partial and full thickness wounds Pressure ulcers, Stage III and some Stage IV (check package insert) Dermal ulcers Donor sites Surgical wounds	Absorbent, non-adherent Biodegradable gel Conforms well May be used in combination with topical agents 1 to 3 day dressing change	Contraindicated for third-degree burns and sensitivities to collagen or bovine products Not recommended for necrotic wounds May require rehydration
Infected wounds Highly colonized wounds	Antimicrobial Can be left on up to 7 days Same advantages as collagen dressings	Sensitive to collagen and silver Will inactivate enzymatic debriding agents Same disadvantages as collagen dressings
	Decreases bacterial load in wound Reduces risk of infection	Contraindicated in patients sensitive to ingredients described
Infected wounds—any type (pressure ulcers, venous, arterial, diabetic, or surgical wounds)		

(continued)

Wound dressing categories (continued)

Generic category	Description/ composition	Trade names
Antimicrobial therapies (continued)		
◆ ◆◆	Controlled release silver powder	Arglaes Powder
◆ ◆◆	Polyhexamethylene Biguanide Impregnated (PHMD)	Kerlix AMD XCell AM
◆◆ ◆◆◆	Methylene Blue and Gentian Violet	Hydrofera Blue
Contact layer with silver ◆ ◆◆ ◆◆◆	Immediate and sustained release of ionic silver in a non-adherent primary dressing	
Contact Layer ◊ ◆ ◆◆ ◆◆◆	Non-adherent primary dressing that allows exudate to pass through	

Indications	Advantages and benefits	Disadvantages
Partial or full thickness wounds Colonized, chronic non-healing wounds		
Inhibits the growth of bacteria and viruses		
Infected wounds Partial or full thickness wounds Colonized, chronic non-healing wounds Under compression wraps/stockings Over grafts or skin substitutes	Inhibits growth of pathogens, especially antibiotic-resistant strains Antimicrobial action effective up to 7 days	Sensitivity to silver Secondary dressing required Must be removed and wound cleansed prior to MRI Not recommended for use in conjunction with topical medications Some may stain or discolor surrounding tissue due to silver turning black when it oxidizes. Contraindicated with enzymatic debriding agents
Partial and full thickness wounds, donor sites, skin grafts	May be used with topical medications Less trauma to the wound bed Prevents the outer dressing from adhering to the wound.	Secondary dressing is required. Impenetrable exudate may macerate.

(continued)

Wound dressing categories (*continued*)

Generic category	Description/ composition	Trade names	
Negative pressure wound therapy ♦♦ ♦♦♦	Noninvasive active therapy using localized negative pressure to promote healing		

ADVANCED WOUND CARE THERAPIES

Skin substitutes	Skin substitutes developed in the laboratory from tissue of human origin or bio-engineered tissue	Apligraf DermaGraft GammaGraft	GraftJacket Orcel TransCyte
Extracellular matrix	Extracellular matrix material derived from the submu-cosal layer of porcine small intestines	Oasis Wound Matrix	

Indications	Advantages and benefits	Disadvantages
Moderate to heavy exuding wounds Partial and full thickness wounds Venous, arterial, diabetic ulcers, and dehisced wounds, Pressure ulcers, Stages III and IV Surgical wounds Flaps and grafts Acute traumatic wounds	Decreases edema Decreases bacterial colonization Increases blood supply and granular tissue formation Generally, dressing changed every 48 to 72 hours (specifics for dressing and equipment vary by manufacturer)	Healthcare worker needs training to apply and operate equipment. Not reimbursed in acute and long term care facilities May adhere to some wounds Not recommended for nondraining wounds or wounds with eschar Contraindicated for wounds with malignancy and untreated osteomyelitis
Partial and full thickness wounds Venous and diabetic ulcers Granular wounds Burns Chronic wounds	Growth factors present in skin equivalent Decreases wound healing time No donor site Decreases pain for many patients	Wound has to be granular. Check manufacturer's directions for storage and shelf life.
Partial and full thickness wounds Diabetic ulcers Second-degree burns Graft sites	Biological dressing Strength and flexibility	Sensitivity to porcine- or bovine-derived products

(continued)

Wound dressing categories (*continued*)

Generic category	Description/ composition	Trade names

ADVANCED WOUND CARE THERAPIES (continued)

Generic category	Description/ composition	Trade names
Autologous platelet-rich plasma (PRP) gel	Autologous point-of-care process where small volume of blood is drawn from the patient; the blood is separated in a centrifuge: the resulting platelet-rich plasma (PRP) gel is extracted and activated. Activation has been shown to cause the platelets to release autologous multiple growth factors; the fibrinogen in the plasma converted to a fibrin matrix scaffold and the liquid forms a gel.	AutoloGel
Miscellaneous wound dressings	Medical-grade active *Leptospermum* honey from New Zealand Available in tube, colloid sheet, or impregnated alginate dressing	ManukaMed MediHoney
	Sodium chlorite dressing: Consists of soft nonwoven material (viscose/polyester) impregnated with sodium chloride	Mesalt

Indications	Advantages and benefits	Disadvantages
Chronic non-healing wounds Exuding wounds Pressure ulcers, Stages III and IV Arterial and venous ulcers Diabetic foot ulcers Mechanically or surgically debrided wounds	Moves stalled wounds out of inflammatory stage Growth factors, cytokines, and chemokines from the patient's own blood are applied topically to the wound bed	Special equipment needed Healthcare worker needs training to apply and operate equipment. Multiple weekly applications
Infected wounds Highly colonized wounds Wounds with slough or necrotic tissue Pressure ulcers, Stages II to IV Partial and full thickness wounds Venous ulcers Diabetic ulcers	Antibacterial barrier Autolytic debridement properties	Allergies to honey Brief stinging sensation
Moderate to heavy exuding wounds of any type Infected wounds of any type	Facilitates cleansing of wounds with exudate, slough, or infection	Should not be used on dry wounds or minimally exuding wounds Should not be allowed to come in direct contact with exposed bone or tendon

(continued)

Wound dressing categories (continued)

Generic category	Description/ composition	Trade names
ADVANCED WOUND CARE THERAPIES (continued)		
♦	Transforming powder dressing with NanoFlex technology Powder interacts with wound exudate and hydrates the wound bed	Altrazeal
	Balsam Peru, Castor Oil USP/NF, Trypsin USP	Allanderm-T Xenaderm Vasolex Ointment Optase

Indications	Advantages and benefits	Disadvantages
Full and partial thickness wounds, surgical wounds, burns, abrasions, donor sites, venous ulcers, pressure and diabetic ulcers	The powder becomes a moist, flexible film over the surface of the wound. For exuding wounds only.	Should not be applied with oil-based products on the wound surface, particularly ointments, salves, or other treatments. These oil-based products will prevent proper hydration and aggregation at the wound surface.
Pressure ulcers, dehisced wounds Radiation injury	Balsam Peru is a capillary bed stimulant and a mild antiseptic that helps prevent bacteria from growing. Castor oil works as a lubricant to protect the tissue. Helps relieve pain. Trypsin is intended for debridement of eschar and other necrotic tissue. Does not require a secondary dressing.	Do not apply to fresh arterial clots. Temporary stinging sensation BID application Prescription is required

(continued)

Wound dressing categories *(continued)*

Generic category	Description/ composition	Trade names
Scar Care	Self-adhesive silicone contained within a gel or flexible sheet. Occludes the skin to hydrate the scar area.	Cica-Care Mepiform
Becaplermin gel	Genetically engineered platelet-derived growth factors produced in yeast and then formulated into a gel	Regranex

The products listed are representative of type and are not meant to be all-inclusive; indications, advantages, and disadvantages are some examples, more suggestions may apply.
Antimicrobials: may be topical or within a dressing component
Surgical, Mechanical, Autolytic or Enzymatic debridement methods
© A. McIntosh and L. (Galvan) Montoya, September 20, 2010

Indications	Advantages and benefits	Disadvantages
Hypertrophic scars, keloids, and closed wounds to prevent hypertrophic and keloid scars.	Re-useable, durable. Conformable	Contraindicated in open or infected wounds Contraindicated over scabs and stitches Takes 2-4 months to see some results
Neuropathic wounds Diabetic ulcers Granular wounds		Can't be used on infected wounds or wounds with necrotic tissue Must be refrigerated

CHAPTER 10

Nutrition and Wound Care

Mary Ellen Posthauer, RD, CD, LD
David R. Thomas, MD, FACP, AGSF, GSAF

Objectives

After completing this chapter, you'll be able to:

- describe the process of screening to identify nutritional problems/concerns
- identify the parameters involved in completing a nutritional assessment
- describe the role of nutrients in wound prevention and healing
- define the role of nutrition management for malnutrition.

Nutrition plays a key role in both the prevention and treatment of wounds. The goal in preventing pressure ulcers is to screen and identify individuals at risk for ulcer development. A nutritional assessment should be completed both for individuals who are at high risk for developing pressure ulcers and for those who currently have one or more wounds, with the data derived from the assessment used to develop a nutrition care plan. The nutrition interventions selected to manage the current condition should be based on standard protocols and reviewed as new research data become available.

NUTRITIONAL SCREENING

A nutritional screening is the process of identifying characteristics that are known to be associated with nutrition problems. Its purpose is to pinpoint individuals who are malnourished or at nutritional risk and then to determine appropriate interventions based on the findings. Depending on the screening tool selected, screening may be completed by any qualified member of the healthcare team, including the dietitian, registered dietetic technician, registered nurse, physician, or other qualified health professional.

A number of nutritional screening tools are available, including the Mini-Nutritional Assessment (MNA), the Malnutrition Universal Screening Tool (MUST), the Malnutrition Screening Tool (MST), and the Subjective Global Assessment (SGA).[1] The MNA has recently been shortened to a six-item tool (MNA short-form).[2] Of the screening tools available, only the MNA has been validated in elderly populations and in long-term care settings. A Simple Nutrition Appetite Questionnaire measures appetite loss in older persons and predicts weight loss over the next 6 months.[3]

A conceptual problem with the use of nutritional assessment instruments is whether the measurement reflects true undernutrition or simply sicker patients. By definition, undernutrition should be responsive to the provision of adequate nutrients. On the contrary, sicker patients with cachexia due to underlying inflammatory disease have been remarkably resistant to nutrition interventions.[4] Some published data suggest that the MNA is sensitive to changes in nutrition status with refeeding,[5] but further research is needed to develop a nutritional assessment instrument that will predict response to nutrition correction.

Significant weight loss without any known medical condition places a patient at risk for undernutrition. Likewise, disease states and conditions (including undernutrition) can increase the risk of pressure ulcer development and impact the healing process. Persons at risk for undernutrition and for the development of pressure ulcers have a number of common factors, including:

- Significant weight loss: 5 lb or more in 1 month, 5% in 30 days, or 10% in 180 days
- Disease states and conditions: diabetes, malabsorption, dementia, chronic obstructive pulmonary disease (COPD), cancer, or renal disease
- Immobility and inactivity: hip fracture, spinal cord injury, stroke
- Chewing and swallowing difficulties (dysphagia) resulting from stroke, Parkinson's disease, and cerebral palsy
- Appetite decline, anorexia, poor food and fluid intake
- Adverse effects of medications

Diabetes

Patients with diabetes frequently have a higher rate of complications, including infections, which can both cause and affect poor wound healing.[6] Hyperglycemia may impair leukocyte function, thus lengthening the inflammatory process and the resolution of infection. For patients with diabetes, a glycosylated hemoglobin (HbA1c) test is the best indicator of glucose status, as it indicates blood glucose control over the previous 3 months. Marston noted that failure to manage uncontrolled HbA1c levels impedes healing of diabetic foot ulcers,[7] but this may not apply to pressure ulcers.

The primary nutritional goal for patients with diabetes is to improve metabolic control of glucose and lipids and provide the appropriate calories. The term *ADA diet* is no longer used because the American Diabetes Association (ADA) does not recommend or endorse any single diet. The Consistent Carbohydrate Diabetes meal plan is now recommended by the ADA and incorporates carbohydrates daily at each meal and at snack time. This plan generally includes 50% of calories from carbohydrates, 20% from protein, and 30% from fat, with an emphasis on monounsaturated and polyunsaturated fats. The consistent carbohydrate approach has been successful in the management of type 2 diabetes in nursing homes.[8]

Renal disease

Patients with renal disease often have multiple medical conditions, such as diabetes or heart disease, which complicates the nutrient parameters of their diet. For example, a renal diet that is limited in calories, protein, potassium, phosphorus, sodium, and fluid often results in poor dietary intake that may not meet the nutrient requirement for a patient with wounds.

Obesity, altered mental status, and functional limitations

An obese patient with wounds should consume a diet adequate in protein and calories to meet wound healing needs instead of a low-calorie diet designed for weight reduction.

Altered mental status often limits patients' abilities to eat independently or to comprehend the importance of consuming a balanced diet. Advanced dementia often results in weight loss, dysphagia, malnutrition, and pressure ulcers. If patients become incapable of responding to caregivers' assistance to nourish them, this may lead to unintentional weight loss and undernutrition, which may increase their risk for pressure ulcer development.

Immobility affects a patient's ability to either prepare meals for themselves or travel to a restaurant for meals, thus resulting in the consumption of a diet lacking in the proper nutrients. For example, hip fracture and spinal cord injury restrict mobility, and hip fracture often results in increased pain that makes it difficult for the patient to concentrate on preparing and/or consuming healthy meals. Functional limitations, such as difficulty chewing or swallowing, affect the patient's ability to ingest adequate calories and fluids. Poor hearing and vision may compromise the patient's communication skills, often resulting in poor intake of meals.

Pressure ulcers

The Centers for Medicare and Medicaid Services (CMS), which regulates long-term-care facilities, has targeted pressure ulcers, inadequate nutrition, and unintended weight loss as key survey issues. The development of a

Definition of high risk for pressure ulcer development

The Centers for Medicare and Medicaid Services has identified the following risk factors for the development of pressure ulcers:

- Impaired/decreased mobility and decreased functional ability
- Comorbid conditions, such as end-stage renal disease, thyroid disease, or diabetes mellitus
- Drugs such as steroids that may affect wound healing
- Impaired diffuse or localized flood flow, for example, generalized atherosclerosis or lower extremity arterial insufficiency
- Resident's refusal of some aspect of care or treatment
- Cognitive impairment
- Exposure of skin to urinary and fecal incontinence
- Undernutrition, malnutrition, and hydration deficits
- A previously healed ulcer

Reprinted from F Tag 314. "Procedures: 483.25(c): Pressure Sores." *Federal Register* 56(187); November 12, 2004.

pressure ulcer in a person who was at low risk is automatically considered a sentinel event. In 2004, the CMS [9,10] revised Federal Tag 314 (F-314), which provides guidance to surveyors as part of the *State Operations Provider Certification Manual* that impacts skilled nursing facilities in the United States. The guidance contains a section on undernutrition and hydration deficits, noting that "continuing weight loss and failure of a pressure ulcer to heal, despite reasonable efforts to improve caloric and nutrient intake, may indicate that the resident is in multisystem failure or in an end-stage or end-of-life condition warranting an additional assessment of the resident's overall condition." The interdisciplinary team should assist in the development of nutrition goals considering the individual's prognosis and projected clinical course. (See *Definition of high risk for pressure ulcer development*.)

NUTRITIONAL ASSESSMENT

Nutritional assessment is a systematic process of obtaining, verifying, and interpreting data in order to make decisions about the nature and cause of nutrition-related problems. It's an ongoing process that involves initial data collection followed by continued reassessment and analysis of the patient's status compared with specific criteria.[11] The assessment reviews the patient's nutritional status using medical, health, and medication history; physical examination; anthropometric measurements; and laboratory data. The assessment also includes interpretation of data from the screening process as well as a review of data from other disciplines (such as speech, occupational, or physical therapy) that may affect the assessment process. Nutritional assessment precedes the implementation of a care plan, intervention, monitoring, and evaluation.

Daily caloric requirements

Estimating a patient's daily caloric requirement is part of the assessment process and assists in determining the appropriate plan for the prevention and/or treatment of wounds. Indirect calorimetry is the gold standard for measuring energy expenditure estimation and quantifies stress due to illness, injury, and other medical conditions.[12] However, indirect calorimetry is not widely used outside the acute care setting. The Harris-Benedict equation measures resting metabolic rate rather than basal energy expenditure, but controversy exists over its accuracy in obese or severely undernourished individuals. The Mifflin-St. Jeor equation is appropriate for healthy adults as well as overweight and obese individuals.[13,14] Activity and injury factors added to the basic equations result in the mean total daily energy requirements.

As part of the nutritional assessment, observation during mealtime gives the healthcare professional the opportunity to determine whether the patient has chewing or swallowing problems that may require either speech or occupational therapy. Adequate intake of food and fluid is a concern for those with swallowing problems, and inadequate intake places them at risk for pressure ulcers. The speech therapist defines the diet texture and also assesses the patient's needs for special feeding techniques, which are implemented by the dining service department. For example, patients may require thickened liquids to prevent aspiration. The occupational therapist determines the appropriate self-help feeding devices that promote eating independence. Likewise, physical therapy sessions often result in the need for both increased calories and fluid, which the dietitian will calculate and arrange to provide at appropriate times.

Signs of malnutrition

Assess the patient's skin condition, checking for loss of subcutaneous fat as evidenced by loose skin in the extremities. Observe for listlessness, muscle wasting, and the presence of peripheral edema in the absence of cardiac disease or circulatory disorder. Dull, dry, sparse hair can signify a possible protein-energy deficiency. (For further signs,[15] see *Physical signs of malnutrition*.)

The older adult is particularly prone to pressure ulcers as a result of decreased mobility, multiple comorbid conditions, poor nutrition, and loss of muscle mass. Nutritional factors thought to contribute to skin breakdown include protein deficiency, which creates a negative nitrogen balance; anemia, which inhibits the formation of red blood cells; and dehydration, which causes dry, fragile skin.

In addition, immune function declines with age, thus increasing the risk of infection. With advancing age also comes decreased skin response to temperature, pain, and pressure. This affects the skin's elasticity and the healing process.

Physical signs of malnutrition

Signs	Possible causes
HAIR	
Dull, dry, lack of natural shine	Protein-energy deficiency
	Essential fatty acid (EFA) deficiency
Thin, sparse, loss of curl, color changes, depigmentation, easily plucked	Zinc deficiency
	Other nutrient deficiencies: manganese, copper
EYES	
Small, yellowish lumps around eyes	Hyperlipidemia
White rings around both eyes	
Angular inflammation of eyelids, "grittiness" under eyelids	Riboflavin deficiency
Pale eye membranes	Vitamin B$_{12}$, folacin, and/or iron deficiency
Night blindness, dry membranes, dull or soft cornea	Vitamin A, zinc deficiency
Redness and fissures of eyelid corners	Niacin deficiency
Ring of fine blood vessels around cornea	General poor nutrition

(continued)

Physical signs of malnutrition (continued)

Signs	Possible causes
LIPS	
Redness and swelling of mouth	Niacin, riboflavin, iron, and/or pyridoxine deficiency
Angular fissures, scars at corner of mouth	Niacin, riboflavin, iron, and/or pyridoxine deficiency
Soreness, burning lips, pallor	Pyridoxine deficiency
GUMS	
Spongy, swollen, bleed easily, redness	Vitamin C deficiency
Gingivitis	Folic acid, vitamin B_{12} deficiency
MOUTH	
Cheilosis, angular scars	Riboflavin, folic acid deficiency, pyridoxine deficiency
Soreness, burning	Riboflavin deficiency
TONGUE	
Sores, swollen, scarlet, raw	Folacin, niacin deficiency
Soreness, burning tongue, purplish color	Riboflavin deficiency
Smooth with papillae (small projections)	Riboflavin, vitamin B_{12}, pyridoxine deficiency
Glossitis	Iron, zinc deficiency, pyridoxine deficiency
TASTE	
Sense of taste diminished	Zinc deficiency
TEETH	
Gray brown spots	Increased fluoride intake
Missing or erupting abnormally	Generally poor nutrition
FACE	
Skin color loss, dark cheeks and eyes, enlarged parotid glands, scaling of skin around nostrils	Protein-energy deficiency, specifically niacin, riboflavin, and pyridoxine deficiencies
Pallor	Iron, folacin, vitamin B_{12}, and vitamin C deficiencies
Hyperpigmentation	Niacin deficiency
NECK	
Thyroid enlargement	Iodine deficiency
Symptoms of hypothyroidism	Iodine deficiency
NAILS	
Fragility, banding	Protein deficiency
Spoon-shaped	Iron deficiency

Physical signs of malnutrition (continued)

Signs	Possible causes
SKIN	
Slow wound healing	Zinc deficiency
Psoriasis	Biotin deficiency
Eczema	Riboflavin deficiency
Scaliness	Biotin deficiency, pyridoxine deficiency
Black and blue marks due to skin bleeding	Vitamin C and/or K deficiency
Dryness, mosaic, sandpaper feel, flakiness	Increased or decreased vitamin A
Swollen and dark	Niacin deficiency
Lack of fat under skin or bilateral edema	Protein-energy deficiency
Yellow colored	Carotene deficiency or excess
Cutaneous flushing	Niacin
Pallor	Iron, folic acid deficiencies
GASTROINTESTINAL	
Anorexia, flatulence, diarrhea	Vitamin B_{12} deficiency
MUSCULAR SYSTEM	
Weakness	Phosphorus or potassium deficiency
Wasted appearance	Protein-energy deficiency
Calf tenderness, absent knee jerks	Thiamin deficiency
Peripheral neuropathy	Folacin, pyridoxine, pantothenic acid, phosphate, thiamine deficiencies
Muscle twitching	Magnesium or pyridoxine excess or deficiency
Muscle cramps	Chloride decreased, sodium deficiency
Muscle pain	Biotin deficiency
SKELETAL SYSTEM	
Demineralization of bone	Calcium, phosphorus, vitamin D deficiencies
Epiphyseal enlargement of leg and knee	Vitamin D deficiency
Bowed legs	Vitamin D deficiency
NERVOUS SYSTEM	
Listlessness	Protein-energy deficiency
Loss of position and vibratory sense, decrease and loss of ankle and knee reflexes, depression, inability to concentrate, defective memory, delirium	Thiamin, vitamin B_{12} deficiencies
Seizures, memory impairment, and behavioral disturbances	Magnesium, zinc deficiencies
Peripheral neuropathy, dementia	Pyridoxine deficiency

An algorithm outlining nutrition guidelines for the prevention of pressure ulcers has been created to guide nutritional assessment and determine appropriate treatment. (See *Algorithm for prevention of pressure ulcers: nutrition guidelines*.)

Medications can influence a patient's nutrition status and have been identified as a cause of weight loss.[16] Drugs may either inhibit or induce metabolism of a nutrient or increase the excretion of a nutrient. Medicine designed to calm and reduce agitation may in turn reduce mobility and activity levels and place patients at risk for pressure ulcer development. Medications may increase or decrease appetite, alter sense of taste or smell, or cause gastric disturbances. Radiation therapy, chemotherapy, and renal dialysis can result in increased nausea and vomiting as well as decreased activity, placing the patient at risk. Drug therapy may trigger adverse effects; for example, antibiotics often cause nausea and gastric disturbances that curtail a patient's food and fluid intake. The list of medications that may influence nutrient intake or interfere with nutrition is very long and complicated.[17] In this context, a consultation with a geriatric pharmacologist may be helpful.

Anthropometric factors

Anthropometry, the measurement of body size, weight, and proportions, is used to evaluate a patient's nutritional status. A change in anthropometric values can signal problems such as wasting or edema, reflecting nutritional excess or deficit. Accurate heights and weights are critical as they are the basis for determining caloric and nutrient requirements. Adjustment or notations should be made for casts and other appliances that alter true weight.

> ### ▶ PRACTICE POINT
>
> Weigh your patient each time on the same scale, at the same time of day, and with minimal clothing.

Body mass index (BMI) is a weight-to-height ratio derived from body weight in kilograms divided by the square of the height in meters:

$$\frac{\text{Weight (kg)}}{\text{Height (m}^2)}$$

or

$$\text{BMI} = \frac{\text{Weight (lb)}}{\text{Height (in}^2)} \times 705$$

A normally hydrated person with a BMI greater than 30 is considered obese.[18] A BMI less than 19 is considered underweight for adults and may place the patient at nutritional risk.[19]

Stress as a result of injury, surgery, burn, fracture, or wounds results in depletion of the nutrient stores required for healing. Protein stores are used as energy sources if adequate carbohydrate and fat aren't provided.

Ideal body weight, sometimes called recommended body weight or desired body weight, can be approximated using specific calculations. However, a more reliable measurement of the severity of undernutrition is any deviation from usual body weight.

$$\frac{\text{Usual Weight} - \text{Current Weight}}{\text{Usual Weight}} \times 100$$
$$= \% \text{ Weight Loss}$$

For example, a usual body weight of 145 lb that decreased to 137 lb in 30 days is a 5.5% loss.

When evaluating the severity of weight variances, it's important to determine possible causes, such as recent surgery, diuretic therapy, or other new treatments, that may affect weight status. Weight loss, especially in older adults, results in undernutrition and increases the risk of mortality. A 5% loss in 30 days or a 10% decline in 6 months increases the risk of death.[20,21]

Biochemical Data

Biochemical tests are evaluated as part of the nutrition assessment process. However, there is no one test specific to nutritional status. (See *Useful lab values to screen for hydration status*, page 248.)

Protein status can be evaluated through a nitrogen-balance study, visceral protein blood levels, and tests of immune function such as total lymphocyte counts.

Algorithm for prevention of pressure ulcers: nutrition guidelines[*]

Trigger Conditions:

- Unintended wt. loss ≤5% in 30 days; ≤10% in 180 days
- BMI[§]< 18.5 (weight (lb) / (height (in) x height (in)) x 703 **or** weight (kg) / (height (m) x height (m)))
- Swallowing Problems /dysphagia
- Receiving enteral or parenteral nutrition
- Poor oral intake
- At risk of developing pressure ulcer (i.e., low score on Braden Scale[Δ])
- Immobility
- Infections (i.e., respiratory, urinary tract, gastrointestinal)
- Decline in ADLs (activities of daily living)
- Other selected conditions per facility

[§]Body Mass Index
[Δ]Braden BJ & Bergstrom N. *Decubitus* 1989;2(3):44

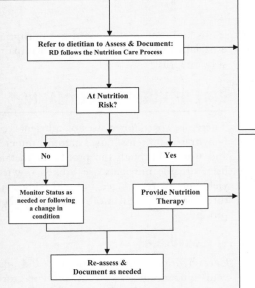

Refer to dietitian to Assess & Document:
RD follows the Nutrition Care Process

At Nutrition Risk?

No   **Yes**

Monitor Status as needed or following a change in condition

Provide Nutrition Therapy

Re-assess & Document as needed

Dietitian Assessment:[1]

- Current weight/height
- Determine deviation from Usual Body Weight.
- Body Mass Index (BMI)
- Interview for food preferences/intolerances
- Determine nutritional needs
  1. Calories (30-35 kcal/kg body wt (BW)s
  2. Protein (1.25-1.5 g/kg)
  3. Fluid (1 mL fluid per calorie intake/d or minimum of 1500 mL/day or per medical condition)
- Compare nutrient intake with nutritional needs: assess adequacy
- Laboratory values (within 30 days)
  1. Serum protein levels may be affected by inflammation, renal function, hydration and other factors and do not reflect nutritional status
  2. Consider lab values as one aspect of the assessment process. Refer to facility policy for specific labs
- Risk factors for pressure ulcer development
  1. Medical history
  2. Validated risk assessment (i.e., Braden Scale)
  3. Malnutrition (use screening tool, e.g. Mini Nutritional Assessment (MNA® for ≥65 years located at www.mna-elderly.com)
  4. Medical Treatments
  5. Medications (review type of medications)
  6. Ability to meet nutritional needs orally (if inadequate, consider alternative method of feeding) consistent with individual's wishes
  7. Oral Problems (e.g. chewing, swallowing) EAT-10: A Swallowing Assessment Tool available through Nestlé Nutrition Institute

Considerations:

- Incorporate fortified foods at meals for weight gain
- Provide supplements between meals as needed
- Vary the type of supplements offered to prevent taste fatigue
- Provide preferred food/food substitutions
- At admission weigh weekly x 30 days and then monthly
- Monitor acceptance of food and/or supplements offered
- Monitor tolerance of oral nutritional supplements, e.g. diarrhea
- Provide a vitamin/mineral supplement, if intake is poor
- Provide assistance at meal time if needed
- Encourage family involvement
- Offer food/fluid at appropriate texture for condition
- Liberalize restrictive diets
- Consult with Pharmacist and provide food and drugs at appropriate times and amounts
- Consider alternative method of feeding and if consistent with individual's wishes and goals of therapy:
  1. Provide tube feeding to meet needs per assessment
  2. Monitor tolerance, if needed recommend a specialty formula
  3. Provide parenteral nutrition when gut is non-functioning

[1] National Pressure Ulcer Advisory Panel and European Pressure Ulcer Advisory Panel. Prevention and treatment of pressure ulcers: clinical practice guideline. Washington DC: National Pressure Ulcer Advisory Panel; 2009.

[*]These are general guidelines based on various clinical references and are not intended as a substitute for medical advice or existing facility guidelines. An individual assessment is recommended.

Useful lab values to screen for hydration status

Test	Normal values	Dehydration	Overhydration
Osmolality	280-303 mOsm/kg	> 303 mOsm/kg > 320 mOsm/kg (critical)	< 280 mOsm/kg
Serum sodium	135-145 mEq/l	> 145 mEq/l	< 130 mEq/l
Albumin	3.4-5.4 g/dl	Higher than normal	Lower than normal
Blood urine nitrogen (BUN)	7-20 mg/dl	> 35 mg/dl	< 7 mg/dl
BUN/creatine ratio	10:1	> 25:1	< 10:1
Urine specific gravity	1.002-1.028 g/ml	> 1.028 g/ml	< 1.002 g/ml

The serum albumin level is dependent on hepatocyte function. The half-life of albumin is 12 to 21 days; so significant changes in liver function specific to albumin synthesis may go undetected. However, serum albumin levels may drop in as few as 8 hours in severe stress or inflammatory conditions such as infection, acute surgery, or cortisone excess, even when protein intake is adequate. For this reason, a decrease in serum albumin is increasingly seen as a poor reflection of nutritional status.[4,19,20,22,23]

Prealbumin (transthyretin and thyroxine-binding albumin) has a half-life of 2 to 3 days. Similar to albumin, prealbumin acts as an acute-phase reactant. Prealbumin level improves as the acute inflammatory response improves and may not be an indicator of nutritional status, metabolic stress, or inflammation.[22,23]

Although some laboratory tests may help clinicians evaluate nutritional issues in patients with pressure ulcers, no laboratory test is patient-specific or sensitive enough to warrant repeated testing. Serum albumin, prealbumin, and cholesterol may be useful to help establish overall prognosis; however, they may not correlate well with clinical observation of nutritional status.[23-26] Low serum protein levels may indicate that the patient is ill and therefore at risk for undernutrition. Frequent monitoring of weight status and oral intake would be appropriate, especially if the patient is at risk for impaired skin integrity.

ROLE OF NUTRIENTS IN HEALING

There are six major classes of nutrients: carbohydrates, proteins, fats, vitamins, minerals, and water. Through the process of metabolism, organic nutrients are broken down to yield energy, rearranged to build body structures, or used in chemical reactions for body processes.

Carbohydrates

Carbohydrates provide energy and prevent gluconeogenesis from protein stores. Carbohydrates should comprise 50% to 60% of an individual's total caloric intake. An inadequate supply of carbohydrates results in muscle wasting (when the body is forced to convert protein stores for energy use), loss of subcutaneous tissue, and poor wound healing. (See *Function and sources of nutrients.*)

Protein and amino acids

Protein is the only nutrient that contains nitrogen in addition to carbon, hydrogen, and oxygen; some protein also contains sulfur and phosphorus. These elements combine to form

Function and sources of nutrients

Nutrient	Function	Source
Calories	Supply adequate energy, prevent weight loss, preserve lean body mass	Carbohydrate, protein, and fat, with carbohydrate and fat the preferred sources
Carbohydrates	Deliver energy, spare protein	Grains, fruits, and vegetables, with complex carbohydrates the preferred source
Proteins	Contain nitrogen, which is essential for wound healing. A component of the immune system that supplies the binding material of skin, cartilage, and muscle	Meats, fish, poultry, eggs, legumes, and dairy products; choose lean meat and reduced-fat or low-fat dairy products.
Fat	Most concentrated energy source carrying the fat soluble vitamins Provides insulation under the skin and padding for bony prominences	Meats, eggs, dairy products, and vegetable oils
Fluids	Solvent for minerals and vitamins, amino acids, and glucose Help maintain body temperature and transport materials to cells and waste products from cells	Water, juices, and other beverages; fruits and vegetables contain approximately 95% water
Vitamin C	Water-soluble, non-caloric organic nutrient essential for collagen formation and iron absorption	Citrus fruits and juices, tomatoes, potatoes, tomatoes, broccoli
Minerals: zinc and copper	Inorganic, non-caloric nutrients Zinc is a co-factor for collagen formation, metabolizes protein, and assists in immune function Copper assists in the formation of red blood cells and is responsible for collagen cross-linking and erythropoiesis	Zinc: meats, liver, eggs, and seafood Copper: nuts, dried fruit, organ meats, dried beans, whole grain cereal

amino acids, the smallest molecular units of protein. Protein is responsible for repair and synthesis of enzymes involved in wound healing, cell multiplication, and collagen and connective tissue synthesis. Protein is a component of antibodies needed for immune system function; 20% to 25% of calories should be obtained from protein sources.

The protein requirement for patients with pressure ulcers is arguable, but it is recognized to be higher than the current adult recommendation of 0.8 g/kg of body weight per day. Aging often leads to a decrease in skeletal muscle as well as a decline in protein turnover, which decreases to 20% or less by age 70. Protein tissue accounts for 30% of whole body turnover prior to age 70. This decline may alter the body's ability to fight infection and heal wounds. Research supports increasing protein for healthy older adults to 1.0 to 1.2 g/kg/day.[27-29] Current recommendations for dietary intake of protein in stressed patients with wounds ranges from 1.2 to 1.5 g/kg/day.[30] Many chronically ill elderly people cannot maintain nitrogen balance at this level. Increasing protein intake beyond 2.0 g/kg/day may not increase protein synthesis and may cause dehydration.[31]

The association of dietary protein intake with wound healing has led to the investigation of specific amino acids. When the body is under stress, glutamine, cysteine, and arginine become conditionally indispensible amino acids. However, although glutamine may function as a fuel source for fibroblasts and epithelial cells, it has not shown noticeable effects on wound healing.[32]

L-arginine is composed of 32% nitrogen, and its function is to stimulate the insulin-like growth factor that is involved in wound healing. Arginine enhances immune function and wound collagen deposition in healthy elderly people.[33] In a study of the tolerability and effect of supplemented oral arginine on immune function in nursing home residents with pressure ulcers, the authors concluded that pharmacologic doses of arginine were well tolerated but didn't enhance lymphocyte proliferation or interleukin (IL)-2 production.[34] Another study evaluated the use of high-calorie supplements containing arginine and found a reduction in the Pressure Ulcer Scale for Healing (PUSH) score for individuals with pressure ulcers who consumed these supplements. However, this was a small, 3-week interventional study that did not measure complete healing rates.[35] Other systematic reviews to date have not found evidence to recommend the use of arginine alone or combined with other nutrients for the healing of pressure ulcers.[36]

A randomized, prospective, controlled, multicenter trial[37] evaluated the use of a concentrated, fortified, collagen protein hydrolysate supplement at 23 long-term care facilities. Ninety residents with stage II, III, or IV pressure ulcers in four states participated in the study. Residents were randomized to receive standard care plus the protein hydrolysate supplement or standard care plus a placebo three times a day for 8 weeks. Standard care meant that residents in the study continued to receive any supplement or fortified foods they received prior to entering the study. By week 8, there was a 50% reduction in PUSH scores in the treatment group compared with the control group. The study concluded that a concentrated, fortified, collagen protein hydrolysate supplement may be associated with a reduction in PUSH scores among residents with pressure ulcers residing in long-term care facilities. Additional research is needed to determine the effectiveness of high-protein supplements fortified with arginine and glutamine.[37]

Fats and fatty acids

Fat is the most concentrated source of energy and provides a reserve source of energy in the form of stored triglycerides in adipose tissue. Fat calories should comprise 20% to 25% of total caloric intake. Lean meats, poultry, fish, low-fat dairy products, and vegetable oils are appropriate sources of fat.

Vitamins
FAT-SOLUBLE VITAMINS

Fat-soluble vitamins A, D, E, and K remain in the liver and fat tissue of the body until used. Because the body does not excrete excess fat-soluble vitamins, the risk of toxicity from overdose exists.

> **PRACTICE POINT**
>
> Look for signs and symptoms of overdose toxicity from fat-soluble vitamins A, D, E, and K if the patient is receiving supplements.

Vitamin A is responsible for epithelium maintenance. It also stimulates cellular differentiation in fibroblasts and collagen formation. Vitamin A deficiency, which is uncommon, may result in delayed wound healing and increased susceptibility to infection.

Vitamin E is an antioxidant and is responsible for normal fat metabolism and collagen synthesis. Vitamin E deficiency does not appear to play an active role in wound healing,[38] and it impedes the absorption of vitamin A by reducing the rate of hepatic retinyl ester hydrolysis.[39]

WATER-SOLUBLE VITAMINS

Water-soluble vitamins C and B play a role in wound healing. Vitamin C is essential for collagen synthesis. Collagen and fibroblasts compose the basis for the structure of a new wound bed. A deficiency of vitamin C prolongs healing time and contributes to reduced resistance to infection.[40] However, there is no clinical evidence that wound healing is improved by providing doses of vitamin C above the dietary reference intake (DRI) of 70 to 90 mg/day. A multicenter, blinded trial of 88 patients with pressure ulcers who were randomized to either 10 mg or 500 mg of vitamin C twice daily failed to demonstrate any improved healing or closure rate between groups.[41] Even supratherapeutic doses of vitamin C have not been shown to accelerate wound healing.[42]

Coenzymes (B vitamins) are necessary for the production of energy from glucose, amino acids, and fat. Pyridoxine (vitamin B_6) is important for maintaining cellular immunity and forming red blood cells. Thiamine and riboflavin are needed for adequate cross-linking and collagenation, but their effect has not been demonstrated in pressure ulcers.

Minerals

Minerals also contribute to a patient's well-being. Zinc, a cofactor for collagen formation, also metabolizes protein, liberates vitamin A from storage in the liver, interacts with platelets in blood clotting, and assists in immune function. Deficiency may occur rapidly through wound drainage or excessive gastrointestinal (GI) fluid loss or from long-term poor dietary intake. Albumin transports zinc through the body, so zinc absorption declines as plasma albumin declines (for example, with infection, sepsis, or trauma).[43] No clinical evidence exists to support supplementation (such as with zinc sulfate 200 to 300 mg daily containing more than 50 mg of elemental zinc). In a small study of patients with pressure ulcers, no effect on ulcer healing was seen at 12 weeks in zinc-supplemented versus non–zinc-supplemented patients.[44] The DRI for zinc is 8 to 11 mg, and the maximum daily intake or tolerable upper intake level (for elemental zinc is 40 mg.[45] High serum zinc levels may inhibit healing, impair phagocytosis, and interfere with copper metabolism.[46,47]

Copper is responsible for collagen cross-linking and erythropoiesis; the DRI for adult men and women is 900 μg/day.

Iron is a constituent of hemoglobin, collagen transport, and oxygen transport. The daily requirement for adult men and women ages 50 to 70 is 8 mg/day. A multivitamin with 100% of the DRI for minerals is the general recommendation if the diet is inadequate or if deficiencies are suspected or confirmed. Many of the oral supplements, enteral formulas, and fortified foods recommended for patients with wounds contain additional micronutrients that should be considered before recommending additional supplementation.

Water

Water constitutes about 60% of the adult body weight. It is distributed in the body in three fluid compartments (intracellular, interstitial, and intravascular). Water serves many vital functions in the body, including:

- aiding in hydration of wound sites and in oxygen perfusion
- acting as a solvent for minerals, vitamins, amino acids, glucose, and other small molecules and enabling them to diffuse into and out of cells
- transporting vital materials to cells and removing waste from cells.

Patients with draining wounds, emesis, diarrhea, elevated temperature, or increased perspiration need additional fluids to replace lost fluid.[48] Patients on air-fluidized beds may require additional fluids daily. Tissue oxygenation is required for proper healing, and data from Stotts and Hopf[49] indicate that improving fluid intake may increase low tissue oxygen levels. The dehydrated patient exhibits weight loss (2%, mild; 5%, moderate; and 8%, severe),

Signs of dehydration

Sufficient hydration is essential for all patients, and no less so for the patient with a wound. Use the following guidelines to prevent dehydration—and to recognize and treat it should it occur.

- If the patient can drink independently, keep water or other beverages at bedside so that they're easily accessible and in a container the patient can handle easily.
- If the patient doesn't consume fluids on his own, offer water at least every 2 hours.

If you suspect dehydration, look for:

- dry skin
- cracked lips
- thirst (often diminished in elderly patients)
- poor skin turgor (The pinch test for skin turgor may be an unreliable indicator of dehydration in elderly patients. If you

use this test, use only the skin on the forehead or sternum, and pinch gently. If well-hydrated, the skin goes back into place in 2 seconds.)
- fever
- appetite loss
- nausea
- dizziness
- increased confusion
- laboratory values (Serum creatinine, hematocrit, blood urea nitrogen, potassium, chloride, and osmolarity are increased. Sodium can be increased, normal, or low, depending on the underlying cause of dehydration.)
- decreased blood pressure
- increased pulse rate
- constipation (Recent diarrhea may explain the dehydrated state, and constipation is common when dehydration exists.)
- concentrated urine.

dry skin and mucous membranes, rapid pulse, decreased venous pressure, subnormal body temperature, low blood pressure, and altered sensation. Total fluid needs are met from the water content of food plus liquids. Food accounts for 19% to 27% of the total fluid intake of healthy adults.[50]

Patients who are at risk of dehydration require careful monitoring, such as daily weights. (See *Signs of dehydration*.) A weight loss of 2 kg in 48 hours indicates a corresponding loss of 2 L of fluid. Elderly patients, whose sense of thirst often declines, should be offered fluids more frequently. The American Medical Directors Association recently published a guideline for the management of dehydration.[48]

NUTRITIONAL INTERVENTIONS

The management of undernutrition is extremely important for patients with wounds such as pressure ulcers. Nutrition status, undernutrition, nutritional support, and

nutrition intake are all critical to this process. The 2009 National Pressure Ulcer Advisory Panel/European Pressure Ulcer Advisory Panel (NPUAP/EPUAP) pressure ulcer prevention and treatment guidelines provide nutrition recommendations that are a resource for practitioners when developing nutrition interventions for individual patients.[30] (See *Nutrition for pressure ulcer prevention*.) Clinical judgment should be used when applying these guidelines as they may not be appropriate in all circumstances.

Does nutrition status influence the incidence, progression, and severity of pressure ulcers? A review of several epidemiological studies supports this concept,[51] including the finding that undernourishment on admission to a healthcare facility is associated with a person's likelihood of developing a pressure ulcer. In one prospective study, high-risk patients who were undernourished (17%) on admission to the hospital were twice as likely to develop pressure ulcers as were adequately

Nutrition for pressure ulcer prevention

1. Offer high-protein mixed oral nutritional supplements and/or tube feeding, in addition to the usual diet, to individuals with nutritional risk and pressure ulcer risk because of acute or chronic diseases or following surgical intervention. (Strength of evidence = A)
   1.1 Administer oral nutritional supplements (ONS) and/or tube feeding (TF) in between the regular meals to avoid reduction of normal food and fluid intake during regular mealtimes. (Strength of Evidence = C)

Role of nutrition in pressure ulcer healing

1. Screen and assess nutritional status for each individual with a pressure ulcer at admission and with each condition change and/or when progress toward pressure ulcer closure is not observed. (Strength of Evidence = C)
   1.1. Refer all individuals with a pressure ulcer to the dietitian for early assessment and intervention for nutritional problems. (Strength of Evidence = C)
   1.2. Assess weight status for each individual to determine weight history and significant weight loss from usual body weight ($\geq$ 5% change in 30 days or $\geq$ 10% in 180 days). (Strength of Evidence = C)
   1.3. Assess the individual's ability to eat independently. (Strength of evidence = C)
   1.4. Assess adequacy of nutrient intake (food, fluid, oral supplements, enteral/parenteral feedings). (Strength of Evidence = C)
2. Provide sufficient calories. (Strength of Evidence = B)
   2.1. Provide 30-35 K calories/kg body weight for individuals under stress with a pressure ulcer. Adjust

formula based on weight loss, weight gain, or level of obesity. Individuals who are underweight or who have had significant unintentional weight loss may need additional K calories to cease weight loss and/or regain lost weight. (Strength of Evidence = C)
   2.2. Revise and modify (liberalize) dietary restrictions when limitations result in decreased food and fluid intake. This is to be done by a dietitian or medical professional. (Strength of Evidence = C)
   2.3. Provide enhanced foods and/or oral supplements between meals if needed. (Strength of Evidence = B.)
   2.4. Consider nutritional support (enteral or parenteral nutrition) when oral intake is inadequate. This must be consistent with individual goals. (Strength of Evidence = C)
3. Provide adequate protein for positive nitrogen balance for an individual with a pressure ulcer. (Strength of Evidence = B)
   3.1. Offer 1.25-1.5 grams protein/kg body weight for an individual with a pressure ulcer when compatible with goals of care, and reassess as condition changes. (Strength of Evidence = C)
   3.2. Assess renal function to ensure high levels of protein are appropriate for the individual. (Strength of Evidence = C)
4. Provide and encourage adequate daily fluid intake for hydration. (Strength of Evidence = C)
   4.1. Monitor individuals for signs and symptoms of dehydration: changes in weight, skin turgor, urine output, elevated serum sodium or calculated serum osmolality. (Strength of Evidence = C)

(continued)

Nutrition for pressure ulcer prevention (*continued*)

4.2. Provide additional fluid for individuals with dehydration, elevated temperature, vomiting, profuse sweating, diarrhea, or heavily draining wounds. (Strength of Evidence = C)

5. Provide adequate vitamins and minerals. (Strength of Evidence = B)

5.1. Encourage consumption of a balanced diet which includes good sources of vitamins and minerals. (Strength of Evidence = B)

5.2. Offer vitamin and mineral supplements when dietary intake is poor or deficiencies are confirmed or suspected. (Strength of Evidence = B)

Adapted with permission: National Pressure Ulcer Advisory Panel and European Pressure Ulcer Advisory Panel, Prevention and treatment of pressure ulcers: clinical practice guidelines. Washington, DC: National Pressure Ulcer Advisory Panel, 2009.

nourished patients (9%).[52,53] In the 12-week retrospective National Pressure Ulcer Long–Term Care Study (NPULS) of 2,420 nursing home residents who were are risk for developing pressure ulcers, 50% of the residents had a 5% weight loss, with the highest percentage of weight loss occurring in those with recent pressure ulcers.[54]

A cohort study of 1,524 residents in 95 nursing homes noted a higher pressure ulcer incidence among frail residents and residents who had more severe illness, low BMI, significant weight loss, and difficulty eating independently.[54,55] This suggests that pressure ulcers occur in ill persons. This same retrospective study found that consumption of an oral nutritional supplement was a predictor of pressure ulcer healing.[54,55] Whether undernutrition and weight loss reflect this ill health or have a causal relationship to pressure ulcers is not clear.[56] The use of pharmacologic agents to stimulate the appetite, or orexigenic agents, has demonstrated weight gain, chiefly in patients with cancer or acquired autoimmune deficiency disease. Clinical studies using oxandrolone have shown weight gain in similar populations. Although it has been hypothesized that weight gain in undernourished patients with wounds would lead to better outcomes in terms of wound healing, there are currently no published studies that test the value of these agents in pressure ulcers or other chronic wounds.[56]

Effects of undernutrition

Undernutrition, or protein-energy malnutrition, is defined as "a wasting and excessive loss of lean body mass resulting from too little energy being supplied to body tissues that can be reversed solely by the administration of nutrients."[57] Protein-energy malnutrition has also been associated with changes in immune function, including increased susceptibility to infection and delayed recovery from illness.

Involuntary weight loss and severe undernutrition are common in the geriatric population and often go unexplained. A common cause may be loss of appetite due to a variety of psychological, GI, metabolic, and nutritional factors.[58]

Cytokine-induced cachexia rather than simple starvation may be the reason that hypercaloric feedings in patients with pressure ulcers aren't effective. Hypercaloric feeding has positive results in all but those who are terminally undernourished. Cytokine-induced cachexia is remarkably resistant to hypercaloric feeding.[59,60]

Cytokine-mediated anorexia and weight loss are common in those who develop pressure ulcers. (See *Associations between cytokines, undernutrition, and chronic wounds.*) Serum IL-1 is elevated in patients with pressure ulcers.[61] Levels of IL-1 are elevated in pressure ulcers but low in acute wound fluid.[62] Circulating serum levels of IL-6, IL-2, and IL-2R are higher in patients with spinal cord injuries compared with normal

Associations between cytokines, undernutrition, and chronic wounds

Proinflammatory cytokines
- Suppressed appetite
- Promotion of or interference with wound healing

Undernutrition
- Poor wound healing
- Increased risk of infection
- Increased incidence of pressure ulcers

Chronic wounds
- Source of cytokines
- Increased association with undernutrition
- Increased serum levels of cytokines

controls and highest in patients with pressure ulcers. In one study, the highest concentration of cytokines was found in patients with the slowest-healing pressure ulcers.[63] In other studies, IL-6 serum levels were increased in patients with pressure ulcers, but IL-1 and tumor necrosis factor levels were not elevated.[64]

Increasing knowledge about the complexity of wound healing has led to the hypothesis that providing hypercaloric feeding in the form of nutritional supplements to patients at risk for undernutrition might reverse undernutrition and prevent the development of pressure ulcers. Indeed, one French trial[65] suggested that the incidence of pressure ulcers may be decreased by nutritional supplements. In this study, 672 people over age 65 and in an acute phase of a critical illness were followed for 15 days or until discharge. At 15 days, the cumulative incidence of pressure ulcers was 40% (118/295) in the nutrition intervention group versus 48% (181/377) in the control group. This equates to a relative risk of developing a pressure ulcer (while taking a supplement) of 0.83 (95% CI, 0.70 to 0.99). The proportion of erythema was 90% for both groups, thus no significant differences in the development of erythema was detected between the two groups.[65] A

retrospective cohort study of 1,524 nursing home residents reported that the consumption of an oral supplement was a predictor of pressure ulcer healing.[54,55]

Providing nutritional support

Nutritional support is available for use when a person can't meet his or her nutritional needs through normal ingestion of food. Support options include such strategies as providing additional oral supplements, adding fortified foods or between-meal snacks to the person's oral diet, feeding through a tube placed into the GI tract or, when the GI tract isn't functional, giving nutrients through the venous system as total parenteral nutrition. (See *Serving supplements*.)

Nutritional support is used to place the patient into positive nitrogen balance (in which the body maintains the same amount of protein in its tissues from day to day) according to the goals of care and whether it's compatible with the patient's and family's wishes. Enteral feeding (tube feeding) may be initiated when the ability to chew, swallow, and absorb nutrients through normal GI route is compromised. This occurs in conditions such as stroke, Parkinson's disease, cancer, and dysphagia or when patients can't meet their nutritional needs orally. Most enteral tube feeding formulas are nutritionally complete and designed for a specific purpose.

Serving supplements

Remember that supplements should be offered between meals and not with a meal.

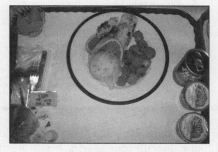

Photo courtesy of Aline Holmes, RN, APNC, MSN, APRN, BC, CNAA, BC

Algorithm for treatment of pressure ulcers: nutrition guidelines[*]

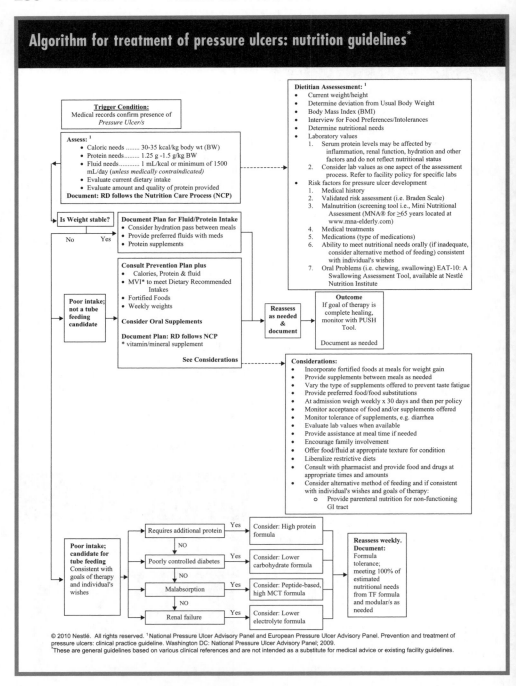

Trigger Condition:
Medical records confirm presence of
Pressure Ulcer/s

Assess: [1]
- Caloric needs .... 30-35 kcal/kg body wt (BW)
- Protein needs......... 1.25 g -1.5 g/kg BW
- Fluid needs............ 1 mL/kcal or minimum of 1500 mL/day (*unless medically contraindicated*)
- Evaluate current dietary intake
- Evaluate amount and quality of protein provided
Document: RD follows the Nutrition Care Process (NCP)

Dietitian Assessment: [1]
- Current weight/height
- Determine deviation from Usual Body Weight
- Body Mass Index (BMI)
- Interview for Food Preferences/Intolerances
- Determine nutritional needs
- Laboratory values
  1. Serum protein levels may be affected by inflammation, renal function, hydration and other factors and do not reflect nutritional status
  2. Consider lab values as one aspect of the assessment process. Refer to facility policy for specific labs
- Risk factors for pressure ulcer development
  1. Medical history
  2. Validated risk assessment (i.e. Braden Scale)
  3. Malnutrition (screening tool i.e., Mini Nutritional Assessment (MNA® for ≥65 years located at www.mna-elderly.com)
  4. Medical treatments
  5. Medications (type of medications)
  6. Ability to meet nutritional needs orally (if inadequate, consider alternative method of feeding) consistent with individual's wishes
  7. Oral Problems (i.e. chewing, swallowing) EAT-10: A Swallowing Assessment Tool, available at Nestlé Nutrition Institute

Is Weight stable? — No / Yes

Document Plan for Fluid/Protein Intake
- Consider hydration pass between meals
- Provide preferred fluids with meds
- Protein supplements

Poor intake; not a tube feeding candidate

Consult Prevention Plan plus
- Calories, Protein & fluid
- MVI* to meet Dietary Recommended Intakes
- Fortified Foods
- Weekly weights

Consider Oral Supplements

Document Plan: RD follows NCP
* vitamin/mineral supplement

See Considerations

Reassess as needed & document

Outcome
If goal of therapy is complete healing, monitor with PUSH Tool.

Document as needed

Considerations:
- Incorporate fortified foods at meals for weight gain
- Provide supplements between meals as needed
- Vary the type of supplements offered to prevent taste fatigue
- Provide preferred food/food substitutions
- At admission weigh weekly x 30 days and then per policy
- Monitor acceptance of food and/or supplements offered
- Monitor tolerance of supplements, e.g. diarrhea
- Evaluate lab values when available
- Provide assistance at meal time if needed
- Encourage family involvement
- Offer food/fluid at appropriate texture for condition
- Liberalize restrictive diets
- Consult with pharmacist and provide food and drugs at appropriate times and amounts
- Consider alternative method of feeding and if consistent with individual's wishes and goals of therapy:
  o Provide parenteral nutrition for non-functioning GI tract

Poor intake; candidate for tube feeding Consistent with goals of therapy and individual's wishes

Requires additional protein	Yes → Consider: High protein formula
Poorly controlled diabetes	Yes → Consider: Lower carbohydrate formula
Malabsorption	Yes → Consider: Peptide-based, high MCT formula
Renal failure	Yes → Consider: Lower electrolyte formula

(NO between each)

Reassess weekly. Document: Formula tolerance; meeting 100% of estimated nutritional needs from TF formula and modular/s as needed

Parenteral nutrition is the delivery of nutrient solutions directly into a vein, bypassing the intestine. This form of feeding is necessary in patients when enteral tube feeding is contraindicated, is insufficient to maintain nutritional status, or has led to serious complications. (See *Algorithm for treatment of pressure ulcers: nutrition guidelines*.)

Does providing enteral feedings prevent pressure ulcers? The answer may lie in the limited number of published studies involving the use of tube feedings in patients with pressure ulcers.

There was no difference in the number or healing of pressure ulcers in 49 long-term care residents with pressure ulcers who received enteral feedings for 3 months.[66] Although pressure ulcers occur frequently in patients with hip fractures, randomized clinical trials of enteral nutrition in this population haven't demonstrated success in preventing pressure ulcer development.[67] It's possible that poor tolerance of the feedings may have contributed to this result. In another study of 135 long-term-care residents with severe cognitive impairment, provision of tube feedings didn't increase survival or have an apparent effect on the prevalence of pressure ulcers.[68] A meta-analysis of high-quality trials found that it was not possible to draw any firm conclusions on the effect of enteral and parenteral nutrition on the prevention and treatment of pressure ulcers.[69]

Ways to enhance nutritional intake

Many elderly people are chronically dehydrated, and ensuring adequate oral fluid intake can be challenging. (See *Beverage consumption*.)

Beverage consumption

The fluid on this tray is untouched; note the tops remain on the coffee, milk, and juice. Employees who deliver trays should open and uncover all liquids and encourage patients to drink beverages. A frail older adult with arthritis, for example, may not be able to open sealed containers.

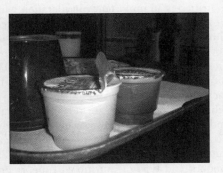

Photo courtesy of Aline Holmes, RN, APNC, MSN, APRN, BC, CNAA, BC

Use creative ways to encourage daily fluid intake. For example, give ice pops in warm climates or hot soup in cooler climates. Avoid beverages with caffeine, alcohol, or high glucose content, as they will act as diuretics, causing fluid loss.

Rather than relying on supplemental shakes to increase calories and nutrients, consider adding powdered milk to foods the patient is already eating, such as pudding or yogurt. Offer small, frequent meals and snacks, such as high-calorie snacks, bars, and other nutrient-rich products. You may also individualize feedings based on the person's preferences to enhance his or her overall food and nutrient intake. To that end, make a contract with your patient to eat or drink some portion or percentage of each meal in return for something he or she loves that doesn't have as much nutritional value. Wilson and colleagues[70] studied the timing of supplements and concluded that consuming supplements between meals resulted in better absorption of nutrients and less interference with meal intake.

Exploring why a patient isn't eating is the first step in helping to meet his or her nutritional needs. (See *Unwanted foods*, page 258.) For example, is there an emotional or physical reason why eating is a problem? Find out if something is bothering the patient that's preventing him or her from eating. Provide an environment that reduces noxious smells, which may decrease appetite, while increasing pleasing aromas of food being prepared or other pleasant smells such as cinnamon. A quiet, unhurried eating environment with frequent cueing is particularly helpful for cognitively impaired persons. Similarly, in evaluating the patient's physical ability to eat, consider the following questions:

- How much time does it take the patient to eat? Fatigue or fear of choking may cause the patient to eat slowly.
- Does the patient have the physical ability to bring the food to the mouth? Can he or she handle eating with utensils? Neuromuscular impairments, fatigue, or decreased endurance can interfere with the patient's ability to eat independently. Consider use of assistive devices and consultation with an occupational therapist. Some patients may prefer "finger" foods. Even with appropriate utensils,

Unwanted foods

The patient ate the main entrée on this tray but left the pasta and broccoli. A survey of the patient's food preferences helps prevent the serving of unwanted foods.

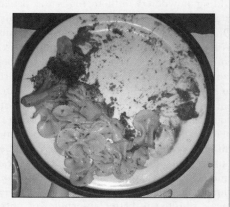

Photo courtesy of Aline Holmes, RN, APNC, MSN, APRN, BC, CNAA, BC

consider whether the patient has the coordination to bring the food to the mouth.
- Can the patient see the food on the tray? Changes in the visual field as a result of stroke, cataracts, glaucoma, or diabetes may alter the ability to see food on all or part of the tray. Arrange food so the patient can see and reach it.
- Can the patient chew? Check on the condition of his or her oral cavity. Provide appropriate mouth care to optimize taste buds and stimulate appetite. Evaluate the patient's oral hygiene and proper fitting or use of any dentures.
- Can the patient swallow? Cranial nerve and other neurologic conditions can cause swallowing difficulties. Evaluate the patient for any signs of abnormal swallowing. Teach the patient to direct food to the unaffected side of the mouth. Consultation from a speech therapist for management of swallowing difficulties and recommendations about food textures may be helpful.
- Is the patient's diet unappealing and unappetizing due to the restrictions of the diet order? Diet restrictions may result in

reduced food and fluid intake. It is the position of the American Dietetic Association that the quality of life and nutritional status of older adults residing in healthcare communities can be enhanced by individualization to less restrictive diets.[71]

Documentation in the medical record

Medical nutrition therapy documentation in the medical record should include:
- amount of food consumed in both quantity (% of meal served) and quality (type of food) related to amount needed
- average fluid consumed with meals
- amount in ounces of liquid supplements or percent of snacks consumed
- ability to eat—assisted, supervised, or independent
- acceptance or refusal of diet, meals, or supplements
- current weight and percentage gained or lost
- new conditions affecting nutritional status, such as introduction of thickened liquids or new diagnosis
- new medications affecting nutritional status
- current laboratory results, if appropriate
- wound condition and stage
- current calorie, protein, or fluid requirements
- recommendation for care plan.

(See *Monthly medical nutrition therapy pressure ulcer progress note.*)

SUMMARY

Nutrition is an important consideration when treating the patient with pressure ulcers, chronic wounds, or diabetic ulcers. Nutrition not only facilitates healing, but it also improves or stabilizes the patient's quality of life. The focus should be on optimal nutrition for each patient, which for some patients may be achieved by a diet that includes supplements and allows the patient to enjoy his or her favorite foods. For others, enteral and parenteral nutritional support may be necessary. The amount and type of nutritional support provided to patients with pressure ulcers should be consistent with both the medical goals and the patient's wishes.[73]

Monthly medical nutrition therapy pressure ulcer progress note

NAME: _____ GENDER: ❏ M   ❏ F

TARGET WEIGHT_____ lb. HEIGHT:_____   AGE: _____ years

DIET ORDER: FLUID INTAKE: _____ % intake _____ ml	DIET ORDER: FLUID INTAKE: _____ % intake _____ ml
SUPPLEMENT TYPE: TIME: _____ _____ % intake	SUPPLEMENT TYPE: TIME: _____ _____ % intake
FORTIFIED FOODS:	FORTIFIED FOODS:
TUBE FEEDING: FLUSH:	TUBE FEEDING: FLUSH:

FEEDING ABILITY Dependent   ❏ Independent ❏
                Limited assist   ❏ Set-up only ❏
                Self-help devices ❏ Type _____
	FEEDING ABILITY Dependent ❏ Independent ❏
	                Limited assist ❏ Set-up only ❏
	                Self-help devices ❏ Type _____

NUTRIENT NEEDS: BEE _____ Activity factor _____ Injury factor _____ Total calories _____ Protein ____ g/kg Total protein _____ Fluid ____ ml/kg Total fluids _____ ml	NUTRIENT NEEDS: BEE _____ Activity factor _____ Injury factor _____ Total calories _____ Protein ____ g/kg Total protein _____ Fluid ____ ml/kg Total fluids _____ ml
CURRENT WEIGHT _____ (lb) ____ % change ❏ 30 days ❏ 90 days ❏ 180 days	CURRENT WEIGHT _____ (lb) ____ % change ❏ 30 days ❏ 90 days ❏ 180 days
PRESSURE ULCER(S) STAGE: I II III IV U sDTI LOCATION: _____ SIZE: _____ Exudate: Light Moderate Heavy Pressure Ulcer Scale for Healing (PUSH) score: _____	PRESSURE ULCER(S) STAGE: I II III IV U sDTI LOCATION: _____ SIZE: _____ Exudate: Light Moderate Heavy Pressure Ulcer Scale for Healing (PUSH) score: _____
PRESSURE ULCER(S) STAGE: I II III IV U sDTI LOCATION: _____ SIZE: _____ Exudate: Light Moderate Heavy Pressure Ulcer Scale for Healing (PUSH) score: _____	PRESSURE ULCER(S) STAGE: I II III IV U sDTI LOCATION: _____ SIZE: _____ Exudate: Light Moderate Heavy Pressure Ulcer Scale for Healing (PUSH) score: _____
RECOMMENDATIONS:	RECOMMENDATIONS:
RD SIGNATURE: _____	RD SIGNATURE: _____

PATIENT SCENARIO

Clinical Data

MT is a 90-year-old woman who is admitted to a long-term-care facility with a hip fracture, stage II pressure ulcer, mild dementia, COPD, and swallowing difficulties. She currently receives physical, occupational, and speech therapy and requires assistance with mobility and supervision at mealtime.

MT's weight at admission is 97 lb; she is 60" tall with a BMI of 19. Her daughter, with whom MT lived before entering the facility, indicates that MT's weight is stable and her appetite has been adequate as long as she eats soft food. However, her daughter rarely served MT vegetables or fruit. MT's score of 8 on the MNA nutrition screen places her at risk for malnutrition, and she is referred to the registered dietitian (RD) for a nutrition assessment.

Case Discussion

The RD estimates that MT's daily caloric requirement is 1,322 to 1,543 Kcal, including 53 g of protein. The RD requests a multivitamin with minerals based on MT's history of eating limited amounts of fruits and vegetables. Since MT's daughter indicated that she served her mother hot cereal daily, her menu includes fortified hot cereal for additional calories and protein. Weekly weights are also part of the interventions for this resident. MT's condition is reviewed weekly by the interdisciplinary wound care team.

After 2 weeks of treatment by the therapy department, MT becomes more confused and resistant to care. Her weight declines to 93 lb, her oral intake is less than 1,200 Kcal/day, and her wound is now at stage III. The speech therapist determines that MT is at high risk for aspiration and orders a mechanical soft diet with nectar thick liquids. The interdisciplinary wound care team, which includes the RD, meets with MT and her daughter to determine a new course of action.

The RD offers MT several types of supplements to determine what type she will accept. Since MT is tiny, her meal plan is adjusted to include supplemental foods between meals so she will still be hungry at meal time. The type of supplements served will be rotated to avoid taste fatigue. MT tastes several types of nectar liquids to determine her preferences. Flavored nectar thick water is offered with MT's medicines to increase hydration. Her caloric and protein requirements are increased based on her declining weight and skin condition. She is offered a minimum of 1,500 Kcal at meals plus 65-g protein supplements. MT and her daughter agree that she should be moved to the restorative dining room where she will receive prompting and encouragement from the staff to finish her meals, including her liquids. The team determines that MT's resistance to care is a result of the pain she experiences during therapy sessions. Her pain medication times are adjusted as appropriate for her therapy session. She will continue to be weighed weekly.

The interdisciplinary team monitors MT's overall condition weekly. Her intake of food and fluids improves, her weight slowly increases, and her wounds begin to heal.

SHOW WHAT YOU KNOW

1. A patient who is 68" tall and weighs 188 lb has a BMI of:
   A. 20.5.
   B. 28.7.
   C. 27.1.
   D. 25.4

   ANSWER: B. *Weight (188 lb) ÷ height (68″²) × 705 = 28.7*

2. A patient who weighs 125 lb with a stage IV pressure ulcer and a poor appetite has a recommended daily protein requirement of:
   A. 57 to 118 g.
   B. 68 to 107 g.
   C. 85 to 113 g.
   D. 68 to 86 g.
   ANSWER: D. *125 ÷ 2.2 = 57 kg × 1.2 − 1.5 = 68.4 g to 85.5 g.*

3. Which of the following NPUAP/EPUAP nutrition guideline for treatment is <u>not</u> correct?
   A. Assess adequacy of total food and fluid intake.
   B. Consider nutrition support (enteral/parenteral) when oral intake is inadequate.
   C. Offer elemental zinc and ascorbic acid twice daily.
   D. Offer 1.25 to 1.5 g protein/kg body weight.
   ANSWER: C. *Elemental zinc is not recommended unless a deficiency is confirmed or suspected.*

4. Which of the following amino acids are considered conditionally indispensable during periods of stress?
   A. Arginine and glutamine
   B. Alanine and glutamine
   C. Valine and arginine
   D. Lysine and glutamic acid
   ANSWER: A. *Arginine and glutamine are conditionally indispensable.*

REFERENCES

1. Thomas, D.R. "Nutritional Assessment in Long Term Care," *Nutrition in Clinical Practice* 23:383-87, 2008.
2. Kaiser, M.J., Bauer, J.M., Ramsch, C., Uter, W., Guigoz, Y., Cederholm, T., et al. "Validation of the Mini Nutritional Assessment Short-Form (MNA-SF): A Practical Tool for Identification of Nutritional Status," *Journal of Nutrition, Health & Aging* 13(9):782-88, 2009.
3. Wilson, M.M., Thomas, D.R., Rubenstein, L.Z., et al. "Appetite Assessment: Simple Appetite Questionnaire Predicts Weight Loss in Community Settings," *American Journal of Clinical Nutrition* 82:1074-81, 2005.
4. Thomas D.R. "Loss of Sskeletal Muscle Mass in Aging: Examining the Relationship of Starvation, Sarcopenia and Cachexia," *Clinical Nutrition* 26(4):389-399, 2007.
5. Lauque, S., Arnaud-Battandier, F., Mansourian, R., et al. "Protein Energy Oral Supplementation in Malnourished Nursing Home Residents: A Controlled Trial," *Age Aging* 29:51-56, 2000.
6. Lioupis, M.D. "Effects of Diabetes Mellitus on Wound Healing: An Update," *Journal of Wound Care* 14(2):84-86, 2005.
7. Marston, W.A. "Risk Factors Associated with Healing Chronic Diabetic Foot Ulcers: The Importance of Hyperglycemia," *Ostomy/Wound Management* 52(3):26-39, 2006.
8. Tariq, S., et al. "The Use of a No-Concentrated-Sweets Diet in the Management of Type 2 Diabetes in the Nursing Home," *Journal of the American Dietetic Association* 101(12):1463-66, December 2001.
9. F Tag 314. "Procedures: 483.25c: Pressure Sores. *Federal Register* 56(187); November 12, 2004.
10. Thomas, D.R. "The New F-tag 314: Prevention and Management of Pressure Ulcers," *Journal of the American Medical Directors Association* 7(8):523-31, 2006.
11. American Dietetic Association. *International Dietetics and Nutrition Terminology (IDNT) Reference Manual: Standardized Language for the Nutrition Care Process*, 3rd ed. Chicago, IL: Author, 2010.
12. Schoeller, D. "Making Indirect Calorimetry a Gold Standard for Predicting Energy Requirements for Institutionalized Patients," *Journal of the American Dietetic Association* 107(3):390-392, 2007.
13. Mifflin, S.T., St. Jeor, et al. "A New Predictive Equation for Resting Energy Expenditure in Healthy Individuals," *Journal of Clinical Nutrition* 51(2):241-47, 1990.

14. Frankenfield D.C., et al. "Comparison of Predictive Equations for Resting Metabolic Rate in Healthy Nonobese and Obese Adults: A Systematic Review," *Journal of the American Dietetic Association* 105:775-89, 2005.

15. *Physical Signs of Malnutrition. Pocket Resource for Nutrition Assessment.* Chicago, IL: Dietetics in Health Care Communities; 2009, pp 65-69.

16. Thomas, D.R. "Anorexia: Aetiology, Epidemiology, and Management in the Older People," *Drugs & Aging* 26:557-70, 2009.

17. Thomas, D.R. "Drug-Nutrient Interactions," in J.E. Morley and D.R. Thomas, eds. *Geriatric Nutrition*, Boca Raton, FL: CRC Press, Taylor and Francis Group; 2007, pp. 469-478.

18. Defining Overweight and Obesity. Available at: *http://www.cdc.gov/obesity/defining.html.* Accessed November 17, 2010.

19. Centers for Disease Control and Prevention. About BMI for Adults. Available at: *http://www.cdc.gov/healthyweight/assessing/bmi/adult_bmi/index.html.* Accessed June 5, 2010.

20. Thomas, D.R. "Unintended Weight Loss in Older Adults," *Aging Health* 4(2):191-200, 2008.

21. Sullivan, D.H., Johnson, L.E., Bopp, M.M., and Roberson, P.K. "Prognostic Significance of Monthly Weight Fluctuations Among Older Nursing Home Residents," *The Journals of Gerontology. Series A, Biological Sciences and Medical Sciences* 59(6):M633-39, 2004.

22. Myron Johnson, A., Merlini, G., Sheldon, J., and Ichihara, K. "Clinical Indications for Plasma Protein Assays: Transthyretin (Prealbumin) in Inflammation and Malnutrition," *Clinical Chemistry and Laboratory Medicine: CCLM/FESCC* 45(3):419-26, 2007.

23. Fuhrman, M.P., Charney, P., Mueller, C.M. "Hepatic Proteins and Nutrition Assessment," *Journal of the American Dietetic Association* 104(8):1258-64, August 2004.

24. Lim, S.H., Lee, J.S., Chae, S.H., Ahn, B.S., Chang, D.J., Shin, C.S. "Prealbumin Is Not a Sensitive Indicator of Nutrition and Prognosis in Critically Ill Patients," *Yonsei Medical Journal* 46(1):21-6, February 28, 2005.

25. Shenkin, A. "Serum Prealbumin: Is It a Marker of Nutritional Status or of Risk of Malnutrition," *Clinical Chemistry* 52(12):2281-5; December 2006.

26. Robinson, M.K., Trujillo, E.B., Mogensen, K.M., Rounds, J., McManus, K., Jacobs, D.O. "Improving Nutritional Screening of Hospitalized Patients: The Role of Prealbumin," *Journal of Parenteral and Enteral Nutrition* 28(4):281, July-August, 2004.

27. Chernoff. "Protein and Older Adults," *Journal of the American College of Nutrition* 23(90006): 601S, 2004.

28. Wolfe, R.R., and Miller, S.L. (2008). "The Recommended Dietary Allowance of Protein: A Misunderstood Concept," *Journal of the American Medical Association* 299(24):2891-93.

29. Campbell, W.W., Trappe, T.A., Wolfe, R.R., Evans, W.J. (2001). "The Recommended Dietary Allowance for Protein May Not Be Adequate for Older People to Maintain Skeletal Muscle," *The Journals of Gerontology. Series A, Biological Sciences and Medical Sciences* 56(6): M373-80.

30. National Pressure Ulcer Advisory Panel and European Pressure Ulcer Advisory Panel. *Prevention and Treatment of Pressure Ulcers: Clinical Practice Guidelines.* Washington, DC: National Pressure Ulcer Advisory Panel, 2009.

31. Long, C.L., et al. "A Physiologic Basis for the Provision of Fuel Mixtures in Normal and Stressed Patients," *Journal of Trauma* 30(9):1077-86, September 1990.

32. McCauley, R., et al. "Effects of Glutamine Infusion on Colonic Anastomotic Strength in the Rat," *Journal of Parenteral and Enteral Nutrition* 15(4):437-39, July-August 1991.

33. Barbul, A., et al. "Arginine Enhances Wound Healing and Lymphocyte Immune Response in Humans," *Surgery* 108(2):331-37, August 1990.

34. Langkamp-Henken, B., Herrlinger-Garcia, K.A., Stechmiller, J.K., Nickerson Troy, J.A., Lewis, B., and Moffatt, L. "Arginine Supplementation Is Well Tolerated but Does Not Enhance Mitogen-induced lymphocyte Proliferation in Elderly Nursing Home Residents with Pressure Ulcers," *Journal of Parentereral and Enteral Nutrition* 24(5), 280-287, 2000.

35. Desneves, K.J., Todorovic, B.E., Cassar, A., and Crowe, T.C. "Treatment with Supplementary Arginine, Vitamin C and Zinc in Patients with Pressure Ulcers: A Randomised Controlled Trial," *Clinical Nutrition* 24(6), 979-987, 2005.

36. Langer, G., Schloemer, G., Knerr, A., Kuss, O., Behrens, J. "Nutritional Interventions for Preventing and Treating Pressure Ulcers," *The Cochrane Database of Systematic Reviews* 1, 2007.

37. Lee, S., et al. "Pressure Ulcer healing with a Concentrated, Fortified, Collagen Protein Hydrolysate Supplement: A Randomized Controlled Trial," *Advances in Skin and Wound Care* 19(2):92-96, March 2006.

38. Waldorf, H., and Fewkes, J. "Wound Healing," *Advances in Dermatology* 10:77-96, 1995.

39. Clark, S. "The Biochemistry of Antioxidants Revisited," *Nutrition in Clinical Practice* 17(1):5-17, February 2002.

40. Ronchetti, I.P., Quaglino, D., Bergamini, G. "Ascorbic Acid and Connective Tissue," *Subcellular Biochemistry, Volume 25: Ascorbic Acid:*

Biochemistry and Biomedical Cell Biology. New York: Plenum Press, 1996.

41. ter Riet, G., et al. "Randomized Clinical Trial of Ascorbic Acid in the Treatment of Pressure Ulcers," *Journal of Clinical Epidemiology* 48(12):1453-60, December 1995.

42. Vilter, R.W. "Nutritional Aspects of Ascorbic Acid: Uses and Abuses," *West J Med* 1980; 133:485-492.

43. Cataldo, C.B., DeBruyne, L.K., and Whitney, E.N. *Nutrition and Diet Therapy, Principles and Practice.* Belmonth, CA: Wadsworth, 2003.

44. Norris, J.R., and Reynolds, R.E. "The Effect of Oral Zinc Sulfate Therapy on Decubitus Ulcers," *Journal of the American Geriatric Society* 19:793, 1971.

45. Institute of Medicine, National Academy of Sciences: *Dietary Reference Intakes: The Essential Guide to Nutrient Requirements.* Washington, DC: Author, 2006

46. Goode, P., and Allman, R. "The Prevention and Management of Pressure Ulcers," *Medical Clinics of North America* 73(6):1511-24, November 1989.

47. Thomas, D.R. "The Role of Nutrition in Prevention and Healing of Pressure Ulcers," *Clinics in Geriatric Medicine* 13(3):497-511, August 1997.

48. Thomas, D.R., Cote, T.R., Lawhorne, L., Levenson, S.A., Rubenstein, LZ., Smith, D.A., et al. "Understanding Clinical Dehydration and Its Treatment," *Journal of the American Medical Directors Association* 9(5), 292-301, 2008.

49. Stotts, N.A., Hopf, H. "The Link Between Tissue Oxygen and Hydration in Nursing Home Residents with Pressure Ulcers: Preliminary Data," *Journal of Wound, Ostomy & Continence Nursing* 30(4):184-190, July 2003.

50. Institute of Medicine, National Academy of Sciences. *Dietary Reference Intakes for Water, Potassium, Sodium, Chloride, and Sulfate.* Washington, DC: Author, 2004.

51. Thomas, D.R. "Improving Outcome of Pressure Ulcers with Nutritional Interventions: A Review of the Evidence," *Nutrition* 17(2):121-25, February 2001.

52. Thomas, D.R, et al. "Hospital Acquired Pressure Ulcers and Risk of Death," *Journal of the American Geriatric Society* 44(12):1435-40, December 1996.

53. Horn S.D., Bender, S.A., Ferguson, M.L., Smout, R.J., Bergstrom, N., Taler, G., Cook, A.S., Sharkey, S.S., Voss, A.C. "The National Pressure Ulcer Long-Term Care Study: Pressure Ulcer Development in Long-term Care Residents," *Journal of the American Geriatrics Society.* 52:359-67, 2004.

54. Bergstrom, N., Horn, S.D., Smout, R.J., Bender, S.A., Ferguson, M.L., Taler, G., et al. "The National Pressure Ulcer Long-Term Care Study: Outcomes of Pressure Ulcer Treatments in Long-term Care," *Journal of the American Geriatrics Society* 53:1721-29, 2005.

55. Thomas, D.R. "Does Pressure Cause Pressure Ulcers? An Inquiry into the Etiology of Pressure Ulcers." *Journal of the American Medical Directors Association* 2010. In press.

56. Demling, R.H., and DeSanti, L. "Oxandrolone, an Anabolic Steroid, Significantly Increases the Rate of Weight Gain in the Recovery Phase After Major Burns," *Journal of Trauma-Injury Infection & Critical Care* 43(1):47-51, July 1997.

57. ASPEN Board of Directors and the Clinical Guidelines Task Force. "Guidelines for the Use of Parenteral and Enteral Nutrition in Adult and Pediatric Patients," *Journal of Parenteral and Enteral Nutrition* 26:22SA-24SA, 2002.

58. Morley, J.E., and Thomas, D.R. "Anorexia and Aging: Pathophysiology," *Nutrition* 15(6):499-503, June 1999.

59. Souba, W.W. "Drug Therapy: Nutritional Support," *New England Journal of Medicine* 336(1):41-48, January 1997.

60. Atkinson, S., et al. "A Prospective, Randomized, Double-blind, Controlled Clinical Trial of Enteral Immunonutrition in the Critically Ill," *Critical Care Medicine* 26(7):1164-72, July 1998.

61. Matsuyama, N., et al. "The Possibility of Acute Inflammatory Reaction Affects the Development of Pressure Ulcers in Bedridden Elderly Patients," *Rinsho Byori-Japanese Journal of Clinical Pathology* 47(11):1039-45, November 1999.

62. Barone, E.J., et al. "Interleukin-1 and Collagenase Activity are Elevated in Chronic Wounds," *Plastic & Reconstructive Surgery* 102:1023-27, 1998.

63. Segal, J.L., et al. "Circulating Levels of IL-2R, ICAM-1, and IL-6 in Spinal Cord Injuries," *Archives of Physical Medicine & Rehabilitation* 78(1):44-47, January 1997.

64. Bonnefoy, M., et al. "Implication of Cytokines in the Aggravation of Malnutrition and Hypercatabolism in Elderly Patients with Severe Pressure Sores," *Age & Ageing* 24(1):37-42, January 1995.

65. Bourdel-Marchasson., I., et al. "A Multi-center Trial of the Effects of Oral Nutritional Supplementation in Critically Ill Older Inpatients, GAGE Group, Groupe Aquitain Geriatrique d"Evaluation," *Nutrition* 16(1):1-5, January 2000.

66. Henderson, C.T., et al. "Prolonged Tube Feeding in Long-term Care: Nutritional Status and Clinical Outcomes," *Journal of the American College of Clinical Nutrition* 11(3):309-25, June 1992.

67. Hartgrink, H.H., et al. "Pressure Sores and Tube Feeding in Patients with a Fracture of the Hip:

A Randomized Clinical Trial," *Clinical Nutrition* 17(6):287-92, December 1998.

68. Mitchell, S.L., et al. "The Risk Factors and Impact on Survival of Feeding Tube Placement in Nursing Home Residents with Severe Cognitive Impairment," *Archives of Internal Medicine* 157(3):327-32, February 10, 1997.

69. Langer, G.,Knerr, A.,Kuss,O., Behrens, J., Schlömer, G.J. "Nutritional Interventions for Preventing and Treating Pressure Ulcers," *Cochrane Database of Systematic Reviews* 4:CD003216. DOI: 10.1002/14651858.CD003216, 2003.

70. Wilson, M.-M.G., Purushothaman, R., and Morley, J.E. "Effect of Liquid Dietary Supplements on Energy Intake in the Elderly," *The American Journal of Clinical Nutrition* 75(5), 944-47, 2002.

71. American Dietetic Association. *Position Paper with Companion Practice Paper of the American Dietetic Association: Individualized Nutrition Approaches for Older Adults in Health Care Communities. Journal of the American Dietetic Association* 1554-1562, October 2010.

72. Thomas, D.R., et al. "Nutritional Management in Long-term Care: Development of a Clinical Guideline. Council for Nutritional Strategies in Long-Term Care," *Journals of Gerontology Series A-Biological Sciences & Medical Sciences* 55(12):M725-34, December 2000.

CHAPTER 11

Pressure Redistribution: Seating, Positioning, and Support Surfaces

David M. Brienza, PhD
Mary Jo Geyer, PT, PhD, FCCWS, CLT-LANA, CPed
Stephen Sprigle, PT, PhD
Karen Zulkowski, DNS, RN, CWS

Objectives

After completing this chapter, you'll be able to:

- demonstrate an understanding of tissue mechanical properties, their measurement, and their relationship to soft tissue–loading tolerance
- identify support surface characteristics related to the maintenance of tissue integrity
- demonstrate an understanding of the categories, functions, and limitations of various support surfaces
- outline an assessment process for selecting an appropriate support surface (seat cushion or horizontal support) and related interventions (positioning).

PREVENTING SKIN BREAKDOWN

Multiple intervention strategies are needed to prevent and treat pressure ulcers. Managing loads on the skin and associated soft tissue is one of these strategies. A comprehensive care plan should include pressure redistribution strategies for individuals both while in bed and when seated. Properly chosen support surfaces, adequate periodic pressure redistribution, protection of especially vulnerable bony prominences such as the heels, and consideration of special patient needs are all essential components of the care plan.

A support surface is a specialized device for pressure redistribution designed for management of tissue loads, microclimate, and other therapeutic functions. Types of surfaces include mattresses, integrated bed systems, mattress replacements, mattress overlays, and seat cushions.[1] Unless specifically identified as a mattress or seat cushion, the term "support surface" will refer to both product categories in this chapter. Achieving a good match between the patient's needs and the performance capabilities of the support surface has a profound, positive impact on a patient's health and well-being; conversely, a poor match has a negative impact. Support surfaces redistribute the body's weight and protect the skin's tissue while providing for proper body alignment, comfort and, as part of a seating system, postural control during functional movement. These effects may conflict and require clinical decision making to strike a balance between protective and functional goals.

Ideally, an algorithm that incorporates an individual's characteristics, conditions, environment, and preferences should be able to guide one to formulate a recommendation for an ideal, personalized support surface. Research in this area has thus far failed to produce strong evidence to justify the selection of one product over another for any given situation. Some guidance is available, but it's not enough to replace good clinical decision making and follow-up evaluations. Existing clinical recommendations need to be updated regularly to reflect new research, technology, and treatment strategies as they become available.

Knowledge of a product's composition and contents is a necessary part of the selection process. Although describing the materials and components of support surface technology may be informative, it isn't always instructive. In terms of selecting a product, the information on the *function* or *performance* of the surface is most critical, regardless of composition. In a study by Krouskop and van Rijswijk,[2] performance

parameters were emphasized when identifying nine key support surface characteristics. (See *Support surface performance parameters*.)

Although function-and-performance-based categorization of seat cushions and support surfaces isn't yet possible, the necessary data from clinical validation studies is being generated. Most significantly, standard tests for cushion and mattress performance have been and are being developed. These tests will provide researchers and industry with the tools needed to differentiate products based on relevant performance measures. This work is a global effort with participants from numerous countries. In the United States, the work is led by the Rehabilitation Engineering and Assistive Technology Association of North America's (RESNA) Wheelchair and Related Seating Standards Committee.[3] The mattress standards development effort is led by the National Pressure Ulcer Advisory Panel's (NPUAP) Support Surface Standard Initiative (S3I) Committee,[4] which is sanctioned by RESNA. The International Organization for Standardization (ISO) coordinates and publishes both cushion and mattress standards for worldwide use. On the clinical validation front, a recent study by Brienza et al.[5] has shown that support surface technology can have a positive effect on preventing pressure ulcers. The best we can do now is to group the devices according to the technologies and materials used in their construction and relate the characteristics of these technologies to the factors believed to have significant effects on the prevention and healing of pressure ulcers.

Support surface performance parameters

Nine parameters must be considered when evaluating the characteristics of a support surface for the patient with a wound:

• Redistribution of pressure
• Moisture control
• Temperature control
• Friction control (between patient and product)
• Infection control
• Flammability
• Life expectancy
• Fail safety
• Product reputation

Adapted with permission from Krouskop, T., and van Rijswijk, L. "Standardizing Performance-Based Criteria for Support Surfaces," *Ostomy/Wound Management* 41(1):34-44, January-February 1995.

SOFT-TISSUE BIOMECHANICS

Human soft tissue consists of a variety of macrostructures, including skin, fat, muscle, vessels, nerves, ligaments, and tendons. The relative amounts and arrangement of tissue macromolecules of the skin and supporting soft tissue are adapted to their specific functions and dictate their biomechanical properties.

In most connective tissue, fibroblasts secrete the macromolecules that make up the extracellular matrix. The matrix is made up of two main classes of macromolecules:

- polysaccharide chains of a class called gly-cosaminoglycans, which are usually found covalently linked to protein in the form of proteoglycans
- fibrous proteins that are either primarily structural (for example, collagen and elastin) or primarily adhesive (for example, fibronectin and laminin).

Glycosaminoglycans and proteoglycans form a highly hydrated, gel-like "ground substance" in which the proteins are embedded. The ground substance is analogous to glue that fills the lattice of collagen and elastin fibers, providing lubrication and shock-absorbing qualities. The polysaccharide gel resists compressive forces on the matrix, while the collagen fibers along with elastin fibers provide tensile strength and resilience.

Tissue mechanical properties

In general, soft tissue is an anisotropic, incompressible biosolid, biofluid mixture.[6] Because soft tissue is largely incompressible, it tends to move slowly from areas of greater pressure to areas of lesser pressure. This slow movement of ground substance and interstitial fluid is responsible for the time-dependent (viscoelastic) behavior of the soft tissue manifested as four phenomena: stress relaxation, creep, hysteresis, and pseudoelasticity (preconditioning).[7]

These phenomena may be graphically represented as stress-strain curves. Stress is represented as the deforming force on the y axis and the tissue strain (deformation) is plotted on the x axis. When soft tissue is suddenly deformed (strained) and the strain is thereafter kept constant, the corresponding stress induced in the tissue decreases over time. This phenomenon is known as stress relaxation. (See *Stress-relaxation phenomenon.*) Alternatively, creep describes the progressive tissue deformation that occurs over time when stress remains constant. (See *Creep phenomenon,* page 268.) During cyclic loading such as that produced by a dynamic, or alternating-pressure mattress, the stress-strain relationship demonstrated during the loading phase is different from that of the recovery, or unloaded, portion of the cycle. This effect is known as hysteresis. Finally, pseudoelasticity is the term associated with an

increase in the repeatability and predictability of a tissue's stress-strain relationship following a defined period of repetitive cyclic loading.

Tissue loading and pressure ulcer formation

Body weight resting on bony prominences, such as the scapula, sacrum, greater trochanters, ischial tuberosities, and heels, can cause significant concentrations of pressure at the skin's surface and in the underlying soft tissue. The pressure peaks and the pressure gradients surrounding these peaks can put the soft tissue at risk for breakdown. However, high pressure alone usually isn't sufficient to cause a pressure ulcer. Research has clearly demonstrated that the damaging effects of pressure are related to both its magnitude and duration. Simply stated, tissue can withstand higher loads for

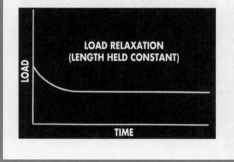

Stress-relaxation phenomenon

The stress vs. strain curve, shown below, illustrates the stress-relaxation phenomenon. With the compression of tissue (strain) held constant, the force (stress) generated in the tissue as a result of that compression reduces over time. The degree of stress relaxation— that is, the amount of reduction in the holding force—can be determined by measuring the distance along the vertical axis between the time when the load is first applied to the time when it reaches steady-state (downward sloping ends).

LOAD RELAXATION
(LENGTH HELD CONSTANT)

LOAD

TIME

Creep phenomenon

Creep reflects the ability of tissue to resist deformation over time when the force causing the deformation remains constant. The creep phenomenon shown here indicates that the tissue progressively deforms over time without any additional force being applied. If creep were zero, the curve would be a flat line, indicating that deformation was constant over time.

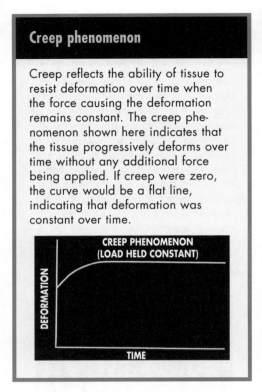

Guidelines for sitting duration

This graph provides guidelines on sitting tolerance based on the magnitude of localized pressure.

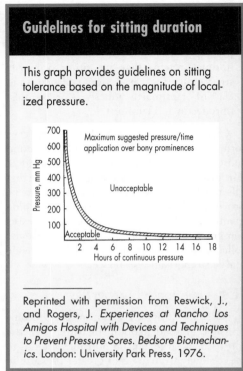

Reprinted with permission from Reswick, J., and Rogers, J. *Experiences at Rancho Los Amigos Hospital with Devices and Techniques to Prevent Pressure Sores. Bedsore Biomechanics.* London: University Park Press, 1976.

shorter periods of time. (See *Guidelines for sitting duration*.)

Recent research has gone beyond assuming that tissue necrosis is a result of ischemia due to external pressure alone. In fact, all of the well-known extrinsic pressure ulcer risk factors (pressure, shear, friction, temperature, and moisture) tend to influence the tissue's ability to withstand loading. Therefore, current investigations are focusing on a variety of physiologic, biochemical, and biomechanical tissue responses to loading.

How pressure, shear, and friction ultimately cause pressure ulcers is complex and not entirely understood. At the cellular level, the three mechanisms most commonly cited describing how external forces result in tissue damage are (1) ischemia resulting from tissue deformation,[8-10] (2) reperfusion injury following pressure relief,[11-13] and (3) mechanical damage to cells caused by excessive deformation.[14,15] Certainly combinations of these factors may be significant. Elevated skin temperature is another factor that appears to be more important than previously believed.[15]

Limitations of interface pressure as a predictor of tissue damage

Tissue interface pressure is the force per unit area that acts perpendicularly between the patient's body and the support surface.[16] It's measured noninvasively by placing a pressure sensor between the patient's skin and the support surface. This measurement is believed to provide an approximation of the pressure on the tissue test site or surrounding area. Single sensors have been used to measure local pressure over a single bony prominence; multiple sensors integrated into a mat may be used to "map" the entire body area in contact with the support surface. (See *color section, Seating, positioning, and support surfaces,* page C18.)

Interface pressure has been used extensively as a tool for predicting the clinical effectiveness of various support surfaces and for comparing products. Many research efforts have been directed toward establishing an interface pressure threshold beyond which pressure ulcers would form. However, what the research has failed to do is to identify a specific threshold at which loads can be deemed harmful across either subject populations or various tissue body sites. This is because a tissue's loading tolerance varies according to its composition, condition, location, age, hydration, and metabolic state. Therefore, while interface pressure may aid in comparing one surface with another based on an individual's relative responses, interface pressure alone isn't sufficient to evaluate the efficacy of a particular device or class of devices.

Clinical implications of aging

The gross morphology of the soft tissue undergoes significant changes due to aging, including decreased moisture content and decreased elasticity manifested as rough, scaly skin with increased wrinkling and laxity. Dry, inelastic skin with larger, more irregular epidermal cells leads to decreased barrier function. These changes are reflected in the tissue biomechanical properties and have been associated with increased risk of tissue injury.

At the microscopic level, flattening of the dermal-epidermal junction (rete ridges) has been observed with the height of the dermal papillae declining by 55% from the third to ninth decade of life. As the space between the well-vascularized dermis and epidermis increases, several functional changes occur. Decreases have been reported in the area available for nutrient transfer, the number of cells within the stratum basale, and the skin's resistance to shearing. A 30% to 50% decrease in epidermal turnover during the third to eighth decade of life has also been reported. This diminution in repair rate has been quantified as both decreased collagen deposition and diminished wound tensile strength. The loss of subcutaneous fat with aging decreases our protection from injury due to pressure and shearing forces between the bony prominences and the support surface. Moreover, decreased sensory perception increases the risk of injury by mechanical forces such as pressure. And, the stiffer, less elastic, drier nature of an elderly

person's skin can result in tissue that tears and bleeds more easily.

SUPPORT SURFACE CHARACTERISTICS

Prevention of pressure ulcers is accomplished primarily by managing tissue loads. Support surfaces have been designed to reduce the effects of tissue loading by controlling the intensity and duration of pressure, shear, and friction. Also, attempts have been made to control the physical factors associated with increased risk through elimination of excess moisture and effective dissipation of heat.

Pressure redistribution

Pressure redistribution is the ability of a support surface to distribute load over the contact areas of the human body. (This term replaces prior terminology of pressure reduction and pressure relief surfaces.[4]) The redistribution of pressure reduces the magnitude of pressure and shear forces, both of which can cause excessive tissue distortion and damage soft tissue. Pressure (stress) is defined as force per unit area; the pressure distribution is influenced by mechanical and physical characteristics of the support surface, mechanical properties of the body's tissue, and weight distribution (posture).

IMMERSION

Immersion is defined as the depth of penetration into a support surface.[4] The fundamental strategy for reducing pressure near a bony prominence is to allow the prominence to be immersed into the support surface. Immersion allows the pressure concentrated beneath a specific bony prominence to be spread out over the surrounding area, including other bony prominences. For example, when a person is sitting on a relatively hard cushion, a disproportionately large portion of his or her body weight is born by the tissue beneath the ischial tuberosities. On a softer surface, the ischial tuberosities and buttocks may immerse more deeply, even to the level of the greater trochanters. With greater immersion, the body weight divided by a greater surface area results in decreased average pressure. This definition of immersion doesn't distinguish between immersion resulting from compression of the support surface and immersion resulting from the displacement of a support surface's fluid components.

The potential for immersion depends on both the force-deformation characteristics of the cushion and its physical dimensions. For fluid-filled support surfaces, immersion depends on the thickness of the surface and the flexibility of the cover. For elastic and viscoelastic support surfaces, immersion depends on their stiffness and thickness. Consider how the thickness of a seat cushion might limit the potential for immersion. If the seat cushion is 1.5" (3.8 cm) in depth and the vertical distance between the ischial tuberosities and greater trochanters is 2" (5 cm), the potential for immersion isn't enough to significantly unload the ischial tuberosities.

ENVELOPMENT

Envelopment is the ability of a support surface to conform to or mold around irregularities in the body.[4] Good envelopment implies that the surface conforms to the body without a substantial increase in pressure. Examples of irregularities are creases in clothing, bedding, or seat covers and protrusions of bony prominences. A fluid support medium would envelop perfectly. However, surface tension plays an important role in envelopment. For example, a fluid-filled support surface such as a waterbed doesn't envelop as well as water alone. The membrane containing the water has surface tension, which has a hammocking effect on irregularities of the interface. Poorly enveloping support surfaces may cause high local peak pressures, thereby potentially increasing the risk of tissue breakdown.

PRESSURE GRADIENT

Pressure gradient, also known as *pressure differential*, is defined as the change in pressure over a distance. Although various distances have been reported in the literature, pressure gradient is expressed most commonly as a change in millimeters of mercury (mm Hg) per square centimeter or square inch. When the pressure across a surface is plotted on a graph, the slope of the curve is the pressure gradient. Because the skin and other soft tissue at risk

for breakdown consist of a mixture of interstitial fluid and ground substance into which structural elements are embedded, a pressure differential between adjacent regions will result in a slow flowing of the tissue's fluid elements from a region of high pressure to one of lesser pressure. This flow is analogous to the movement produced when one compresses the surface of a bucket of wet sand with one's hand.

Several investigators have hypothesized that the flow of interstitial fluid caused by pressure gradients is the primary factor in the development of pressure ulcers.[17-19] The flow of ground substance and interstitial fluids from an area of high pressure is believed to increase the likelihood of intercellular contact, resulting in cellular ruptures.[18,19] This theory is consistent with the classic experimental results of several researchers showing a relationship between duration of pressure application and the magnitude of pressure that results in the formation of a pressure ulcer.[17,20]

Pressure gradient is intimately linked to pressure and is affected by immersion and envelopment in a similar manner. Under certain circumstances, it's possible to have pressure gradients without high pressure, and vice versa. For example, the boundary of the contact area on a support surface necessarily demonstrates a significant pressure gradient where the pressure magnitude transitions from zero outside the area of support to a nonzero value in the supported region. Despite these significant gradients, boundary areas are typically areas of lower risk for pressure ulcer development, suggesting that pressure gradient only becomes an important factor when combined with high pressure. Further research is needed to test and investigate this hypothesis.

Shear and friction reduction

Shear is an action or stress resulting from applied forces that causes or tends to cause two contiguous internal parts of the body to deform in the transverse plane. The term *shear* is commonly used to refer to the effect of a loading condition in which the skin surface remains stuck to a support surface while the underlying bony structure moves in a direction tangential to the surface. For example, when the head of a bed is raised or lowered, if the skin over the sacrum does not slide along the surface of the bed, or the bed does not absorb the resulting shear force by deforming in the horizontal direction, the effect will be a shearing of the soft tissue between the sacrum and the support surface. In engineering terms, the resulting shearing or deformation of the soft tissue would be referred to as "shear strain." The characteristics of the support surface affecting this potentially harmful situation are the coefficient of friction of the surface and the ability of the surface to deform horizontally. Some support surface technologies protect the skin from shear better than others. Shear as a contributing factor for pressure ulcers is currently a topic of international discussion. A task force is looking at ways to measure shear and quantify its effects on skin.[4]

Friction is the resistance to motion of the external tissue sliding in a parallel direction relative to the support surface resulting in external tissue damage.[4] Friction refers to the force acting tangential to the interface that opposes shear force. For example, when someone is pulled across a bed sheet during transfer, the frictional force prevents the person from sliding off the surface. In a static condition (when a person is not sliding along the surface), the friction force is equivalent to the shear force at the surface. (See *Friction and shear forces*.)

The maximum friction is determined by the coefficient of friction of the support surface and the pressure. This is why surfaces with high coefficients of friction have the potential for producing high shear. Friction and shear are local phenomena and are affected by moisture on the skin. Moist or wet skin usually has a higher coefficient of friction and, as will be discussed below, is more susceptible to damage caused by shearing. Ironically, friction is necessary to prevent a person from simply sliding off the bed surface or wheelchair cushion. For optimal prevention of pressure ulcers, the friction necessary to prevent sliding should be applied in low-risk regions of the support surface and minimized near high-risk areas surrounding bony prominences.

Temperature control

One of the extrinsic factors in pressure ulcer development, temperature, has not been

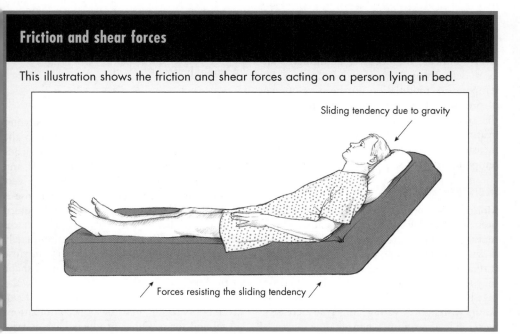

Friction and shear forces

This illustration shows the friction and shear forces acting on a person lying in bed.

Sliding tendency due to gravity

Forces resisting the sliding tendency

definitively investigated. However, some clinical trials have shown that the application of repetitive surface loading alone induces an elevated skin temperature of 41° F or greater.[21] In addition, peak skin temperatures have been found to be proportional to the magnitude and duration of the applied pressure.[21,22] The conclusions of research vary depending upon the amount and duration of pressure that's simultaneously applied with varying temperatures.[23,24]

In addition, higher ambient temperatures have been shown to cause an increase in tissue metabolism and oxygen consumption on the order of 10% for every 1.8° F increment.[25] Thus, patients with compromised tissue already at risk for pressure ulcers may have increased demands for oxygen in excess of their metabolic capabilities. Any increase in temperature in combination with pressure is believed to increase the susceptibility of the tissue to injury either from ischemia or reperfusion when the pressure is relieved.[26]

Also, it has been shown that increased temperature causes an exponential increase in blood perfusion, which has been associated with an increase in either core body temperature or local skin temperature.[27,28] For example, in a study of operatively acquired pressure ulcers, the single greatest predictor of pressure ulcer development was the use of a warming blanket under the patient.[29] These findings clearly indicate the need for additional studies to definitively determine the effects of skin temperature modulation on the development of pressure ulcers. Therefore, when choosing the right support surface for the patient, its heat transfer rate is an objective performance measurement related to its ability to control temperature effects.

Moisture control

Moisture is another key extrinsic factor in pressure ulcer development. The sources of skin moisture that may predispose the skin to breakdown include perspiration, urine, feces, and fistula or wound drainage. Excessive moisture may lead to maceration of the skin.[30] Increases may be due to the slight increase in friction that occurs with light sweating[31] or to the increase in bacterial load resulting when alkaline sources of moisture neutralize the protection provided by the normal acid mantle of the skin.

The detrimental effect of an increase in moisture adjacent to the skin has been demonstrated by tensile tests on excised skin strips in a controlled humidity environment. In a study by Wildnauer et al.[32] the tensile strength of the strips decreased by 75% with an increase in relative humidity from 10% to 98%. Skin with such reduced strength may be more prone to mechanical damage from shear stress and could easily be abraded.[33-35]

MATERIALS AND COMPONENTS USED IN SUPPORT SURFACE SYSTEMS

The components and materials described here are the most commonly used in support surface systems and may be used alone or in combination. They include foam, gel and gel pads, fluid-filled bladders, viscous fluid, and elastomers.

Foam

Foam may be elastic or viscoelastic and may be comprised of open or closed cells. Open-cell foam is defined as a permeable structure in which there's no barrier between cells, and gases or liquids can pass through the foam. Closed-cell foam is defined as a non-permeable structure in which there's a barrier between cells, preventing gases or liquids from passing through the foam.

ELASTIC FOAM

Elastic foam is a type of porous polymer material that conforms in proportion to the applied load.[4] Consequently, greater loads result in predictably greater deformations, and vice versa. If time is a factor in the load versus deformation characteristic, the response is considered to be viscoelastic, which is discussed separately. The response of support surfaces made from resilient foam is predominately elastic. Foam is said to have "memory" because of its tendency to return to its nominal shape or thickness.

Foam products typically consist of foam layers of varying densities or combinations of gel and foam. Other products have a series of air-filled chambers covered with a foam structure or are available as multidensity, closed-cell products and may be 4″ to 10″ deep with deflectable tips. For these types of products, "memory" is not total because only the foam components will return to their unloaded shape. Several seat cushion products have this construction. A degree of postural stability can be achieved by adding a resilient shell to support surfaces consisting of a combination of fluid-filled bladders and resilient foam, and envelopment can be improved with a fluid or viscous fluid–filled layer at the interface.

An ideal combination of characteristics for an elastic support surface is resistance that adjusts to the magnitude of compressive forces.[36,37] The support surface should have a high enough compression resistance to fully support the load (prevent bottoming-out) without providing too high a reactive force (memory) so that the interface pressure remains low. Over time and with extended use, foam degrades and loses its resilience. This decreased ability results in higher interface pressures. Krouskop et al.[37] estimate that a foam mattress wears out after approximately 3 years of use, and the compressive forces are transferred to the underlying structure used to support the foam. In other words, the mattress "bottoms out."

Foams of varying densities may be combined or cut to relieve or conform to bony landmarks to enhance pressure distribution and even reduce shear forces. For example, multi-density, closed-cell foam products with deflectable tips provide some shear protection. Many pressure-reducing mattresses have loose-fitting covers to reduce friction.

The stiffness and thickness of foam limit its ability to immerse and envelop; soft foams will envelop better than stiffer foams but will necessarily be thicker to avoid bottoming out. Foam seat cushions are typically contoured to improve their performance. Precontouring the seat cushion to provide a better match between the buttocks and the cushion increases the contact area and immersion, thereby reducing average pressure and pressure peaks.[38-40] (See *Elastic foam seat cushions*.)

Foam tends to increase skin temperature because its materials and the air they entrap are poor heat conductors. Moisture doesn't increase

Elastic foam seat cushions

These photos show four different types of elastic foam seat cushions.

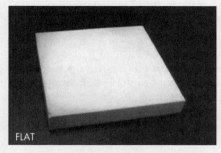

FLAT

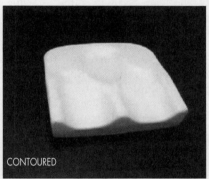

CONTOURED

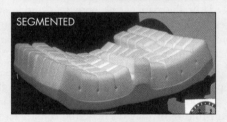

SEGMENTED

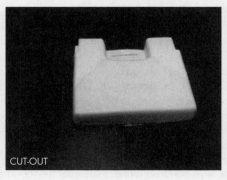

CUT-OUT

as much on foam products with a porous cover because the open-cell structure of the cover provides a pathway through which moisture can diffuse. Patient movement can also increase heat transfer rates. Mean temperature increases of 6.1° F (3.4° C) and a 10.4% increase in moisture at the skin surface have been recorded on foam products after 1 hour of contact.[41]

VISCOELASTIC FOAM

Viscoelastic foam is a type of porous polymer material that conforms in proportion to the applied load and to the rate of loading.[4] Viscoelastic foam products consist of temperature-sensitive, viscoelastic open-cell foam. At temperatures near that of the human body, the foam becomes softer, allowing the layer of foam nearest to the body to provide improved pressure distribution through envelopment and immersion when compared with high resilient foam. Viscoelastic foam acts like a self-contouring surface because the elastic response diminishes over time, even after the foam is compressed. However, the desirable temperature and time-sensitive responses of viscoelastic foam may not be realized when the ambient temperature is too low. The properties of viscoelastic foam products vary widely and must be chosen according to the specific needs of the patient for both seat and mattress applications. Solid gel products respond similarly to viscoelastic foam products and are included in this category.

Mean temperature increases of 5° F have been reported for viscoelastic foam.[41] Solid gel products tend to maintain a constant skin-contact temperature or may decrease the contact temperature. (See *Viscoelastic gel seat cushion*.)

Gel pads have higher heat flux than foam due to the high specific heat (ability to conduct heat) of the gel material. However, in Stewart et al.'s study,[41] the heat transfer decreased after 2 hours. This indicates that the heat reservoir was indeed filling, which suggests that the temperature may increase during longer periods—for example, more than 2 hours—of unrelieved sitting. Moisture increased 22.8% over a 1-hour period.[41] The relative humidity of the skin surface increases considerably because of the nonporous nature of the gel pads.

Viscoelastic gel seat cushion

The photo shows a viscoelastic gel seat cushion. Viscoelastic products are also available in other shapes.

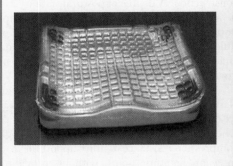

Fluid-filled bladders and compartments

Fluid-filled products may consist of small or large chambers filled with air, water, or other viscous fluid materials, such as silicon elastomer, silicon, or polyvinyl. The "fluid" flows from chamber to chamber or within a single chamber in response to movement and requires no supplemental power. The term "air-flotation" is sometimes used to describe interconnected multi-chamber surfaces. (See *Fluid-filled products*.)

PRACTICE POINT

Be careful to maintain the correct levels of inflation in air cushions to achieve optimal pressure reduction. Under-inflation causes bottoming out and over-inflation increases the interface pressure. For viscous fluid–filled surfaces, such as seat cushions, it's important to monitor the distribution of viscous material and manually move it back to the areas under bony prominences if it has moved away from these areas.

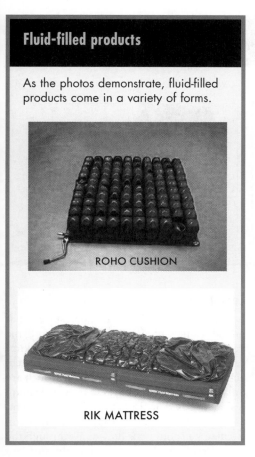

As the photos demonstrate, fluid-filled products come in a variety of forms.

ROHO CUSHION

RIK MATTRESS

Most fluid-filled products permit a high degree of immersion, allowing the body to sink into the surface. The surface conforms to bony prominences, effectively increasing the surface-pressure distribution area and lowering the interface pressure by transferring the pressure to adjacent areas. These products are capable of achieving small to modest deformations without large restoring shear forces. In a direct comparison of interface pressures with air-fluidized and low-air-loss beds, the RIK mattress was shown to relieve pressure as effectively as the air-fluidized and low-air-loss surfaces used in the study.[31]

Skin temperature is affected by the specific heat (ability to conduct heat) of the fluid material contained in the support device. Air has a low specific heat, and water has a high specific heat. The viscous material used in the RIK mattress also has a high specific heat,

and skin temperature decreases have been demonstrated with this product.[42]

Given the large variety of materials used as covers in products falling into the fluid-filled category, it's difficult to generalize on the moisture control characteristics of these products. However, the insulating effects of rubber and plastic used in some fluid-filled products have been shown to increase the relative humidity due to perspiration.[41]

FEATURES OF SUPPORT SURFACES

The features covered in this section can be used alone or in combination with other features. They include air-fluidized, low-air-loss, alternating-pressure, and lateral rotation products.

Air-fluidized

A support surface with an air-fluidized feature provides pressure redistribution via a fluid-like medium created by forcing air through beads and characterized by immersion and envelopment.[4] These beds were originally developed in the late 1960s for use with burn patients. These products consist of granular materials such as silicon beads encased in a polyester or Gore-Tex sheeting. The granular material takes on the characteristics of a fluid when pressurized air is forced through them. In some models, the fluidization feature is variable, permitting individualization based on the patient's needs. Feces and other body fluids flow freely through the sheet; to prevent bacteriologic contamination, the bed must be pressurized at all times and the sheet must be properly disinfected after use by each patient and at least once per week with long-term use by a single patient.[43]

Air-fluidized beds use fluid technology to decrease pressure through the principle of immersion while simultaneously reducing shear. Air-fluidized products permit the highest degree of immersion currently available among support surfaces. The surface conforms to bony prominences by permitting deep immersion into the surface—almost two-thirds of the body may be immersed.[44] The immersion effectively lowers the interface pressure by increasing the surface-pressure distribution area. The greater deformations

Air-fluidized and low-air-loss beds

AIR-FLUIDIZED BED

LOW-AIR-LOSS BED

possible with this technology enable the transfer of pressure to adjacent body areas and other bony prominences. Envelopment and shear force are minimized. A loose but tightly woven polyester or Gore-Tex cover sheet is used to reduce surface tension. Low surface tension enhances envelopment and minimizes shear forces.

The pressurized air in these products is generally warmed to a temperature level of 82.4° to 95° F (28° to 35° C); however, warming may be beneficial or harmful depending on the patient's needs. For example, heat may be harmful to patients with multiple sclerosis but beneficial for patients in pain. The beneficial effects must be balanced against the increasing metabolic demands of the tissue.

The high degree of moisture-vapor permeability of the air-fluidized system is effective in managing body fluids; in patients with severe burns, air-fluidized beds have been known to cause dehydration. (See *Air-fluidized and low-air-loss beds.*)

PRACTICE POINT

Air-fluidized beds are advantageous for burn patients due to their effectiveness in managing body fluids.

Low-air-loss

Low-air-loss is a feature of a support surface that provides a flow of air to assist in managing the heat and humidity (microclimate) of the skin.[4] Low-air-loss systems use a series of connected, air-filled cushions or compartments, which are inflated to specific pressures to provide loading resistance based on the patient's height, weight, and distribution of body weight. An air pump circulates a continuous flow of air through the device, replacing air lost through the surface's pores. The inflation pressures of the cushions vary with the patient's weight distribution; some systems have individually adjustable sections for the head, trunk, pelvic, or foot areas.[45] As with other fluid-filled surfaces, the temperature of the skin is affected by the specific heat of the fluid material. However, the constant air circulation and evaporation tend to keep the skin from overheating.

In low-air-loss systems, the patient lies on a loose-fitting, waterproof cover placed over the cushions. The waterproof covers are designed to let air pass through the pores of the fabric and are usually made of a special nylon or polytetrafluoroethylene fabric with high moisture-vapor permeability. Manufacturers have addressed the problem of skin dehydration by altering the number, size, and configuration of the pores in the covers.[45] The material is very smooth, with a low coefficient of friction;

in addition, it's impermeable to bacteria and easy to clean.[44] Low-air-loss devices have been shown to prevent buildup of moisture and subsequent skin maceration.[44]

Alternating pressure

Alternating pressure is a feature of a support surface that provides pressure redistribution via cyclic changes in loading and unloading as characterized by frequency, duration, amplitude, and rate of change parameters over the "active area" of the surface.[4] These systems contain air-filled chambers or cylinders arranged lengthwise or in various other patterns. Air or fluid is pumped into the chambers at periodic intervals to inflate and deflate the chambers in opposite phases, thereby changing the pressure distribution. The frequency of the alternating-pressure feature can have an effect on its use. For example, very short peak inflation and cycling time appear to have a dramatic effect on increasing lymphatic flow.[6,45,46]

Rather than increasing the surface area for distribution through immersion and envelop-ment, alternating-pressure devices distribute the pressure by shifting the body weight to a different surface-contact area. This may increase the interface pressure of that area during the inflation phase.

Alternating-pressure technology has the same potential as any other fluid-filled support surface to influence temperature at the interface; thus care must be taken to maintain the correct levels of inflation. The skin moisture control and temperature control characteristics of alternating-pressure surfaces also depend on the characteristics of the cover and supporting material. (See *Alternating-pressure integrated cushions*.)

Lateral rotation

Lateral rotation is a feature of a support surface that moves the patient in a regular pattern around a longitudinal axis as characterized by degree of patient turn, duration, and frequency.[4] Although these devices have been used for several decades for other medical purposes, such as pulmonary therapy, research

Alternating-pressure integrated cushions

The illustration shows the characteristics of alternating-pressure integrated cushions.

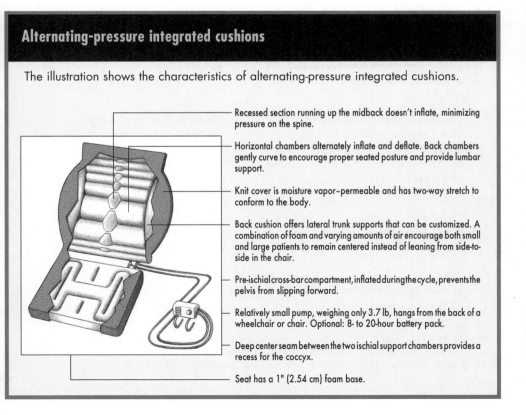

Recessed section running up the midback doesn't inflate, minimizing pressure on the spine.

Horizontal chambers alternately inflate and deflate. Back chambers gently curve to encourage proper seated posture and provide lumbar support.

Knit cover is moisture vapor–permeable and has two-way stretch to conform to the body.

Back cushion offers lateral trunk supports that can be customized. A combination of foam and varying amounts of air encourage both small and large patients to remain centered instead of leaning from side-to-side in the chair.

Pre-ischial cross-bar compartment, inflated during the cycle, prevents the pelvis from slipping forward.

Relatively small pump, weighing only 3.7 lb, hangs from the back of a wheelchair or chair. Optional: 8- to 20-hour battery pack.

Deep center seam between the two ischial support chambers provides a recess for the coccyx.

Seat has a 1" (2.54 cm) foam base.

is conflicting on their use for pressure ulcer treatment.[47] Lateral rotation may be continuous (that is, on an automatic timed cycle) or manual (that is, the bed is rotated and locked in a given position). The therapy works by positioning the patient in such a way so that one lung is higher than the other to prevent pneumonia. This therapy is not intended for patients with cervical or spinal fracture, intracranial pressure instability, or long-bone fractures.

According to the NPUAP, "Whenever lateral rotation features are used, the risk for shear injury exists. Shear force tangentially strains the skin (through stretching) and interrupts blood flow of the skin. Unless the individual is properly positioned and bolstered, shearing can occur with every rotation, causing a new ulcer or worsening existing ulcers."[1] (See *Recommendations for lateral rotation.*)

MATCHING SUPPORT TO PATIENT NEEDS

Although widely used, support surfaces have neither performance standards nor criteria for function that can be tested against clinical out-

---

Recommendations for lateral rotation

(Strength of Evidence = C)

Lateral rotation in individuals without pressure ulcers	**Lateral rotation in individuals with pressure ulcers**
• Secure the individual with bolster pads (provided by the manufacturer) to prevent sacral shearing when lateral-rotation features are selected for individuals without pressure ulcers. The individual should be aligned properly in the center of the surface.	• Consider alternative methods of pressure redistribution (or avoid lateral-rotation beds) in individuals with sacral or buttocks pressure ulcers.
• Continue to turn the individual and assess skin for pressure and shear damage. Discontinue lateral rotation at the first sign of tissue damage, and re-evaluate the individual and the support surface.	• Offload the pressure ulcer(s) in individuals undergoing lateral-rotation therapy.
• Change lateral-rotation support surface to a support system with improved pressure redistribution, shear reduction, and microclimate control and without rotation when there is evidence of shear injury. Position the individual off the area as much as possible.	• Inspect the pressure ulcer and the periulcer skin for shear injury with every dressing change. Shear injury may appear as deterioration of the ulcer edge, undermining, and/or as increasing inflammation of periulcer skin or the ulcer.

Adapted with permission: National Pressure Ulcer Advisory Panel and European Pressure Ulcer Advisory Panel. "Prevention and Treatment of Pressure Ulcers: Clinical Practice Guideline." Washington, DC: National Pressure Ulcer Advisory Panel; Special Populations: p 71, 2009.

comes. Indeed, the basis for effective function isn't known, or is poorly understood, for such common products as wheelchair seat cushions and horizontal support surfaces intended for skin protection and healing of wounds. Despite this, clinicians must have some basis for decision making regarding the selection of these products. The following key questions should be used to guide the decision-making process.

What are the patient's specific load management needs?

Regardless of body position, the first step in determining an individualized protective intervention is to perform a general physical assessment and functional evaluation. Much of this information will then be used to assess the patient's risk for pressure ulcer development.

GENERAL PHYSICAL EXAMINATION AND FUNCTIONAL EVALUATION

Patient evaluation is described elsewhere in this text; however, several additional items are germane to the selection of a support surface. These include assessing the capability of the patient for specific bed mobility (movement on the surface, ingress and egress, and ability to place supportive devices), the number of available turning surfaces, the time spent in lying in bed or sitting per day, the number of devices or pillows needed for positioning, the patient's body weight and its distribution, and the presence of contractures.

Wheelchair cushion selection

For selection of wheelchair cushions, the evaluation is quite extensive because cushions are part of the total seating system that also includes the wheelchair. Indeed, no cushion can perform effectively in the prevention of pressure ulcers if the wheelchair isn't properly fitted. Therefore, it's recommended that a trained seating specialist perform the seat cushion evaluation and selection.

The seating evaluation should also include a mat examination to determine the functional postural limitations of the spine, pelvis, and extremities and to determine appropriate measurements for wheelchair fitting. An extensive functional examination is also required to consider the seating and mobility needs of the

individual in the immediate, intermediate, and community environments.[48-50]

Strategies for maintaining tissue integrity can be extremely complicated for spinal cord–injured patients, elderly people, and other populations with degenerative neuromuscular conditions or diseases. For example, a patient's ability to sit unsupported can be characterized by the amount of external support needed to maintain posture: hands-free, hands-dependent, or prop-sitting with external support only.[50] This capability has significant implications for compensatory functional postures, ability to reposition, and the method used for intermittent pressure relief. Figures 11-1, 11-2, and 11-3 (page 280) illustrate three common and effective strategies for intermittent pressure relief.

Specialty mattress selection

When selecting a specialty mattress, a patient's weight and the distribution of that weight are important factors. Indeed, each mattress overlay, replacement, or integrated bed unit has weight limits. For heavier patients, bariatric (bari) beds should be used. However, for patients approaching the manufacturer's recommended weight limit, the distribution of the weight should be examined. For example, patients who are heavier in the hip region but who don't exceed the manufacturer's weight limit may need to be placed on a bariatric product in order to achieve effective pressure redistribution. Patients with contractures may have their weight dispersed unevenly. For example, contractures could pull the heels toward the groin or increase flexion between other body parts, creating special needs for tissue management beyond what a mattress can provide.

ASSESSING RISK

The most commonly used risk assessment scales for prediction of pressure ulcer incidence are the Braden, Norton, and Waterlow Scales.[51-53] The sensitivity and specificity of these scales vary depending on the population setting and the position of the patient's body. For example, different Braden cut-off scores are associated with different settings (nursing home versus intensive care unit), and in a recent study of risk assessment scales for general inpatients versus wheelchair users, the Waterlow Scale outper-

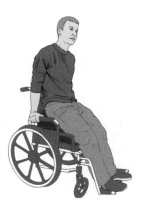

Figure 11-1. A push-up pressure relief can completely off-load the buttocks but requires sufficient arm strength and trunk control.

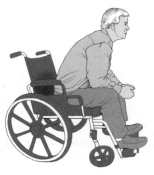

Figure 11-2. A forward lean can unweight the ischial tuberosities.

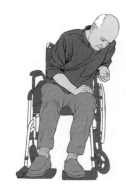

Figure 11-3. A side lean pressure relief off-loads the contralateral side and so must be done in both directions.

formed the Braden Scale.[54-56] Risk assessment scales specifically designed for wheelchair users are currently being developed.

Bergstrom and colleagues[56] reported that mattress selection based on categorizing patients via a pressure ulcer risk assessment scale produced both efficacious and cost-effective results. Patients of a large tertiary care hospital scoring nine or lower on the Braden pressure ulcer risk assessment scale were provided a group 2 support surface (low-air-loss mattress) as a preventive measure. Those scoring above nine were evaluated and provided with the most appropriate surface according to individual patient needs. Results indicated that not only did pressure ulcer incidence and prevalence drop by more than 50% when patients were categorized according to pressure ulcer risk, but costs associated with overlays, replacement mattresses, and low-air-loss beds also decreased.

Similar results have been realized by studies that selected wheelchair cushions from a set of cushion alternatives based on risk assessment. Krouskop and colleagues[57] described how a seating clinic assigned risk to their clients with spinal cord injury by using such factors as gender, interface pressure, lifestyle, and stability. In 80% to 90% of the clients, cushions were selected from three alternatives, with the remaining clients being provided with other cushion types.

When assessing risk, remember that proper follow-up care is necessary to prevent pressure ulcers regardless of the cushion or bed prescribed. Skin redness often occurs because of positioning and use and doesn't necessarily indicate that a poor surface choice was made.

Clinical judgment

Clinicians should know how to evaluate bed or cushion performance, which includes an assessment of how adequately the product provides pressure redistribution, or if the patient is "bottoming out" or actually having soft tissue in close proximity to the hard undersurface. Clinicians should also observe any powered products for loss of power, sensor malfunctions, or disconnected hoses. Frequently checking the product's performance is especially important for patients who are unable to express their discomfort due to cognitive or communication impairment.

INTERFACE PRESSURE-MAPPING

Interface pressure-mapping—comparison of a patient's relative responses from one surface to another—can be an effective clinical tool to aid in the selection of a support surface for a specific patient. Pressure-mapping may also be used to determine the relative effectiveness of modifications to the wheelchair and other positioning devices or to obtain information about pressure relief for patients with spinal cord injuries. For example, Henderson and colleagues[58] used a pressure-mapping system to compare three methods of relieving pressure in seated individuals with spinal cord injuries. The positions studied were tilted back 35 degrees, tilted back 65 degrees, and forward-leaning seated posture. The results indicated that the greatest pressure relief over the ischial tuberosities was seen in the forward-leaning position, followed by the 65-degree backward-tilt position.[58] Observing the change in pressure distribution on the mapping display allows patients without sensation to observe the effects of various weight-shifting methods and learn to consciously integrate them into their seated behavior.

USING CLINICAL PRACTICE GUIDELINES

Clinical practice guidelines offer recommendations, based on scientific evidence and the professional judgment of expert panels, about how healthcare professionals can provide quality care. Historically, the two most commonly referenced clinical practice guidelines with regard to support surface selection are:

- Agency for Health Care Policy and Research Clinical Practice Guideline Number 15, "Treatment of Pressure Ulcers"[59]
- Consortium for Spinal Cord Medicine Clinical Practice Guideline, "Pressure Ulcer Prevention and Treatment Following Spinal Cord Injury."[60]

The recently published NPUAP-EPUAP guideline "Prevention and Treatment of Pressure Ulcers"[1] serves as an update for these older documents.

How does the product function and how well does it perform?

Answers to what the product does and how it performs should be sought from a variety of sources. Sources of information for support surfaces include marketing materials, controlled clinical trials, and objective indirect data from laboratory testing or clinical studies (interface pressure and other physiological responses).

LABORATORY TESTING

What a support surface does has been largely determined by studies using laboratory methods to measure variables believed to be clinically relevant in pressure ulcer formation. For example, Krouskop's[61] study of foam mattress overlays provided the following recommended specifications for selection based on the results of independent laboratory testing:

- a thickness of 3″ to 4″ (7.5 to 10 cm)
- a density of 1.3 to 1.6 lb per cubic foot as an indicator of the amount of foam in the product
- a 25% indentation load deflection (ILD) equal to about 30 lb (the amount of force required to compress the foam to 75% of its thickness as an indicator of the foam's compressibility and conformability)
- a modulus of 2.5 or greater (the ratio of 60% ILD to 25% ILD).

SUPPORT SURFACE AND CUSHION STANDARDS

Standards have been developed for wheelchair seat cushions and are under development for other support surfaces. Publishing national or international standards for support surfaces requires that uniform test methods be developed to quantify clinically relevant characteristics. Simply stated, to make valid comparisons among products, characteristics and properties need to be measured using the same test and under the same conditions. Testing conditions should model clinically relevant parameters as closely as possible. The requirement that the tests be repeatable across laboratories in different countries means that standardized tests typically use models rather than human subjects. Clinicians, therefore, must consider test results as relative measures.

The results of standard tests often don't include pass-fail criteria. Just as there are valid reasons to purchase an automobile with an engine that only gets 15 mpg over another with a fuel-efficient engine that gets 25 mpg, so are there reasons to purchase support surfaces with, for example, a lower pressure distribution characteristic but higher moisture dissipation ability over a product with a higher pressure distribution characteristic but lower moisture dissipation ability. The primary objectives of the standard tests are to characterize their different functional properties and to permit comparisons of performance among products with similar functions.

The range of products on the market places a heavy burden on clinicians to keep abreast of new technology; therefore, patients, clinicians, vendors, manufacturers, third-party payers, and researchers all benefit from standard terminology, definitions, and test methods. Clinicians benefit from a mechanism to objectively match a seat cushion's or support surface's characteristics to the needs of their patients.[32] Vendors benefit by being able to clearly describe products from different manufacturers in a manner understood by clinicians and patients. Testing standards aid manufacturers by guiding new product development and assisting in the redesign of existing products. In addition, standards promote quality assurance within manufacturing processes. The final potential beneficiaries of standards are third-party payers because the seat cushion and support surface market is a payer's market; that is, payer reimbursement drives the market. A validated system to test and objectively characterize support surfaces will give funding agencies an objective means for making funding decisions. In fact, standards form the basis for certain tests used by funding agencies to classify or categorize products.

SEAT CUSHION STANDARDS

Standards for seat cushions are being developed by the ISO. In the United States, the effort is organized through RESNA as an accredited standards organization for the American National Standards Institute.[34,35] One of the four interrelated working groups focuses on tissue integrity management and has developed test methods that address key performance features of cushions, including load deflection

and hysteresis, frictional properties, lateral and forward stiffness, sliding resistance, impact damping, recovery, loaded contour depth and overload deflection, water spillage, and biocompatibility.[62] Additional tests are being developed that measure heat and water vapor transmissibility and stability of properties with use (fatigue). Although all these tests have clinical relevance, a subset is described below. And, even though tests have been designed for seat cushions, the constructs are described in relation to both cushions and horizontal support surfaces to illustrate key concepts.

Load deflection

Materials used in mattresses and cushions support the body by compression (foam and air), deflection (gel and viscous fluid), or tension (bladder material and fabric). Material stiffness impacts how materials deform to accommodate the body. Load deflection tests typically involve loading a cushion or support surface with a standardized indenter that mimics a part(s) of the body. Deflection into the support surface is measured as the weight on the indenter is increased.

Clinically, materials can be too stiff or too soft. When too stiff, the body does not immerse, and high pressures or instability can result. When too soft, materials can "bottom-out," leading to poor support and high pressures. Foams are made with different stiffness ratings, called indentation force deflection. Many products use a combination of foam with a softer material positioned on top of a more stiff material. This configuration permits deflection of the top surface while protecting against bottoming-out through the use of the stiffer bottom layer.

Because the amount of air impacts the stiffness of a support surface or cushion, products that use air are often adjustable. Too much air leads to an overly stiff surface, and too little air can lead to bottoming-out. In addition to body weight, the amount of tissue, the type of tissue (hypotonic, normal, hypertonic), and a person's posture or position all influence how stiff a surface must be to adequately support a person.[63]

Frictional properties

Friction is the result of a relationship between materials; so standardized tests for friction measure the sliding forces of one material on another. In terms of cushions and support surfaces, these standardized tests concentrate on cover materials, such as fabrics and bed linens.

Sliding resistance

Unlike friction tests, which focus on cover material, sliding resistance tests measure the influence of the entire system, including the cover and all support materials. All users of support surfaces and cushions have to transfer onto and off the bed or wheelchair. For people who can't fully transfer, certain materials and designs facilitate easier transfers. However, if a support is too easy to slide on, stability on that surface can be compromised. Standardized tests of sliding resistance involve loading the surface with an indenter modeled on the human body or buttocks and pulling it forward or sideways. The force required to slide the indenter on the surface is measured and reflects sliding resistance.

Loaded contour depth and overload test

This test measures the immersion of a standardized indenter into a cushion surface. Clinically, the test provides two key pieces of information about seat cushions: the initial contour of a cushion and the amount of deflection that may occur when someone sits on it. The overload portion of the test adds 33% more weight and measures additional immersion of the indenter. A cushion that has "bottomed-out" will not deflect further under the additional weight. A support surface should maintain a margin of safety that allows additional cushioning during overload conditions. Certain functional movements and postural adjustments, such as leaning and reaching, impart an overload condition on the surface.

As noted, several standardized tests have been developed for wheelchair cushions by the ISO. The NPUAP S3I Committee[63] is developing standards for mattresses. At this time there are draft U.S. national standards for terms and definitions, immersion, and heat and water vapor transmission characteristics.

PRODUCT EFFECTIVENESS

The effectiveness of a support surface product is measured by two methods: its efficacy in

use by patients and its efficacy in comparison with similar products. Several articles provide an overview of support surface research.[64-67] Rather than basing comparisons on functional classification, most studies compared classes of products based on the product's ability to redistribute pressure.

Considering the limitations ascribed to interface pressure measurement, it may be more useful to categorize devices according to their ability to evenly distribute pressure over the contact surface area rather than ascribe any significance to the magnitude of pressure measured at a particular location.[68] However, the most common comparison has been the use of interface pressure to compare a product against a "standard" hospital bed or mattress. When reviewing this literature, remember that the "standard" support surface probably varies from study to study. Most studies also vary with regard to patient population (for example, orthopedic or neurologic) and setting (for example, acute care, intensive care, long-term care, or home care). All three independent variables (products compared, subject population, setting) affect both study outcomes and the interpretation of results. Finally, when comparing performance studies, remember that treatment studies, in which subjects already have ulcers, are fundamentally different from prevention studies.

PREVENTION EFFECTIVENESS

Generally, studies have shown that nonpowered, constant low-pressure supports (foam, air, gel, and combinations of these materials) are more effective in preventing pressure ulcers than a "standard" hospital mattress. Generalization of the results of studies comparing different pressure redistribution products is difficult. Most comparative studies of various constant low-force products have demonstrated no differences in the prevention of pressure ulcers.[69,70]

Conclusions from research investigating the more complex technology, including low-air-loss and alternating-pressure products, are similar. Evidence suggests that both low-air-loss and alternating-pressure surfaces are more effective than "standard" mattresses, but comparative studies of the performance of low-air-loss and alternating-pressure products are inconsistent regarding the clinical superiority of one over the other. Moreover, comparisons of alternating-pressure and constant low-pressure products have not produced definitive differences.

Because the evidence is not definitive, clinicians must carefully read the original study to generalize the results to a specific clinical situation. When considering a product's clinical applicability, the characteristics of the population, setting, and products must closely match one's clinical situation and the limitations of the study must be known. For example, consider the design of alternating-pressure products where such variables as cell height or bladder thickness and cycle timing and frequency can significantly affect product performance. One can't necessarily generalize the performance of one alternating-pressure product against another. Similarly, the results of a support surface study within acute care might not produce similar results in a home care setting using the same support surfaces.

Evidence about specific cushions and their respective effectiveness is insufficient. Contradictions also exist in the literature regarding the clinical benefits of cushions designed to reduce the risk of sitting-acquired pressure ulcers. Most research has used indirect outcomes, such as interface pressure or blood flow. Relatively few studies have measured direct outcomes related to specific types of cushions,[33,71-73] but these have not resulted in definitive findings of efficacy of one product over another. One facility performed two studies targeting elderly wheelchair users. The first study found no difference in the incidence of pressure ulcers in users of flat foam compared with custom-contoured foam cushions, and a subsequent study found that more users of flat foam (41%) developed ulcers compared with users of a contoured foam-viscous fluid cushion (25%), but this difference did not reach statistical significance. In a study tracking interface pressure and wheelchair cushions in elderly users, Brienza and colleagues[73] found that interface pressures were higher for subjects who developed sitting-acquired pressure ulcers compared with those who didn't

develop ulcers. No definitive relationship was found between interface pressures and cushion types across these subjects.

TREATMENT EFFECTIVENESS

Widely varying subject populations and care settings have complicated the ability to compare results across studies investigating the effectiveness of support surfaces in the treatment of pressure ulcers. Furthermore, a number of treatment outcome measures have been used to judge effectiveness, such as the relative or actual reduction in ulcer size (area or volume), the percentage of ulcers healed within a specified time period, and the time until wound closure. Different operational definitions have also been used for wound status, such as "healed" and "closure," making it difficult to compare equitably. Adding to the confusion, the terms "healed" and "closed" are used interchangeably in the Centers for Medicare and Medicaid Services Resident Assessment Instrument (RAI) Manual Version 3.0 in Section M, Skin Conditions.[74]

Generally, studies targeting support surfaces for ulcer treatment have produced results similar to those targeting prevention. Low-air-loss and air-fluidized surfaces have been shown to improve treatment outcomes more effectively compared with "conventional" treatment[75,76] and nonpowered foam alternatives.[65,66] Results of alternating-pressure surface studies are inconsistent with some studies showing a treatment effect and others showing none. No clinically significant treatment differences have been shown among similar products.

What other patient needs must be met?

While load management and product function are critical areas to consider in matching patient support needs, other pressure redistribution options must also be considered. These options include repositioning, heel protection, managing heel pressure, encouraging ambulation, and managing skin microclimate.

TURNING AND REPOSITIONING SCHEDULES

The frequency of repositioning required to prevent ischemia is variable and unknown, yet regular repositioning is believed to help deter the deleterious effects of pressure by decreasing the duration of exposure. Through the process of repositioning, the body's weight is redistributed, and new pressure areas are introduced. To provide effective pressure relief, both pressure and time must be considered. For example, in 1961, Kosiak recommended that repositioning be done in intervals of 1 to 2 hours based on the interface readings from healthy subjects.[77]

Turning schedules have been studied empirically and experimentally. Bliss[78] studied turning schedules in a spinal injury ward and found that 2 hours was adequate for some, whereas others required more frequent, and some less frequent, turning. Two important aspects of these findings are that some patients exhibited redness after 2 hours and that many patients disliked frequent turning.

In an experimental study by Knox and colleagues,[79] variables such as temperature, pressure, and redness were monitored while people rested on a mattress for 60, 90, and 120 minutes. Some subjects exhibited redness after each of the intervals, leading the researchers to conclude that a 2-hour turning schedule might not be sufficient.

Such theoretical evidence points directly to the duration of loading as the way to maintain tissue integrity. If, however, the above experiment is only one example of patients experiencing redness after less than a 2-hour turning schedule, then it cannot be construed as the answer for all clinical practices.

While the every-2-hour turn schedule has traditionally been entrenched in clinical practice, new research has challenged this long-held belief. Recent findings from two randomized controlled trials have provided evidence that the frequency of repositioning for persons who are on a viscoelastic foam mattress may be extended for longer than every 2 hours without increasing the incidence of pressure ulcers. In a study of 838 nursing home patients who were turned every 4 hours on a viscoelastic mattress, DeFloor et al.[80] reported a reduction in stage II and more severe pressure ulcers. Vanderwee et al.[81] also studied nursing home patients who were also on a viscoelastic foam mattress ($n = 235$). The time in lateral position of 2 hours was compared with 4 hours

in a supine position. Turning these patients every 2 hours did not result in fewer pressure ulcers compared with the group turned every 4 hours.

In addition, no knowledge exists as to how turning schedule should be affected by support services. Therefore, the best approach is to evaluate and reevaluate each patient to best determine an appropriate turning schedule.

POSITIONING

In addition to the NPUAP-EPUAP Guidelines[1] for repositioning, a number of recommendations exist with regard to positioning for management of tissue loads. (See *Repositioning for the prevention of pressure ulcers,* page 286.)

The following eight positions are commonly used to reposition patients on horizontal surfaces:

- a prone position with rotation of 30 degrees to the right or left
- a supine position with 30 degrees of rotation to the right or left
- a supine position with slight right or left sacral relief[68]
- a supine position with the head of the bed elevated 30 degrees or less and the feet blocked
- a supine position with the head of the bed elevated 30 degrees or less and the knees flexed with the bed. (See *Horizontal positioning,* page 287.)

In all of these positions, the heels must be elevated with pillows or other devices. Note the use of pillows and towels to separate and protect bony prominences. Additional positioning technique includes blocking the feet and knees in a flexed position to prevent shear forces created when the patient slides down in bed.

Small shifts in weight can also be accomplished by positioning. For instance, foam wedges or pillows, used to position the patient on his or her side, can be altered slightly every 15 minutes. Pulling them out gradually over 1 to 1½ hours shifts the weight slightly. A patient who is in a wheelchair still requires shifts in his or her body weight. If possible, this patient should be taught to shift his or her weight every 15 minutes with repositioning every hour.

Repositioning for the prevention of pressure ulcers

- Repositioning should be undertaken to reduce the duration and magnitude of pressure over vulnerable areas of the body. Strength of evidence = A
- Repositioning frequency will be determined by the individual's tissue tolerance, his/her level of activity and mobility, his/her general medical condition, the overall treatment objectives, the support surface used, and assessments of the individual's skin condition. Strength of Evidence = C
- Repositioning should be undertaken using the 30-degree tilted side-lying position (alternately, right side, back, left side) or the prone position if the individual can tolerate this and her/ his

medical condition allows. Avoid postures that increase pressure, such as the 90-degree side-lying position or the semi-recumbent position. Strength of Evidence = C
- If sitting in bed is necessary, avoid head-of-bed elevation and a slouched position that places pressure and shear on the sacrum and coccyx. Strength of Evidence = C
- Position the individual so as to maintain his/her full range of activities. Strength of Evidence = C
- Additional recommendations are available in the repositioning for prevention of pressure ulcer section of the NPUAP/EPUAP Guidelines

Adapted with permission: National Pressure Ulcer Advisory Panel and European Pressure Ulcer Advisory Panel. "Prevention and Treatment of Pressure Ulcers: Clinical Practice Guideline." Washington, DC: National Pressure Ulcer Advisory Panel; Repositioning for prevention of pressure ulcers, p 33-35, 2009.

HEEL PROTECTION

The heel presents unique challenges for pressure-reducing interventions due to its small radius of curvature and its thin layer of subcutaneous tissue between the skin and calcaneal structures.[1,82] This small contact area affords minimal protection from the pressure exerted by the weight of the foot and, frequently, a portion of the lower limb. The lower limb is approximately one-sixth of the total body weight, so even if a small proportion of this rests on the heel, high interface pressure may result, even on air support systems.

Existing clinical practice guidelines recommend the use of pillows to suspend the heels.[1,4,82] However, pillows don't protect against footdrop and, due to patient movement, pillows require time and diligent positioning to maintain proper suspension. To provide continuous heel suspension via heel protective devices, clinicians must consider proper fit and placement of the device, patient position, the presence of additional equipment, as well as

the performance characteristics of the product. When elevated, the heel should be positioned completely off the bed surface. (See *Floating heels off the bed*, page 288.) The weight of the leg needs to be distributed to avoid putting pressure on the Achilles tendon. The knee should be slightly flexed, avoiding hyperextension.[83]

Clinical recommendations[83] for pressure-reducing heel protection include:

- reducing pressure, friction, and shear
- separating and protecting the ankles
- suspending the heels
- permitting repositioning without increasing pressure in other areas
- preventing footdrop
- enhancing patient comfort
- reassessing at least daily

EVIDENCE FOR MANAGING HEEL PRESSURE

Although relatively few studies of heel protection devices have been completed in the past decade, the majority of those that have been published

Horizontal positioning

The following photos show how to position patients properly on horizontal surfaces.

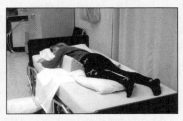 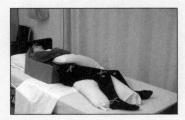

30-degree rotation from prone and supine positions, respectively

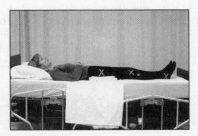 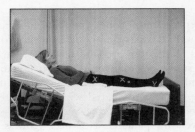

Head of the bed elevated 30 degrees or less with unilateral sacral relief and feet blocked, respectively

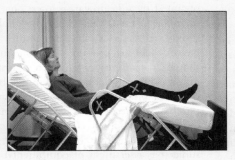

Head of the bed elevated 30 degrees with knees flexed to prevent shearing at the sacrum

have examined the pressure distribution capabilities of heel wraps, heel dressings, pillows, water-filled gloves, and various specialty heel products using interface pressure or pressure ulcer incidence as the primary outcomes. We will examine these devices here.[84]

As with other support surfaces, most heel protection products consist of a combination of materials and incorporate multiple strategies to optimize their therapeutic function. The distribution of pressure on a heel support surface depends on the relative fit between the heel and the surface, the mechanical properties of the heel tissue and the device, and the distribution of weight in the body part (heel). An ideal pressure distribution is one in which soft-tissue shape isn't altered relative to its unloaded condition.[85]

In a study designed by Zernike to investigate the efficacy of clinically "familiar" heel devices, the preventive use of routine nursing care, hydrocolloid dressings, egg-crate foam,

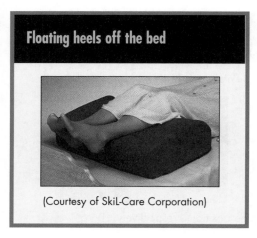

Floating heels off the bed

(Courtesy of SkiL-Care Corporation)

polyester-filled heel boots, and foam footdrop splints were compared in geriatric orthopedic patients at risk for pressure ulcers.[86,87] In a second study, a combination of 4 × 4″ gauze pads and an absorbent pad held in place with a gauze roll was compared with a laminated foam boot (Lunax Boot, Bio-Sonics) in at-risk intensive care patients with heel redness.[88] Although the statistical analyses of both studies were limited, the egg-crate boot and laminated foam boot were more effective in preventing pressure ulcers. Other methods in these studies either increased incidence or, as with the footdrop splints, proved too uncomfortable despite their ability to effectively suspend the heel. What's notable about Zernike's study is that deterioration of the heel tissue ensued despite routine nursing care (heel observation every 2 to 3 hours and direct pressure relief and repositioning of patients' heels). In a similar study, however, the prompt reporting of heel discomfort by patients to the nursing staff, with subsequent simultaneous use of heel elevation with a pillow or bath blanket under the calf and a Spenco Silicore quilted heel protector, resulted in zero incidence of pressure ulcers in 30 hip replacement patients.[89]

Flemister[90] also examined heel interface pressures with use of both a foam and polyester heel protector in seven patients assessed to be at moderate to high risk for pressure ulcer development. The foam heel protector marginally reduced heel interface pressures (1.3 mm Hg),

whereas the polyester protector actually resulted in a significant increase in interface pressure.

While a variety of heel protective devices are available commercially, their effectiveness seems to vary across the board. The few studies that have been performed suggest that while matching the device to the patient may be challenging, with careful consideration of patient needs and characteristics, it can be done.

What's available in this setting?

A patient's needs can change over the course of his or her illness. A product that's appropriate for acute care use may not work in the patient's home. Clinical judgment should consider therapy goals (ease of getting into or out of the bed for therapy or mobility), ability of the patient to move himself or herself in the bed, other complications (heel breakdown, pulmonary complications), and body weight and weight distribution.

WHAT'S PRACTICAL?

The issue of practicality relates to the overall care plan, the goals of load management (prevention versus treatment), how complicated the product is to use, and whether it will be operated by a healthcare professional, family member, or the patient. Many hospitals, long-term care facilities, and home care agencies have developed product selection guidelines that are usually presented as an algorithm[5] or graph. These guidelines are typically based on the availability of equipment from previous purchases in accordance with other published guidelines. Another common method used in selection and purchasing decisions is the subjective assessment of equipment based on a trial use in the clinical setting. This gives the staff a chance to use the equipment in a variety of situations and judge its performance.

HOW EASY IS THE PRODUCT TO USE?

Equipment that's easy to use has been associated with successful compliance. Awkward design or difficult assembly may cause the patient and his or her family to abandon using the equipment or increase the likelihood of misuse. Directions must be clear and obvious. For example, if the product is powered, it should have a battery backup to facilitate transferring patients to other locations as needed.

WHAT SERVICE AND MAINTENANCE ARE AVAILABLE?

A 24-hour call service with on-site repair or replacement is essential.

WHAT TYPE OF ALARM SYSTEM DOES THE PRODUCT HAVE?

Visual alarms are rarely sufficient, especially if the alarm is obscured under the bed. In the home-care setting, visible alarms are of little value unless there's constant attendance.

IS THE EQUIPMENT EASILY MAINTAINED?

If the equipment must be deflated for storage, reinflation time may be critical as well as the ability to deflate the equipment in the event of a cardiac arrest. Additionally, if the product isn't a personal use item, one must consider how long it takes to clean and ready the item for subsequent use.

WHAT OPERATING MECHANISM AND SPACE REQUIREMENTS DOES THE PRODUCT HAVE?

If the product has some form of movement, is cessation possible to facilitate such procedures as bedpan usage and hygiene care? Is the product the correct size for the home or setting where it will be used? Is the floor structure sound and capable of holding the weight of the bed? Will the bed fit through the door?

HOW MUCH DOES THE PRODUCT COST?

Technology has produced some innovative treatment products, but costs are high for patients, insurance companies, and hospitals. Prevention is more cost-effective than any other treatment. Available technology (support surfaces) may provide solutions when used correctly by properly educated staff. Indeed, one study demonstrated that educated staff can reduce the number of pressure ulcers better than noneducated staff. The same study indicated

that the cost of care is significantly less under the supervision of educated staff.[91]

The cost of support surfaces varies. Third-party reimbursement (Medicare may provide coverage), rental versus purchase, and cost-benefit issues need to be evaluated carefully. Some devices are only available on a rental basis. Although reimbursement is an issue in any setting, operational costs are of particular importance if the product is used in the home care setting where costs may be absorbed by the patient.

Consideration should also be given to the projected number of days that a support surface will be in use. More patients are being placed on advanced technology surfaces for considerably longer periods of time. Cost-effectiveness may be measured by relating the cost of the product to its efficacy.

When managing the allocation of specialty mattress and bed systems, a continuous process of evaluation and reevaluation should be employed to ensure that the patient's needs are reassessed on a regular basis.

SUMMARY

Understanding the nature of pressure ulcer etiology, the factors affecting pressure redistribution, and other physical factors associated with the use of specific support surface products and heel protection products is a necessity for nursing and other health-care personnel involved with tissue integrity management. As standardized test methods are developed and used for support surface

PRACTICE POINT

Consider these patient factors before purchasing support surfaces:

- Ease of use
- Operational costs of the equipment
- Service contracts and backup service
- Alarm systems
- Daily maintenance
- Operating mechanisms and space requirements

products, the clinical validation of specialized protective devices and the development more specific clinical practice guidelines will be possible. Until then, matching products to patient needs is a challenging process and must be based on the available evidence regarding the performance characteristics of existing support surfaces.

PATIENT SCENARIO

Clinical Data

Ms. CM is a 35-year-old woman with a T11-14 spinal cord injury. She lives alone, works full-time, and drives her own car. She presents in clinic with a right ischial pressure ulcer that will not heal and requests a new cushion. Inspection confirms an ischial ulcer that appears clean and well dressed.

Postural evaluation revealed a flexible left pelvic obliquity and minimal to moderate posterior pelvic tilt. Interface pressures measured on her current cushion were consistent with her posture, with higher pressure under the left ischial tuberosity and lesser pressure under the right ischial tuberosity, where the ulcer exists. Overall, the pressure profile was deemed acceptable. Subsequent discussion revealed that Ms. CM spends between 12 and 14 hours per day in her wheelchair and is able to achieve full pressure relief using a pushup technique. Ms. CM reported doing a pushup a couple times per day. A request to demonstrate a transfer showed good technique, adequate clearance of the buttocks over the drive wheels, and acceptable impact when landing. Ms. CM also reported that she sits on her Jay wheelchair cushion while driving.

A decision was made to try to increase pressure relief frequency and to change the technique from a pushup to a forward lean. By using a forward lean, Ms. CM was able to maintain pressure relief for a greater period of time. Her clinician asked her to limit her sitting to 9 hours per day with pressure relief every 30 minutes. This suggestion allowed Ms. CM to continue working while attempting to reduce her sitting time.

When Ms. CM returned for follow-up in 2 weeks, inspection showed little change in the appearance of the pressure ulcer.

In her description of a typical day, Ms. CM stated: " . . . and then I usually go upstairs to bed." This statement prompted the clinician to ask if her bedroom was on the second floor and how she got up the stairs. Ms. CM responded: "I bump my way up and down the stairs." This was obviously a significant finding as this technique can repeatedly load the buttocks in a dangerous manner. Several interventions were discussed, including the use of a protective cushion during stair ascent and home modification to install a stair lift.

Case Discussion

This case highlights several important issues. A postural assessment done in concert with interface pressure mapping revealed that the side opposite of a pelvic obliquity was the site of an ulcer. This is typically not the case as the lower side usually receives higher pressures. Weight shift technique and frequency were addressed, but they did not have an impact. Nonetheless, it was an important intervention that may prove beneficial in the future. Finally, investigating all the places that Ms. CM "sits" proved to offer the key piece of information. Because highly functional wheelchair users may sit on a variety of surfaces, clinicians cannot presuppose that the cushion or wheelchair is always the causative factor in pressure ulcer formation.

SHOW WHAT YOU KNOW

1. The feature of a support surface primarily indicated for pulmonary therapy that provides rotation about a longitudinal axis as characterized by degree of patient turn, duration, and frequency is called:
   A. low-air-loss.
   B. alternating pressure.
   C. air-fluidized.
   D. lateral rotation.

   ANSWER: D. *Lateral rotation moves the patient side to side to aid pulmonary function, but unless a second feature is present such as low-air-loss, it's not appropriate for pressure ulcer prevention.*

2. The selection of an appropriate support surface depends on:
   A. the clinical condition of the patient.
   B. the characteristics of the support surface.
   C. the characteristics of the care setting.
   D. all of the above.

   ANSWER: D. *All are important considerations. A patient at home may have different needs than one in an acute care setting.*

3. Support surfaces are designed to:
   A. lower pressure.
   B. eliminate pressure.
   C. redistribute pressure.
   D. relieve pressure.

   ANSWER: C. *Support surfaces redistribute pressure.*

4. The ability of a support surface to distribute load over the contact areas of the human body is:
   A. immersion.
   B. envelopment.
   C. pressure gradient.
   D. pressure redistribution.

   ANSWER: D. *This is the revised NPUAP definition of pressure redistribution. Immersion is the depth of penetration into a support surface. Envelopment is the ability of a support surface to conform to the body irregularities. Pressure gradient is a change in pressure over a distance.*

REFERENCES

1. National Pressure Ulcer Advisory Panel and European Pressure Ulcer Advisory Panel. "Prevention and Treatment of Pressure Ulcers: Clinical Practice Guideline." Washington, DC: National Pressure Ulcer Advisory Panel, 2009.

2. Krouskop, T., and van Rijswijk, L. "Standardizing Performance-Based Criteria for Support Surfaces," *Ostomy Wound Management* 41(1):34-44, January-February 1995.

3. Rehabilitation Engineering and Assistive Technology Association of North America (RESNA) Wheelchair and Related Seating Standards Committee. Available at *www.resna.org*. Accessed October 5, 2010.

4. National Pressure Ulcer Advisory Panel (NPUAP) Support Surface Standard Initiative Committee. "Terms and Definitions Related to Support Surfaces." January 2007. Available at: *http://www.npuap.org/NPUAP_S3I_TD.pdf*. Accessed December 10, 2010.

5. Brienza, D., Kelsey, S., Karg, P., et al. "A Randomized Clinical Trial on Preventing Pressure Ulcers with Wheelchair Seat Cushions," *Journal of the American Geriatrics Society* 58:2308–14, 2010. doi: 10.1111/j.1532-5415.2010.03168.x

6. Cochran, G. "Identification and Control of Biophysical Factors Responsible for Soft Tissue Breakdown," *RSA Progress Report,* 1979.

7. Silver-Thorn, M. "In Vivo Indentation of Lower Extremity Limb Soft Tissues," *IEEE Transactions on Rehabilitation Engineering* 7(3): 268-77, September 1999.

8. Salcido, R., Fisher, S.B., Donofrio, J.C., Bieschke, M., Knapp, C., Liang, R., et al. "An Animal Model and Computer-Controlled Surface Pressure Delivery System for the Production of Pressure Ulcers." *Journal of Rehabilitation Research and Development* 32(2):149-161, 1995.

9. Bader, D.L. "The Recovery Characteristics of Soft Tissues Following Repeated Loading," *Journal of Rehabilitation Research and Development* 27(2): 141-150, 1990.

10. Newson, T.P., & Rolfe, P. "Skin Surface PO2 and Blood Flow Measurements over the Ischial Tuberosity," *Archives of Physical Medicine and Rehabilitation* 63(11):553-56, 1982.

11. Peirce, S.M., Skalak, T.C., & Rodeheaver, G.T. "Ischemia-Reperfusion Injury in Chronic Pressure Ulcer Formaion: A Skin Model in the Rat," *Wound Repair and Regeneration* 8(1):68-76, 2000.

12. Tsuji, S., Ichioka, S., Sekiya, N., & Nakatsuka, T. "Analysis of Ischemia-Reperfusion Injury in a Microcirculatory Model of Pressure Ulcers," *Wound Repair and Regeneration* 13(2):209-15, 2005.

13. Bouten, C.V., Knight, M.M., Lee, D.A., & Bader, D.L. "Compressive Deformation and Damage of Muscle Cell Subpopulations in a Model System," *Annals of Biomedical Engineering* 29:153-63, 2001.

14. Breuls, R.G.M., Bouten, C.V., Oomens, C.W., Bader, D.L., & Baaijens, F.P. "Compression Induced Cell Damage in Engineered Muscle Tissue: An in Vitro Model to Study Pressure Ulcer Aetiology," *Annals of BiomedicalEngineering* 31:1357-64, 2003.

15. Sae-Sia, W., Wipke-Tevis, D.D., Williams, D.A. "Elevated Sacral Skin Temperature (T(s)): A Risk Factor for Pressure Ulcer Development in Hospitalized Neurologically Impaired THAI Patients," *Applied Nursing Research* 18(1):29-35, February 2005.

16. Agency for Health Care Policy and Research. "Pressure Ulcers in Adults: Prediction and Prevention. AHCPR Clinical Practice Guideline No. 3." Publication No. 92-0047. Rockville, MD: Author; 1992.

17. Reswick, J., and Rogers, J. *Experiences at Rancho Los Amigos Hospital with Devices and Techniques to Prevent Pressure Sores. Bedsore Biomechanics.* London: University Park Press; 1976.

18. Krouskop, T.A. "A Synthesis of the Factors That Contribute to Pressure Sore Formation," *Medical Hypotheses* 11(2):255-67, June 1983.

19. Reddy, N.G., et al. "Interstitial Fluid Flow as a Factor in Decubitus Ulcer Formation," *Journal of Biomechanics* 14(12):879-81, December 1981.

20. Daniel, R.D., et al. "Etiologic Factors in Pressure Sores: An Experimental Model," *Archives of Physical Medicine and Rehabilitation* 62(10):492-98, October 1981.

21. Vistnes, L. "Pressure Sores: Etiology and Prevention," *Bulletin of Prosthetic Research* 17: 123-25, 1980.

22. Verhonick, P.D., et al. "Thermography in the Study of Decubitus Ulcers," *Nursing Research* 21:233-37, May-June 1972.

23. Patel, S.C., et al. "Temperature Effects on Surface Pressure-Induced Changes in Rat Skin Perfusion: Implications in Pressure Ulcer Development," *Journal of Rehabilitation Research and Development* 36(3):189-201, May-June 1999.

24. Kokate, J.K., et al. "Temperature-Modulated Pressure Ulcers: A Porcine Model," *Archives of hysical Medicine and Rehabilitation* 76(7):666-73, July 1995.

25. Brown, A., and Brengelmann, G. *Energy Metabolism. Physiology and Biophysics.* Philadelphia: W.B. Saunders Co.; 1965.

26. Fisher, S.T., et al. "Wheelchair Cushion Effect on Skin Temperature," *Archives of Physical Medicine and Rehabilitation* 59(2):68-72, February 1978.

27. Johnson, J.M., and Park, M. "Reflex Control of Skin Blood Flow by Skin Temperature: Role of Core Temperature," *Journal of Applied Physiology* 47(6):1188-93, December 1979.

28. Johnson, J.M., et al. "Reflex Regulation of Sweat Rate by Skin Temperature in Exercising Humans," *Journal of Applied Physiology* 56(5): 1283-88, May 1984.

29. Aronovitch, S. "A Comparative Study of an Alternating Air Mattress for the Prevention of Pressure Ulcers in Surgical Patients," *Ostomy Wound Management* 45(3):34-44, March 1999.

30. Yarkony, G. "Pressure Ulcers: A Review," *Archives of Physical Medicine and Rehabilitation* 75(8): 908-17, August 1994.

31. Sulzberger, M., et al. "Studies on Blisters Produced by Friction: Results of Linear Rubbing and Twisting Techniques," *Journal of Investigational Dermatology* 47(5):456-65, November 1966.

32. Wildnauer, R.H., et al. "Stratum Corneum Biomechanical Properties: Influence of Relative Humidity on Normal and Extracted Human Stratum Corneum," *Journal of Investigational Dermatology* 56(1):72-78, January 1971.

33. Geyer, M.J., et al. "A Randomized Control Trial to Evaluate Pressure-Reducing Seat Cushion for Elderly Wheelchair Users," *Advances in Skin & Wound Care* 14(3):120-29, May-June 2001.

34. Cochran, G.V., and Palmieri, V. "Development of Test Methods for Evaluation of Wheelchair Cushions," *Bulletin of Prosthetics Research* 33:9-30, Spring 1980.

35. Sprigle, S.L., et al. "Development of Uniform Terminology and Procedures to Describe Wheelchair Cushion Characteristics," *Journal of Rehabilitation Research and Development* 38(4): 449-61, July-August 2001.

36. Noble, P.C., et al. "The Influence of Environmental Aging Upon the Load-Bearing Properties of Polyurethane Foams," *Journal of Rehabilitation Research and Development* 21(2):31-38, July 1984.

37. Krouskop, T., et al. "Evaluating the Long-Term Performance of a Foam-Core Hospital Replacement Mattress," *Journal of Wound, Ostomy and Continence Nursing* 21(6):241-46, November 1994.

38. Sprigle, S., et al. "Reduction of Sitting Pressures with Custom Contoured Cushions," *Journal of Rehabilitation Research and Development* 27(2): 135-40, Spring 1990.

39. Brienza, D.M., et al. "A System for the Analysis of Seat Support Surfaces Using Surface Shape Control and Simultaneous Measurement of Applied Pressures," *IEEE Transactions on Rehabilitation Engineering* 4(2):103-13, June 1996.

40. Brienza, D.M., and Karg, P.E. "Seat Cushion Optimization: A Comparison of Interface Pressure and Tissue Stiffness Characteristics for Spinal Cord Injured and Elderly Patients," *Archives of Physical Medicine and Rehabilitation* 79(4):388-94, April 1998.

41. Stewart, S., et al. "Wheelchair Cushion Effect on Skin Temperature, Heat Flux and Relative Humidity," *Archives of Physical Medicine and Rehabilitation* 61(5):229-33, May 1980.

42. Wells, J., and Karr, D. "Interface Pressure, Wound Healing and Satisfaction in the Evaluation of a Non-Powered Fluid Mattress," *Ostomy Wound Management* 44(2):38-54, February 1998.

43. Peltier, G., et al. "Controlled Air Suspension: An Advantage in Burn Care," *Journal of Burn Care Research* 8(6):558-60, November-December 1987.

44. Holzapfel, S. "Support Surfaces and their Use in the Prevention and Treatment of Pressure Ulcers," *Journal of Enterostomal Nursing* 20(6): 251-60, November-December 1993.

45. Weaver, V., and Jester, J. "A Clinical Tool: Updated Readings on Tissue Interface Pressure," *Ostomy Wound Management* 40(5):34-43, June 1994.

46. Gunther, R., and Brofeldt, B. "Increased Lymphatic Flow: Effect of a Pulsating Air Suspension Bed System," *Wounds: A Compendium of Clinical Research and Practice* 8(4):134-40, 1996.

47. Anderson, C., and Rappl, L. "Lateral Rotation Mattress for Wound Healing," *Ostomy Wound Management* 50(4): 50-4, 56, 58, April 2004.

48. Engstrom, B. Seating for Independence. *Ergonomic Seating and Propulsion Improves Performance.* Presentation, Pittsburgh, PA, August 1997.

49. Waugh, K. *Therapeutic Seating I: Principles and Assessment.* Pittsburgh, PA: RESNA, 1997.

50. Minkel, J. "Seating and Mobility Considerations for People with Spinal Cord Injuries," *Physical Therapy* 80(7):701-709, July 2000.

51. Braden, B.J., and Bergstrom, N. "Clinical Utility of the Braden Scale for Predicting Pressure Sore Risk," *Decubitus* 2(3):44-46, 50-51, August 1989.

52. Norton, D. "Norton Scale for Decubitus Prevention," [German] *Krankenpflege* 34(1):16, 1980.

53. Waterlow, J. "Pressure Sores: A Risk Assessment Card," *Nursing Times* 81(48):49-55, November 27-December 3, 1985.

54. Braden, B., and Bergstrom, N. "Predictive Validity of the Braden Scale for Pressure Sore Risk in a Nursing Home Population," *Research in Nursing and Health* 17(6):459-70, December 1994.

55. Anthony, D., et al. "An Evaluation of Current Risk Assessment Scales for Decubitus Ulcer in General Inpatients and Wheelchair Users," *Clinical Rehabilitation* 12(2):136-42, April 1998.

56. Bergstrom, N., et al. "Using a Research-Based Assessment Scale in Clinical Practice," *Nursing Clinics of North America* 30(3):539-50, September 1995.

57. Krouskop, T.A., et al. "Custom Selection of Support Surfaces for Wheelchairs and Beds: One Size Doesn't Fit All," *Dermatology Nursing* 4(3):191-94, 204, June 1992.

58. Henderson, J.L., et al. "Efficacy of Three Measures to Relieve Pressure in Seated Persons with Spinal Cord Injury," *Archives of Physical Medicine and Rehabilitation* 75(5):535-39, May 1994.

59. Agency for Health Care Policy and Research. "Treatment of Pressure Ulcers," Publication No. 95-0652, 1994. Available at: *http://www.ncbi.nlm.nih.gov/books/NBK12202/*. Accessed December 10, 2010.

60. Consortium for Spinal Cord Medicine. *Pressure Ulcer Prevention and Treatment Following Spinal Cord Injury: A Clinical Practice Guideline for Health-Care Professionals.* Washington, DC: Paralyzed Veterans of America, 2000.

61. Krouskop, T. "Scientific Aspects of Pressure Relief." IAET Annual Conference, Washington, DC, 1989.

62. ISO/CD 16840-3: *Wheelchair Seating-Part 3: Postural Support Devices.* Committee Draft, International Organization for Standardization, June 2002.

63. National Pressure Ulcer Advisory Panel. *NPUAP's Research tab, Support Surface Standards Initiative*

(S3I). April 2003. Available at *www.npuap.org.* Accessed December 30, 2010.

64. Whittemore, R. "Pressure-Reduction Support Surfaces: A Review of the Literature," *Journal of Wound, Ostomy and Continence Nursing* 25(1):6-25, January 1998.

65. Cullum, N. "Evaluation of Studies of Treatment or Prevention Interventions. Part 2: Applying the Results of Studies to Your Patients," *Evidence-Based Nursing* 4(1):7-8, January 2001.

66. Cullum, N., et al. "Beds, Mattresses, and Cushions for Pressure Sore Prevention and Treatment," *Nursing Times* 97(19):41, May 10-16, 2001.

67. Thomas, D.R. "Issues and Dilemmas in the Prevention and Treatment of Pressure Ulcers: A Review," *Journals of Gerontology, Series A, Biological Sciences and Medical Sciences* 56(6):328-40, 2001.

68. Rithalia, S.V., and Kenney, L. "Mattresses and Beds: Reducing and Relieving Pressure," *Nursing Times* 96(36 Suppl):9-10, September 7, 2000.

69. Cullum, N., et al. "Preventing and Treating Pressure Sores," *Quality in Health Care* 4(4): 289-297, December 1995.

70. Lazzara, D.J., and Buschmann, M.T. "Prevention of Pressure Ulcers in Elderly Nursing Home Residents: Are Special Support Surfaces the Answer?" *Decubitus* 4(4):42-48, November 1991.

71. Lim, R., et al. "Clinical Trial of Foam Cushions in the Prevention of Decubitus Ulcers in Elderly Patients," *Journal of Rehabilitation Research and Development* 25(2):19-26, Spring 1988.

72. Conine, T., et al. "Pressure Ulcer Prophylaxis in Elderly Patients Using Polyurethane Foam or Jay Wheelchair Cushions," *International Journal of Rehabilitation Research* 17(2):123-37, June 1994.

73. Brienza, D.M., et al. "The Relationship Between Pressure Ulcer Incidence and Buttock-Seat Cushion Interface Pressure in At-Risk Elderly Wheelchair Users," *Archives of Physical Medicine and Rehabilitation* 82(4):529-33, April 2001.

74. Centers for Medicare and Medicaid Services. "Nursing Home Quality Initiative: MDS 3.0 for Nursing Homes and Swing Bed Providers." Available at *http://www.cms.hhs.gov/ Nursinghomequalityinits/25_NHQIMDS30.asp.* Accessed December 10, 2010.

75. Allen, V. et al. "Air-Fluidized Beds and Their Ability to Distribute Interface Pressures Generated Between the Subject and the Bed Surface," *Physiological Measurement* 14(3):359-64, August 1993.

76. Munro, B.H., et al. "Pressure Ulcers: One Bed or Another?" *Geriatric Nursing* 10(4):190-92, July-August 1989.

77. Kosiak, M. "Etiology of Decubitus Ulcers," *Archives of Physical Medicine and Rehabilitation* 42(1):19-28, January 1961.

78. Bliss, M.R. "Pressure Sore Management and Prevention," in Brocklehurst, J.C., et al., eds., *Textbook of Geriatric Medicine and Gerontology,* 4th ed. London: Churchill Livingstone, 1992.

79. Knox, D.M., et al. "Effects of Different Turn Intervals on Skin of Healthy Older Adults," *Advances in Wound Care* 7(1):48-56, January 1994.

80. Defloor, T., Grydonck, M., De Bacquer, D. "The Effect of Various Combinations of Turning and Pressure Reducing Devices on the Incidence of Pressure Ulcers," *International Journal of Nursing Studies* 4(3):422-50, 2005.

81. Vanderwee, K., Grypdonck, M.H., De, B.D., Defloor, T. "Effectiveness of Turning with Unequal Time Intervals on the Incidence of Pressure Ulcer Lesions," *Journal of Advanced Nursing* 57(1):59-68, 2007.

82. Wound, Ostomy and Continence Nurses Society (WOCN). *Guideline for Prevention and Management of Pressure Ulcers.* Glenview, IL: Author, 2003.

83. Cuddigan, J.E., Ayello, E.A., Black, J. "Saving Heels in Critically Ill Patients," *World Council of Enterostomal Therapists Journal* 28(2):16-24, 2008.

84. Abu-Own, A., et al. "Effects of Compression and Type of Bed Surface on the Microcirculation of the Heel," *European Journal of Vascular and Endovascular Surgery* 9(3):327-34, April 1995.

85. Petrie, L.A., and Hummel, R.S. III. "A Study of Interface Pressure for Pressure Reduction and Relief Mattresses," *Journal of Enterostomal Therapy* 17(5):212-16, September-October 1990.

86. Zernike, W. "Preventing Heel Pressure Sores: A Comparison of Heel Pressure Relieving Devices," *Journal of Clinical Nursing* 3(6):375-80, November 1994.

87. Zernike, W. "Heel Pressure Relieving Devices: How Effective Are They?" *Australian Journal of Advanced Nursing* 14(4):12-19, June-August 1997.

88. Cheneworth, C.C., et al. "Portrait of Practice: Healing Heel Ulcers," *Advances in Wound Care* 7(2):44-48, March 1994.

89. Cheney, A.M. "Portrait of Practice: A Successful Approach to Preventing Heel Pressure Ulcers After Surgery," *Decubitus* 6(4):39-40, July 1993.

90. Flemister, B.G. "A Pilot Study of Interface Pressure with Heel Protectors Used for Pressure Reduction," *Journal of Enterostomal Nursing* 18(5):158-61, September-October 1991.

91. Moody, B., et al. "Impact of Staff Education on Pressure Sore Development in Elderly Hospitalized Patients," *Archives of Internal Medicine* 148(10):2241-243, October 1988.

CHAPTER 12

Pain Management and Wounds

Linda E. Dallam, MS, RN-BC, GNP-BC, CWCN-AP
Christine Barkauskas, BA, RN, CWOCN, APN
Elizabeth A. Ayello, PhD, RN, ACNS-BC, CWON, MAPWCA, FAAN
Sharon Baranoski, MSN, RN, CWCN, APN-CCRN, DAPWCA, FAAN
R. Gary Sibbald, BSc, MD, MEd, FRCPC (Med Derm), MACP, FAAD, MAPWCA

Objectives

After completing this chapter, you'll be able to:

- define and identify the components of wound-associated pain
- describe the similarities and differences of pain associated with various types of chronic wounds
- utilize two validated tools for your patients to rate their pain related to a chronic wound
- assess the advantages and disadvantages of wound pain treatment modalities.

ETIOLOGY AND DEFINITIONS OF PAIN

Pain has an element of blank;
It cannot recollect
When it began, or if there were
A day when it was not.
— EMILY DICKINSON

As clinicians, we have a tendency to identify certain types of wounds as having pain of a specific type or amount. However, pain is what the patient states it is—not what we believe it to be. Our responsibility as clinicians is to assess the patient's pain accurately and treat it adequately, without judging the patient or doubting that the pain is as described. Pain is often more important to patients than it is to clinicians, with surveys indicating that pain is the most important parameter for many patients but is often only the third or fourth priority for clinicians.

There are several definitions of pain in the literature. Both the 1979 International Association for the Study of Pain (IASP) Subcommittee on Taxonomy[1] and the Agency for Healthcare Research and Quality (AHRQ, formerly the Agency for Healthcare Policy and Research, or AHCPR)[2] support a common definition of pain. They have defined pain as *"an unpleasant sensory and emotional experience associated with actual or potential tissue damage or described in terms of such damage."*[1,2]

Another commonly used pain definition is that of McCaffery and colleagues,[3,4] who state that "pain is whatever the experiencing person says it is and exists whenever he says it does." This definition of pain encompasses the subjective component and acknowledges the patient as the best judge of his or her own pain experience. Experts in the field of pain have come to accept that the patient's self-reporting of pain, including its characteristics and intensity, encompasses the most reliable assessment. This belief that the patient in pain is his or her own best judge is also accepted as the basis for pain assessment and management by such regulatory agencies as the Joint Commission, formerly known as the Joint

295

Commission on Accreditation of Healthcare Organizations[5] as well as such professional organizations as the American Pain Society (APS).[6]

TYPES OF PAIN

Pain can be nociceptive, neuropathic, or have components of both as commonly experienced with wound-associated pain. Nociceptive pain can result from ongoing activation of primary afferent neurons by noxious stimuli, with an intact nervous system. Neuropathic pain is initiated or caused by a primary lesion or dysfunction of the nervous system.[7]

The two types of nociceptive pain are somatic and visceral. Somatic pain arises from bone, skin, muscle, or connective tissue. It's usually gnawing, aching, tender, or throbbing and well localized. Pressure ulcer pain is usually somatic in nature. Visceral pain arises from the visceral organs such as the gut or from an obstruction of a hollow viscous organ, as occurs with a blockage of the small bowel. Visceral pain is poorly localized and is commonly described as cramping. Both types of nociceptive pain respond well to non-opioid and opioid pain medication.

In neuropathic pain, there's abnormal processing of the sensory input by the peripheral or central nervous system (CNS). The pain is typically described as having burning, stabbing, stinging, shooting, or electrical characteristics. Diabetic neurotrophic foot ulcer pain and the pain of shingles are examples of neuropathic pain. Neuropathic pain responds more readily to adjuvant agents, including tricyclic antidepressants or anticonvulsant therapy. Tricyclic antidepressants, such as amitriptyline, nortriptyline, or desipramine, are good choices because of their high anti-noradrenaline activity.

Amitriptyline is a first-generation tricyclic agent with almost equal anti-noradrenalin, anti-histamine, anti-serotonin, and anti-adrenergic actions. Nortriptyline is a second-generation tricyclic that has higher anti-noradrenalin activity at a lower dose, with fewer side effects such as double vision, dry mouth, and urinary retention. Desipramine has the same advantages as noradrenalin with less drowsiness. If tricyclic agents are not tolerated or provide inadequate relief of neuropathic pain at reasonable dosages, then anticonvulsants, such as gabapentin and its derivative pregabalin, should be considered. Indeed, gabapentin has been shown to be useful in treating neuropathic pain.[8] Pregabalin has also proved to be useful in the treatment of neuropathic pain, with studies demonstrating a benefit in painful post-herpetic neuropathy[9] and painful diabetic neuropathy.[10] Both gabapentin and pregabalin require dose adjustments in patients with renal disease.

Pain can also be acute or persistent (chronic). Acute pain has a distinct onset, with an obvious cause and short duration, and is usually associated with acute wounds, subsiding as healing takes place. Chronic pain can be from a chronic wound or other long-term disease, such as cancer. If it persists for 3 months or more, chronic pain is usually associated with functional and psychological impairment. Chronic pain can fluctuate in character and intensity.

The American Geriatric Society (AGS)[11] supports the terminology of "persistent" pain rather than "chronic" pain to circumvent the negative stereotypes that have been associated with the word "chronic." The AGS Clinical Practice Guideline, "The management of persistent pain in older persons," states: "Unfortunately, for many elderly persons, chronic pain has become a label associated with negative images and stereotypes commonly associated with long-standing psychiatric problems, futility in treatment, malingering, or drug-seeking behavior. Persistent pain may foster a more positive attitude by patients and professionals for the many effective treatments that are available to help alleviate suffering."[11]

Persistent and acute wound-associated pain can occur at the same time; similarly, nociceptive and neuropathic pain may occur simultaneously. Wound pain is often a combination of nociceptive and neuropathic pain. It may be compounded by an inflammatory process that occurs from local tissue damage due to surgery, infection, trauma, or other inflammatory conditions. Inflammation is characterized by redness, heat, and swelling and has been associated with an increased sensitivity to pain in and around the wound site.[12-14] This pain usually resolves when the condition that provoked the inflammation is controlled. Ischemic changes have also been implicated as a contributing factor to incisional pain.[12] All types of pain can be associated with functional or psychosocial losses and can affect quality of life or the quality of spiritual, social, emotional, and physical decline associated with dying. Pain can be debilitating and can also cause suffering beyond its physical component.

PRACTICE POINT

Reframing the phrase "patient complains of pain" to "patient reports pain" may help to foster a more positive and objective way for practitioners and caregivers to connect with the patient's experience of pain. Use the term *persistent pain* rather than *chronic pain*.

The persistent (chronic) pain experience

Krasner[15-17] has conceptualized pain in chronic wounds as the chronic wound pain experience. Within this model, pain is divided into three categories: noncyclic, cyclic, and chronic pain. *Noncyclic* or *incident* pain is defined as a single episode of pain that might occur, for example, after wound debridement. *Cyclic* or *episodic* pain recurs as the result of repeated treatments, such as dressing changes or turning and repositioning. *Chronic* or *continuous* pain is persistent and occurs without manipulation of the patient or the wound. For example, the patient may feel that the wound is throbbing even when he or she is lying still in bed and with no treatment occurring at the local wound site. (See *Practice Point: Interventions for noncyclic wound pain*. See also *Practice*

PRACTICE POINT
Interventions for Noncyclic Wound Pain

- Identify and develop a pain treatment plan for potentially painful procedures.
- Administer topical or local anesthetics.
- Consider an operating room procedure under general anesthesia rather than bedside debridement for large, deep ulcers.
- Administer opioids and/or nonsteroidal anti-inflammatory drugs before and after procedures.
- Assess and reassess for pain before, during and after procedures.
- Avoid using wet-to-dry dressings.
- Consider alternatives to surgical/sharp debridement, such as transparent dressings, hydrogels, hydrocolloids, hypertonic saline solutions, or enzymatic agents.[14]

Point: Interventions for cyclic wound pain, page 298, and Practice Point: Interventions for persistent [chronic] wound pain, page 298.)

Pain and wound types

The type of pain a patient experiences depends largely on the type of wound present. Pain can occur in patients with acute and chronic wounds and can be related or unrelated to the wound or its cause. Clinicians should determine whether pain is generalized, regionalized, or related directly to the wound bed. Regional pain often relates to the wound cause. Localized wound pain may relate to local wound manipulation, treatment modalities, or infection.[18] Gardner and Frantz[18] identified increased wound-associated pain as a potential symptom of infection. This section discusses various types of wounds and the types of pain that accompany them.

PRESSURE ULCER PAIN

Pain at the site of a pressure ulcer is supported by pressure ulcer experts and anecdotal reports by clinicians, although few studies concerning pressure ulcer pain have been published.

PRACTICE POINT

Interventions for Cyclic Wound Pain

- Perform interventions at a time of day when the patient is less fatigued.
- Provide analgesia 30 to 60 minutes before dressing change.
- Assess the patient for pain before, during, and after dressing changes.
- Provide analgesia 30 to 60 minutes before whirlpool.
- If the patient's dressing has dried out, thoroughly soak the dressing— especially the edges—prior to removal.
- Observe the wound for signs of local infection.
- Gently and thoroughly cleanse or irrigate the wound to remove debris and reduce the bacterial bioburden, which can cause contaminated wounds to become infected. Infection will increase the inflammation and pain at the wound site.
- Avoid using cytotoxic topical agents.

- Avoid aggressive packing. (Fluff; do not stuff!)
- Avoid drying out the wound bed and wound edges.
- Protect the periwound area with sealants, ointments, or moisture barriers.
- Minimize the number of daily dressing changes.
- Select pain-reducing dressings that include moisture balance and avoid aggressive adhesives.
- Avoid using tape on fragile skin.
- Splint or immobilize the wounded area as needed.
- Utilize pressure-reducing devices in bed or chair.
- Provide analgesia as needed to allow positioning of patient.
- Avoid trauma (shearing and tear injuries) to fragile skin when transferring, positioning, or holding a patient.

PRACTICE POINT

Interventions for Persistent (Chronic) Wound Pain

- Use all of the interventions listed for non-cyclic and cyclic wound pain.
- Control edema.
- Control infection.
- Monitor wound pain while the patient is at rest (at times when no dressing change is taking place).
- Control pain to allow healing and positioning.
- Provide regularly scheduled analgesia, including opioids, patient-controlled analgesia, and topical preparations such as lidocaine gel 2%, depending on the severity of pain.
- Attend to non-wound associated pain from:
  - co-morbid pain syndromes such as contractures and diabetes

  - iatrogenic device insertions, such as central lines, venous puncture sites, catheters, feeding tubes, blood gas drawing, or other equipment or procedures.

- Address the emotional component of the pain or the patient's suffering:
  - What does the wound represent to the patient?
  - What does pain mean? Is it associated with loss of function?
  - Has the wound altered the patient's body image?
  - Did unrelieved pain alter the patient's mental status or behavior?

At its first conference in 1989, the National Pressure Ulcer Advisory Panel (NPUAP) stated that "pressure ulcers are serious wounds that cause considerable pain, suffering, disability, and even death."[19] Van Rijswijk and Braden[20] reevaluated the AHCPR Treatment of Pressure Ulcer guidelines in light of studies published after the guidelines were released in 1994[21] and reaffirmed the panel's first recommendation about assessing pressure ulcer patients for pain. Based on additional evidence from studies supporting pain reduction with the use of moisture-retentive dressings, however, van Rijswijk and Braden[20] proposed that the 1994 AHCPR recommendations concerning pain and pressure ulcers be rewritten.

The etiology of pain in patients with pressure ulcers isn't known. Pieper[22] quotes the work of Rook[23] and suggests that the common sources of pressure ulcer pain are from the "release of noxious chemicals from damaged tissue, erosion of tissue planes with destruction of nerve terminals, regeneration of nociceptive nerve terminals, infection, dressing changes, and debridement." In stage III or IV pressure ulcers, this pain may come from ischemic necrosis of the tissue triggered by a deep tissue injury or shear forces. Superficial stage II ulcers may be associated with skin surface pain from moisture, friction, or shear injuries.

According to a study by Szors and Bourguignon,[24] pressure ulcer pain depends not only on the stage of the ulcer but also on whether a dressing change is taking place at the time the assessment is made. The majority of patients in their study (88%) reported pressure ulcer pain with dressing changes; a lower number of patients (84%) had persistent pain at rest. Patients rated the pain from sore to excruciating. Seventy-five percent rated their pain as mild, discomforting, or distressing; 18% rated their pain as horrible or excruciating. Clinicians need to ensure adequate pain control for patients with persistent pain with long-acting pain and breakthrough medication; they must also time the breakthrough medication so that it is effective against the pain experienced at dressing change. In addition, appropriate cleansing and debridement methods and suitable dressings need to be chosen that will minimize pain and trauma at the time of removal and reapplication.

ARTERIAL ULCER PAIN

Pain associated with peripheral vascular disease can be due to intermittent claudication or to rest pain with advanced disease that may be more prominent at night with leg elevation. Intermittent claudication pain results from physical exertion or exercise-induced ischemia and has been described as cramping, burning, or aching. The blood flow with exertion is inadequate to meet the needs of tissues. Patients can employ several tactics to relieve pain. The most important are to stop smoking, start gradual and regular exercises, lose weight, and have vascular risk factors treated.

Nocturnal pain may have the same symptoms but usually precedes the occurrence of rest pain. Rest pain occurs—even without activity—when blood flow is inadequate to meet the needs of tissues in the extremities. These types of pain are described as a sensation of burning or numbness aggravated by leg elevation where gravity no longer can facilitate local blood flow. The pain is constant and intense, and isn't easily relieved by pain medications. Pain can sometimes be alleviated by stopping the activity or exercise and placing the legs in a dangling or dependent position.

VENOUS ULCER PAIN

Venous ulcer pain can have several possible sources:

- Edema due to extravasated fluid from the capillaries
- Inflammation of woody fibrosis: acute or subacute lipodermatosclerosis
- Bacterial damage:
  - Superficial increased bacterial burden (NERDS©[25])
  - Deep and surrounding skin cellulitis (STONES©[25])
- Inflammation of the veins: superficial and deep phlebitis

The range of venous ulcer pain is extensive; the patient may report mildly annoying pain, a dull ache, or sharp, deep muscle pain. Pain is more intense at the end of the day secondary to edema resulting from the legs being in a dependent position and is often aggravated by standing, sitting, or crossing the legs. The pathophysiology of venous disease is related to reduction or occlusion of blood return to the heart. Incompetent superficial, perforating, or deep veins can cause pooling of fluid in the legs leading to pitting edema and resultant pain. To minimize pain, patients should be instructed to elevate the legs when sitting and encouraged to wear support stockings. Stocking selection is based on accurate individualized measurement, and their effectiveness relies on putting them on before the legs are placed on the floor in the morning. Other clinical management goals that help to minimize venous disease–related edema include the avoidance of prolonged sitting, weight reduction, and smoking cessation.

Thrombus formation in the deep veins can lead to leg swelling and pain, mimicking an infection or superficial phlebitis. The patient may report localized tenderness and pain over the long and short saphenous veins. Increased bacterial burden in the superficial wound bed can lead to delayed healing and localized pain. Clinicians should look for NERDS©—non-healing wounds; increased exudate; red, friable granulation tissue; new debris or slough on the surface; and an unpleasant smell or odor. (For more information about NERDS and STONES, see chapter 7, Wound bioburden and infection, and *color section, NERDS*©, page C7, and *STONES*©, pages C8–C9.)

When venous disease has been present for a long period of time, the veins become leaky with fibrin extravasation into the dermis (woody fibrosis). In addition, red blood cells can leak into the tissue, causing staining that's often referred to as hemosiderin and hyperpigmentation. The woody fibrosis does not go away at the end of the day, and patients can have acute and chronic inflammatory changes within the woody fibrosis, leading to acute and chronic lipodermatosclerosis-type pain.

NEUROPATHIC ULCER PAIN

Neuropathy is the most common complication of diabetes. The amount of pain present depends on the severity of the neuropathy.

Unlike stimulus-dependent nociceptive pain, neuropathic pain is spontaneous. The patient may state that the pain interferes with his or her entire life—especially the ability to sleep. The affected extremity may feel like it's asleep ("a block of wood") or have the "pins and needles" pain that occurs after a part of the body has "fallen asleep" and starts to wake up. The quality of pain can be burning, stinging, stabbing, or shooting and may include increased skin sensitivity to non-noxious stimuli (allodynia) and itching. True pain relief is accomplished primarily with pharmacologic intervention. All pain needs to be assessed adequately to ascertain the most effective treatment modality. If a patient reports excessive pain in a neuropathic limb that hasn't had pain before, an infection or acute Charcot joint changes may be developing.

Patients with diabetes lose protective sensation after 10 to 15 years. This loss of protective sensation allows these individuals to undergo sharp surgical debridement without nociceptive pain, although they may have referred pain in the leg or foot. If persistent nociceptive pain develops in a neuropathic limb, it usually means there's disruption of the deeper structures. In a person with a foot ulcer, clinicians should check for underlying osteomyelitis. If a patient has a tender, swollen foot without ulceration and an increase in skin surface temperature, there's a strong possibility of a Charcot joint. Occasionally, a patient may have both osteomyelitis and a Charcot joint.

> ### ▶ PRACTICE POINT
>
> Determining whether pain results from neuropathy or is associated with peripheral vascular disease is extremely important because patients with diabetes have a high incidence of peripheral vascular disease. In addition, pain in a painless foot usually indicates disruption of the deeper structures and a strong possibility of associated osteomyelitis, Charcot foot, or even both conditions co-existing.

UNDERSTANDING WOUND PAIN

Most of our understanding of wound pain comes from literature about other diseases.[26] Clinicians are increasingly acknowledging that pain is a major issue for patients suffering from many different types of wounds.[26] (See *Practice Point: Pain: what we know, what we don't know.*) Several consensus statements and other documents regarding wound pain during dressing changes are available to help clinicians manage this type of pain properly.

International guidelines

The European Wound Management Association (EWMA)[27] has developed a position document on wound pain titled "Pain at wound dressing changes." The document is subdivided into three sections:

- Understanding wound pain and trauma from an international perspective[28]
- The theory of pain[29]
- Pain at wound dressing changes: A guide to management[30]

In the first section of the document, Moffat and colleagues[27] surveyed 3,918 healthcare professionals from the United States and 10 countries in Western and Eastern Europe. The survey respondents indicated that pain prevention was the second highest ranking

---

PRACTICE POINT

Pain: what we know, what we don't know

McCaffery and Robinson[4] reported on nurses' self-evaluation of their knowledge about pain.

- Observable changes in vital signs must be relied upon to verify a patient's report of severe pain: False (answered correctly by 88.4%).
- Pain intensity should be rated by the clinician, not the patient: False (answered correctly by 99.1%).
- A patient may sleep in spite of moderate or severe pain: True (answered correctly by 90.6%).
- Intramuscular (IM) meperidine is the drug of choice for prolonged pain: False (answered correctly by 85.6%).
- Analgesics for chronic pain are more effective when administered as needed rather than around the clock: False (answered correctly by 92.7%).
- If the patient can be distracted from the pain, he has less pain than he reports: False (answered correctly by 94.7%).
- The patient in pain should be encouraged to endure as much pain as possible before resorting to a pain relief measure: False (answered correctly by 98.4%).
- Respiratory depression (less than 7 breaths per minute) probably occurs in at least 10% of patients who receive one or more doses of an opioid for

relief of pain: False (answered correctly by 60.5%; clinicians tend to exaggerate the risk of respiratory depression with opioid use; according to McCaffery and Robinson, the risk is less than 1%).
- Vicodin (hydrocodone 5 mg and acetaminophen 500 mg) is approximately equal to the analgesia of one-half of a dose of meperidine 75 mg IM: False (correctly answered by 48.3%).
- If a patient's pain is relieved by a placebo, the pain isn't real: False (answered correctly by 86.1%).
- Beyond a certain dose, increasing the dosage of an opioid such as morphine won't increase pain relief: False (answered correctly by 57.2%).
- Research shows that promethazine reliably potentiates opioid analgesics: False (correctly answered by 35.1%).
- When opioids are used for pain relief under the following circumstances, what percentage of patients is likely to develop opioid addiction?
  - Patients who receive opioids for 1 to 3 days: Answer is less than 1% (correctly answered by 82.8%).
  - Patients who receive opioids for 3 to 6 months: Answer is less than 1% (correctly answered by 26.7%).

consideration at dressing change, with trauma prevention being first.[27] Pain from leg ulcers was ranked as the most severe pain compared with other wound types, and dressing removal caused the greatest pain.[23]

A copy of this EWMA position document can be found on the Internet and is available in Dutch, English, French, German, Italian, and Spanish. (See *EWMA suggestions for preparing the wound pain environment*.)

Another international consensus statement was developed by the World Union of Wound Healing Societies (WUWHS).[31] This document, entitled "Principles of best practice: Minimizing pain at wound dressing related procedures," outlines common pain management challenges, myths, and misunderstandings that are useful for improved clinical practice during wound dressing changes. (See *Dispelling myths about wound pain*.) This

document also includes helpful suggestions for care planning and treatment interventions. (See *WUWHS procedural wound pain interventions*, page 304.)

Lastly, a third international document (not a consensus statement), addresses the management of pain associated with burns. This document is titled "The management of pain associated with dressing changes in patients with burns" and can be found in the electronic wound care journal, *World Wide Wounds*.[32]

Pain research: pressure ulcers

NURSING MANAGEMENT

Nursing management of patients with pressure ulcers sometimes does not adequately address the component of pain management. Hollingworth[26] determined that nurses' assessment, management, and documentation of pain after completing a wound dressing change was inadequate. Likewise, in a qualitative study that examined the reflections of 42 general and advanced practice nurses, Krasner[33] identified three distinct patterns nurses used to address pressure ulcer pain in their patients—nursing expertly, denying the pain, and confronting the challenge of pain:

1. Nursing expertly
   • Reading the pain
   • Attending to the pain
   • Acknowledging and empathizing with the patient
2. Denying the pain
   • Assuming that it doesn't exist
   • Not hearing the cries
   • Avoiding failure
3. Confronting the challenge of pain
   • Coping with frustration
   • Being with the patient.[33]

Krasner[16,17,33] suggested that clinicians use this information to provide more patient-centered sensitive care for patients with pressure ulcer pain.

THE PATIENT'S PAIN EXPERIENCE

Few studies (four quantitative and five qualitative) have been published concerning the pain experience of patients with pressure ulcers. Variability in pain perceptions can be influenced by many contextual and psychological

---

EWMA suggestions for preparing the wound pain environment [27-30]

Prepare, plan, prevant

• Choose an appropriate non-stressful environment, close windows, turn off mobile phones, etc.
• Explain to the patient in simple terms what will be done and the method used.
• Assess the need for skilled or unskilled assistance, such as help with simple hand holding.
• Be thoughtful in positioning the patient to minimize discomfort and avoid unnecessary contact or exposure.
• Avoid prolonged exposure of the wound, (e.g., waiting for specialist advice).
• Avoid any unnecessary stimulus to the wound and handle wounds gently, being aware that any slight touch can cause pain.
• Involve the patient throughout; frequent verbal checks and use of pain tools offer real-time feedback.
• Consider preventive analgesia.

Dispelling myths about wound pain

In its international consensus statement,[31] WUWHS outlines several myths related to wound pain.

- **Myth:** Wet-to-dry dressing are still the gold standard for wound care.
- **Fact:** Adherent gauze can disrupt delicate healing tissue and provoke severe pain.
- **Myth:** Transparent films are the best dressing for treating and reducing the pain of skin tears and other minor acute wounds.
- **Fact:** The misuse of transparent films is a common cause of skin tears.
- **Myth:** Using paper tape is the least painful way to secure a dressing.
- **Fact:** Heightened nerve sensation in a wide area around a wound can make adhesive tape painful to remove.
- **Myth:** Pulling a dressing off faster rather than slower reduces pain at dressing changes.
- **Fact:** This method has the potential to inflict tissue damage and traumatic pain.

- **Myth:** Using a skin sealant on periwound skin reduces the risk of pain and trauma.
- **Fact:** Skin sealants only create a thin topical layer and do not protect deeper dermal layers.
- **Myth:** People with diabetic foot wounds do not experience pain.
- **Fact:** There may be some loss of peripheral nerve sensation, but sensitivity in the area can be heightened.
- **Myth:** Pain comes from the wound. The surrounding tissue nerves play little role.
- **Fact:** Spinal-cord responses to incoming pain signals can give rise to abnormal sensitivity in the surrounding area (allodynia).
- **Myth:** The only way to treat wound pain is by oral analgesic, 30 to 60 minutes before dressing changes.
- **Fact:** An oral analgesic can give some relief but should not be seen as a single solution. A full pain assessment must be used to evaluate and fine-tune any prescribed therapy.

(patient-centered) factors. Woo[34] examined 96 patients with chronic wounds to determine whether anxiety or anticipatory pain played a role in the intensity of pain experienced at dressing changes. He uncovered a direct relationship between anxiety related to impending pain that subsequently intensified the experienced pain intensity. With heightened anxiety, environmental and somatic signals are brought to the patient's attention, sharpening the degree of sensory receptivity and reducing pain tolerance. Woo documented that certain individuals who are insecure in their relationship with others were susceptible to experiencing anxiety and intensified pain.[34]

The first study to quantify pain by pressure ulcer stage was completed by Dallam and colleagues,[14] who studied the perceived intensity and patterns of pressure ulcer pain in hospitalized patients. The study population was diverse, with 66% being white (non-Hispanic)

and the remainder being black (non-Hispanic), Hispanic, or Asian. Of the 132 patients enrolled in the study, 44 (33.3%) were respondents and 88 (66.7%) were non-respondents because they couldn't communicate responses to the instruments (language and other cognitive barriers). Two different scales were used to measure pain intensity: the Visual Analog Scale (VAS) and the Faces Pain Rating Scale (FPRS). (See the next section for additional discussion of these pain scales.) The authors found a high degree of agreement between the two pain scales. They also noted that the FPRS was easier to use for patients who were cognitively impaired or for whom English was their second language.

The major findings of this important study include the following[14]:

- The majority of patients with pressure ulcers had pain (68% of respondents reported some type of pain).

WUWHS procedural wound pain interventions

The following planning and treatment suggestions from WUWHS[31] can be helpful in caring for patients with wound pain:

- Be aware of the current status of pain.
- Know pain triggers, and avoid them where possible.
- Know and use pain reducers (when possible and not contraindicated).
- Avoid unnecessary manipulation of the wound.
- Explore with the patient simple distraction techniques, such as counting up and down, focusing on the breath entering and leaving the lungs, or listening to music.
- Reconsider management choices if pain becomes intolerable, and document as an adverse event.
- Observe the wound and surrounding skin for evidence of infection, necrosis, or maceration.
- Consider the temperature of the product before applying it to the wound.
- Avoid excessive pressure from a dressing, bandage, or tape.
- Follow the manufacturer's instructions when using a dressing or technology.
- After the procedure, assess comfort of intervention and/or dressing/bandages applied.

Ongoing evaluation and modification of the management plan and treatment intervention is essential as wounds change over time. More advanced nonpharmacologic techniques that require specialist training or skilled personnel, such as the use of hypnosis or therapeutic touch, may be considered.

- Most patients didn't receive analgesics for pain relief; only 2% (n = 3) of patients in this population were given analgesics for pressure ulcer pain within 4 hours of the pain measurement.
- Patients who couldn't express pain or respond to pain scales may still have had pain.
- Patients with deeper pressure ulcer stages (stages III and IV) had more pain.

Some procedures, such as surgical debridement or wet-to-dry dressing changes, may increase pain. While the study didn't identify the interventions that might be most effective in controlling pain, patients whose beds had static air mattresses rather than regular hospital bed mattresses and those whose wounds were dressed with hydrocolloid dressings had significantly less pain.[14] The study also demonstrated that patients are able to differentiate between ulcer site pain, generalized pain, and other local pain sites such as IV and catheter sites.[14] Some cognitively impaired patients were able to indicate the presence of pain and respond to pain intensity scales.

Both Dallam et al.[14] and Szors and Bourguinon[24] found that many patients suffer with untreated or undertreated pressure ulcer pain. Dallam and colleagues[14] determined that only 2% of patients with pressure ulcer pain received analgesia. Four years later, Szors and Bourguinon[24] found little improvement in the administration of pain-relieving medication: only 6% of patients with pressure ulcer pain had analgesics prescribed to address their pain.

Both studies reflect the need for clinicians to realize the potential for pain from pressure ulcers. Because only 44 of the 132 patients with pressure ulcer pain could respond to pain scales, Dallam and colleagues[14] recommend that pressure ulcer pain should be suspected even when the patient can't report pain. Both studies recommend further research to identify interventions that can relieve pressure ulcer pain and the associated suffering.

Franks and Collier[35] conducted a study in the United Kingdom in which they compared home-care patients with (n = 75) and without

SKIN: AN ESSENTIAL ORGAN

Classification of skin tears

PAYNE-MARTIN	STAR (AUSTRALIA)	

Category Ia: Linear
Epidermis is pulled apart as if an incision has been made.

Category 1a
Skin tear edges <u>can</u> be realigned to the normal anatomical position, and the skin flap <u>is not</u> pale, dusky, or darkened.

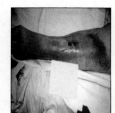

Category Ib: Flap
Epidermal flap completely covers the dermis to within 1 mm of the wound margin.

Category 1b
Skin tear edges <u>can</u> be realigned to the normal anatomical position, and the skin or flap color <u>is</u> pale, dusky, or darkened.

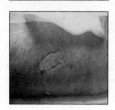

Category IIa: Scant tissue loss
25% or less of epidermal flap is lost.

Category 2a
The edges of the tear <u>cannot</u> be realigned to the normal anatomical position, and the skin or flap color <u>is not</u> pale, dusky, or darkened.

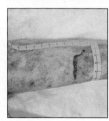

Category IIb: Moderate to large tissue loss
More than 25% of epidermal flap is lost.

Category 2b
The edges <u>cannot</u> be realigned to the normal anatomical position, the skin or flap color is pale, dusky, or darkened

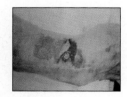

Category III: Complete epidermal tissue loss
Epidermal flap is absent.

Category 3
The skin flap is completely absent.

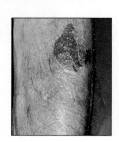

Used with permission: Payne-Martin, OWN 39(5):June 1993; STAR, Skin Tear Audit Research, Silver Chain Nursing Association, Curtin University of Technology, 2007.

SKIN: AN ESSENTIAL ORGAN (continued)

Senile purpura

Example of senile purpura in the elderly

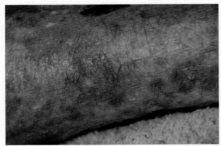

Courtesy of B. Beck, RN, CWOCN

WOUND ASSESSMENT

Hemosiderin deposit

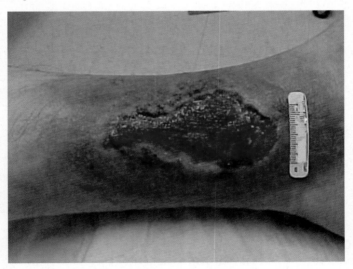

Geography of chronic wounds: Location, location, location

A + B + C + = the total wound
A is the wound bed; B is the wound edge; and C is the surrounding skin.

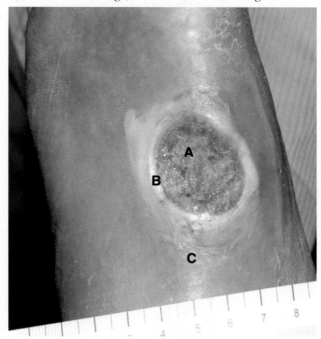

Photo: M. Tomic Cane. Used with permission.

Maceration

This photograph shows maceration of the surrounding skin caused by an overwhelmed dressing.

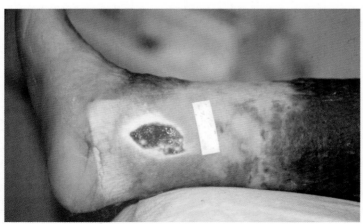

Wound edges with epithelialization
In this photograph, wound edges are attached and epithelialization present.

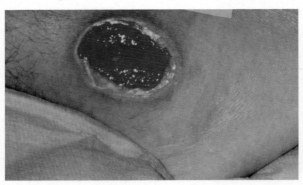

Rolled edges
Wound edges rolled inward

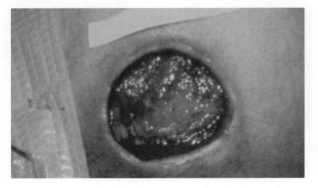

Wound Terminology

Using current terminology is imperative for accurate assessment. The photograph below labels this wound's characteristics as well as its length and width.

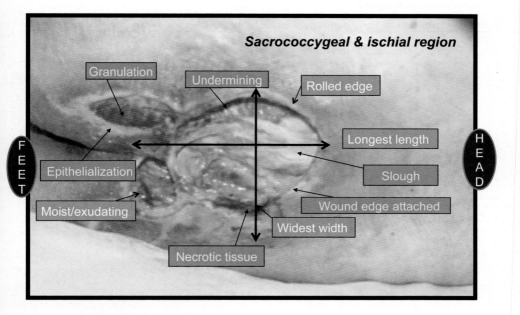

DIAGNOSING INFECTION

Progression of bacterial balance to bacterial damage in a chronic wound

Contaminated or colonized

Bacteria are present on the wound surface (contaminated). A steady state of replicating organisms are attaching to the wound tissue and multiplying, but they aren't associated with tissue damage or delayed healing (colonization).

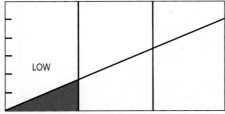
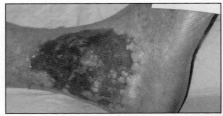

Critically colonized
(local infection, covert infection, increased bacterial burden)

- The bacterial burden in the wound bed is increasing, initiating an immune response (inflammation).
- The wound is no longer healing at the expected rate: wound size isn't decreasing
- Look for the signs outlined in the enabler NERDS©.

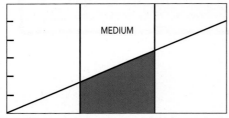
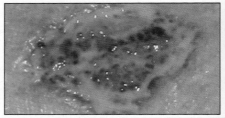

Infected

- Bacteria are present within the wound and have spread to the deeper and surrounding tissue; they're multiplying and causing tissue damage.
- There's an associated host inflammatory response that has now spread to the deeper tissue and surrounding skin.
- The wound is painful and may increase in size with potential satellite areas of breakdown.
- Look for the signs outlined in the enabler STONES©.

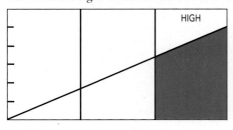
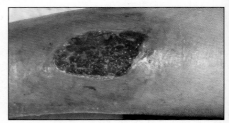

NERDS©: Superficial increased bacterial burden

Letter	Key information to know	
NONHEALING WOUND 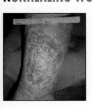	• The wound is nonhealing despite appropriate interventions (healable wound with the cause treated and patient-centered concerns addressed). • Bacterial damage has caused an increased metabolic load in the chronic wound, creating a proinflammatory wound environment that delays healing.	• To determine a healing trajectory, the wound size should decrease 20% to 40% after 4 weeks of appropriate treatment to heal by week 12. • If the wound does not respond to topical antimicrobial therapy, consider a biopsy after 4 to 12 weeks to rule out an unsuspected diagnosis, such as vasculitis, pyoderma gangrenosum, or malignancy
EXUDATIVE WOUND 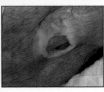	• An increase in wound exudates can be indicative of bacterial imbalance and leads to periwound maceration. • Exudate is often clear before it becomes purulent or sanguineous.	• Increased exudates needs to trigger the clinician to assess for subtle signs of infections. • Protect periwound area using the LOWE© memory jogger (Liquid film-forming acrylate; Ointments; Windowed dressings; External collection devices) for skin barrier to wound margins.
RED AND BLEEDING WOUND 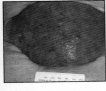	• When the wound bed tissue is bright red with exuberant granulation tissues and bleeds easily, bacterial imbalance can be suspected.	• Granulation tissue should be pink and firm. The exuberant granulation tissue that is loose and bleeds easily reflects bacterial damage to the forming collagen matrix and an increased vasculature of the tissue.
DEBRIS IN THE WOUND 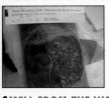	• Necrotic tissue and debris in the wound is a food source for bacteria and can encourage a bacterial imbalance.	• Necrotic tissue in the wound bed will require debridement in the presence of adequate circulation. • Debridement choice needs to be determined based on wound type, clinician skill, and resources.
SMELL FROM THE WOUND 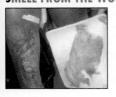	• Smell from bacterial byproducts caused by tissue necrosis associated with the inflammatory response is indicative of wound-related bacterial damage. *Pseudomonas* has a characteristic sweet smell/green color; anaerobes have a putrid odor due to the breakdown of tissue.	• Clinicians need to differentiate the smell of bacterial damage from the odor associated with the interaction of exudates with different dressing materials, particularly some hydrocolloids. Odor may come from superficial or deep tissue damage, and this should not be relied on along with exudates alone as the only signs of increased superficial bacterial burden.

STONES©: Deep compartment infection

Letter	Key information to know
SIZE IS BIGGER 	• Size as measured by the longest length and widest width at right angles to the longest length. Only very deep wounds need to have depth measured with a probe. • An increased size may be due to deeper and surrounding tissue damage by bacteria or alternately because the cause has not been treated or there is a systemic or local host factor impairing healing.
TEMPERATURE INCREASED 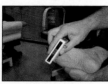	• With surrounding tissue infection, temperature is increased. This may be performed crudely by touch with a gloved hand or by using an infrared thermometer or scanning device. There should be a high index of suspicion for infection if > 3° F difference in temperature exists between 2 mirror-image sites.
OS (PROBES TO OR EXPOSED BONE) 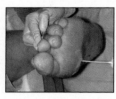	• There is a high incidence of osteomyelitis if bone is exposed or if the clinician can probe to the bone in a person with a neurotrophic foot ulcer. • An MRI is probably the most discriminating diagnostic test and considered necessary for diagnostic dilemmas.
NEW AREAS OF BREAKDOWN 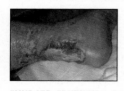	• Note the satellite areas of skin breakdown that are separated from the main ulcer. • It is important to remember this may be due to the cause of the wound, infection, or local damage being left uncorrected.
EXUDATE, ERYTHEMA, EDEMA 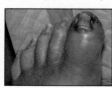	• All of the features here are due to the inflammatory response. With increased bacterial burden, exudates often increases in quantity and transforms a clear or serous texture to frank purulence and may have a hemorrhagic component. The inflammation leads to vasodilatation (erythema), and the leakage of fluid into the tissue will result in edema.
SMELL 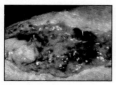	• Bacteria that invade tissue have a "foul" odor. There is an unpleasant sweet odor from *Pseudomonas* Gram-negative organisms, and anaerobe organisms can cause a putrid smell from the associated tissue damage.

© 2006 Sibbald, Ayello

Comments

- Clinicians need to have a consistent approach to measurement.
- An increased size from bacterial damage is due to the bacteria spreading from the surface to the surrounding skin and the deeper compartment. This indicates that the combination of bacterial number and virulence has overwhelmed the host resistance.

It is important to distinguish between infection and the other 2 potential causes of temperature change:
- A difference in vascular skin supply (decreased circulation; is colder).
- Inflammatory conditions are not usually as warm, but they can demonstrate a marked increase temperature with extensive deep tissue destruction (acute Charcot joint).

- Radiographs and bone scans are less reliable for diagnosis of osteomyelitis with loss of bone mass that occurs with neuropathy. Radiographs of well-calcified bone, such as pressure ulcers of the pelvis, may be more reliable. The majority of ulcers that probe to bone in other locations are less likely to be associated with osteomyelitis.

- Search for the cause of the satellite areas of breakdown and the need to correct the cause.
- Check for local damage and consider infection, increased exudates, or other sources of trauma.

- For exudates control, determine the cause and then match the absorbency of the dressing (non, low, moderate, heavy) to the amount of exudates from the wound.
- Assess surrounding skin to evaluate for maceration. Again, use the LOWE© memory jogger (Liquid film-forming acrylate; Ointments; Windowed dressings; External collection devices) for skin barrier for wound margins.
- For erythema and edema control, the cause or the tissue infection needs to be treated.

- Make sure the smell is from organisms and not from the normal distinct odor from the interaction of exudates with some of the dressing material.
- Systemic antimicrobial agents are indicated that will treat the causative organisms, and devitalized tissue should be aggressively debrided in wounds with the ability to heal.

WOUND DEBRIDEMENT

Eschar

In a wound that has become dehydrated, necrotic tissue turns thick, leathery, and black. This tissue is referred to as *eschar*.

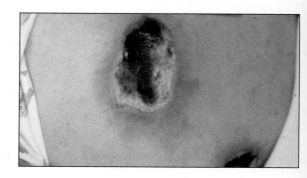

Slough

Necrotic tissue that's moist, stringy, and yellow (devitalized tissue) is referred to as *slough*.

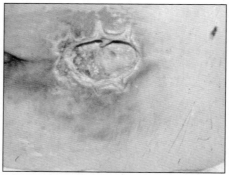

Differentiating tendon from slough

Performing debridement requires knowing where and what to cut. For example, tendon and slough both are yellow— the clinician must be able to distinguish between them.

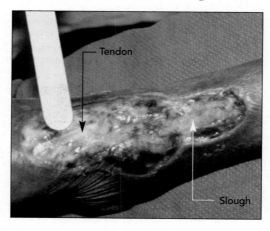

The wound "bar code" (gene expression pattern)

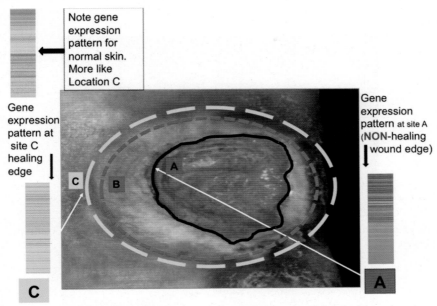

Note gene expression pattern for normal skin. More like Location C

Gene expression pattern at site C healing edge

Gene expression pattern at site A (NON-healing wound edge)

Cells at Location A multiply at a higher rate than usual (hyperproliferative), yet they are unable to migrate into the wound to close it as would be expected from normally activated keratinocytes. Instead, these cells form thickened layers around the edge, much like a callus or corn. When looking at the edge of a chronic wound (*solid black outline*), most clinicians would readily identify the "stalled" rounded (rolled) edge (i.e., callus) that indicates that debridement is needed to facilitate wound healing. However, research indicates that debriding only to this edge may be inadequate, leaving impaired cells behind at the wound edge boundary at Location B (*dashed blue line*). What would be helpful is a way to clearly and easily distinguish the non-healing edge of Location A (non-migrating cells) from the healing edge of Location C (migrating cells); this "margin of response" is indicated by the *broken yellow line*. Using gene activity (expression pattern), the healing and non-healing edges can be graphically depicted by a color patterns that produces a "bar code" similar to the bar code found on products or an airplane boarding pass.

Research has shown that the color patterns of gene expression of the wound edges at Locations A and C are very different from each other, while the gene pattern at Location C is more like that of unwounded skin. This means that during the debridement procedure, one can identify the specific bar code of the location before and after debridement to determine whether the extension of debridement was sufficient.

(Figure adapted from Tomic-Canic, M., Ayello, E.A., Stojadinovic, O., Golinko, M.S., Brem, H. "Using Gene Transcription Patterns (Bar Coding Scans) to Guide Wound Debridement and Healing." *Advances in Skin & Wound Care* 21(10):487-92, 2008.)

Surgical wound debridement case series

This pressure ulcer with slough and eschar requires surgical debridement because of advancing cellulitis.

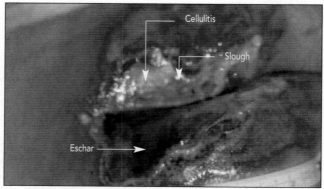

The same pressure ulcer after surgical debridement. Note the absence of eschar. Cellulitis is still present.

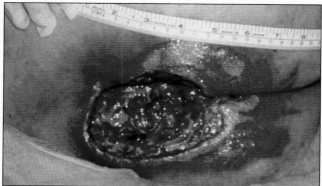

The same pressure ulcer after 7 days of treatment shows minimal necrotic tissue and significant amounts of granulation tissue. Note the change in the cellulitis surrounding the wound.

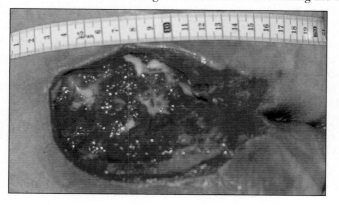

Sharp debridement at the bedside

Small wounds may be débrided at the bedside, as shown here.

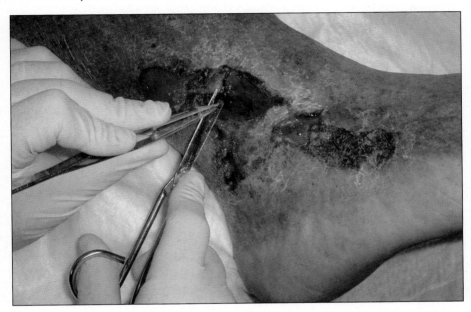

Notice the increased size of this ulcer after debridement.

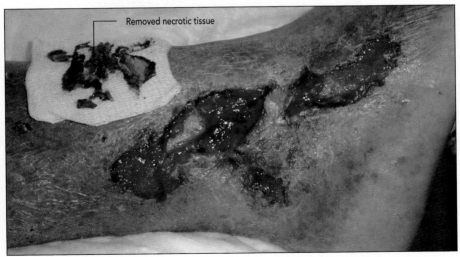

Removed necrotic tissue

Photos courtesy of Steven Black, MD

Maggot therapy

This photo shows a heel ulcer with osteomyelitis on a middle-aged woman with diabetes who was on immunosuppressants following a kidney transplant 27 years earlier.

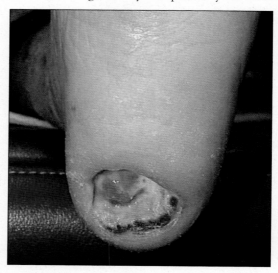

The same ulcer with sterile maggots placed in the wound for the purpose of debridement.

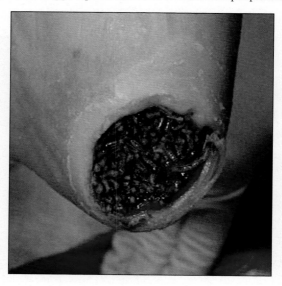

The same ulcer after removal of the first application of maggots.

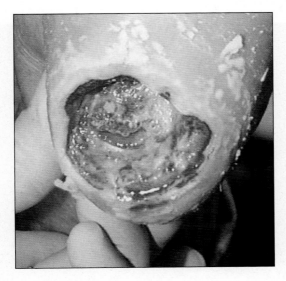

The same ulcer, healed.

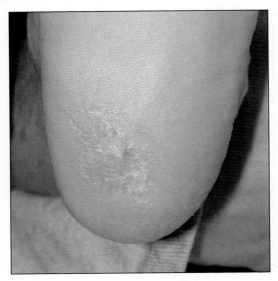

Photos courtesy of Pamela Mitchell, BTER Foundation

WOUND HEALING BIOLOGY

Electromagnetic spectrum

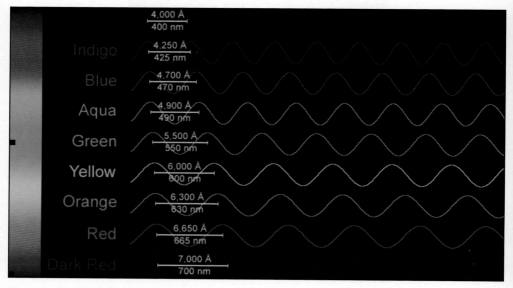

Artwork by Randy Russell

Scar management

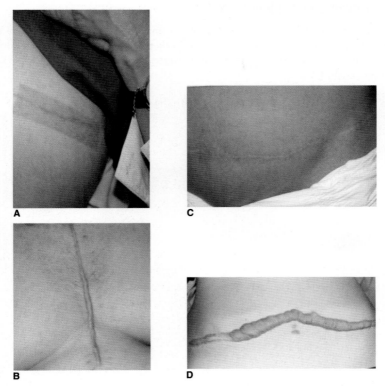

Figure 9-15. (A) Tape applied longitudinally along the direction of the scar. White or flesh-tone tape may be used, with the same effect. **(B)** Untreated hypertrophic scar in the presternal area; multiple vector forces are working against this scar. **(C)** The mature treated abdominal scar is flat, white, and non-reactive (note that it is normal for most scars to become hypopigmented to some extent). Compare this scar with the untreated scar. **(D)** Keloid scarring, which grows like a tumor and flows over the scar boundary, occurs wherever the skin is breached. Its pathogenesis and treatment are different from those of hypertrophic scars.

Photos used with permission of World Council of Enterostomal Therapists (WCET). From Widgerow, A. D. "Scar Management: The Principles and Their Practical Application." *WCET* 31(1):18-21, 2011

PRESSURE REDISTRIBUTION

Seating, positioning, and support surfaces

Multiple sensors integrated into a mat may be used to "map" the entire body area that comes in contact with the support surface. This pressure map of a patient lying face up on a horizontal support surface shows varying degrees of pressure exerted by the patient's heels, calves, thighs, buttocks, shoulders, and head.

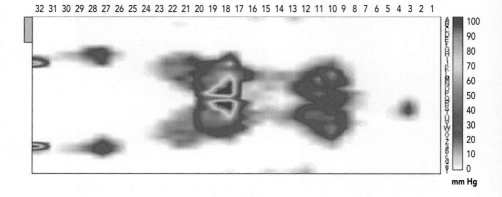

PRESSURE ULCERS

Pressure ulcers are commonly staged using the International NPUAP/EPUAP classification system described briefly here.

Suspected deep tissue injury

Purple or maroon localized area of discolored intact skin or blood-filled blister due to damaor underlying soft tissue from pressure and/or shear. The area may be preceded by tissue that is painful, firm, mushy, boggy, warm, or cooler as compared with adjacent tissue.

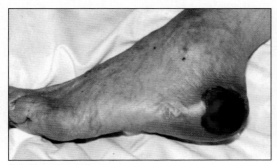

© J. M. Levine, MD

Suspected deep tissue injury on the buttocks in an ICU patient.

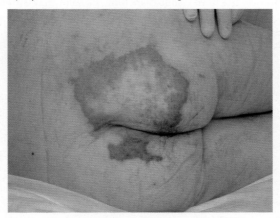

Photo courtesy of Janet E. Cuddigan, PhD, RN, CWCN

Unstageable pressure ulcer

Full-thickness tissue loss in which the base of the ulcer is covered by slough (yellow, tan, gray, green, or brown) and/or eschar (tan, brown, or black) in the wound bed.

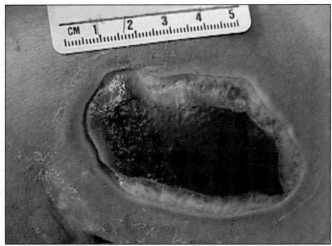

© 2006 by Elizabeth A. Ayello

Stage I

Intact skin with non-blanchable redness of a localized area usually over a bony prominence. Darkly pigmented skin may not have visible blanching; its color may differ from the surrounding area.

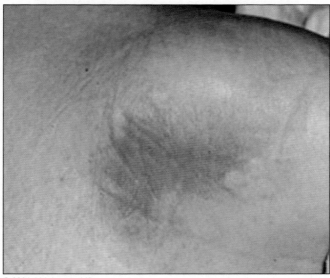

© 2006 J.M. Levine, MD

Stage II

Partial thickness loss of dermis presenting as a shallow open ulcer with a red pink wound bed, without slough. May also present as an intact or open/ruptured serum-filled blister.

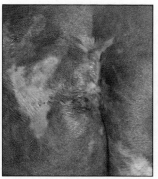

© 2007 H. Brem, MD

Stage III

Full-thickness tissue loss. Subcutaneous fat may be visible but no bone, tendon, or muscle is exposed. Slough may be present but does not obscure the depth of tissue loss. May include undermining and tunneling.

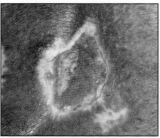

© 2007 H. Brem, MD

Stage IV

Full-thickness tissue loss with exposed bone, tendon, or muscle. Slough or eschar may be present on some parts of the wound bed. Often includes undermining or tunneling.

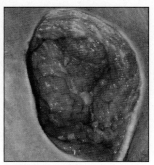

© 2007 H. Brem, MD

VASCULAR ULCERS

Vascular ulcers include wounds resulting from arterial, venous, and lymphatic conditions.

Venous ulcer

This photograph shows a venous ulcer. Venous ulcers are typically moist with irregular edges and firm, fibrotic, and indurated surrounding skin.

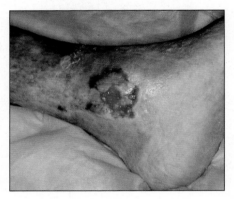

Arterial ulcer

This photograph shows a necrotic great toe with blisters on the toes and foot, representing arterial insufficiency.

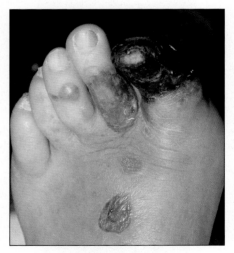

Lymphedema

Top photograph shows lymphedema with fibrosis and scarring.

- Aplasia/dysplasia or damage to lymphatic vessels or nodes
- Proliferation of fibroblasts
- Disturbance of local metabolism, chronic inflammation
- Increased infections (cellulitis)

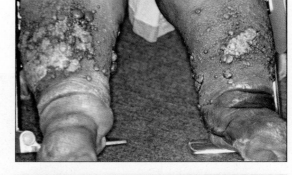

Failure to identify lymphedema leads to improper treatment.

- Pain
- Further damage to lymphatics
- Increased risk of complications
- Functional limitations and disability

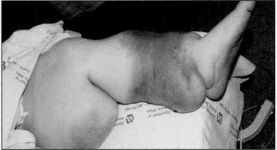

© 2007 Mary Jo Geyer

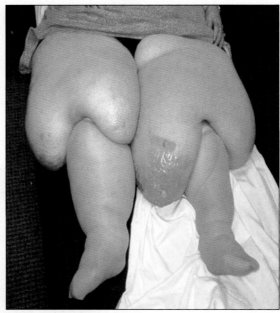

© 2007 Mary Jo Geyer

DIABETIC FOOT ULCERS

Ulcer on the sole

Repetitive, moderate pressure can cause skin breakdown and ulcers in the neuropathic foot, as shown here.

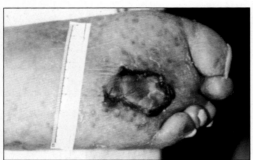

Charcot's foot with infection

This photograph shows Charcot's foot with infection present. Treatment of such wounds may include administration of parenteral antibiotics and surgical debridement of necrotic and infected tissue.

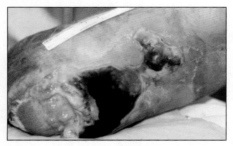

Callus with thick rim of tissue

Diabetic ulcers typically have a thick rim of keratinized tissue surrounding the wound, as shown here.

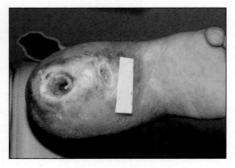

ULCERS IN SICKLE CELL DISEASE

Sickle cell ulcer

Sickle cell ulcer with fibrinous material covering the ulcer bed

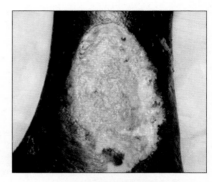

Predebridement

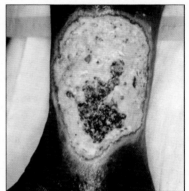

Postdebridement

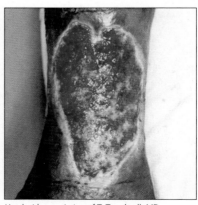

Used with permission of T. Treadwell, MD

Recurrent sickle cell ulcer

Recurrent sickle cell ulcer treated with tissue-engineered skin

Healed 8 weeks post application

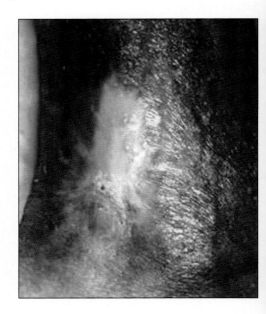

Ulcer remains healed 8 months later—note improved scar

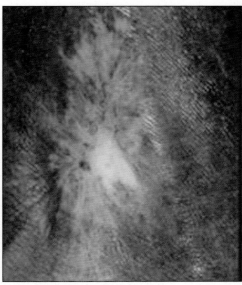

Used with permission of T. Treadwell, MD

SURGICAL WOUNDS

Surgical closure of a pressure ulcer

This photograph shows markings made for gluteal fasciocutaneous flaps for surgicalclosure of a stage II pressure ulcer.

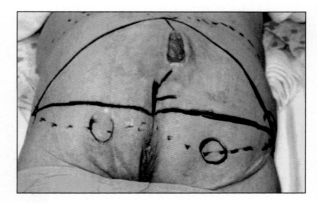

Shown here is surgical closure of the same ulcer.

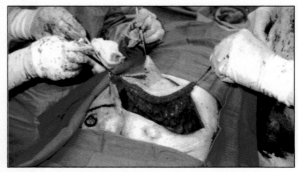

Photos courtesy of S. Black, MD

ATYPICAL WOUNDS

Wounds with uncommon etiologies are called atypical wounds.

Vasculitis

This photograph shows reticulated erythema and necrotic ulcers on the thighs of a patient with vasculitis.

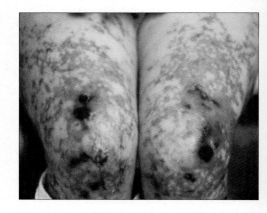

Pyoderma gangrenosum

In a patient with inflammatory bowel disease and pyoderma gangrenosum, this ulcer on the lateral leg shows areas of cribriform scarring.

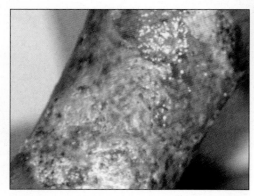

Peristomal pyoderma gangrenosum in a patient with Crohn's disease

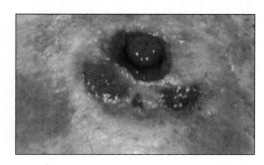

Hansen's disease

Shown here are the leg and foot of a patient with Hansen's disease caused by *Mycobacterium leprae*. In addition to neuropathic changes of the toes and plantar aspect of the foot, this patient has a large lateral leg ulcer.

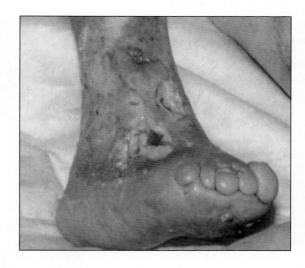

Buruli ulcer

This photo shows extensive sloughing and massive ulceration, typically leading to contractures and extensive disability and disfigurement.

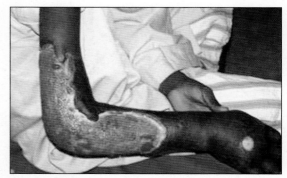

© 2007 E. Ampadu, MD

Necrotizing fasciitis

Necrotizing fasciitis of the abdomen

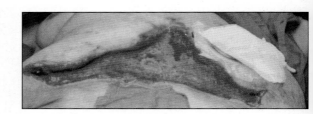

Cryofibrinogenemia

This patient has painful punctate ulcers on the feet and legs secondary to cryofibrinogenemia.

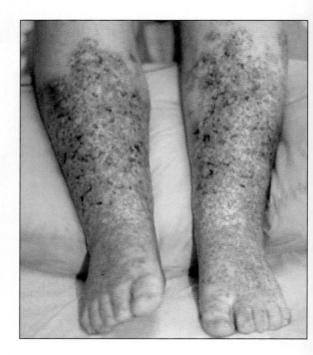

Calciphylaxis

Shown here is necrotic plaque with livedo reticularis in a dialysis patient with end-stage renal disease and calciphylaxis.

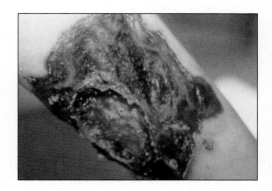

This photograph shows calciphylaxis of both extremities in a patient with end-stage renal failure. Despite aggressive local wound care, the wounds never healed, and the patient died of sepsis.

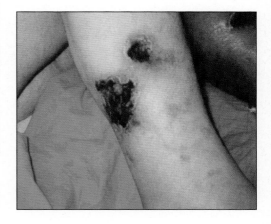

Calcific uremic arteriopathy (CUA)

CUA with livedo reticularis pattern

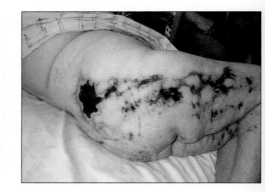

CUA of the thigh

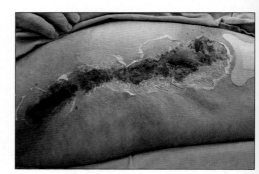

CUA of bilateral extremities

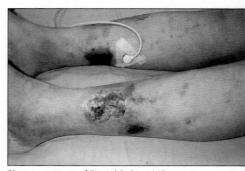

Photos courtesy of Daniel Beless, MD

Malignancies

Shown here is a right medial leg ulcer in a venous distribution secondary to T-cell lymphoma.

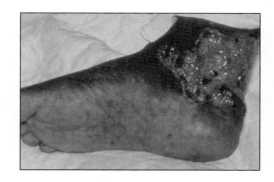

Marjolin ulcer

Shown here is a chronic wound that developed malignant changes (squamous cell carcinoma).

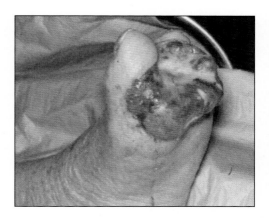

Loxoscelism

Bite from a brown recluse spider (*Loxosceles reclusa*). Note the deep purple plaque surrounded by a clear halo and erythema, the so-called red, white, and blue sign.

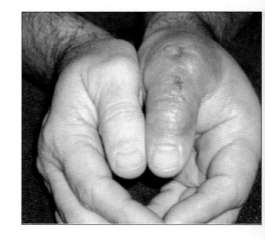

Factitial dermatitis

This photograph shows an angulated factitial ulcer on the breast. The term *factitial* denotes a self-imposed injury.

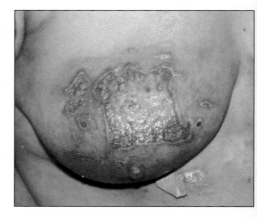

Extravasation

Extravasation can cause tissue loss that may evolve into extensive wounds, as shown in this I.V. site 24 hours after infiltration of calcium chloride.

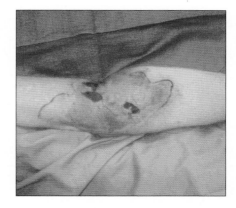

The same site 48 hours after wound debridement.

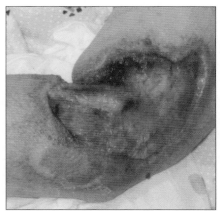

The same site after surgical debridement down to viable tissue.

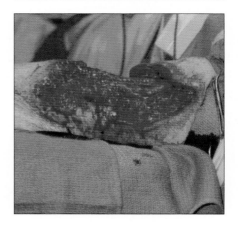

SPECIAL POPULATIONS: HIV/AIDS

Kaposi's sarcoma

Kaposi's sarcoma on the sole of the foot

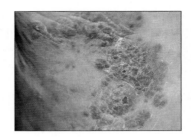

SPECIAL POPULATIONS: BARIATRIC PATIENTS

Skin folds

Skin folds on back of neck

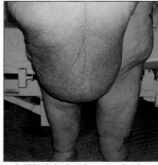

Pannus

Grade 5 abdominal pannus

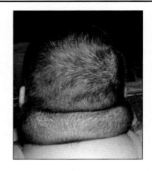

Photos © 2006 Coloplast Corp. Used with permission.
Photographer: K.L. Kennedy-Evans, RN, CS, FNP

Grade 5 pannus with intertrigo.

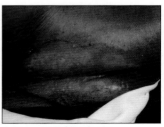

Photo courtesy of C. Fife, MD.

SPECIAL POPULATIONS: BARIATRIC PATIENTS (continued)

Acanthosis nigricans

This photo shows a patient with brown velvety hyperpigmentation of the skin often seen in bariatric patients.

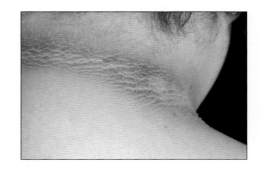

Plantar hyperkeratosis

Hyperkeratosis results from chronic excessive pressure or friction to the epidermis, as seen here on the plantar aspect of the foot.

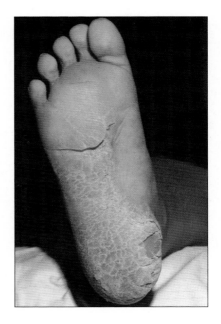

SPECIAL POPULATIONS: BARIATRIC PATIENTS (continued)

Intertrigo

Intertrigo between the skin folds of the breast of a femal patient with a body mass index of 60. Note the fissure at the base of a skin fold.

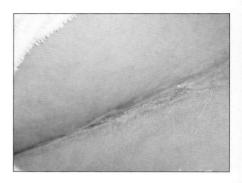

Intertrigo with erythema, erosion, and denudation

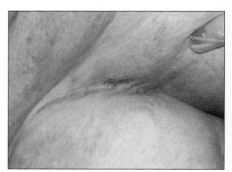

© 2006 Coloplast Corp. Used with permission
Photographer: K.L. Kennedy-Evans, RN, CS, FNP

Candida intertrigo in a skin fold

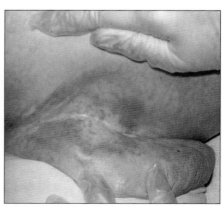

© 2006 Coloplast Corp. Used with permission.
Photographer: K.L. Kennedy-Evans, RN, CS, FNP

NEONATAL AND PEDIATRIC PRESSURE ULCERS

Occiput pressure ulcer

Critically ill infant with stage IV occipital pressure ulcer

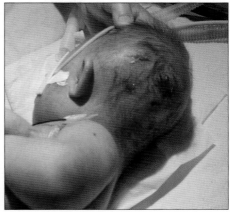

Photo courtesy of Dr. Mona Baharestani

PATIENT SCENARIOS

Chapter 4—Skin: An Essential Organ

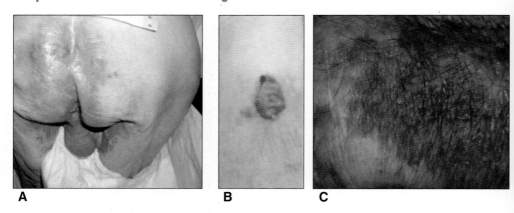

Figure 4-1. (A) Incontinence-associated dermatitis. **(B)** Skin tear. **(C)** Senile purpura. (View C, courtesy of B. Beck, RN, WOCN.)

Chapter 5—Acute and Chronic Wound Healing

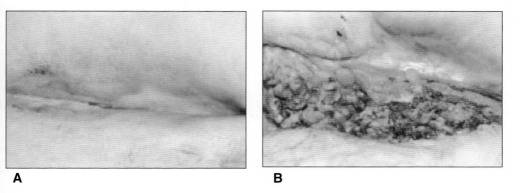

A   **B**

Figure 5-1. (A) Wound appearance (right groin) 2 weeks post surgery. **(B)** Wound appearance at week 3.

Chapter 7—Wound Bioburden and Infection

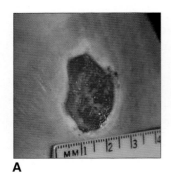 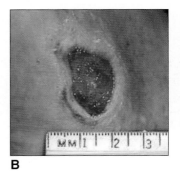

A   **B**

Figure 7-1. (A) Baseline photo. **(B)** The appearance of the wound after 2 weeks of topical antibiotic therapy.
(Photos courtesy of S. Gardner.)

Chapter 8—Wound Debridement

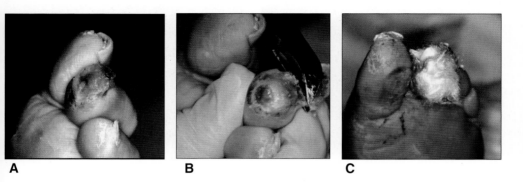

A   **B**   **C**

Figure 8-1. (A) Keratotic cap on the left second toe. **(B)** A small ulcer probing to bone was revealed when the nail and callus were removed. **(C)** Calcium alginate dressing applied for hemostasis after debridement.

Chapter 14—Venous Disease and Lymphedema Management

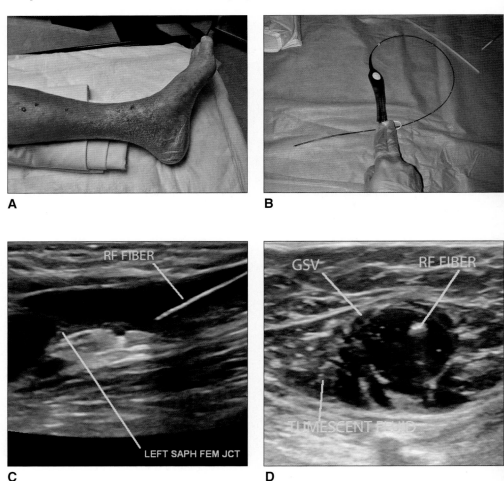

Figure 14-3. (A) Macerated skin due to multiple recurrent superficial ulcers in the medial aspect of the left ankle region. **(B)** Radiofrequency fiber. **(C)** Placement of the radiofrequency fiber approximately 2 cm distal to the junction of the common femoral vein. **(D)** Tumescent fluid infused around the GSV.

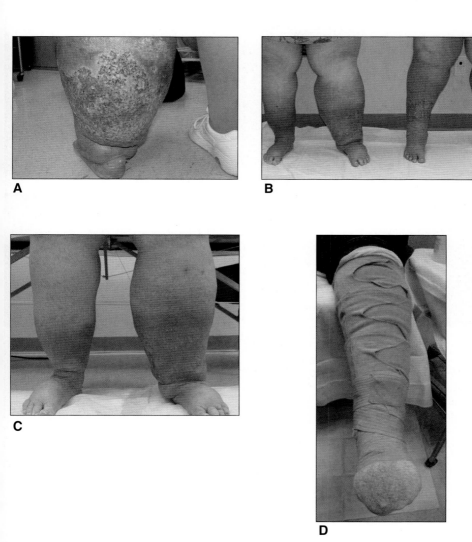

Figure 14-4. (A) Diffuse areas of skin breakdown in an obese patient with lymphedema in the left leg. **(B)** Skin breakdown due to cellulitis also seen in the patient's husband. **(C)** Resolution of ulcerations in the patient following antibiotic treatment. **(D)** Semirigid Velcro strap device used to control lymphedema.

Courtesy of C. Fife, MD

Chapter 16—Diabetic Foot Ulcers

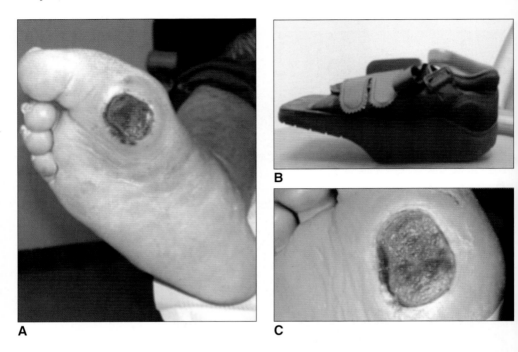

A   **B**   **C**

Figure 16-16. Neuropathic diabetic ulcer sub–first metatarsal. **(A)** The wound on initial presentation. **(B)** The off-loading device prescribed initially. **(C)** The wound following debridement and cleansing.

Courtesy of J. McGuire, DPM, PT

Chapter 18—Surgical Reconstruction of Wounds

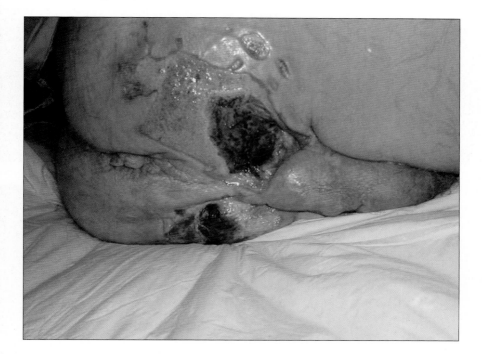

Figure 18-1. Extensive pressure ulcers throughout the perineum in a 22-year-old paraplegic man.

Chapter 19—Tube, Drain, and Fistula Management

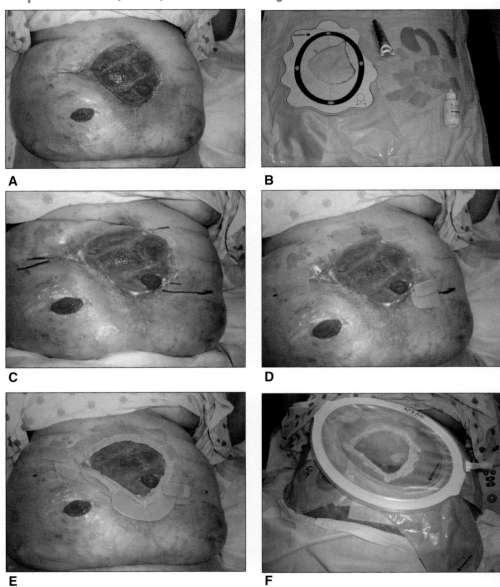

Figure 19-1 (A) The patient's skin condition when she arrived at the hospital. Irritant dermatitis resulted from frequent leakage of effluent. **(B)** Pouch equipment used. **(C)** The contour of the abdomen was checked with the patient in a sitting position. Deep creases around the wound were marked. **(D)** Creases were filled with CMC skin barrier wedges. **(E)** The "petaling" method was used to build up the wound edges. **(F)** Finished pouching product.

Courtesy of P. Erwin-Toth MSN, CWOCN, CNS

($n = 100$) pressure ulcers. Interestingly, they found that patients with pressure ulcers had less pain than those who did not have pressure ulcers. The authors speculated that perhaps pressure ulcer pain might not be the problem, as previously presumed, or that pain control was somehow more effective for patients receiving home care. An alternative explanation is that the home-care patients with pressure ulcers did not have the same co-morbid conditions as previously reported in hospital populations.

In a quantitative pain study of 128 chronic wound patients, Ayello and colleagues[36] found that more than half of the patients with venous ulcers had pain (54%), almost one-third with diabetic ulcers had pain (30%), and one-quarter of those with pressure ulcers (25%) had pain.

Langemo and colleagues[37] published a qualitative phenomenological study about pain in pressure ulcer patients. They interviewed eight adults, half with active pressure ulcers at the time of the study and the other half with healed pressure ulcers. Seven themes were identified:

1. the perceived etiology of the pressure ulcer
2. life impact and changes
3. psychospiritual impact
4. extreme painfulness associated with the pressure ulcer
5. the need for knowledge and understanding
6. the need for and stress related to numerous treatments
7. the grieving process

The fourth theme—extreme pain—was subdivided into three categories: intensity of pain, duration of pain, and analgesic use. Patients commonly referred to the intensity of pain from pressure ulcers with descriptors such as "it burned," "feeling like being stabbed," "sitting on a bunch of needles," or "stinging." Some examples of statements by actual study respondents include a woman with a stage II pressure ulcer who said, "I felt like somebody was getting a knife and really digging in there good and hard." In the words of another male respondent, "They [pressure ulcers] are very painful because no matter what way you put your bottom, it hurts."[37]

Respondents also commented on the duration of the pain, with statements such as "the majority of the time, even when I was lying down, it hurt." Pain continued to be a problem even after the pressure ulcer had healed. As one respondent stated, "Every now and again, it still hurts. But there is nothing there. This time there is nothing really there." The fear of addiction resulting from analgesic use was expressed by some respondents. One respondent with a stage IV pressure ulcer on the buttock commented, "I was constantly in pain and was taking morphine and other types of painkillers to try and ease the pain."

Another qualitative study reported about the pain of 10 pressure ulcer patients.[38] Although Rastinehad identified 22 themes, lack of communication and painful treatment interventions were the two most common complaints.[38] Some patients related accounts of communication failures that contributed to stress, tension, and anxiety.[38]

The European Pressure Ulcer Advisory Panel (EPUAP) funded a phenomenological study by Hopkins et al.,[39] who identified endless pain as one of the three main themes in older people living with pressure ulcers. The eight patients in this study were all over age 65 and had stage III or IV pressure ulcers for more than 1 month. None had spinal cord injuries, as suggested by Langemo and colleagues[37] for future qualitative pressure ulcer pain studies. The four subthemes of endless pain were constant pain presence, keeping still, equipment pain, and treatment pain. For some patients, keeping still reduced their pain: "I don't dare move because everything then gets worse. I lie very still." For others, pain was exacerbated by pressure-relieving equipment as well as dressing changes. All but one of the patients described their endless pain in a graphic way. "You put a bit of weight on your heel and (it) feels as though it's burst open."[39]

Chronic wound studies[40,41] and the studies cited in this chapter emphasize the importance of adequate pain assessment and treatment.

PAIN ASSESSMENT

Despite the APS's identification of pain as "the fifth vital sign,"[6] it isn't always included in the assessment of a patient's pressure ulcer. Dallam and colleagues[14] urged that pain be added to the assessment of pressure ulcers and that a patient's pain status be assessed during dressing changes as well as when the patient is at rest. They also cautioned clinicians to remember that the absence of a response or an expression of pain doesn't mean that the patient doesn't have pain. Despite research about the pain experience,[14,37,38,40-42] assessment of pain in persons with pressure ulcers continues to be underreported.[36] Documentation of pain assessment may vary by chronic wound type, as patients with venous ulcers (63%) and diabetic foot ulcers (53%) in one study were more likely to have their pain assessment recorded compared with those with pressure ulcers (45%).[36]

Two assessment guides include pain as part of pressure ulcer assessment. The AHCPR[21] treatment guidelines include an example of a sample pressure ulcer pain assessment guide in which there is a place to check either yes or no regarding the presence of pain. Ayello's[43,44] ASSESSMENT mnemonic asks the clinician to quantify the patient's pain experience, including the presence of pain, when the pain occurs (for example, is it episodic or constant), and if the patient is receiving measures for pain relief. The caregiver checks one of the following boxes under T = tenderness to touch or pain:

• no pain
• pain present on touch, anytime
• pain only when performing ulcer care.[43,44]

The mnemonic PQRST, which outlines the specific questions to ask the patient, is another useful tool for assessing a patient's pain.[14] (See *Essential pain assessment elements*.)

Essential pain assessment elements

Use the PQRST mnemonic (shown below) to assess your patient's pain.

P = Palliative/provocative factors
• What makes the pain worse?
• What makes it better?

Q = Quality of pain
• What kind of pain are you experiencing?
• Would you describe it as:
  • gnawing, aching, tender, throbbing (nociceptive)?
  • burning, stinging, shooting, stabbing (neuropathic)?
  • or any combination thereof?
• Do you have other symptoms with the pain, such as fever, chills, nausea, or vomiting?

R = Region and radiation of pain
• Where is the pain?
• Does the pain travel or remain in the same spot?

S = Severity of pain
• Would you describe your pain as none, mild, moderate, severe, or excruciating?
• Rate your pain on a scale from 0 to 10, with 0 representing "no pain" and 10 being "the worst imaginable pain."
• How would you rate the pain intensity at its worst, best, and now?

T = Temporal aspects of pain
• Is the pain better or worse at any particular time of the day or night?
• When does it start or when does it stop?
• Is it intermittent or constant, or does it occur only when you're moving?

A complete and thorough pain assessment enables the clinician to develop an effective pain treatment regimen and evaluate its effectiveness. (See *Additional pain assessment elements*.) The American Society for Pain Management Nursing offers a position statement and clinical practice recommendations for pain assessment in specific patient populations—groups that clinicians may not always identify as needing pain assessment. These groups include patients with advanced dementia, infants and preverbal toddlers, and intubated and/or unconscious patients.[45] The Hartford Institute for Geriatric Nursing has produced a series on pain assessment called "Try This." These one-page (front and back) documents provide a succinct summary that covers the important points on pain assessment in older adults and in patients with dementia.[46]

PRACTICE POINT

Pain is the fifth vital sign.

Pain intensity scales

Pain intensity scales use a simple verbal, visual, or numeric measure to help determine how much pain the patient is experiencing. The gold standard for assessing pain intensity is self-report and the utilization of standard pain intensity instruments.[47,48] Pain intensity scales are unidimensional, quantitative measures designed to measure the sensory aspect of a patient's pain and to obtain a more objective approximation of pain by minimizing inaccuracies.[48]

The use of pain intensity scales to quantify pain levels and determine patients' responses to pain treatments has been mandated by The Joint Commission for use in all hospitals.[5] Two of the most widely accepted and utilized pain assessment scales are the Numeric Pain Intensity Scale and the Faces Pain Rating Scale (FPRS).[49] Another commonly used scale is the Visual Analog Scale (VAS), which consists of a 10-cm line that has no numbers on it. At one end is the term "no pain," and at the other end is the phrase "pain as bad as it could possibly be."[2]

NUMERIC PAIN INTENSITY SCALE

The Numeric Pain Intensity Scale is considered the gold standard for pain assessment for adults and children over age 7.[2,49] This scale is a 10-cm line with the words "no pain" at one end, "worst possible pain" at the other end, and the numbers 0 to 10 running from one end of the scale to the other. (See *Numeric Pain Intensity Scale*, page 308.) The patient is asked to select the number on the scale that represents the level of pain he or she is experiencing. Zero indicates no pain, 5 indicates moderate pain, and 10 indicates the worst possible pain.[2] The Numeric Pain Intensity Scale is sometimes presented verbally[2,49]; however, visual presentation may help to standardize the process of pain assessment and assist hearing-impaired patients. In addition, the scale has been translated into many languages.[7]

Additional pain assessment elements

Include the following additional elements in your initial assessment plan and treatment:

- detailed history consisting of:
  - medication usage
  - treatment history
  - previous surgeries and injuries
  - impact on quality of life and activities of daily living.
- physical examination, emphasizing the body system involved in the pain complaint (for example, the musculoskeletal or neurologic system).
- psychosocial assessment, including family history of depression or chronic pain.
- appropriate diagnostic workup to determine the cause of pain and to rule out any contributing, treatable causes.

A thorough pain assessment enables the clinician to develop an effective pain treatment regimen and evaluate its effectiveness.

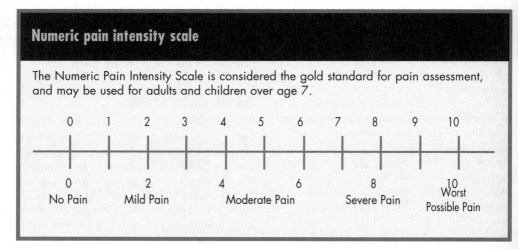

Numeric pain intensity scale

The Numeric Pain Intensity Scale is considered the gold standard for pain assessment, and may be used for adults and children over age 7.

```
0   1   2   3   4   5   6   7   8   9   10

0       2       4       6       8       10
No Pain  Mild Pain   Moderate Pain   Severe Pain   Worst
                                              Possible Pain
```

The Numeric Pain Intensity Scale aids in the adequate assessment and treatment of pain. It also helps clinicians choose the appropriate classification of pain medication recommendations based on any given patient response.[19,49,50] The scale can also help determine whether the patient has a response to the interventions if the numbers show a downward trend on repeated assessments.

FACES PAIN RATING SCALE (FPRS)

The FPRS[51] consists of six faces that range from a happy, smiling face (no pain) to a crying, frowning face (worst pain). The first face on the scale, which is numbered 0, represents the absence of pain; the next face, numbered 1, represents very little pain; and so forth. The last face on the scale indicates extreme/worst pain. The patient is asked to choose the face that most closely reflects his or her own pain at that point in time. (See *FACES Pain Rating Scale*.) The FPRS is preferred over other pain intensity scales for use with children.[49] The word "hurt," which appears on the FPRS, is the preferred word to use when assessing children, as children may not respond to the word "pain." In an older person, the word "ache" may be more useful in obtaining a response, as some older persons may be stoic and not admit to "pain." The validity and reliability of this scale in adult patients haven't been established, although in a geriatric population a high degree of agreement was found between the FPRS and the VAS ($r = 92; p < 0.5$).[52] The

FPRS has been used with cognitively impaired patients and with those for whom English is their second language. A high degree of consistency has been noted between the VAS and FPRS when utilized in any population.

After the initial pain assessment has been completed, reassessment should be performed at regular intervals. Reassess the patient after administration of pain medication or nondrug pain-relieving interventions to ensure that optimal pain relief has been achieved.

PAIN MANAGEMENT

Accurate and continuous pain assessment is the foundation of successful pain management.[7,47] However, evidence supports the fact that pain is poorly assessed. Of physicians with patient care responsibilities in oncology, 76% rated poor pain assessment as the number one barrier to adequate pain management.[8] Donovan et al.[53] found that of the 58% of hospitalized patients reporting excruciating pain, fewer than half had a member of the healthcare team ask them about their pain or note the pain in their records. The use of pain assessment measures has been shown to improve pain management for patients.[52,54] However, problems using the pain assessment scales in everyday practice persist. One problem includes the lack of clinicians' knowledge and familiarity in the use of pain rating scales. Training is required for clinicians to administer pain scales and offer adequate patient

FACES pain rating scale

The FACES Pain Rating Scale may be used for children ages 3 and older, for cognitively impaired patients, and for non-native speakers of English. This scale is not always culturally or gender appropriate, as not everyone with a pain score of 10 will cry.

Do you have:

0	2	4	6	8	10
No pain/hurt?	Very little pain/hurt?	Some pain/hurt?	A lot of pain/hurt?	Terrible pain/hurt?	Worst pain/hurt?

From Hockenberry-Eaton, M., and Wilson, D. *Wong's Essentials of Pediatric Nursing*, 8th ed. St. Louis: Mosby, 2009. © Mosby, Inc. Reprinted with permission.

instructions on the possible responses to the pain scale questions.

After pain has been identified, its cause should be determined and treated. "The goal of pain management in the pressure ulcer patient is to eliminate the cause of pain, to provide analgesia, or both."[20] Practical ways of treating pain, depending on the specific chronic wound etiology, have been described by McCaffery and Robinson[4] and Freedman and colleagues.[55]

Dressing changes, debridement, wound edema, infection, turning, and positioning are some of the factors that can cause wound-associated pain. An appropriate plan of action can be implemented after the specific cause of pain has been identified. For example, if the pain results from dressing changes, administering pain medication prior to dressing changes or switching to a different type of dressing may be indicated. According to Bergstron and colleagues,[21] "Besides medications, pain may be treated with physical and occupational therapy to decrease muscle spasms, decrease contractures, and aid in selecting less painful methods of wound debridement and cleaning. Proper seating, positioning, and adaptive equipment may also help to decrease pain." The optimal way to treat the pain associated with pressure ulcers requires more research, but clinicians can look at the cause of the ulcer, patient-centered concerns, and all the components of local wound care to minimize pain at each step in their care plan.

PRACTICE POINT

Pain management should include interventions that:

- treat the cause
- address patient-centered concerns
- educate the patient
- improve activities of daily living (ADLs) and quality of life
- minimize pain and trauma by incorporating local wound care measures for cleansing, debridement, and moist interactive dressings
- provide palliation to the dying patient
- decrease or eliminate pain with minimal adverse effects
- minimize the patient's dependency on healthcare workers and family members.

Pain medication

The World Health Organization[56] (WHO) developed a three-step analgesic ladder for the treatment of cancer pain that has been accepted for use in patients with nonmalignant pain.[8] (See *WHO analgesic ladder*.) The WHO approach advises clinicians to match the patient's reported pain intensity of 0 to 10 with the potency of the analgesic to be prescribed, starting with non-opioid analgesics and progressing to stronger medications if pain isn't relieved. For example, a patient who reports a pain score of 1 to 3 (mild pain) should receive a non-opioid with or without an adjuvant. If the patient reports a score of 4 to 6 (moderate pain), an appropriate low-dose single or combination opiate, with or

without an adjuvant, should be administered. Any opioid may be potent or may cause harm if used at doses that are inappropriate to the patient's tolerance level. The terms "combination opioid" (immediate and sustained release) and "low-dose single opioid" are used to replace "weak opioid" where applicable. If the patient's pain score is 7 to 10 (severe pain), he or she should be given a strong opioid with or without an adjuvant.

An adjuvant medication is a drug that has a primary indication other than pain but is analgesic for some painful conditions.[7] Examples of adjuvant medications are anticonvulsants or tricyclic antidepressants. (See *Adjuvant agents*.) Adding an adjuvant medication is most useful in addressing the burning, stinging, shooting, or stabbing symptoms of neuropathic pain. Using a combination of drugs such as an opioid and a non-opioid can enhance pain relief because the two drugs work synergistically. The opioid works on the CNS to alter the perception of pain, and the non-opioid works on the periphery to block painful impulses. Using a combination method may decrease the need for higher doses of opioids.

STEP 1: NON-OPIOID ANALGESICS

Acetaminophen or nonsteroidal anti-inflammatory drugs (NSAIDs) should be initiated as first-line therapy. They should be administered on a regular rather than an as-needed basis to increase their effectiveness and maintain a constant level of the medication in the blood. If one group of NSAIDs doesn't work, try another group. (See *Examples of non-opioid analgesics*, page 312.)

NSAID groups include:

- salicylates: aspirin, diflunisal, choline magnesium trisalicylate, salsalate
- propionic acids: naproxen, ibuprofen, fenoprofen, ketoprofen, flurbiprofen, suprofen
- acetic acids: indomethacin, tolmetin, sulindac, diclofenac,
- oxicams: piroxicam.

Clinicians must remember that NSAIDs have increased side effects in elderly people, including gastrointestinal bleeding, decreased

---

WHO analgesic ladder

This analgesic ladder, developed by the World Health Organization (WHO)[56] for pain management in patients with cancer, may be used as a guideline to manage mild through severe wound pain.

Freedom from cancer pain

3 — Opioid for moderate to severe pain ± non-opioid ± adjuvant

Pain persisting or increasing

2 — Opioid for mild to moderate pain ± non-opioid ± adjuvant

Pain persisting or increasing

1 — Non-opioid ± adjuvant

PAIN

© World Health Organization, 2003.
Reprinted with permission.

Adjuvant agents

Drug class	Drug name	Indications
Tricyclic antidepressants	Amitriptyline Desipramine Nortriptyline	• Multi-purpose • Any chronic pain • Lower level of sedation • Neuropathic pain
Anticonvulsants	Carbamazepine Clonazepam Gabapentin Pregabalin Valproic acid	• Burning, neuropathic, lancinating pain
Systemic local anesthetics	Lidocaine Mexiletine	• Burning pain
Topical anesthetics	Capsaicin EMLA cream Lidocaine gel Lidocaine 1% Lidocaine 4% Lidocaine patch 5%	• Analgesic for intact skin (use on wound periphery prior to dressing changes) • Before changing vacuum-assisted-closure dressing (instill solution through the tubing, with the pressure at 50 mm Hg, and clamp tubing for 15 to 20 minutes)* • Saturate gauze for 15 to 20 minutes prior to dressing change • Post-herpetic neuralgia, stump pain

*Systemic absorption and toxicity can occur in moderate to large wounds. Lidocaine products should not be used in patients who are taking class 1 antiarrhythmic drugs such as tocaine or mexiletine.

renal function, and aggravation of congestive heart failure, and so should be used with caution in persons over age 65. NSAIDs should also be avoided in patients on anticoagulation therapy. All NSAIDs, including gels and patches, carry a black box warning. The warning is as follows:

NSAIDs may cause an increased risk of serious cardiovascular thrombotic events, myocardial infarction, and stroke, which can be fatal. This risk may increase with duration of use. Patients with cardiovascular disease or risk factors for cardiovascular disease may be at greater risk.

Low-dose, single-agent opioids such as oxycodone (5 mg) may be safer for patients with moderate pain who cannot take NSAIDs because of their side effect profile.

Examples of non-opioid analgesics

- Acetaminophen
- Aspirin
- Tramadol*
- Nonsteroidal anti-inflammatory drugs
  - Celecoxib
  - Ibuprofen
  - Keterolac
  - Salsalate

---

*Tramadol is not classified as an opioid, but it is centrally acting. It may cause any of the side effects experienced with opioids, including abuse potential and withdrawal. Dose adjustments must be made for those who have renal impairment and/or liver disease. It also lowers seizure thresholds.

Tricyclic antidepressants, such as amitriptyline, imipramine, nortriptyline, and desipramine, have been shown to relieve neuropathy and post-herpetic neuralgia but are contraindicated in patients with coronary disease (although they may be taken cautiously in coronary disease patients at low doses of 10 to 30 mg in a daily night-time dosage).[8] Hydroxyzine has analgesic, antiemetic, and mild sedative properties as well as antihistamine effects. These drugs may help to induce sleep in patients with chronic pain and ordered along with other neuropathic agents as adjuvants for nociceptive pain. Diabetic patients with neuropathic pain or other patients with conditions arising from peripheral nerve syndromes may benefit from the use of certain anticonvulsants, such as gabapentin, pregabalin[9,10] phenytoin, carbamazepine, sodium valproate, or clonazepam.[8] Clonazepam, although pharmacologically classified as a benzodiazepine, not as an anticonvulsant, has anticonvulsant, muscle relaxant, and anxiolytic properties.

Opioids vary in strength from mild to very strong and are available in different forms, including oral, oral–transmucosal, rectal, transdermal, subcutaneous, IV, and IM.[57,58] The oral form is preferred for long-term use. However, for pre-procedural use or for some patients with post-procedural pain from debridement, the IV route may allow for better pain control and an ability to increase the dosage more quickly as needed. Whether an oral or IV route is used, doses should be scheduled on a regular basis to avoid breakthrough pain. If breakthrough pain occurs when the patient is on a long-acting (sustained-release) opioid regimen, a short-acting (immediate-release) opioid may be given in conjunction with the long-acting opioid to provide pain relief. Breakthrough pain can occur spontaneously but is most likely to occur when the patient is moved, if a dressing change is required, if tubes are being manipulated, or if the patient has an increase in activity. When using opioids around the clock, the clinician should assess the patient for pain caused by an "analgesic gap" or "end of dose failure." An example of this type of pain is when a patient is on a rescue dose for breakthrough pain every 6 hours as needed, but the medication only provides relief for 4 hours because of its pharmacologic properties. Shortening the interval at which the rescue dose can be used to every 4 hours as needed may correct this problem. Note also that approximately 15% of patients who are on long-acting opioid preparations require dosing every 8 hours rather than every 12 hours. (See *Evidence-Based Practice: Avoiding addiction: The four A's of opioid treatment*.)

Constipation can be one of the most common side effects with the use of opioid analgesics. This side effect can be easily remedied by taking stool softeners and laxatives and increasing fiber and fluid intake (especially water). It's better to anticipate constipation and treat it before it happens.

Other common side effects of opioids include sedation, nausea, vomiting, itching, urinary retention, and sensory or motor deficits. Many clinicians undertreat pain because they fear respiratory depression. While respiratory depression may occur with the use of opioids, it is uncommon in patients who are appropriately dosed and monitored. Patients

Evidence-Based Practice
Avoiding Addiction: The Four A's of Opioid Treatment

Caregivers tend to underutilize opioid analgesics because of the fear of addiction. Caregiver education in this area is very important, especially in the home-care setting where the caregiver is the one deciding when to give the patient pain medication. Addiction to opioids should be a concern, but the fear of addiction has been greatly exaggerated. Studies have shown that the incidence of addiction in patients who take an opioid for acute pain relief is about 1%. The length of time on the analgesic and the amount given are irrelevant to the risk for addiction.[23]

While the incidence of addiction is low, the potential for abuse does exist. Therefore, clinicians should remain diligent in monitoring patients who are taking opioids to assess their risk for abuse. Patients with a history of non-opioid substance abuse, including cigarettes and alcohol, and mental health disorders are at higher risk of developing opioid abuse.[58] An indication that abuse is developing is if the patient begins to crave the drug for reasons other than pain relief. When patients are using opioids, it is important to for the clinician to assess and document the 4 A's of opioid treatment as follows:

1. Analgesia (Is the pain score going down?)
2. Activities of daily living (Is there improvement in functional ability, positioning?)
3. Adverse effects (Are there mental status changes, such as confusion, or other effects, such as sedation, jerky motions, etc.?)
4. Aberrant behaviors (Does the patient report lost prescriptions, lost pills?)

at risk for developing respiratory depression include those with advanced disease states and/or comorbid conditions such as frailty, chronic obstructive pulmonary disease, congestive heart failure, sleep apnea, and kidney and/or liver disease. Respiratory depression can be decreased or eliminated with the use of lower initial doses that are increased gradually while monitoring the patient's vital signs, especially the quality and rate of respiration and the patient's sedation status.

Meperidine is not recommended for the management of persistent (chronic) pain. Disadvantages include the hazards of the normeperidine metabolite of meperidine. Repeated doses of meperidine can lead to an accumulation of normeperidine, which causes CNS excitability and toxicity. This toxicity will be manifested in the patient by twitching, numbness, seizures, and hallucinations.[2] Coma and death are also possible. According to the APS,[8] "although the oral doses of meperidine have about one quarter of the analgesic effectiveness of similar parenteral doses, they produce just as much of this toxic metabolite." The APS also warns that patients with compromised renal function are particularly at risk for the accumulation of this toxic metabolite.

STEP 2: OPIOIDS FOR MILD TO MODERATE PAIN

Opioids combined with an NSAID, or acetaminophen, or low-dose single-agent opioids, such as oxycodone immediate release 5 mg, may be used if step 1 is ineffective. (See *Examples of combination opioid,* page 314.) Propoxyphene and combined propoxyphene drugs are step 2 drugs, but these agents should be avoided in elderly patients because the drug metabolite, norproxyphene, may cause CNS and cardiac toxicity. Codeine may cause excessive constipation, nausea, and vomiting.[50,59]

Examples of combination opioids

- Acetaminophen with codeine
- Hydrocodone with acetaminophen
- Hydrocodone with ibuprofen
- Oxycodone with acetaminophen
- Oxycodone with ibuprofen
- Propoxyphene with acetaminophen

Note that there is a maximum recommended acetaminophen dose to decrease the risk of hepatotoxicity:
- Short-term use (<10 days): 4,000 mg/day
- Long-term use: 2,500 mg/day.

Examples of opioids: morphine and morphine-like agents

- Morphine
- Methadone
- Fentanyl
- Hydromorphone
- Levorphanol
- Oxycodone

STEP 2: OPIOIDS FOR MODERATE TO SEVERE PAIN

Opioids, including morphine and morphine-like agents, may be used when steps 1 and 2 are ineffective. (See *Examples of opioids: morphine and morphine-like agents* and *Practice Point: Helpful hints for using opioids.*)

Morphine is one of the drugs of choice for chronic pain largely because it is more cost-effective than meperidine, may be administered via many different routes, and is easily titrated. It has predictable and treatable side effects. The side effects of nausea and constipation

are usually treated with antiemetic drugs and laxatives, respectively. Other side effects are usually dose-related and can be resolved with dose adjustments.[7] Some patients cannot tolerate the side effects of morphine even with dose adjustments, and some experience significant side effects such as a skin rash or changes in mental status; the drug should be discontinued in these patients and a pain management consultation should be sought to determine an appropriate alternative analgesic.

Morphine is not for use in patients with renal disease (glomerular filtration rate < 30 mL/min) owing to the rapid accumulation of non-dialyzable metabolite that can be neurotoxic.[60] Patients who have liver disease may also be sensitive to the effects of morphine because it takes longer for the damaged liver to metabolize and eliminate the drug. Patients with asthma may have increased wheezing with morphine use and should be monitored carefully. Any patient whose daily dose of narcotic agents exceeds the equivalent of 120 mg of morphine should have a specialized pain consultation.[57]

Although studies are limited, some researchers are exploring the effects of topical opioids in the treatment of painful skin ulcers. In their report on nine patients with open skin ulcers caused by a variety of medical conditions, Twillman and colleagues[61] found that pain at the ulcer site was decreased when a morphine-infused gel dressing was used. The researchers reported remarkable efficacy in eight of the nine patients studied and believe further research is needed in this area because so many patients stand to gain pain relief.

Nonpharmacologic treatment modalities

Management of pain from wounds can require a combination of pharmacologic and nonpharmacologic treatments; the latter may include the use of music, massage, and relaxation techniques. Pain associated with dressing changes and debridement can be minimized by allowing patients to call "time-outs." Many other nonpharmacologic treatments can also be used prior to, and in conjunction with, medications. These

PRACTICE POINT

Helpful hints for using opioids

- Fentanyl
  - Oral–transmucosal fentanyl works in 10 minutes, which is good for dressing changes, but its use for this purpose is considered off-label. This drug is FDA approved only for cancer-related pain. Oral–transmucosal fentanyl should only be used in patients who are opioid tolerant (patients whose total dose of opioids is equal to 60 mg of morphine a day, for a total of 1 week or longer).
  - Fentanyl patches should be started at the lowest dose for patients who are opioid naïve (have never used opioids). Opioid naive patients need careful monitoring. In frail patients, even the lowest dose may cause sedation or other unwanted side effects.
  - It will take 18-24 hours for the first patch to reach maximum effect. If immediate pain relief is required, a short-acting opioid can be used along with the patch and then discontinued, if needed, when the patch begins to reach its maximum effect. A rescue dose of a short-acting opioid may still be needed for breakthrough pain once the long-acting dose has been titrated.
- Use short-acting agents (at 10% to 15% of total daily dose) for breakthrough pain.
- Titrate up to long-acting agents if the patient needs more than three breakthrough doses on a normal day.
- Don't wait for constipation to begin. Start the patient on stool softeners and laxatives to avoid this common adverse effect.
- To taper or discontinue opioid analgesics, decrease the dose by 25% every 2 to 3 days. Monitor for pain or withdrawal symptoms, as these would indicate that the tapering is too rapid.

PRACTICE POINT

Symptoms of withdrawal or abstinence from opioids include:

- tachycardia
- hypertension
- insomnia
- diaphoresis
- piloerection
- enlarged pupils
- nausea and diarrhea
- abdominal pain
- body aches
- increased sensitivity to pain
- yawning
- runny nose
- anxiety

The presence of these symptoms may indicate that the opioid medication is being tapered too quickly, and not necessarily that the patient is addicted to it.

include physical and occupational therapy, repositioning the patient, providing support surfaces, and optimizing local wound care with materials that minimize pain.

PHYSICAL AND OCCUPATIONAL THERAPY

Physical and occupational therapy services may be a valuable asset to utilize in conjunction with pharmacologic therapy. Passive and active range-of-motion exercises should be taught to the patient and his or her caregivers. Additional measures include the following:

- Patients with peripheral vascular disease may benefit from a walking program to facilitate development of collateral circulation in the lower extremities.
- Application of a transcutaneous electrical nerve stimulation unit may help to decrease pain, particularly in patients with chronic or acute wounds. It's believed that the electrical stimulation provided by the

unit helps to inhibit pain transmission cells.

- Hot or cold packs can be applied to decrease spasms in the affected area.
- Stretching exercises help to decrease contractures.
- Exercise helps to decrease muscle spasms with massage.

LOCAL PAIN MANAGEMENT

The use of appropriate dressings and dressing techniques can help to relieve pain during and between dressing changes. The international survey conducted by Moffatt et al.[28] highlights the importance of low-pain dressing changes. All respondents agreed that gauze dressings cause the most pain, while pain is noticeably less severe with the use of hydrogels, hydrofibers, alginates, and soft silicone dressings.

When administering wound care, choose products carefully to provide the patient with a pain-free experience. (See chapter 9, Wound treatment options.) Patients who express discomfort despite careful product selection should be given medication prior to dressing changes.

Moist wound dressings can be left in place for a longer period of time than wet-to-dry dressings. This reduces the frequency of dressing changes, thereby decreasing the opportunities for the patient to experience pain associated with dressing changes.

The following interventions will ease the dressing change process and manage pain for your patients.

Treating the cause/aggravating factors
- Provide pressure redistribution for your patients.
- Keep the patient's heels off the bed at all times.
- Control edema to avoid decreased blood flow to the wound, which may lead to additional pain.
- Eliminate or decrease pain from other possible pain sources.

Addressing patient-centered concerns
- Keep in mind that pharmacologic management is the gold standard for moderate to severe pain. Give pain medication around the clock, if necessary, to keep the pain under control.
- Instruct the patient and his or her family regarding pain management to alleviate fear of addiction with the use of opioids.
- Explain the role that pain control plays in improved wound healing.
- Explain dressing change procedures to the patient before proceeding with dressing changes.
- Allow the patient to select the time for dressing changes, if appropriate.
- Assess for pain and medicate the patient before and after dressing changes or debridement.
- Allow the patient or his family members to participate in dressing changes, as indicated.
- Offer the patient distraction techniques, such as conversation, television, and videos during dressing changes.
- Inform the patient that he or she may call a "time-out" if pain is present during dressing changes.
- Ensure that the patient has adequate rest and sleep. Lack of rest and sleep will decrease the patient's pain threshold, decrease his or her mental performance, and increase the emotional response to pain.
- Teach the patient to substitute worry beads, a pet rock, bean bag, tapping, rubbing, or gentle slapping for scratching.
- Instruct the patient in relaxation techniques and the use of visual imagery when encountering a potentially pain-provoking situation.
- Reevaluate the pain management plan when needed. Document the effectiveness of the analgesic or other treatments for pain relief with a pain score. This will help to assess whether the pain management program is working.
- Address other factors, such as loss of function, inability to perform ADLs, and possible changes in body image to help the patient deal with ancillary problems that might contribute to his pain.

Cleansing and debridement
- Assess pain when the patient is at rest to provide adequate pain control.

PRACTICE POINT

Wet-to-dry dressings can desiccate a wound, thus causing pain on removal. (Removing viable stuck tissue from the wound surface leads to bleeding, trauma, pain and delayed wound healing.) Avoid these dressings in favor of moisture-retentive dressings to promote a healing environment and patient comfort.

- Use warm normal saline solution or low cytotoxicity wound cleaners to clean wounds. (Cytotoxic solutions such as Betadine or hydrogen peroxide not only deter wound healing, but they may cause burning, adding to the patient's discomfort.)
- Use moist wound therapy to enhance autolytic debridement as an alternative to surgical or sharp debridement to eliminate pain associated with sharp debridement.
- Change dressings in a timely manner. Excess exudate on periwound skin or dressings that are allowed to dry on a wound may increase the patient's pain.
- Protect the periwound skin with skin barrier wipes, film-forming liquid acrylates, or ointment (petrolatum or zinc oxide) to prevent excoriation, trauma, maceration, or dermatitis that can delay wound healing, increase wound size, and increase patient discomfort. Avoid using strong adhesive tape on elderly patients or patients with fragile skin.

Alternative pain management methods

Many natural pain control methods and therapies may be implemented to ease pain, stress, and anxiety. These methods can improve one's outlook, attitude, and quality of life. Alternative therapies, when used in conjunction with pain medications, may enhance the beneficial effects of pain medication.

Laughter. Laughter helps you breathe deeper, lowers your blood pressure, and changes your mood.

Acupuncture. The application of needles to specific areas of the body may decrease or eliminate pain and has been used for more than 2,500 years.

Environment. Having the room at a comfortable temperature, avoiding bright lights, and keeping the room quiet may help to decrease pain.

Distraction. Playing cards, watching television, visiting with friends, petting an animal, and writing about his or her feelings can help the patient focus attention on something other than the pain.

Music. Music increases blood flow to the brain and increases energy, which in turn causes an increase in the production of endorphins (a natural body chemical similar to morphine) that work to decrease or eliminate pain and anxiety.

Magnets. Magnets may effect changes in cells or body chemistry that can produce pain relief. The use of magnets, which dates back to ancient Egypt and Greece, is popular with athletes, who report their effectiveness in controlling pain.

Capsaicin. Capsaicin, a chemical found in chili peppers, is the primary ingredient in many pain-relieving creams for the treatment of neuropathic pain. The local burning sensation it produces replaces the pain sensation.

SUMMARY

Pain scores derived from patient-completed validated pain assessment scales can be useful as the basis for assessing and treating chronic wound-associated pain. The scales enable the clinician to accurately assess the patient's pain, thereby facilitating effective treatment modalities to help decrease the wound-associated pain. Pain is detrimental for patients because it can exhaust them, reduce their ability to perform ADLs, add to feelings of decreased worth as a person, affect their interactions with loved ones and friends, deter wound healing and, overall, diminish quality of life and as well as quality of death for patients who are in the process of dying. As clinicians, we are obligated to provide adequate pain relief for our patients by selecting appropriate pain-control treatment modalities.

PATIENT SCENARIO

Clinical Data

Ms. CB is a 54-year-old woman who is hospitalized for severe pain associated with a right thigh ulcer. Her self-reported pain level is 10/10 with sustained-release morphine 15 mg and "12/10" without medication. The pain extends beyond the wound and increases with dressing changes ("horrible aching and burning that leaves me breathless" even at rest).

The right thigh ulcer started some months ago with a dark purple, burning, itching skin patch that became progressively larger, deeper, and more painful, affecting Ms. CB's ability to transfer and perform limited ADLs. Physical examination reveals a 5 × 5 × 5 cm tender ulcer on the right medial anterior thigh, exposing full-thickness skin loss and fibrous tissue at 12 to 1 o'clock over 10% of the wound. The remainder of the wound (90%) consists of black, leathery, odorous eschar with serosanguineous exudate.

Ms. CB lives alone and has a home health aide 8 hours a day, 7 days a week. She has been a pack-a-day smoker for 30 years and participates in a methadone maintenance program for intranasal heroin abuse. She denies current IV street drug use, alcohol use, and suicidal ideations. She has a past history of nonadherence to medical treatments. Ms. CB is on dialysis due to end-stage renal disease, receives highly active antiretroviral therapy due to AIDS, and has sarcoidosis with multiple medical complications, including anemia. Her analgesic use history is as follows:

- Oxycodone once daily without pain relief
- Tramadol 400 mg/day (maximum) without pain relief
- Acetaminophen with codeine frequently with pain relief in past
- Oxycodone 5 mg with acetaminophen 325 mg (Percocet) every 4 hours with pain relief and without adverse effects.

Ms. CB has a well-demarcated non-healing, painful, deep necrotic ulcer with exposed muscle. The clinical picture is consistent with calciphylaxis versus Coumadin-induced necrosis.

Case Discussion

Initial Pain Assessment and Treatment Rationale

Ms. CB should discontinue morphine and avoid codeine because its non-dialyzable metabolite can accumulate in patients with renal disease and because morphine may cause respiratory depression and neurotoxicity. Likewise, she should avoid NSAIDs because they can aggravate the renal disease.

The recommended treatment for this patient to control her pain is Percocet every 4 hours; the patient may refuse the medication if it is not needed. If her pain score remains at 5/10 or higher, the dose can be doubled and given every 4 hours, and again the patient may refuse the medication. The medication should be withheld if the patient becomes sedated.

To ameliorate the burning sensation in the ulcer, treatment should include a tricyclic antidepressant (amitriptyline, nortriptyline, or desipramine) 10–30 mg at bedtime or gabapentin (Neurontin) 100 mg at bedtime for 3 nights, followed by 100 mg twice daily for 3 days, followed by 200 mg twice daily. Titrate to maximum dose of 300 mg twice daily (dose for renal disease patients based on glomerular filtration rate).

A laxative will prevent constipation. Start with Lactulose 15–30 ml daily; if no bowel movement occurs, add Colace 100 mg three times daily, two Senna tablets as needed at bedtime, and Dulcolax 10 mg at bedtime .

Follow-Up Pain Assessment and Treatment

The patient was given two Percocet tablets every 4 hours (for a maximum of 60 mg of oxycodone daily) with good pain control and no side effects. An additional two Percocet tablets were given a half-hour prior to dressing changes, again with good pain control and no side effects. Opioid-induced constipation was controlled with a combination of Colace, Senna, Dulcolax.

A skin biopsy should be performed to diagnose the cause of the wound. Wounds in patients with calciphylaxis or Coumadin-induced necrosis should not be debrided surgically until the cause is corrected (renal and metabolic improvement in calciphylaxis and discontinuation of Coumadin in Coumadin necrosis).

The best local wound care is conservative, avoiding saline wet-to-dry dressings and strong adhesive dressings (or tape) because these will increase pain at dressing change. Cleansing can be facilitated with normal saline. If surgical debridement cannot be performed, the wound can be treated with an enzymatic ointment, calcium alginate, or hydrogel to facilitate autolytic debridement.

SHOW WHAT YOU KNOW

1. Which of the statements listed below most accurately defines pain? Pain is:
   A. an objective finding based on prolonged elevation of the patient's blood pressure and pulse rate.
   B. a state of discomfort evidenced by the person being unable to sleep.
   C. a physical consequence of wound care.
   D. whatever the experiencing person says it is.

   ANSWER: D. *McCaffery's classic definition of pain is that it's whatever the experiencing person says it is.[7] A is incorrect as research has shown that sudden, severe pain may elevate vital signs, but this only occurs for a short time.[7] B is incorrect as research has shown that patients can sleep even though they have moderate or severe pain.[7] C is incorrect because even though pain may be a consequence of wound care, this isn't a definition of pain.*

2. Which of the following statements best describes the Numeric Pain Intensity Scale? It's a:
   A. 10-cm line with the words "no pain" at one end and "worst possible pain" at the other end.
   B. series of faces ranging from smiling to frowning.
   C. rainbow of colors starting with green and ending with red.
   D. decision tree for determining which medications to give to a person experiencing pain.

   ANSWER: A. *The Numeric Pain Intensity Scale is a 10-cm line with the words "no pain" at one end and "worst possible pain" at the other end. B refers to the Faces Pain Rating Scale. C doesn't describe a pain scale. D refers to the WHO analgesic ladder.*

3. According to the WHO analgesic ladder, which medications should you use initially for relief of mild pain?
   A. None
   B. Non-opioid with or without an adjuvant
   C. Opioid with or without an adjuvant
   D. Opioid

   ANSWER: B. *A non-opioid is the drug recommended initially for mild pain. An adjuvant can be added if there is neuropathic and/or nociceptive pain. A is wrong as drugs are part of the WHO analgesic ladder. C and D are incorrect as they are part of step 2 in the ladder.*

REFERENCES

1. "Pain Terms. A List with Definitions and Notes on Usage Recommended by the IASP Subcommittee on Taxonomy," *Pain* 6(3):249-252, June 1979.

2. Acute Pain Management Guideline Panel. *Acute Pain Management: Operative or Medical Procedures and Trauma, Clinical Practice Guideline,* No.3. Rockville, Md.: AHCPR, 1992.

3. McCaffery, M., and Beebe, A. *Pain: Clinical Manual for Nursing Practice.* St. Louis, Mo.: Mosby–Year Book, Inc., 1989.

4. McCaffery, M., and Robinson, E.S. "Your Patient Is in Pain, Here's How You Respond," *Nursing* 32(10):36-45, October 2002.

5. Dahl, J.L., and Gordon, D.B. "Joint Commission Pain Standards: A Progress Report," *APS Bulletin* 12(6), 2002.

6. American Pain Society. (1995). Pain: The Fifth Vital Sign. Retrieved October 12, 2010, from *www.ampainsoc.org/advocacy/fifth.htm*.

7. McCaffery, M., and Passero, C. *Pain: Clinical Manual,* 2nd ed. St. Louis, Mo.: Mosby–Year Book, Inc.1999.

8. American Pain Society. *Principles of Analgesic Use in the Treatment of Acute Pain and Cancer Pain,* 6th ed. Glenview, Ill.: Author, 2008.

9. Lesser, H., et al. "Pregabalin Relieves Symptoms of Painful Diabetic Neuropathy: a randomized controlled trial," *Neurology* 63(11):2104-10, December 14, 2004.

10. Dworkin, R.H., et al. "Pregabalin for the Treatment of Postherpetic Neuralgia: a Randomized, Placebo-controlled Trial," *Neurology* 60(8):1274-83, April 2003.

11. American Geriatric Society. "The Management of Persistent Pain in Older Persons," *AGS Panel on Persistent Pain in Older Persons* 50(6 Suppl):S205-S224, June 2002.

12. Arroyo-Novoa, C.M., Figueroa-Ramos, M.I., Miaskowski, C., et al, "Acute Wound Pain: Gaining a Better Understanding," *Advances in Skin & Wound Care* 322(8):373-80, 2009.

13. Polomano, R. C., "Neurophysiology of Pain," in Core *Curriculum for Pain Management Nursing,* 2nd ed. Edited by St. Marie, B. Philadelphia: WB Saunders Company, 2002.

14. Dallam, L., et al. "Pressure Ulcer Pain: Assessment and Quantification," *Journal of Wound, Ostomy, and Continence Nursing* 22(5):211-17, September 1995.

15. Krasner, D. "The Chronic Wound Pain Experience: A Conceptual Model," *Ostomy/Wound Management* 41(3):20-29, April 1995.

16. Krasner, D. "Caring for the Person Experiencing Chronic Wound Pain," *in Chronic Wound Care: A Clinical Source Book for Healthcare Professionals,* 3rd ed. Edited by Krasner, D.L. Wayne, Pa.: HMP Communications, 2001.

17. Krasner, D. "Managing Wound Pain in Patients with Vacuum-Assisted Closure Devices," *Ostomy/Wound Management* 48(5):38-43, May 2002.

18. Gardner, S.E., Frantz, R.A., Doebbeling, B.N. The validity of the clinical signs and symptoms used to identify localized chronic wound infection. *Wound Repair Regen* 9:178-86, 2001.

19. National Pressure Ulcer Advisory Panel. "Pressure Ulcer Prevalence, Cost, and Risk Assessment: Consensus Development Conference Statement," *Decubitus* 2(2):24-28, May 1989.

20. Van Rijswijk, L., and Braden, B.J. "Pressure Ulcer Patient and Wound Assessment: An AHCPR Clinical Practice Guideline Update," *Ostomy/Wound Management* 45(1A Suppl):56S-67S, January 1999.

21. Bergstrom, N., et al. *Pressure Ulcer Treatment: Clinical Practice Guideline #15.* Rockville, Md.: AHCPR, 1994.

22. Pieper, B. "Mechanical Forces: Pressure, Shear and Friction," *in Acute and Chronic Wounds: Nursing Management,* 2nd ed. Edited by Bryant, R.A. St. Louis, Mo.: Mosby–Year Book, Inc., 2000.

23. Rook, J.L. "Wound Care Pain Management," *Advances in Wound Care* 9(6):24-31, November-December 1996.

24. Szors, J.K., and Bourguignon, C. "Description of Pressure Ulcer Pain at Rest and Dressing Change," *Journal of Wound, Ostomy, and Continence Nurses* 26(3):115-20, May 1999.

25. Sibbald, R.G., Woo, K, Ayello, E.A. "Increased Bacterial Burden and Infection: The Story of NERDS and STONES," *Advances in Skin and Wound Care* 19(8): 447-462, 2006.

26. Hollingworth, H. "Nurse's Assessment and Management of Pain at Wound Dressing Changes," *Journal of Wound Care* 4(2):77-83, February 1995.

27. European Wound Management Association. *EWMA Position Document: Pain at Wound Dressing Changes, London,* UK: MEP Ltd., 2002.

28. Moffatt, C.J., Franks, P.J., Hollinworth, H. "Understanding Wound Pain and Trauma: An International Perspective," *in EWMA Position Document: Pain at Wound Dressing Changes* (pp 2-7). London, UK: MEP Ltd., 2002.

29. Wulf, H, and Baron, R. "The Theory of Pain," *in EWMA Position Document: Pain at Wound Dressing Changes* (pp 8-11). London, UK: MEP Ltd., 2002.

30. Briggs, M., Torra I Bou, J.E. "Pain at Wound Dressing Changes: a Guide to Management," *in EWMA Position Document: Pain at Wound Dressing Changes* (pp 12-17). London, UK: MEP Ltd., 2002.

31. Briggs, M., Ferris, F.D., et al. *Principles of Best Practice: A World Union of Wound Healing Societies' Initiative. Minimizing pain at wound dressing-related procedures: A consensus document.* London, UK: MEP Ltd., 2004.

32. Latarjet, J. "The Management of Pain Associated with Dressing Changes in Patients with Burns," *World Wide Wounds* (Electronic journal), November 2002.

33. Krasner, D. "Using a Gentler Hand: Reflections on Patients with Pressure Ulcers Who Experience Pain," *Ostomy/Wound Management* 42(3):20-29, April 1996.

34. Woo K. *Wound-Related Pain and Attachment in the Older Adults.* Saarbrucken, Germany: Lambert Academic Publishing, 2002.

35. Franks, P.J., and Collier, M.E. "Quality of Life: The Cost to the Individual," *in The Prevention of Pressure Ulcers.* Edited by Morrison, M.J. St. Louis, Mo.: Mosby–Year Book, Inc., 2001.

36. Ayello, E.A., et al. "Is Pressure Ulcer Pain Documented? Paper presented at the Clinical Symposium on Advances in Skin and Wound Care, Las Vegas, NV; 2006.

37. Langemo, D.K., et al. "The Lived Experience of Having a Pressure Ulcer: A Qualitative Analysis," *Advances in Skin & Wound Care* 13(5):225-35, September-October 2000.

38. Rastinehad, D. "Pressure Ulcer Pain," *Journal of Wound Ostomy and Continence Nursing* 33(3):252-57, May/June 2006.

39. Hopkins, A., et al. "Patient Stories of Living with a Pressure Ulcer," *Journal of Advanced Nursing* 56(4):1-9, April 2006.

40. Roth, R.S., Lowery, J.C., Hamill, J.B. "Assessing Persistent Pain and Its Relation to Affective Distress, Depressive Symptoms, and Pain Catastrophizing in Patients with Chronic Wounds: A Pilot Study," *American Journal of Physical Medicine & Rehabilitation* 83(11):827-34, November 2004.

41. Shukla, D., Tripathi, A.K., et al. "Pain in Acute and Chronic Wounds: A Descriptive Study," *Ostomy Wound Management* 51(11):47-51, November 2005.

42. Fox, C. "Living With a Pressure Ulcer: A Descriptive Study of Patients' Experiences," *British Journal of Community Nursing* 7:10-22, July 2002.

43. Ayello, E.A. "Teaching the Assessment of Patients with Pressure Ulcers," *Decubitus* 5(4):53-54, July 1992.

44. Ayello, E.A. "A Pressure Ulcer ASSESSMENT Tool," *Advances in Skin & Wound Care* 13(5):247, September-October 2000.

45. Herr, K., et al. "Pain Assessment in the Nonverbal Patient: Position Statement with Clinical Practice Recommendations," *Pain Management Nursing* 7(2):44-52, June 2006.

46. Hartford Institute for Geriatric Nursing. Try This. Retrieved Oct 31, 2010 from www.hartfordign.org.

47. Fink, R., and Gates, R. "Pain Assessment," in *Textbook of Palliative Nursing.* Edited by Ferrell, B.R., and Coyle, N. New York: Oxford University Press, 2001.

48. Keele, K.D. "The Pain Chart," *The Lancet* 48(2):6-8, February 1948.

49. Wong, D.L., and Baker, C.M. "Pain in Children: Comparison of Assessment Scales," *Pediatric Nursing* 14(1):9-17, January-February 1988.

50. Flaherty, S.A. "Pain Measurement Tools for Clinical Practice and Research," *Journal of the American Association of Nurse Anesthetists* 64(2):133-140, April 1996.

51. Hockenberry-Eaton, M., and Wilson, D. *Wong's Essentials of Pediatric Nursing*, 8th ed. St. Louis: Mosby, 2009.

52. Simon, W., and Malabar, R. "Assessing Pain in Elderly Patients Who Can't Respond Verbally," *Journal of Advanced Nursing* 22(4):663-669, October 1995.

53. Donovan, M., et al. "Incidence and Characteristics of Pain in a Sample of Medical-Surgical Patients," *Pain* 30(1):69-78, July 1987.

54. Faires, J.E., et al. "Systematic Pain Records and Their Impact on Pain Control: A Pilot Study," *Cancer Nursing* 12(6):306-13, December 1991.

55. Freedman, G., et al. "Practical Treatment of Pain in Patients with Chronic Wounds: Pathogenesis-guided Management," *The American Journal of Surgery* 188(suppl):31S-35S, July 2004.

56. World Health Organization. *Cancer Pain Relief,* 2nd ed., Geneva: Author, 1996.

57. Washington State Agency Medical Directors Group. *Interagency Guideline on Opioid Dosing for Chronic Non-cancer Pain: An Educational Pilot to Improve Care and Safety with Opioid Treatment.* Olympia, Wash.: Author, 2010.

58. Edlund, M.J., et al. "Risk Factors for Clinically Recognized Opioid Abuse and Dependency among Veterans using Opioids for Non-cancer Pain," *Pain* 129(3):355-362. June 2007.

59. Derby, S., and O'Mahony, S. "Elderly Patients," in *Textbook of Palliative Nursing.* Edited by Ferrell, B.R., and Coyles, N. New York: Oxford University Press, 2001.

60. Osborne R, et al. "The Pharmacokinetics of Morphine and Morphine Glucuronides in Kidney Failure," *Clinical Pharmacology & Therapeutics* 54:158-67, 1993.

61. Twillman, R.K., et al. "Treatment of Painful Skin Ulcer with Topical Opioids," *Journal of Pain and Symptom Management* 17(4):288-92, April 1999.

PART II

Wound Classifications and Management Strategies

CHAPTER 13

Pressure Ulcers

Elizabeth A. Ayello, PhD, RN, ACNS-BC, CWON, MAPWCA, FAAN
Sharon Baranoski, MSN, RN, CWCN, APN-CCRN, DAPWCA, FAAN
Courtney H. Lyder, ND, GNP, FAAN
Janet E. Cuddigan, PhD, RN, CWCN
Wendy S. Harris, BSHS

Objectives

After completing this chapter, you'll be able to:

- discuss the significance of pressure ulcers as a healthcare problem
- describe the etiology of a pressure ulcer
- explain how to complete a risk assessment tool
- discuss strategies for pressure ulcer prevention
- define pressure ulcer classification systems
- discuss strategies for treating a patient with pressure ulcers
- state how to determine pressure ulcer prevalence and incidence.

PRESSURE ULCERS AS A HEALTHCARE PROBLEM

Pressure ulcers are a global healthcare concern and require an interdisciplinary approach to care and management.[1,2] All clinicians need to be responsible for the prevention and treatment of pressure ulcers.

Over the centuries, pressure ulcers have been referred to as decubitus ulcers, bedsores, and pressure sores. The term *pressure ulcer* has become the preferred name because it most closely describes the etiology and resultant ulcer. In 2009, the National Pressure Ulcer Advisory Panel (NPUAP), in collaboration with the European Pressure Ulcer Advisory Panel (EPUAP), released this common definition: "A pressure ulcer is a localized injury to the skin and/or underlying tissue usually over a bony prominence, as a result of pressure, or pressure in combination with shear. A number of contributing or confounding factors are also associ-

ated with pressure ulcers; the significance of these factors is yet to be elucidated."[1] Pressure ulcers are usually located over bony prominences (such as the sacrum, coccyx, hips, heels) and are classified according to the extent of the type of observable tissue damage.[1] Relying just on *depth* of tissue damage rather than tissue type may be misleading because pressure ulcers in locations where there is little adipose tissue, such as the ear, may be shallow but still extend through the subcutaneous tissue.[1] (See *International NPUAP/EPUAP Pressure Ulcer Classification System*. See also *color section*, *Pressure Ulcers*, pages C19–C21.)

The incidence and prevalence of pressure ulcers are truly enigmatic. Pressure ulcers aren't a reportable event in all healthcare settings, so data are speculative at best. We do know, however, that the numbers are significant enough to warrant national healthcare initiatives in the United States as well as other countries. As early as 1989, the US federal

International NPUAP/EPUAP pressure ulcer classification system

Category/Stage I: Non-blanchable Erythema

- Intact skin with non-blanchable redness of a localized area, usually over a bony prominence. Darkly pigmented skin may not have visible blanching; its color may differ from the surrounding area.
- The area may be painful, firm, soft, warmer or cooler as compared to adjacent tissue. Category/Stage I may be difficult to detect in individuals with dark skin tones. May indicate "at risk" persons (a heralding sign of risk).

Category/Stage II: Partial Thickness Skin Loss

- Partial-thickness loss of dermis presenting as a shallow open ulcer with a red pink wound bed, without slough. May also present as an intact or open/ruptured serum-filled blister. Presents as a shiny or dry shallow ulcer without slough or bruising.* This Category/Stage should not be used to describe skin tears, tape burns, incontinence associated dermatitis, maceration, or excoriation.

Category/Stage III: Full Thickness Skin Loss

- Full-thickness tissue loss. Subcutaneous fat may be visible, but bone, tendon, or muscle are *not* exposed. Slough may be present but does not obscure the depth of tissue loss. *May* include undermining and tunneling.
- The depth of Category/Stage III pressure ulcer varies by anatomical location. The bridge of the nose, ear, occiput, and malleolus do not have subcutaneous tissue, and category/stage III ulcers can be shallow. In contrast, areas of significant adiposity can develop extremely deep Category/Stage III pressure ulcers. Bone/tendon is not visible or directly palpable.

Category/Stage IV: Full Thickness Tissue Loss

- Full-thickness tissue loss with exposed bone, tendon, or muscle. Slough or eschar may be present on some parts of the wound bed. Often includes undermining and tunneling.
- The depth of a Category/Stage IV pressure ulcer varies by anatomical location. The bridge of the nose, ear, occiput, and malleolus do not have subcutaneous tissue, and these ulcers can be shallow. Category/stage IV ulcers can extend into muscle and/or supporting structures (e.g., fascia, tendon, or joint capsule), making osteomyelitis possible. Exposed bone/tendon is visible or directly palpable.

Unstageable: Depth Unknown

- Full-thickness tissue loss in which the base of the ulcer is covered by slough (yellow, tan, gray, green, or brown) and/or eschar (tan, brown, or black) in the wound bed.
- Until enough slough and/or eschar is removed to expose the base of the wound, the true depth, and therefore Category/Stage, cannot be determined, Stable (dry, adherent, intact without erythema or fluctuance) eschar on the heels serves as "the body's natural (biological) cover" and should not be removed.

(continued)

International NPUAP/EPUAP pressure ulcer classification system (continued)

Suspected Deep Tissue Injury: Depth Unknown

- Purple or maroon localized area of discolored intact skin or blood-filled blister due to damage of underlying soft tissue from pressure and/or shear. The area may be preceded by tissue that is painful, firm, mushy, boggy, or warmer or cooler as compared to adjacent tissue.
- Deep tissue injury may be difficult to detect in individuals with dark skin tones. Evolution may include a thin blister over a dark wound bed. The wound may further evolve and become covered by thin eschar. Evolution may be rapid, exposing additional layers of tissue even with optimal treatment.

---

*Bruising indicates suspected deep tissue injury.

National Pressure Ulcer Advisory Panel and European Pressure Ulcer Advisory Panel. *Prevention and Treatment of Pressure Ulcers: Clinical Practice Guideline.* Washington, DC: National Pressure Ulcer Advisory Panel, pp. 19-20. 2009. Used with permission.

government focused its attention on pressure ulcers with the appointment of a panel charged with developing the Agency for Health Care Policy and Research (AHCPR) guidelines.[3,4] Since that time, clinical practice guidelines regarding pressure ulcers have been released by several other organizations, including the Wound, Ostomy & Continence Nurses Society (WOCN),[5] the Registered Nurses' Association of Ontario (RNAO),[6] and the Wound Healing Society (WHS).[7]

Long-term care in the United States has long been regulated regarding pressure ulcers as mandated by Federal Tag (F-Tag) 314.[8] In addition, the Agency for Healthcare Research and Quality (AHRQ; formerly AHCPR) stated in its 2008 statistical brief report that there was nearly an 80% increase in hospital stays in which pressure ulcers were noted, even though the total number of hospitalizations for the reported time period (1993–2006) increased by only 15%.[9] Given the attention from regulatory and quality improvement agencies on pressure ulcer occurrence, preventing pressure ulcers should be a priority of patient care across all care settings.

The financial cost associated with pressure ulcers to all institutions and facilities isn't precisely known. According to the Centers for Medicare and Medicaid Services (CMS), the average cost of pressure ulcers for hospitalized patients in 2007 was $43,180.[9] Published estimates of treatment costs vary across hospital, long-term care, and home care settings; the one certainty is that pressure ulcers do create a financial burden for the facility, patient, and family alike. Pressure ulcers cost institutions valuable staff time, supplies, and reputation.

Pressure ulcer practices should be evidenced based. However, adequate research-based, randomized clinical studies to support all of our current practices do not exist. For example, in the NPUAP/EPUAP clinical practice guideline, there are seven recommendations at the A level of evidence for pressure ulcer prevention and only one A-level recommendation for treatment.[1] Wound care interventions and modalities have often been based on an "it works for me" attitude. We need to encourage healthcare providers to participate in research studies so that we'll have the evidence in the future to direct and improve our clinical decision making process, thereby improving patient outcomes.

WOUND ETIOLOGY

How do pressure ulcers occur? This is an interesting and challenging question. Literature reviews demonstrate several etiologies of pressure ulcers. Earlier reviews focused on a model of pressure ulcer development caused by pressure-induced capillary closure cutting off blood supply and leading to tissue ischemia, injury, and death. More recent research, using techniques such as magnetic resonance imaging (MRI), has documented cellular distortion and damage from pressure. There is also a renewed appreciation for the effects of shear in damaging deeper tissue and microclimate (moisture and temperature) in rendering tissue less tolerant of the effects of pressure.[10]

PRACTICE POINT

Muscle tissue dies first from pressure. Look at a variety of extrinsic and intrinsic factors that could put your patient at risk for pressure ulcers.

The recent international NPUAP/EPUAP clinical practice guideline states that "pressure ulcers develop as a result of the internal response to external mechanical load."[1] The pressure gradient[1,4,11–14] has been used to explain how pressure translates into tissue death. (See *Pressure gradient*.) External pressure is transmitted from the epidermis inward toward the bone as well as by counter-pressure from the bone. As a result, the loaded soft tissues, including skin and deeper tissues (adipose tissue, connective tissue, and muscle), will deform, resulting in strain and stress within the tissues."[1]

Body tissues differ in their ability to tolerate pressure. The blood supply to the skin originates in the underlying muscle. Muscle is more sensitive to pressure damage than is skin tissue.[1,15] Tissue tolerance is further compromised by extrinsic and intrinsic factors. Extrinsic factors include moisture, friction, and irritants. Numerous intrinsic factors affect the ability of the skin and supporting structures to respond to pressure and shear forces, including age, spinal cord injury, nutrition, and steroid administration; these factors are believed to affect collagen synthesis and degradation.[16] Other intrinsic factors affect tissue perfusion, including systemic blood pressure, extracorporeal circulation, serum protein, smoking, hemoglobin and hematocrit, vascular disease, diabetes mellitus, vasoactive drugs, and increases in body temperature.[16]

A recent comprehensive review of risk factor research helps explain the complex interaction between increased pressure intensity/

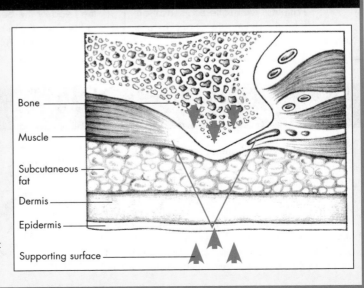

Pressure gradient

In this illustration, the V-shaped pressure gradient results from the upward force (upward arrowheads) exerted by the supporting surface against downward force (downward arrowheads) exerted by the bony prominence. Pressure is greatest on tissues at the apex of the gradient and lessens to the right and left of this point.

Bone

Muscle

Subcutaneous fat

Dermis

Epidermis

Supporting surface

duration and the extrinsic and intrinsic factors that affect tissue tolerance to pressure.[1] Activity and mobility limitations create the necessary conditions for pressure ulcers to develop (i.e., unrelieved pressure). Individuals who are bedbound or chairfast and unable to effectively reposition themselves fall into these risk factor categories and should be considered at risk. Epidemiological studies show that limitations in activity and mobility are independently predictive of pressure ulcers. Changes in sensory perception may further impair movement.

Once the conditions for increased pressure intensity and duration are established, intrinsic and extrinsic factors affecting tissue tolerance contribute to pressure ulcer development. According to epidemiological evidence, these factors fall under several categories: (1) poor nutritional status (e.g., decreased intake of nutrients—especially protein, weight loss, lower albumin); (2) skin moisture (e.g., urinary or fecal incontinence, excessive sweating or wound drainage); (3) advanced age; (4) factors affecting perfusion and oxygenation (e.g., hypotension, hemodynamic instability, peripheral vascular disease, diabetes, vasopressor drugs, need for supplemental oxygen); (5) friction and shear; (6) poor general health status; and (7) increased body temperature.[1]

Friction and shear are also mechanical forces contributing to pressure ulcer formation. The tissue injury resulting from friction may look like a superficial skin insult. Shear has the potential to damage deeper tissue. Shear and friction are two separate phenomena, yet they often work together to create tissue ischemia and ulcer development.

Shear is a "mechanical force that acts on an area of skin in a direction parallel to the body's surface. It's affected by the amount of pressure exerted, the coefficient of friction between the materials contacting each other, and the extent to which the body makes contact with the support surface."[4] The NPUAP includes definitions of shear stress and shear strain in its international guideline.[1] You can think of shear stress and strain as pulling the bones of the pelvis in one direction and the skin in the opposite direction. (See *Shearing force.* See also *Effects of shear on tissue.*) The deeper fascia slides downward with the bone, while the superficial fascia remains attached to the dermis. This insult and compromise to the blood supply creates ischemia, reperfusion injury, lymphatic impairment, and mechanical deformation of tissue cell[17,18] and

> ### ◤ PRACTICE POINT
>
> Patients with altered sensation are at risk for the development of pressure ulcers.

> ### ◤ PRACTICE POINT
>
> You won't see shear injury at the skin level because it occurs underneath the skin. You will see friction injury. Elevation of the head of the bed increases shear injury in the deep tissue and may account for the number of sacral ulcers we see in practice.

Shearing force

Shear injury is a mechanical force parallel, rather than perpendicular, to an area of tissue. In this illustration, gravity pulls the body down the incline of the bed. The skeleton and attached deep fascia slide within the skin, while the skin and superficial fascia, attached to the dermis, remain stationary, held in place by friction between the skin and the bed linen. This internal slide compromises blood supply to the area and deforms or distorts tissue.

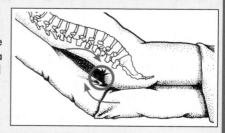

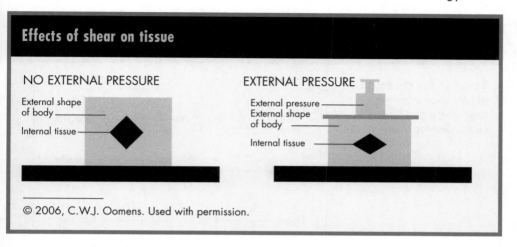

Effects of shear on tissue

NO EXTERNAL PRESSURE

External shape of body

Internal tissue

EXTERNAL PRESSURE

External pressure
External shape of body

Internal tissue

© 2006, C.W.J. Oomens. Used with permission.

leads to cellular death and tissue necrosis. Shear and friction go hand in hand—you'll rarely see one without the other.

Friction was originally defined by the AHCPR as the "mechanical force exerted when skin is dragged across a coarse surface such as bed linens."[4] The NPUAP defines friction or frictional force as "the resistance to motion in a parallel direction relative to the common boundary of two surfaces."[1] Simply stated, friction or frictional force results when two surfaces move across one another. A skin insult caused by friction looks like an abrasion or superficial laceration. Friction, however, isn't a primary factor in the development of pressure ulcers. It can contribute to an insult or stripping of the epidermal layer of the skin, creating an environment conducive to further insult. An alteration in the coefficient of friction increases the skin's adherence to the outside surface (for example, the bed). Friction then combines with shearing forces, and the ultimate outcome may be a pressure ulcer. Tissue subjected to friction is more susceptible to pressure ulcer damage.[19] The three mechanical forces (pressure, friction, and shear) may act in concert to create tissue damage. Other patients at risk for pressure ulcers from friction are elderly people, those with uncontrollable movements such as spastic movements, and those who use braces or appliances that rub against the skin.[11]

Exactly what causes pressure ulcers remains controversial.[20] Theories on the etiology of pressure ulcers need continued research. Those described here may be correct, but addi-tional research and basic science will hold the answers to many unanswered questions.

Most pressure ulcers occur in the lower part of the body over bony prominences such as the sacrum, coccyx, ischial tuberosities, greater trochanters, heels, iliac crests, and lateral and medial malleoli.[11,21] (See *Pressure ulcer sites,* page 330.) Other areas, where pressure ulcers may be overlooked, include the occiput (especially in infants and toddlers, see chapter 22, Pressure ulcers in neonatal and pediatric populations), elbows, scapulae, and ears (especially in patients using nasal oxygen cannulas).

Several national surveys demonstrated that the most common site for pressure ulcers among patients in acute care facilities is the sacrum, with the heels being second.[21] The incidence of heel ulcers has increased incrementally over the past decade, creating a need for prevention protocols targeting the heels. The HEELS© mnemonic[22] can be used to care for heels at risk for pressure ulcers. (See *HEELS© mnemonic,* page 330.) A growing clinical problem is pressure ulcers caused by medical devices. In a recent survey of 86,932 patients in acute care facilities, 9.1% of all pressure ulcers identified were device related, with the ear being the most common site (20%).[21] Devices that are commonly associated with pressure ulcers include oxygen tubing (ears), endotracheal tubes (mouth and lips), continuous positive airway pressure (CPAP) masks (bridge of nose, face), cervical collars (neck and head), and splints, braces, heel lifts, thromboembolic deterrent (TED) hose, and compression devices (lower extremities). Any tube under pressure can create pressure

Pressure ulcer sites

Shown in this illustration are the most common sites where pressure ulcers develop.

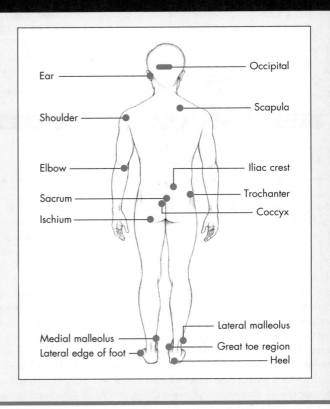

HEELS© mnemonic

H ave foot or leg movement?
E valuate heels and sensation.
E valuate foot drop risk.
L imit friction.
S uspend heels with devices as needed.

© 2005, Ayello, Cuddigan, and Black. Used with permission. From Cuddigan, J., Ayello, E.A., and Black, J. "Saving Heels in Critically Ill Patients," *World Council of Enterostomal Therapists Journal* 28(2):16-24, 2008.

damage. Edematous patients are at particularly high risk.[23]

 PRACTICE POINT

Careful observation of the sacrum/coccyx and heels is warranted because these are the most frequent sites of pressure ulcers.

PREVENTION

Preventing pressure ulcers is of vital importance. Elements of pressure ulcer prevention include identifying individuals at risk for developing pressure ulcers, preserving skin integrity, treating the underlying causes of the ulcer, relieving pressure, paying attention to the total state of the patient to correct any deficiencies, and educating the patient and his or her family about pressure ulcers.

Risk factors and risk assessment

Risk assessment is used to identify:

- patients at risk
- the level of risk
- the type of risk.

Identifying individuals at risk for pressure ulcers enables clinicians to make decisions about when to begin using preventive measures. This is important for the most effective use of resources because the level of risk guides the intensity and cost of preventive interventions. Risk assessment is governed by the regulations in effect in a particular setting. For example, the Outcome and Assessment Information Set (OASIS-C) guidelines for home care recommend that a structured approach to risk assessment be conducted on all home care clients.[24] MDS 3.0 describes several methods for determining a long-term-care resident's pressure ulcer risk, including a formal assessment instrument, a clinical assessment conducted by the clinician, an existing stage 1 or higher pressure ulcer, a scar over a bony prominence, or a non-removable dressing or device.[25–28]

Many validated pressure ulcer risk assessment tools are available, including the Norton Scale,[29] the Gosnell Scale,[30] the Braden Scale,[31] and the Waterlow Scale.[32] Deciding which scale to use can be challenging. Reviewing the reliability (consistency) and validity (accuracy) of each scale should always be the first step in the decision-making process. Reliability for risk assessment scales is usually described in terms of inter-rater reliability. According to Ayello and Braden,[33] "a common measure of inter-rater reliability for a risk assessment tool is percentage agreement, which looks at the percentage of instances in which different raters assign the same score to the same patients. Validity, or accuracy, is measured by the ability of the tool to correctly predict who will or won't develop a pressure ulcer."

Predictive validity is dependent on the sensitivity and specificity of the tool. Sensitivity is "the percentage of individuals who develop a pressure ulcer who were assessed as being at risk for a pressure ulcer. A tool has good sensitivity if it correctly identifies true positives while minimizing false negatives. Specificity is the percentage of individuals who don't develop a pressure ulcer who were assessed as being not at risk for developing an ulcer. A tool has good specificity if it identifies true negatives and minimizes false positives."[33,34] Because of the amount of clinical research supporting their reliability and validity, the Norton,[29] Braden,[31] and Waterlow[32] Scales are mentioned in the NPUAP/EPUAP clinical practice guideline[1] as appropriate to use to determine pressure ulcer risk assessment. One study that compared four of the risk assessment scales found that the Gosnell Scale[30] was the most appropriate for patients with neurologic and orthopedic conditions.[35]

BRADEN SCALE

The Braden Scale is the most commonly used pressure ulcer assessment tool in the United States. Available in many languages (English, French, Portuguese)[36–38] and used worldwide, this copyrighted tool was created in 1987 by Barbara Braden and Nancy Bergstrom[31] and is available at http://www.bradenscale.com/images/bradenscale.pdf .[38] The Braden Scale has six subscales: sensory perception, moisture, activity, mobility, nutrition, and friction/shear.[31,38] (See *Braden Scale: predicting pressure sore risk*, pages 332 and 333.) The scale is based on the two primary etiologic factors of pressure ulcer development—intensity and duration of pressure and tissue tolerance for pressure. "Sensory perception, mobility, and activity address clinical situations that predispose a patient to intense and prolonged pressure, while moisture, nutrition, and friction/shear address clinical situations that alter tissue tolerance for pressure."[33]

Each subscale contains a numerical range of scores, with 1 being the lowest score possible.[38] The sensory perception, moisture, activity, mobility, and nutrition subscales have scores ranging from 1 to 4. Friction/shear is the only

Braden Scale: predicting pressure ulcer risk

SENSORY PERCEPTION Ability to respond meaningfully to pressure-related discomfort	**1. Completely limited:** Unresponsive (doesn't moan, flinch, or grasp) to painful stimuli due to diminished level of consciousness or sedation OR limited ability to feel pain over most of body surface.	**2. Very limited:** Responds only to painful stimuli. Can't communicate discomfort except by moaning or restlessness OR has a sensory impairment that limits the ability to feel pain or discomfort over half of body.
MOISTURE Degree to which skin is exposed to moisture	**1. Constantly moist:** Skin is kept moist almost constantly by perspiration or urine. Dampness is detected every time patient is moved or turned.	**2. Often moist:** Skin is often but not always moist. Linen must be changed at least once per shift.
ACTIVITY Degree of physical activity	**1. Bedfast:** Confined to bed.	**2. Confined to chair:** Ability to walk severely limited or nonexistent. Can't bear own weight and must be assisted into chair or wheelchair.
MOBILITY Ability to change and control body position	**1. Completely immobile:** Doesn't make even slight changes in body or extremity position without assistance.	**2. Very limited:** Makes occasional slight changes in body or extremity position but unable to make frequent or significant changes independently.
NUTRITION Usual food intake pattern NPO: Nothing by mouth IV: Intravenously TPN: Total parenteral nutrition	**1. Very poor:** Never eats a complete meal. Rarely eats more than one-third of any food offered. Eats two servings or less of protein (meat or dairy products) per day. Takes fluids poorly. Doesn't take a liquid dietary supplement OR is NPO or maintained on clear liquids or I.V. fluids for more than 5 days.	**2. Probably inadequate:** Rarely eats a complete meal and generally eats only about half of any food offered. Protein intake includes only three servings of meat or dairy products per day. Occasionally will take a dietary supplement OR receives less than optimum amount of liquid diet or tube feeding.
FRICTION AND SHEAR	**1. Problem:** Requires moderate to maximum assistance in moving. Complete lifting without sliding against sheets is impossible. Frequently slides down in bed or chair, requiring frequent repositioning with maximum assistance. Spasticity, contractures, or agitation leads to almost constant friction.	**2. Potential problem:** Moves feebly or requires minimum assistance. During a move, skin probably slides to some extent against sheets, chair, restraints, or other devices. Maintains relatively good position in chair or bed most of the time but occasionally slides down.

Used with permission from Barbara Braden, PhD, RN, FAAN, and Nancy Bergstrom, PhD, RN, FAAN. © 1988.

3. Slightly limited:

Responds to verbal commands but can't always communicate discomfort or need to be turned

OR

has some sensory impairment that limits ability to feel pain or discomfort in one or two extremities.

4. No impairment:

Responds to verbal commands. Has no sensory deficit that would limit ability to feel or voice pain or discomfort.

3. Occasionally moist:

Skin is occasionally moist, requiring an extra linen change approximately once per day.

4. Rarely moist:

Skin is usually dry; linen only requires changing at routine intervals.

3. Walks occasionally:

Walks occasionally during day, but for very short distances, with or without assistance; spends majority of each shift in bed or chair.

4. Walks frequently:

Walks outside the room at least twice per day and inside room at least once every 2 hours during waking hours.

3. Slightly limited:

Makes frequent though slight changes in body or extremity position independently.

4. No limitations:

Makes major and frequent changes in position without assistance.

3. Adequate:

Eats over half of most meals. Eats a total of four servings of protein (meat, dairy products) each day. Occasionally will refuse a meal, but will usually take a supplement if offered

OR

is on a tube feeding or TPN regimen that probably meets most nutritional needs.

4. Excellent:

Eats most of every meal and never refuses a meal. Usually eats a total of four servings of meat and dairy products. Occasionally eats between meals. Doesn't require supplementation.

3. No apparent problem:

Moves in bed and in chair independently and has sufficient muscle strength to lift up completely during move. Maintains good position in bed or chair at all times.

subscale in which scores range from 1 to 3. Definitions of each subscale as to what patient characteristics to evaluate are given for each numerical ranking. The Braden Scale score is derived from totaling the numerical ratings from each of the six subscales. Six is the lowest possible score, and 23 is the highest possible score.

A low numerical score indicates that the patient is at high risk for developing pressure ulcers. The original at-risk score was 16.[31] Subsequent research is the basis for the recommendation to use 18 as the risk score for elderly,[39] black, and Hispanic patients.[40,41] Braden and Bergstrom[33,34,38] suggest the following levels of risk based on total Braden Scale scores: 15 to 18, at risk; 13 to 14, moderate risk; 10 to 12, high risk; and 9 or below, very high risk. In practice, however, many clinicians have only two categories—patients who are at risk for pressure ulcers and those who aren't.

It's important that nurses perform ulcer risk assessments accurately. In one recent study, online education was found to be more helpful for new nurse users of the Braden Scale than it was for more experienced nurses.[42] Nurses were best at identifying patients at either extreme, high, or low levels of risk. Persons at "mild risk" were least likely to have correct nurse ratings.[43] Nurses also had the least agreement about which preventive interventions to use for patients with Braden scores of 13–18.[42] Determining the risk level is helpful in deciding on appropriate prevention strategies. Clinical judgment should play a part in interpreting the total Braden Scale score because not all risk factors are quantified on the scale.

After the total Braden Scale score is computed, a patient's risk and need for preventive protocols can be determined. Recommendations for pressure ulcer prevention management by level of risk are available on the Braden website.[38] However, the individualized plan of care for any particular patient needs to be based on his or her specific risk factors and needs. (See *Braden score interventions.*) Questions have surfaced regarding when to assess patients for pressure ulcer risk and when to reassess risk. These two aspects

of care are both very important. The NPUAP/EPUAP clinical practice guideline on pressure ulcer prevention recommends that initial pressure ulcer risk be assessed upon admission as well as at periodic intervals, especially when there is any change in the patient's condition.[1] (See *Pressure ulcer risk assessment recommendations,* page 336.) However, the guideline doesn't provide specific time frames for reassessments. Reassessment intervals should be based on the acuity of the individual for whom the pressure ulcer risk is being calculated.[1] Studies by Bergstrom and Braden[39,44] found that in skilled nursing facilities, 80% of pressure ulcers develop within 2 weeks of admission and 96% develop within 3 weeks of admission.[33,34,44] The following recommendations listed below for assessment and reassessment are based on this research.

ACUTE CARE

While most guidelines agree that risk assessment should be completed on admission, there is no consensus on how often a reassessment should be completed. The NPUAP/EPUAP clinical practice guideline[1] recommends that reassessment be conducted regularly and based on the acuity of the patient. Although the guideline recommends frequent skin assessment for shear injury in critically ill individuals,[1] no guidance is given as to what "frequently" means. The WOCN guidelines[5] recommend reassessment on a regularly scheduled basis or when there is a significant change in the individual's condition such as surgery or decline in health status. The Institute for Healthcare Improvement (IHI) recommends that pressure ulcer risk assessment be done every 24 hours.[45] The World Union of Wound Healing Societies[46] recommends that assessments be performed daily in the intensive care unit and every second day on general medical/surgical floors.

LONG-TERM CARE

Assess initially upon admission, then reassess weekly for the first 4 weeks, monthly to quarterly after that, and whenever the resident's condition changes.[39] Pressure ulcer

Braden score interventions

- At risk: 15 to 18—Consider a protocol of frequent turning, facilitating maximal remobilization, protecting the patient's heels, providing a pressure-reducing support surface if the patient is bedridden or confined to a chair, and managing moisture, nutrition, and friction and shear. If other major risk factors are present (advanced age, fever, poor dietary intake of protein, diastolic blood pressure below 60 mm Hg, or hemodynamic instability), advance to the next level of risk.
- Moderate risk: 13 to 14—Consider a protocol of frequent turning, facilitating maximal remobilization, protecting the patient's heels, providing a pressure-reducing support surface, providing foam wedges for 30-degree lateral positioning, and managing moisture, nutrition, and friction and shear. If other major risk factors are present, advance to the next level of risk.
- High risk: 10 to 12—Consider a protocol that increases the frequency of turning, supplements turning with small shifts in position, facilitates maximal remobilization, protects the patient's heels, provides a pressure-reducing support surface, provides foam wedges for 30-degree lateral positioning, and manages moisture, nutrition, and friction and shear.
- Very high risk: 9 or below—Consider a protocol that incorporates the points for high-risk patients. Add a pressure-relieving surface if the patient has intractable pain, severe pain exacerbated by turning, or additional risk factors such as immobility and malnutrition. A low-air-loss bed is no substitute for a turning schedule.
- Managing moisture—Use a commercial moisture barrier, and use absorbent pads or diapers that wick and hold moisture. Address the cause of the moisture if possible, and offer a bedpan or urinal and a glass of water in conjunction with turning schedules.
- Managing nutrition—Consult a dietitian and act quickly to alleviate nutritional deficits. Increase the patient's protein intake and increase his or her calorie intake if needed. Provide a multivitamin containing vitamins A, C, and E.
- Managing friction and shear—Elevate the head of the bed no more than 30 degrees and have the patient use a trapeze when indicated. Use a lift sheet to move the patient. Protect the patient's elbows, heels, sacrum, and back of head if he's exposed to friction.
- Other general care issues—Don't massage reddened bony prominences and don't use donut-type devices. Maintain good hydration and avoid drying out the patient's skin.

Adapted with permission from Ayello, E.A., and Braden, B. "How and Why to Do a Pressure Ulcer Risk Assessment," *Advances in Skin & Wound Care* 15(3):125-32, May-June 2002.

risk assessment is now required under MDS 3.0 Section M, Skin Conditions.[25–28] Under section M0100 of the MDS tool, the clinician can use *any* of the following criteria to determine risk:

- M0100A: Stage I or higher ulcer, scar over a bony prominence, or non-removal dressing or device in place[25–28]
- M0100B: Formal assessment instrument or tool (i.e., Braden, Norton, or others)[25–28]

Pressure ulcer risk assessment recommendations

1. Establish a risk assessment policy in all health care settings. (Strength of Evidence = C)
2. Educate health care professionals on how to achieve an accurate and reliable risk assessment. (Strength of Evidence = B)
3. Document all risk assessments. (Strength of Evidence = C)

Risk Assessment Practice

4. Use a structured approach to risk assessment to identify individuals at risk of developing pressure ulcers. (Strength of Evidence = C)
5. Use a structured approach to risk assessment that includes assessment of activity and mobility. (Strength of Evidence = C)
6. Use a structured approach to risk assessment that includes a comprehensive skin assessment to evaluate any alterations to intact skin. (Strength of Evidence = C)

   6.1 Consider individuals with alterations to intact skin to be at risk of pressure development.

7. Use a structured approach to risk assessment that is refined through the use of clinical judgment informed by knowledge of key risk factors. (Strength of Evidence = C)
8. Consider the impact of the following factors on an individual's risk of pressure ulcer development
   a) Nutritional indicators
   b) Factors affecting perfusion and oxygenation
   c) Skin moisture
   d) Advanced age
9. Consider the potential impact of the following factors on an individual's risk of pressure ulcer development:
   a) Friction and shear (Subscale Braden Scale)
   b) Sensory perception (Subscale Braden Scale)
   c) General health status
   d) Body temperature
10. Conduct a structured risk assessment on admission, and repeat as regularly and as frequently as required by patient acuity. Reassessment should also be undertaken if there is any change in patient condition. (Strength of Evidence = C)
11. Develop and implement a prevention plan when individuals have been identified as being at risk of developing pressure ulcers. (Strength of Evidence = C)

National Pressure Ulcer Advisory Panel and European Pressure Ulcer Advisory Panel. *Prevention and Treatment of Pressure Ulcers: Clinical Practice Guideline.* Washington, DC: National Pressure Ulcer Advisory Panel, 2009.

- M0100C: Comprehensive clinical assessment of the resident since this will include factors other than what is on formal tools.[25–28]

Based on the determination of pressure ulcer risk by some method in section M0100, in M0150 the clinician must check Yes or No to indicate whether the resident is at risk for developing pressure ulcers.[25–28] Further details about MDS 3.0 section M skin conditions can be found on the CMS website[25,26] or in the literature.[27,28]

HOME HEALTH CARE

The plan of care needs to address the areas of risk for home care patients. A Braden Scale for the home care setting is available online[38] and in the literature.[36] Risk assessment tools complement clinical judgment, as patients with the same risk score may have differing actual risks. Section M1300, Pressure Ulcer Assessment of OASIS C, identifies whether the home health agency providers assessed the patient's risk of developing pressure ulcers by either evaluation of clinical factors or use of a standardized tool. CMS does not require the use of standardized tools, nor does it endorse one particular tool.[24] Section M1302 addresses the question of whether the patient is at risk for developing pressure ulcers, with the answer being either No or Yes. Reassessment of risk should be performed with each home visit by a nurse.

> ### PRACTICE POINT
>
> CMS requires a pressure ulcer risk assessment in both long-term and home care settings. It *does not* mandate the use of a standardized risk tool (e.g., Braden, Norton).[24–26]

Patient care to prevent pressure ulcers

Preventing pressure ulcers can best be accomplished by using a multidisciplinary approach.[31,33,47,48] Several pressure ulcer prevention protocols and guidelines exist,[1,2,4–6,47–50] most of which advocate taking a holistic approach to pressure ulcer prevention. Any good prevention program begins with assessing the patient's skin. The skin should be assessed and its condition documented daily in acute and long-term care settings and at each home care visit. Careful attention to preventing skin injury during performance of activities of daily living is paramount. The bathing schedule should be individualized based on the patient's age, skin texture, and dryness or excessive oiliness of the skin. Use of nondrying products to clean the skin is recommended. One study found that the incidence of stage I and II pressure ulcers could be reduced by educating the staff about using body wash and skin protectant products.[51] In another study by Carr and Benoit, the incidence of pressure ulcers

decreased from 7.14% at baseline to 0% at the end of the study through education of nonlicensed staff about the use of protective skin barriers and implementation of a comprehensive interventional patient hygiene bathing and incontinence management program.[52] Avoid excessive friction and hot water when cleaning. Use nonalcoholic moisturizers after bathing. A daily bath may not be needed for all patients; elderly patients, for example, may benefit from "lotion" baths.

For the incontinent patient, moisture barriers and ointments should be considered as treatment options. Soiled skin should be cleaned immediately and products to protect the skin applied. If containment products are used, follow the correct methods of application. Reasons for incontinence should always be determined and appropriate measures to address the cause of the incontinence should be implemented.

The skin should be protected from injury. Pad bony prominences using dressings, such as films, hydrocolloids, foams, stockinettes, or roller gauze. In a study of 93 high-risk patients in a surgical trauma intensive care unit, the use of intervention bundles that included a prophylactic soft silicone dressing product resulted in 0 pressure ulcers.[53] Although a review of the literature suggests that one type of massage may be beneficial for at-risk patients,[54] most clinical guidelines recommend against massaging reddened bony prominences because this can lead to further tissue damage.[1,2,4] Keep the patient's heels off the bed[55]; use pillows, wedges, and foot elevation devices as indicated. (See *HEELS© mnemonic,* page 330). A folded bath blanket under the calves can "float the heels," completely relieving heel pressure in a bedridden patient. Flex the knee when elevating the leg to avoid pressure injury to the Achilles tendon.[1] Best practices for preventing heel pressure ulcers in orthopedic population are published.[56]

>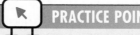
> ### PRACTICE POINT
>
> Keep the patient's heels off the mattress!

Be careful not to drag your patient during transfers or position changes. Use appropriate devices, such as a turn sheet or mechanical lifting device, to prevent friction injuries to the patient's skin. Use the 30-degree lateral position for patients in bed. Keep the head of the bed below 30 degrees to prevent shearing injuries, unless contraindicated due to the patient's clinical condition.

The role of nutrition in pressure ulcer interventions has been controversial. The NPUAP/EPUAP has made the following recommendation with the strength of evidence at the A level: "Offer high-protein mixed oral nutritional supplements and/or tube feeding, in addition to the usual diet, to individuals with nutritional risk and pressure ulcer risk because of acute or chronic diseases, or following a surgical interventions."[1] In a large prospective cohort study, Bergstrom and Braden[39] found that nursing home residents who developed pressure ulcers had a significantly lower intake of protein. Clinicians need to ensure that a patient's caloric, protein, vitamin, and mineral needs are met. Recommendations from the dietitian can be an important source of assistance in helping patients to get their required nutrients.

Physical and occupational therapists are important members of the pressure ulcer team, a valuable resource for maximizing patient mobility. Their expertise in selecting appropriate-size wheelchairs and evaluating seating angles and postural alignment can't be over-emphasized. Patients who are confined to a chair should be repositioned every hour, with small shifts in weight made every 15 minutes. Although most clinicians consider turning and repositioning bedridden patients every 2 hours to be a standard of care, the appropriate turning interval for all patients has yet to be determined by research. A 2-hour interval may be too long for some patients, whereas for others every 2 hours may not be necessary, such as for palliative care patients in whom frequent repositioning would cause more pain and suffering than benefit. Because there is no standard time interval or frequency for repositioning all patients, a repositioning schedule needs to be individualized for each patient. The most recent NPUAP/EPUAP guideline[1] provides evidence that repositioning frequency may be influenced by the type of support surface being used. Contrary to the earlier AHCPR (AHRQ) recommendation for every-2-hour turning/repositioning,[3,4] new evidence from Defloor et al.[57] and Vanderwee et al.[58] found that turning a patient every 4 hours on a viscoelastic mattress resulted in a significant reduction in the incidence of pressure ulcers.

> **PRACTICE POINT**
>
> Repositioning schedules should take into consideration the condition of the patient and the support surface in use.[1]

Appropriate pressure-relieving devices and surfaces need to be used. Rastinehad reported that using support surfaces can decrease the incidence of pressure ulcers in at-risk oncology patients.[59] Devices such as "donuts" shouldn't be used. The results of a preliminary Canadian study have led to a model for support surface selection.[60] See the NPUAP website (www.npuap.org) to review the latest definitions of physical concepts related to support surfaces as developed by the NPUAP Support Surface Standards Initiative.[61] (Also see chapter 11, Pressure redistribution: Seating, positioning, and support surfaces.)

Ongoing monitoring and documentation are essential. In a pilot study, Horn et al.[62] found that establishing a multidisciplinary team and redesigning documentation processes for certified nursing assistants in several long-term-care facilities throughout the United States resulted in a decrease in the required facility documentation. For the seven facilities in the study, there was a combined 33% reduction in pressure ulcers.[62]

Milne et al.[63] decreased facility-acquired pressure ulcer prevalence from 41% to 4.2% in a 108-bed long-term acute care hospital (LTACH) by developing policies that were supported by published clinical practice guidelines and incorporating them into the facility's plan of care. They established a wound care team, improved documentation methods, and educated the staff. They also reviewed the facility's wound products and revised its electronic record. All of these efforts resulted in care improvement outcome.[63]

Communication of the prevention plan to all members of the healthcare team, including patients and their families, is imperative. Supplement your verbal teaching with one of the prevention booklets designed for use by the consumer, such as pamphlets available from wound care companies as well as the AHRQ. The AHRQ[64] also has a pressure ulcer patient guide available in Spanish.

PRESSURE ULCER STAGING

A comprehensive wound assessment includes many parameters, one of which is staging. (See chapter 6, Wound assessment.) Once the wound etiology is known, the correct classification system to describe the wound can be selected. For example, arterial and venous ulcers are described by their characteristics. Diabetic or neuropathic ulcers are classified by the American Diabetes Association, Wagner Grading System for Vascular Wounds, or San Antonio Diabetic Wound Classification System. The NPUAP staging system was designed specifically for pressure ulcers. An outcome of the first NPUAP consensus conference[65] was the NPUAP staging system for pressure ulcers, which was based on staging systems by Shea[66] and the International Association of Enterostomal Therapists[67] (now called WOCN). In February 2007, NPUAP once again revised its staging system.[68] The latest revision of the pressure ulcer classification system to include six categories or stages was included in the 2009 NPUAP/EPUAP international pressure ulcer guideline.[1]

Pressure ulcer staging is a classification system to describe the level of tissue destroyed. It provides practitioners with a common language to communicate with each other what the pressure ulcer looks like clinically. This staging system should only be used to describe pressure ulcers and not other types of skin or wound injuries. NPUAP states that mucous membrane pressure ulcers should not be staged using its pressure ulcer staging system.[69] Mucous membrane pressure ulcers

(MPrU) are "pressure ulcers found on mucous membranes with a history of a medical device in use at the location of the ulcer."[69] Staging is only part of the total assessment of an ulcer; a comprehensive assessment also includes factors such as the state of surrounding skin and presence of infection, among others. (See chapter 6, Wound assessment.)

After the present on admission (POA) indicator went into effect in the acute care setting, confusion existed as to whether nurses could continue to stage pressure ulcers. An NPUAP position statement[70] as well as information in the literature from the American Nurses Association (ANA) reaffirms that pressure ulcer staging is within the scope of practice for RNs.[71,72]

NPUAP classification of pressure ulcers staging definitions

"Pressure ulcers are classified according to the amount of visible tissue loss."[1] Necrotic ulcers cannot be staged numerically because visualization of the wound bed is necessary to determine the level of tissue involvement; therefore, necrotic ulcers are classified as unstageable pressure ulcers. Numerical staging of necrotic wounds should be done after the necrotic tissue is removed. (See chapter 8, Wound debridement.)

A few of the most widely used pressure ulcer staging definitions, the NPUAP/EPUAP classification system for staging or categories of pressure ulcers, are described below. (Also see color photos of staging, pages C20–C21.)

STAGE I

The original definition of a stage I pressure ulcer was "non-blanchable erythema of intact skin, the heralding lesion of skin ulceration."[65] Given the diversity of people with different skin pigmentation, detecting stage I pressure ulcers can be a challenge if clinicians only use color as an indicator. In 1997, to provide a more culturally sensitive definition, NPUAP revised the definition of a stage I ulcer to include indicators that went beyond color. NPUAP continued to refine this definition to include "intact skin with non-blanchable redness of a localized area usually over a bony prominence."

In darkly pigmented skin, the area may not have visible blanching and its color may differ from surrounding skin. (See *International NPUAP/EPUAP Pressure Ulcer Classification System,* pages 325 and 326, and color photos, pages C20–C21.)

Persons with darkly pigmented skin have the lowest prevalence of stage I pressure ulcers.[73,74] The incidence of pressure ulcers was higher in people with darkly pigmented skin in several studies conducted by Lyder and colleagues.[40,41] Sprigle and colleagues[75] found that warmth or coolness was present in 85% of patients with stage I pressure ulcers.

STAGING CONCEPTS

Staging competency

Accuracy in staging pressure ulcers is a challenge. Nurses have reported being less confident in identifying stage III ulcers.[76–79] Clinicians can test their ability to classify pressure ulcers by taking the ePUCLAS$_2$ staging test (available in English and other languages) on the EPUAP website (www.epuap.org)[80] or the quiz on the National Database of Nursing Quality Indicators (NDNQI) educational modules.[81]

Staging healing ulcers—Reverse staging controversy

It is only appropriate to use pressure ulcer staging to define the maximum depth of pressure ulcer tissue "wounded." Some clinicians have erroneously used it in reverse order to describe improvement in a pressure ulcer,[82] while those in long-term-care facilities were mandated to use it previously when MDS 2.0 was in effect.[83] This is no longer the case since MDS 3.0 went into effect on October 1, 2010.[25–28] Use of the NPUAP staging system to describe healing is physiologically inaccurate and shouldn't be done. When stage IV pressure ulcers heal to progressively more shallow depth, they don't replace lost muscle, subcutaneous fat, and dermis before they re-epithelialize. Instead, the wound is filled with granulation tissue. Thus, the ulcer doesn't heal from a stage IV to III, II to I. More information on why clinicians shouldn't follow this inaccurate practice of "reverse staging" can be found in the NPUAP position statement on reverse staging.[16,84]

With the implementation of MDS 3.0, CMS no longer requires reverse staging and in fact prohibits it.[25–28]

SUSPECTED DEEP TISSUE INJURY

Clinicians often struggle with the concept of suspected deep tissue injury (sDTI)[85] that presents as a purplish color, most often seen in the heel area. Typically, these wounds appear as dusky, boggy, or discolored areas of purple ecchymosis. (See color photos on page C17.) Sometimes they appear a few days after surgery as a discolored area on the sacrum and may be misidentified as a burn.[86] Often these areas deteriorate rapidly from intact skin to deep open wounds. sDTI can now be coded on MDS 3.0 under section M0300G.[25–28]

What is sDTI?[87,88] Can these pressure ulcers be prevented and, if so, how? What is the best treatment? Clinicians have sought guidance about this particular type of pressure ulcer. Baharestani reported that 36% of her sDTI cases resolved and 90% of these patients had anemia.[88] Initially, sDTI lesions have the appearance of a deep bruise and may herald the subsequent development of a stage III or IV pressure ulcer even with optimal management. (See *International NPUAP/EPUAP Pressure Ulcer Classification System,* pages 325 and 326, for a description of this evolving stage.)

EARLY DETECTION OF sDTI

The pressure ulcer staging system relies on visual inspection of the skin. Newer technologies may hold the promise of early detection for pressure ulcer injury *before* visible signs of tissue destruction can be seen. One study reported on the pre-ulcerative changes in long-term residents using diagnostic ultrasound.[89]

PRESSURE ULCER TREATMENT

Avoidable pressure ulcers

As a result of an international consensus conference in February 2010, NPUAP issued a revised definition of unavoidable pressure ulcers that was applicable across all care settings.[90] It is based on the CMS definition of "unavoidable" from Long Term Care F-Tag 314.[8]

Although the debate continues as to whether all pressure ulcers are avoidable,[90,91] several guidelines are now available for clinicians to use in planning treatment.[1–7,47–50] Clinical guidelines provide the foundation for establishing evidence-based pressure ulcer management.

The wound bed preparation model has been applied to pressure ulcer prevention and treatment (Fig. 13-1).[92] A pressure ulcer won't heal unless the underlying causes are effectively managed. A general assessment should include identifying and effectively managing the patient's medical diseases, health problems (such as urinary incontinence), nutritional status, individual concerns (such as pain level),[93] and psychosocial health. Unless these major areas are effectively addressed, the probability of the pressure ulcer healing is unlikely.

The comprehensive local management of pressure ulcers includes cleaning, controlling infections, debridement, dressings that promote a moist wound environment (if a healable wound), nutritional support, and redistribution of pressure (repositioning and use of support surfaces). (See chapter 11, Pressure redistribution: seating, positioning, and support surfaces.) The use of adjunctive therapies to heal pressure ulcers should be considered for recalcitrant ulcers. Options are discussed later in the chapter.

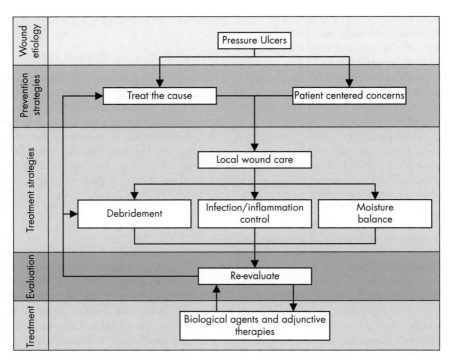

Figure 13-1. Pressure ulcer treatment and prevention using the wound bed preparation model. (Used with permission from Dr. David Keast.)

> **PRACTICE POINT**
>
> Unstageable pressure ulcers are those covered with necrotic (slough and eschar) tissue. Until the necrotic tissue is removed, the ulcer can't be visualized accurately and is therefore unstageable in patients in all care settings.

Monitoring healing

Because reverse staging of pressure ulcers to monitor healing is inappropriate, several instruments have been developed and validated to assess the healing of pressure ulcers.

TOOLS THAT MEASURE HEALING

The two most widely used tools to measure healing in pressure ulcers are the Pressure Sore Status Tool (PSST)[94] and the Pressure Ulcer Scale for Healing (PUSH).[95] The PSST is comprised of 13 variables that provide a numerical indicator of the status of the pressure ulcer (healing or deteriorating).[94] The score ranges from 1, which indicates tissue health (or healed), to 65, which indicates wound degeneration. The variables that comprise the PSST score include wound size (length and width), depth, edges, undermining, necrotic tissue type, necrotic tissue amount, exudate type, exudate amount, skin color of surrounding wound, peripheral tissue edema, peripheral tissue induration, granulation tissue, and epithelialization. The PSST provides a comprehensive assessment of pressure ulcers[94] and is currently being evaluated for use with other wound types.

The PUSH tool[95,96] uses only three variables—surface area (length and width), exudate amount, and tissue appearance—to derive a numerical indicator of the status of the pressure ulcer. (See *NPUAP PUSH tool.*) A score of 0 indicates that the pressure ulcer has healed, while the highest score of 17 indicates wound degeneration. The PUSH tool intentionally takes a "minimalist approach." Using research databases in its development, the PUSH tool seeks to select the minimum number of assessment parameters needed to monitor ulcer healing or deterioration. Its brevity and accuracy in monitoring make the PUSH tool ideal for quality assurance monitoring of large groups of patients and identifying patients who are deteriorating and require reassessment and possibly treatment changes. The PUSH tool isn't intended to provide a comprehensive assessment of pressure ulcers and hasn't yet been validated for other types of wounds, although it is being tested in research studies and clinical use. A survey of 103 respondents found the PUSH tool reliable and easy to use.[97]

Although tools exist for measuring pressure ulcer healing, more evidence is needed to determine pressure ulcer healing rates.[98–101] Among chronic wounds, pressure ulcers have the slowest healing rate—0.077 mm/day, with 2.156 mm of healing expected at 4 weeks.[100]

Recently, the use of high-frequency portable ultrasound to measure wound healing has been introduced. The use of this technology, which can capture three-dimensional measurements, has been shown to be quite beneficial in objectively monitoring healing. Ultrasound is also "color blind"; that is, it can detect stage I pressure ulcers in darkly pigmented skin.[102]

Principles of local wound care

After addressing the cause and patient-centered concerns, healing a pressure ulcer using the wound bed preparation model requires attention to determining the wound prognosis (healable, maintenance or non-healable wound)[103] and applying the principles of local wound care (debridement, infection management, moisture balance before attention to the edge). (See *NPUAP/EPUAP Clinical Practice Guideline at Strength of Evidence = A,* page 344.)

CLEANSING

Cleaning the pressure ulcer to remove devitalized tissue and decrease bacterial burden is often recommended. NPUAP/EPUAP also recommends cleansing the surrounding skin.[1] Pressure ulcers can exhibit delayed healing in the presence of high levels of bacteria.[104] Solutions that don't traumatize the healing ulcer should be used.[1,105] Normal saline solution (0.9%) is usually recommended because it

NPUAP PUSH tool

PATIENT NAME: PATIENT ID. #

ULCER LOCATION: DATE:

Directions

Observe and measure the pressure ulcer. Categorize the ulcer with respect to surface area, exudate, and type of wound tissue. Record a subscore for each of the ulcer characteristics. Add the subscores to obtain the total score. A comparison of total scores measured over time provides an indication of the improvement or deterioration in pressure ulcer healing.

LENGTH	**0** 0 cm²	**1** <0.3 cm²	**2** 0.3–0.6 cm²	**3** 0.7–1.0 cm²	**4** 1.1–2.0 cm²	**5** 2.1–3.0 cm²	**Blank**
× WIDTH		**6** 3.1–4.0 cm²	**7** 4.1–8.0 cm²	**8** 8.1–12.0 cm²	**9** 12.1–24.0 cm²	**10** >24.0 cm²	**Sub-score**
EXUDATE AMOUNT	**0** None	**1** Light	**2** Moderate	**3** Heavy			**Sub-score**
TISSUE TYPE	**0** Closed	**1** Epithelial Tissue	**2** Granulation Tissue	**3** Slough	**4** Necrotic Tissue		**Sub-score**
							Total score

LENGTH × WIDTH

Measure the greatest length (head to toe) and the greatest width (side to side) using a centimeter ruler. Multiply these two measurements (length × width) to obtain an estimate of surface area in square centimeters (cm²). Do not guess! Always use a centimeter ruler and always use the same method each time the ulcer is measured.

EXUDATE AMOUNT

Estimate the amount of exudate (drainage) present after removal of the dressing and before applying any topical agent to the ulcer. Estimate the exudate as none, light, moderate, or heavy.

TISSUE TYPE

This refers to the types of tissue that are present in the wound (ulcer) bed. Score as a "4" if any necrotic tissue is present. Score as a "3" if any amount of slough is present and necrotic tissue is absent. Score as a "2" if the wound is clean and contains granulation tissue. Score as a "1" if the wound is superficial and reepithelializing. Score as a "0" if the wound is closed.

4–Necrotic tissue (eschar): Black, brown, or tan tissue that adheres firmly to the wound bed or ulcer edges and may be either firmer or softer than surrounding tissue.
3–Slough: Yellow or white tissue that adheres to the ulcer bed in strings or thick clumps or is mucinous.
2–Granulation tissue: Pink or beefy-red tissue with a shiny, moist, granular appearance.
1–Epithelial tissue: For superficial ulcers, new pink or shiny tissue (skin) that grows in from the edges or as islands on the ulcer surface.
0–Closed/resurfaced: The wound is completely covered with epithelium (new skin).

PUSH Tool version 3.0, ©1998 National Pressure Ulcer Advisory Panel. Used with permission.

NPUAP/EPUAP Clinical Practice Guideline at Strength of Evidence = A

Prevention

1. Offer high-protein mixed oral nutritional supplements and/or tube feeding, in addition to the usual diet, to individuals with nutritional risk and pressure ulcer risk because of acute or chronic disease following a surgical intervention. (Strength of Evidence = A)
2. Repositioning should be undertaken to reduce the duration and magnitude of pressure over vulnerable areas of the body. (Strength of Evidence = A)
3. Frequency of repositioning will be influenced by variables concerning the individual (Strength of Evidence = C) and the support surface in use. (Strength of Evidence = A)
4. Repositioning frequency should be influenced by the support surface used. (Strength of Evidence = A)
5. Use high-specification foam mattresses rather than standard hospital foam mattresses for all individuals assessed as being at risk for pressure ulcer development. (Strength of Evidence = A)
6. There is no evidence of the superiority of one higher-specification foam mattress over an alternative higher-specification foam mattress. (Strength of Evidence = A)
7. Alternating-pressure active support overlays and replacement mattresses have a similar efficacy in terms of pressure ulcer incidence. (Strength of Evidence = A)

Treatment

1. Consider the use of direct contact (capacitative) electrical stimulation (ES) in the management of recalcitrant Category/Stage II as well as Category/Stage III and IV pressure ulcers to facilitate wound healing. (Strength of Evidence = A)

National Pressure Ulcer Advisory Panel and European Pressure Ulcer Advisory Panel. *Prevention and Treatment of Pressure Ulcers: Clinical Practice Guideline.* Washington, DC: National Pressure Ulcer Advisory Panel, 2009.

isn't cytotoxic to healthy tissue.[1,4] Although the active ingredients in newer wound cleaners may be noncytotoxic (surfactants), the inert carrier may be cytotoxic to healthy granulation tissue. Review of all ingredients is warranted. Hellewell et al.[106] found that antiseptic cleaners were the most cytotoxic to granulation tissue. An in vitro study found relative toxicity indexes ranging from 0 to 100,000 with saline and Shur-clens to be least toxic to fibroblasts, while Dial antibacterial soap and Ivory liquid-gel were most toxic.[107] Least toxic to keratinocytes were Biolex, Shur-clens, and Techni-Care, while hydrogen peroxide, modified Dakin's solution, and povidone (10%) were most toxic.[107]

The mechanical method used to deliver the cleaning agent must provide enough pressure to remove debris without presenting trauma to the ulcer bed.[1] Optimal pressure to clean an ulcer is between 4 and 15 pounds per square inch (psi).[108] A 35-ml syringe with a 19-gauge needle creates an 8 psi irrigation pressure stream,[1] which was found to be more effective in removing bacteria than other irrigation pressures.[109] It should be noted that irrigation pressures exceeding 15 psi can cause trauma to the ulcer bed and may drive bacteria into the tissue.[110] New technology such as battery-powered, disposable irrigation devices can provide an alternative to the syringe and needle system to loosen wound debris.

DEBRIDEMENT

The presence of necrotic devitalized tissue promotes the growth of pathologic organisms and prevents wounds from healing.[111] Therefore, debridement is a very important step in the local management of pressure ulcers. There's no optimal debridement method; selection should be based on the goals of the patient, absence or presence of infection, amount of necrotic tissue present, and economic considerations for the patient and the facility.

Many types of debridement, including surgical, autolytic, enzymatic, mechanical, biological, and laser, are available. (See chapter 8, Wound debridement.) However, surgical (or sharp laser) debridement is considered by many to be the most effective form of debridement because it involves the cutting away (with a scalpel) of necrotic tissue.[112] In addition, surgical debridement is relatively quick and can be done at the bedside. Surgical debridement is essential when cellulitis or sepsis is suspected.[113] Autolytic debridement involves the use of a semi-occlusive or occlusive dressing (e.g., hydrocolloids, hydrogels) and employs the body's own natural enzymes to digest necrotic tissue. Autolytic debridement takes much longer than sharp debridement. Watch closely for signs and symptoms of infection. Enzymatic debridement uses proteolytic enzymes to remove necrotic tissue. In the United States, papain urea and trypsin are no longer available for use; only collagenase can be used for enzymatic debridement. Mechanical debridement uses wet-to-dry gauze to adhere to the necrotic tissue, which is then removed. Upon removal of the gauze dressing, necrotic tissue and wound debris are removed. However, healthy granulation tissue is also removed, which can delay wound healing.[112]

PRESSURE REDISTRIBUTION

The use of support surfaces is an important consideration in redistributing pressure. (See chapter 11, Pressure redistribution: seating, positioning, and support surfaces.) The NPUAP Support Surface Standards Initiative redefined the physical concepts related to support surfaces.[61] CMS has divided support surfaces into three categories for reimbursement purposes. Group one devices are those support surfaces that are static; they don't require electricity. Static devices include air, foam (convoluted and solid), gel, and water-overlay mattresses. They redistribute pressure, may decrease shearing, and are relatively inexpensive. If foam is used, it should weigh 1.3 lb per cubic foot and be more than 3″ (7.5 cm) thick.

Group two devices are powered by electricity or a pump and are considered dynamic in nature. These devices include alternating air mattresses and low-air-loss mattresses. The advantages of alternating air mattresses include portability, redistribution of pressure, reduced shearing, and moderate cost. The disadvantage of some of these mattresses is their inability to reduce heat accumulation on the patient's body. The advantages of low-air-loss mattresses are pressure redistribution, low moisture retention, and reduced heat accumulation.

Group three devices are also considered dynamic in nature. This classification includes only air-fluidized beds, which are electric and contain silicone-coated beads. They are often recommended for patients at very high risk for pressure ulcers as well as after flap or graft surgery. They're often used for patients with non-healing full-thickness pressure ulcers or those with numerous truncal full-thickness pressure ulcers. The advantages of air-fluidized beds are that they redistribute pressure and reduce heat accumulation, moisture retention, and shearing forces. The patient's ability to move in a fluidized bed is hampered, however, which is considered a disadvantage of this product.

Few studies demonstrate significant differences within the support surface classifications and preventing or healing pressure ulcers. Therefore, the level and type of risk factors should guide the level and type of support surface selected. The NPUAP/EPUAP clinical practice guideline recommends that a patient should not be positioned directly on a pressure ulcer and that an individualized turn and reposition schedule be established based on the characteristics of the support surface, the person's response, and the clinical goals.[1]

DRESSINGS

The use of moist wound therapy dressings is a major component in managing a healable pressure ulcer. (See chapter 9, Wound treatment options.) At present, it's conservatively estimated that thousands of different dressings are available for pressure ulcer management. Dressings can be broken down into several classifications: gauze, non-adherent gauze, transparent films, hydrocolloids, foams, alginates, hydrogels, collagens, antimicrobials, composites, and combinations. Matching the dressing to the wound bed characteristics is essential. A guiding principle is to maintain a moist environment for a healable wound.

Although nongauze dressings are usually more expensive than gauze dressing, less frequent dressing changes, faster healing rates, and decreased rates of infection can make nongauze-based dressing more cost-effective over time.[114–117] It's also important to note that wet-to-dry gauze dressings are a form of debridement and shouldn't be used on ulcers with good granulation tissue. CMS specifically states that use of wet-to-dry dressings should be limited in long-term-care patients.[8] No specific dressing heals all pressure ulcers within an ulcer classification. Consequently, a careful assessment of the pressure ulcer, the patient's needs, and environmental factors (frequency of dressing changes to increase adherence) must be considered. (See chapter 9, Wound treatment options.)

NUTRITION

Nutrition is important to maintain the body in positive nitrogen balance,[1] thereby increasing wound healing. Patients should be assessed and screened for nutritional status, including weight, weight history (e.g., significant weight loss), and adequacy of nutrient and fluid intake.[1] It's important to provide protein (30 to 35 calories/kg body weight) for malnourished patients with pressure ulcers.[1] Always check renal status to make sure that the patient's kidneys can handle the protein load.[1] Although dietary supplementation of vitamins and minerals in the absence of deficiency remains controversial,[118–121] the NPUAP/EPUAP recommends "vitamin and mineral supplements when dietary intake is poor or deficiencies are confirmed or suspected (Strength of Evidence = B)."[1] The use of enteral and parental nutritional support should always be considered when the patient is unable to meet caloric needs.[1]

CONTROL OF INFECTIONS

All pressure ulcers will become colonized with both aerobic and anaerobic bacteria; therefore, pressure ulcers aren't sterile wounds. (See chapter 7, Wound bioburden and infection.) Avoid swab-culturing the surface of a pressure ulcer to diagnosis infection. Clean technique is customarily used when treating pressure ulcers. If an ulcer may be infected (independent of a puncture biopsy), most experts assess for the amount of drainage and odor and examine the surrounding tissue for cellulitis. It should be noted that some infected ulcers may not demonstrate the typical signs and symptoms associated with infection; rather, they may appear as non-healing ulcers.

A pressure ulcer will not heal until infection is controlled. The use of topical agents such as silver sulfadiazine (Silvadene) and oral antibiotics for a 1- or 2-week period may be useful. Non-healable or infected wounds may benefit from short-term use of 1% povidone-iodine. Clearly, additional research is needed to examine the role of topical antibiotics in decreasing bacterial loads in pressure ulcers. Systemic antibiotics should only be used when a systemic infection is suspected.

ADJUNCTIVE THERAPIES

The use of adjunctive therapies is the fastest-growing area in pressure ulcer management. Adjunctive therapies include electrical stimulation, hyperbaric oxygen, radiant heat, growth factors, and skin equivalents. Except for electrical stimulation, published research substantiating the effectiveness of adjunctive therapies in healing pressure ulcers is scarce.

The only NPUAP/EPUAP Clinical Practice Guideline recommendation at the A level of evidence is on electrical stimulation.[1] Electrical stimulation is the use of electrical current to stimulate a number of cellular processes, such as increasing fibroblasts, neutrophils, macrophages, collagen synthesis, DNA synthesis, and increasing the number of receptor sites for specific growth factors.[122] Electrical stimulation appears to be most effective on stage III and IV pressure ulcers[1] that are unresponsive to traditional methods of healing. Although there are much data to suggest that electrical stimulation is effective in healing pressure ulcers, the optimal electrical charge needed to stimulate pressure ulcer healing remains unclear. The literature suggests that an optimal electrical charge of 300 to 500 uA/sec produces positive effects on the pressure ulcer.[123] However, additional research is needed to determine the optimal electrical charge based on the characteristics of pressure ulcers (for example, stage, depth, and amount of drainage).

Hyperbaric oxygen is believed to promote wound healing by stimulating fibroblasts, collagen synthesis, epithelialization, and control of infection.[124] However, controlled clinical studies couldn't be found regarding the association of hyperbaric oxygen and the healing of pressure ulcers. The limited literature that does exist suggests that topical hyperbaric oxygen doesn't increase tissue oxygenation beyond the superficial dermis.[125] NPUAP/EPUAP concluded that there was insufficient evidence to recommend hyperbaric or topical oxygen therapy for the treatment of pressure ulcers.[1]

Growth factors and skin equivalents are emerging methods of healing pressure ulcers. The use of cytokine growth factors (for example, recombinant human platelet-derived growth factor-BB [rhPDGF-BB]), basic fibroblast growth factor (bFGF), and skin equivalents are currently being studied. Only one multicenter, randomized, double-blind study examining the use of rhPDGF-BB was found.[126] This study enrolled 45 patients with stage III or IV pressure ulcers who were randomized to either treatment group 1 (300 μg/ml of rhPDGF), treatment group 2 (100 μg/ml rhPDGF), or treatment group 3 (placebo). After 4 weeks of treatment, patients in group 1 had a 40% reduction in ulcer area, group 2 had a 71% reduction in ulcer area, and group 3 had a 17% reduction in pressure ulcer area. From these results, it is clear that the use of growth factors may have a crucial impact on the future of wound healing. However, additional research is needed to evaluate the efficacy of specific growth factors in healing pressure ulcers. The NPUAP/EPUAP Clinical Practice Guideline notes that PDGF-BB may improve healing of pressure ulcers, but because the available evidence is insufficient the guideline does not recommend this treatment for routine use.[1]

PREVALENCE AND INCIDENCE

It has been said, "what can be measured can be managed." To improve pressure ulcer care, the number of patients with pressure ulcers must be accurately determined. Doing so will require careful attention to prevalence and incidence data. The data represent the percentage of patients with pressure ulcers among all those surveyed in a setting (prevalence) and the percentage of patients who developed pressure ulcers after admission to the setting (incidence).

In 1989, at its first consensus conference, NPUAP brought attention to the pressure ulcer problem in the United States by reporting prevalence and incidence data.[65] The group set a national goal to reduce the incidence of pressure ulcers by 50% by the year 2000.[65] During the next decade, NPUAP engaged in an active program to improve pressure ulcer practice through education, research, and public policy.

At the close of the 20th century, NPUAP assessed the progress toward this goal through its Pressure Ulcers Challenge 2000 project. This 2-year project included a Medline database search for all articles on pressure ulcer incidence and prevalence published and indexed between January 1, 1990 and December 31, 2000. More than 300 studies were found. Pressure ulcer incidence and prevalence data were analyzed across care settings and in specific populations, such as people with spinal cord injuries, elderly patients, infants and children, patients with hip fractures, people of color, and those at the end of life receiving palliative or hospice care.[127]

Study data presented in the NPUAP monograph detailing the results of the project indicate a wide variation in the range of incidence rates from 1990 to 2000 (acute care, 0.4% to 38%; long-term care, 2.2% to 23.9%; and home care, 0% to 17%).[127] Prevalence rates from 1990 to 2000 ranged from 10% to 18% in general acute care,[1,127] 2.3% to 28% in long-term care,[1,127] and 0% to 29% in home care.[127] Inconsistencies in the methodologies used and in the populations studied contribute to these differences and make comparisons and analyses of trends problematic.[127,128] However, many positive developments in the prevention and treatment of pressure ulcers have occurred over the past decade, including development of evidence-based practice guidelines, standardization of risk assessment, and improved technologies for prevention and treatment.[127,128] NPUAP estimates that pressure ulcer prevalence in acute care is 15%, with incidence of 7%.[127,128] Although methodological issues require caution in interpreting the data, these estimates are based on several large studies conducted from 1990 to 2000.

Large U.S. surveys in 2009 of pressure ulcer incidence and prevalence have revealed an overall pressure ulcer prevalence of 12.3% and facility-acquired prevalence of 5.0%.[21] (See *Pressure ulcer prevalence in the United States by facility type.*)

Most pressure ulcers, regardless of setting, are partial-thickness (stages I and II) and are located on the sacrum or coccyx.[129] Heels are the second most common location.

Pressure ulcer prevalence in the United States by facility type

	2006	2009
All US facilities		
Overall prevalence	13.5%	12.3%
Facility-acquired prevalence	6.2%	5.0%
Acute care		
Overall prevalence	13.3%	11.9%
Facility-acquired prevalence	6.4%	5.0%
Long-term acute care		
Overall prevalence	32.9%	29.3%
Facility-acquired prevalence	9.0%	3.8%
Long-term care		
Overall prevalence	12.1%	11.8%
Facility-acquired prevalence	5.6%	5.2%
Rehabilitation		
Overall prevalence	16.3%	19.0%
Facility-acquired prevalence	4.0%	4.7%

From Van Gilder, C., Amlung, S., Harrison, P., Meyer, S. "Results of the 2008-2009 International Pressure Ulcer Prevalence™ Survey and a 3-year, Acute Care, Unit-specific Analysis." *Ostomy Wound Management* 55(11):39-45, 2009.

The proportion of sDTI pressure ulcers has increased threefold to 9% in 2009.[129] The heels (41%), sacrum (19%), and buttocks (13%) are the locations for 73% of all sDTI ulcers. This is in a different order than the most frequent locations for all pressure ulcers (sacrum, heels, etc).[129]

Prevalence and incidence definitions and formulas

Lack of clarity and consistency in definitions and calculation formulas impedes our understanding of pressure ulcer prevalence and incidence. Standardization of definitions and formulas will enhance comparability of data among future studies. NPUAP recommends the adoption of consistent definitions and formulas for determining pressure ulcer prevalence and incidence.[127,130]

NPUAP suggests that prevalence should be defined as a "cross-sectional count of the number of cases at a specific point in time, or the number of people with pressure ulcers who exist in a patient population at a given point in time. In assessing prevalence, it doesn't matter in what setting the pressure ulcer was acquired."[127,130] Suggested standard formulas for obtaining prevalence are:

- Pressure ulcer *point* prevalence

$$\frac{\text{Number of people} \atop \text{with a pressure ulcer} \times 100}{\text{Number of people in a polulation} \atop \text{at a particular point in time}}$$

- Pressure ulcer *period* prevalence

$$\frac{\text{Number of people} \atop \text{with a pressure ulcer} \times 100}{\text{Number of people in a polulation} \atop \text{at a particular period in time}}$$

NPUAP recommends using the following definition of incidence: "the number of new cases appearing in a population indicates the rate at which new disease occurs in a population previously without disease."[127,131] Several approaches to measuring incidence have been used. NPUAP defines cumulative incidence as "the rate of new pressure ulcers in a group of patients of fixed size, all of whom are observed over a period of time."[127,131,132] The formula is as follows:

- Pressure ulcer cumulative incidence

$$\frac{\text{Number of people developing a} \atop \text{new pressure ulcer} \times 100}{\text{Total number of people in a population} \atop \text{at beginning of time period}}$$

A problem with using this approach is that it doesn't count pressure ulcers that occur in people admitted to the setting after the study population has been defined. Therefore, it may not be indicative of the true incidence of new ulcers in that setting.

Another way to calculate prevalence is to measure the number of new cases of pressure ulcers that occur in a changing population. In this case, the people who are being studied have varying lengths of stay. Incidence is calculated as the number of people developing pressure ulcers per 1,000 patient-days and is called *incidence density*. Calculate this by using the following suggested formula:

- Pressure ulcer incidence density

$$\frac{\text{Number of people developing a} \atop \text{new pressure ulcer} \times 1000}{\text{Total patient days free of pressure ulcers}}$$

$$= \frac{\text{Number of people developing a pressure ulcer}}{1000 \text{ patient-days}}$$

Using the NPUAP recommended standard formulas alone may not be enough to avoid errors in prevalence and incidence calculations. (See *Pitfalls to calculating prevalence and incidence,* page 350.)

COMPETENCIES AND CURRICULUM

Accurate and current knowledge is essential for clinicians to prevent and treat pressure ulcers. Pressure ulcer knowledge varies among members of the wound care team. For example, physicians in two studies were found to have low levels of pressure ulcer knowledge.[133,134] In addition, some nurses believe that their basic education is insufficient regarding wound care.[76-79] What's more, high pressure ulcer prevalence rates have

Pitfalls to calculating prevalence and incidence

Be sure to avoid the following pitfalls when calculating pressure ulcer prevalence and incidence for your facility.

- Define the population and apply the definition consistently throughout the study.
- Count the number of patients with pressure ulcers — not the number of pressure ulcers.
- Count only pressure ulcers, not other wounds.
- Define the stages of the pressure ulcers you count to include and assess them accurately.

Adapted with permission from Ayello, E.A., et al. "Methods for Determining Pressure Ulcer Prevalence and Incidence," in *Pressure Ulcers in America: Prevalence, Incidence, and Implications for the Future,* edited by Cuddigan, J., et al. Reston, VA: National Pressure Ulcer Advisory Panel, 2001.

been linked to poor knowledge.[132,135-137] Several initiatives are under way to decrease pressure ulcers by increasing the knowledge level of clinicians; these initiatives include the IHI[45] and the New Jersey Hospital Association's "No Ulcers" project.[138]

As knowledge about pressure ulcers has increased, their occurrence has decreased across care settings.[138] AHRQ is pilot testing a pressure ulcer tool kit to assist hospitals in decreasing the incidence of pressure ulcer.[139] Certification has made a difference in pressure ulcer knowledge. In one study, nurses who had received any wound care certification from the WOCN Society, the American Academy of Wound Management, or the National Alliance of Wound Care had higher scores on a standardized 47-item pressure ulcer test.[140]

Suggestions to improve both pressure ulcer prevention practice and the characteristics of pressure ulcer incidence reduction initiatives have been reported in the literature.[141,142] For example, after introduction of the Canadian Association of Wound Care Pressure Ulcer Awareness Program, the pressure ulcer prevalence and incidence rates in Canada decreased by 57% and 71%, respectively.[143] In long-term care, Horn and colleagues achieved a 33% reduction in pressure ulcers in seven facilities by implementing a real-time optimal care plan for nursing home quality initiative in which the number of documentation forms was reduced from 6.2 to 2.8.[62] Citing the limited literature on pressure ulcer injury in patients undergoing procedures in diagnostic and interventional ancillary units such as radiology, renal dialysis, and cardiac and vascular procedure laboratories, Messer[144] stresses the importance of focusing on prevention in these areas. The NPUAP has updated its competency-based curriculum on pressure ulcer prevention[145-147] for registered nurses. (See *NPUAP registered nursing competency base curriculum: Pressure ulcer prevention.*)

Building knowledge about pressure ulcer care is vital. While many experts believe that all pressure ulcers cannot be prevented,[148] it's been shown that education can reduce pressure ulcer incidence and expedite treatment.[149] A variety of continuing education programs, symposia, and national conferences as well as company-sponsored online learning programs exist to facilitate this knowledge building. Interactive computer-based testing on pressure ulcer risk assessment using the Braden Scale, as described by Maklebust and colleagues,[43] as well as the EPUAP-endorsed ePUCLAS$_2$ pressure ulcer staging module[80] are just two of the resources available. The John A. Hartford Institute for Geriatric Nursing also has several one-page quick references in its "Try This" series, one of which is using the Braden Scale.[150] The National Database of Nursing Quality Indicators offers four online modules covering several aspects of pressure ulcer care in which clinicians can acquire knowledge as well as measure their learning through interactive testing.[81] With all this information available, the challenge for clinicians is to put this knowledge into practice in order to prevent or treat pressure ulcers.

NPUAP registered nursing competency base curriculum: Pressure ulcer prevention

- Identify etiologic factors contributing to pressure ulcer occurrence.
- Conduct a structured risk assessment on admission, and repeat regularly and as frequently as required by patient acuity and setting.
- Ensure that a complete skin assessment is part of the risk assessment screening policy in place in all healthcare settings.
- Develop and implement an individualized program of skin care.
- Demonstrate proper positioning/repositioning for pressure ulcer prevention/treatment.

- Choose appropriate support surface for a patient based on risk and the patient's attributes.
- Implement nutritional interventions as appropriate to prevent pressure ulcers.
- Accurately document results of risk assessment, skin assessment, and prevention strategies.
- Apply critical thinking skills to clinical decision making regarding the impact of changes in the individual's condition on pressure ulcer risk.
- Make referrals to other healthcare professionals based on client assessment.

Pieper, B., and Ratliff, C. "National Pressure Ulcer Advisory Panel Registered Nurse Competency-based Curriculum: Pressure Ulcer Prevention." Available at http://www.npuap.org/NPUAP%20RN%20Curr%20landscape%5B1%5D.pdf. Accessed January 14, 2011.

SUMMARY

Pressure ulcers are a common healthcare problem throughout the world. Intensity and duration of pressure as well as tissue tolerance are the etiologic factors that lead to pressure ulcer development. Incorporation of clinical practice guidelines provides a basis for evidence-based pressure ulcer prevention and treatment practice. Results of a pressure ulcer risk assessment using a validated tool can serve as the foundation for developing a pressure ulcer prevention protocol based on the level and type of risk the individual demonstrates. After determining the pressure ulcer stage and other wound characteristics, a comprehensive plan to treat the pressure ulcer that uses a combination of local wound care, debridement, moist wound healing, cleaning, and pressure relief needs to be implemented. A multidisciplinary approach to patient care that includes patient and family education as well as staff education is essential. Use of the standardized formulas as proposed by NPUAP will provide a basis for universal comparison of prevalence and incidence data. Many educational resources are available to clinicians to increase their knowledge level so as to decrease pressure ulcer incidence and enhance treatment.

PATIENT SCENARIO

Clinical Data

Mrs. VP is a 79-year-old woman who fractured her right hip. Following open reduction and internal fixation of the fracture, she was non-compliant with ambulation during her hospitalization and developed a sacral stage II pressure ulcer as well as pneumonia. She is now being cared for in her daughter's home with the assistance of home care services. Her prior dietary intake was inadequate as she had lost 5 lb in 4 weeks while hospitalized. She nibbles at her food and eats less than half of her meals. Mrs. VP is able to respond to commands. She is very reluctant to get up and walk as her "bottom is painful," so she sits in her bed, which has a standard mattress, most of the day. She wears adult incontinence briefs because it is too difficult to get her to the commode, so her skin in the pelvic area is moist. The skin on her extremities is pale, thin, and dry.

Case Discussion

Mrs. VP has several risk factors for developing pressure ulcers, including her age, poor dietary intake, recent weight loss, immobility and inactivity, and moist skin from incontinence. Her plan of care included consultation with a dietician to review innovative ways of getting protein and nutrients into her diet. Protein supplements were added to the foods she likes to ingest (coffee, soups, and puddings).

She was referred to a certified wound and incontinence nurse for management of her incontinence, pressure ulcer, and skin care needs. The use of incontinence pads was discontinued and alternative strategies taught to her daughter. Because moist skin needs less pressure to break down and Mrs. VP is immobile, a pressure redistribution mattress and chair cushion were acquired for use on her bed and chair, respectively. Mrs. VP's daughter was educated about the importance of frequent repositioning, including the use of pillows, and why support surfaces should be used to promote healing and prevent further tissue insult. A schedule was developed to aid in implementing the home care strategies for Mrs. VP. Appropriate wound dressings were placed to support healing of the stage II pressure ulcer. Physical and occupational therapists were consulted for increased ambulation and muscle strengthening exercises.

SHOW WHAT YOU KNOW

1. A pressure ulcer is a lesion caused by:
   A. incontinence.
   B. unrelieved pressure.
   C. heat.
   D. diabetes mellitus.

   ANSWER: B. *Unrelieved pressure is the cause of tissue death in pressure ulcers. Incontinence and diabetes mellitus are patient characteristics that may put a patient at risk for pressure ulcers but in and of themselves don't cause pressure ulcers. Heat causes burns, not pressure ulcers.*

2. A patient is dragged across the bed when transferring to a stretcher. Which one of the following forces that contribute to pressure ulcer development has occurred?
   A. Electrical stimulation
   B. Shear
   C. Friction
   D. Maceration

   ANSWER: C. *Friction has occured. Electrical stimulation is an adjunct therapy used to heal pressure ulcers. Shear is a type of mechanical trauma caused by tissue layers sliding against each other. Maceration is not a mechanical force caused by dragging the skin across a surface.*

3. A patient has a 2 × 3–cm sacral pressure ulcer that has some depth and extends into the subcutaneous tissue with some undermining; no bone is palpable nor visible. There's a small amount of slough seen in one corner of the wound. Using the NPUAP staging classification system, this pressure ulcer is:
   A. stage I.
   B. stage II.

C. stage III.
D. stage IV.

ANSWER: C. *In this ulcer the tissue destroyed is into the subcutaneous tissue. The newly revised NPUAP classification system now includes that category/stage III pressure ulcers are full-thickness wounds that may have some slough and undermining/tunneling, but bone or muscle is not visible or palpable. The ulcer isn't a stage I because the epidermis is no longer intact. It isn't a stage II because the tissue destroyed is deeper than superficial level (partial thickness) and is well into the subcutaneous tissue. It isn't a stage IV because in this ulcer muscle or bone is not palpable or visible.*

4. Which of the following Braden Scale scores for an elderly black man would indicate pressure ulcer risk?
   A. 23
   B. 21
   C. 19
   D. 17

   ANSWER: D. *The research-based cut score for onset of pressure ulcer risk for older patients and blacks is 18. With the Braden Scale, scores at or lower than the cutoff score indicate risk for pressure ulcer development. Answers A, B, and C are all wrong answers because they're higher than the cutoff score of 18. With the Braden Scale, low numerical scores indicate a risk for pressure ulcers.*

5. Which one of the following should be included in a care plan to prevent pressure ulcers?
   A. Turn and reposition every 5 hours.
   B. Clean skin daily using hot water and soap.
   C. Encourage the patient who's confined to a chair to relieve pressure every hour.
   D. Limit fluids to 10 ml/kg of body weight daily.

   ANSWER: C. *It is recommended that pressure lifts be done every hour for chairbound patients. Answer A is incorrect. The exact frequency of turning a patient is not yet known but needs to be individualized. Turn the patient at least every 2 to 4 hours as his or her condition warrants. B is incorrect. Don't use hot water, but rather warm water, and avoid soaps that dry the skin. D is incorrect as there's no need to limit the patient's fluids.*

6. Which one of the following parameters is <u>not</u> part of the NPUAP PUSH tool?
   A. Depth
   B. Exudate
   C. Tissue type
   D. Length × width

   ANSWER: A. *Depth is not on the PUSH tool to measure pressure ulcer healing. Exudate, tissue type, and length × width are the three variables measured.*

7. The best current estimate for pressure ulcer prevalence in acute care in the United States is:
   A. 20%.
   B. 15%.
   C. 7%.
   D. 0.8%.

   ANSWER: B. *According to NPUAP, prevalence rates over the past decade ranged from 10% to 18% in general acute care. The best estimate of incidence according to NPUAP is 7%, and 0.8% is the target number as identified in the initiative Healthy People 2010.*

REFERENCES

1. National Pressure Ulcer Advisory Panel and European Pressure Ulcer Advisory Panel. "Prevention and Treatment of Pressure Ulcers: Clinical Practice Guideline." Washington, DC: National Pressure Ulcer Advisory Panel, 2009.
2. Bolton, L. "Pressure Ulcers," in Macdonald, J.M., Geyer, M.J., eds. *Wound and Lymphedema Management* (pp 95-101). Geneva: World Health Organization, 2010.
3. Panel on the Prediction and Prevention of Pressure Ulcers in Adults. "Pressure Ulcers in Adults: Prediction and Prevention." Clinical Practice Guideline No. 3. AHCPR Publication No. 92-0047. Rockville, MD: Agency for Health Care Policy and Research, 1992.
4. Bergstrom, N., et al. "Treatment of Pressure Ulcers in Adults." Clinical Practice Guideline Number 15. Rockville, MD: Public Health Service, U.S. Department of Health and Human Services; Agency for Health Care Policy and Research publication 95-0652, December 1994.
5. Wound, Ostomy and Continence Nurses Society. "Guideline for Prevention and Management of Pressure Ulcers." *WOCN Clinical Practice Guideline Series 2.* Mount Laurel, NJ, June 1, 2010.
6. Registered Nurses' Association of Ontario. "Best Practice Guidelines for Risk Assessment and the Prevention of Pressure Ulcers." Toronto, ON: Author, 2005.
7. Whitney, J., Phillips, L., Aslam, R., et al. "Guidelines for the Treatment of Pressure Ulcers," *Wound Repair and Regeneration* 14:663-79, 2006.
8. CMS Manual System. "State Operations, Provider Certification, Transmittal 4. Guidance to Surveyors for Long Term Care Facilities." Publication 100-07. November 12, 2004. Available at www.cms.hhs.gov/manuals/pm_trans/R4SOM.pdf. Accessed January 14, 2011.
9. Russo, C.A., Steiner, C. Spector, W. "Hospitalizations Related to Pressure Ulcers Among Adults 18 Years and Older, 2006, Healthcare Cost and Utilization Project." Agency for Healthcare Research and Quality, Rockville, MD. December 2008. Available at *http://www.hcup-us.ahrq.gov/reports/statbriefs/sb3.pdf.* Accessed January 4, 2011.
10. "Pressure Ulcer Prevention: Pressure, Shear, Friction and Microclimate in Context. A Consensus Document." London: Wounds International, 2010. Available at http://www.woundsinternational.com/article.php?issueid=0&contentid=127&articleid=8925&page=1. Accessed January 4, 2011.
11. Maklebust, J., and Sieggreen, M. *Pressure Ulcers: Guidelines for Prevention and Management,* 3rd ed. Philadelphia: Lippincott Williams & Wilkins, 2001.
12. Gefen, A. "Reswick and Rogers Pressure-time Curve for Pressure Ulcer Risk. Part 2." *Nursing Standard (Royal College of Nursing Great Britain)* 23(46):40-44, 2009.
13. Linder-Ganz, E., Engelberg, S., Scheinowitz, M., and Gefen, A. "Pressure-time Cell Death Threshold for Albino Rat Skeletal Muscles as Related to Pressure Sore Biomechanics," *Journal of Biomechanics* 39(14), 2725-32, 2006.
14. Stekelenburg, A., Oomens, C.W.J., Strijkers, G.J., Nicolay, K., and Bader, D.L. "Compression-induced Deep Tissue Injury Examined with Magnetic Resonance Imaging and Histology," *Journal of Applied Physiology* 100(6):1946, 2006.
15. Parish, L.C., et al. *The Decubitus Ulcers.* New York: Masson Publishing, 1983.
16. Dyson, M., and Lyder, C. "Wound Management-physical Modalities," in: Morison, M., ed. *The Prevention and Treatment of Pressure Ulcers.* Edinburgh: Harcourt Brace/Mosby International, 2001.
17. Kottner, J., Balzer, K., Dassen, T., Heinze, A. "Pressure Ulcers: A Critical Review of Definitions and Classifications," *Ostomy Wound Management* 55(9):22-29, 2009.
18. Gefen, A. "Deep Tissue Injury from a Bioengineering Point of View," *Ostomy Wound Management* 55(4):26-36, 2009.
19. Dinsdale, S.M. "Decubitus Ulcers: Role or Pressure and Friction in Causation," *Archives of Physical Medicine and Rehabilitation* 55(4):147-52, April 1974.
20. Maklebust, J. "Pressure Ulcers: The Great Insult," *Nursing Clinics of North America* 40(2):365-89, 2005.
21. Van Gilder, C., Amlung, S., Harrison, P., Meyer, S. "Results of the 2008-2009 International Pressure Ulcer Prevalence™ Survey and a 3-year, Acute Care, Unit-specific Analysis," *Ostomy Wound Management* 55(11):39-45, 2009.
22. Cuddigan, J., Ayello, E.A., Black, J. "Saving Heels in Critically Ill Patients," *WCET Journal* 28(2):16-24, 2008.
23. Black, J.M., Cuddigan, J.E., Walko, M.A., Didier, L.A., Lander, M.J. Kelpe, M.L. "Medical Device Related Pressure Ulcers in Hospitalized Patients," *International Wound Journal* 7(5)358-65, October 2010.
24. Centers for Medicare and Medicaid Services. "Home Health Quality Initiatives: OASIS-C." Available at *www1.cms.gov/HomeHealthQualityInits/06_OASISC.asp.* Accessed January 3, 2011.
25. Centers for Medicare and Medicaid Services. "Home Health Quality Initiatives MDS 3.0

Overview." Available at http://www.cms.hhs.gov/NursingHomeQualityInits/01_Overview.asp#TopOfPage. Accessed January 4, 2011.

26. Centers for Medicare and Medicaid Services. "Home Health Quality Initiatives MDS 3.0 for Nursing Hones and Swing Bed Providers." RAI Manual Version 3.0 and MDS Forms are downloadable at http://www.cms.hhs.gov/Nursinghomequalityinits/25_NHQIMDS30.asp. Accessed January 4, 2011.

27. Levine, J.M., Roberson, S., Ayello, E.A. "Essentials of MDS 3.0, Section M, Skin Conditions," *Advances in Skin & Wound Care* 23(6):273-84; quiz 285-6, 2010.

28. Ayello, E.A., Levine, J.M., Roberson, S. "CMS Updates on MDS 3.0 Section M: Skin Conditions—Change in Coding of Blister Pressure Ulcers," *Advances in Skin & Wound Care.* 2010:23(9):394, 396-7.

29. Norton, D., et al. *An Investigation of Geriatric Nursing Problems in Hospital.* London: National Corporation for the Care of Old People, 1962.

30. Gosnell, D.J. "An Assessment Tool to Identify Pressure Sores," *Nursing Research* 22(1):55-59, January-February 1973.

31. Bergstrom, N., et al. "The Braden Scale for Predicting Pressure Sore Risk©," *Nursing Research* 36(4):205-10, July-August 1987.

32. Waterlow, J. "Pressure Sores: A Risk Assessment Card," *Nursing Times* 81(48):49-55, November 27-December 3, 1985.

33. Ayello, E.A., and Braden, B. "How and Why to do Pressure Ulcer Risk Assessment," *Advances in Skin & Wound Care* 15(3):125-32, May-June 2002.

34. Ayello, E.A., and Braden, B. "Why Is Pressure Ulcer Risk Assessment So Important?" *Nursing* 31(11):75-79, November 2001.

35. Jalali, R., and Rezaie, M. "Predicting Pressure Ulcer Risk: Comparing the Predictive Validity of 4 Scales," *Advances in Skin & Wound Care* 18(2):92-97, 2005.

36. Braden, B. "Translating the Braden Scale for Predicting Pressure Sore Risk©: The Challenge Continues," *WCET Journal* 30(2):29-33, 2010.

37. Braden, B. "Translating the Braden Scale for Predicting Pressure Sore Risk©. Brazilian Portugese," *WCET Journal* 30(3):43, 2010.

38. "Braden Scale for Predicting Pressure Sore Risk." Available at *www.bradenscale.com.* Accessed January 20, 2011.

39. Bergstrom, N., and Braden, B. "A Prospective Study of Pressure Sore Risk Among Institutionalized Elderly," *Journal of the American Geriatric Society* 40(8):747-58, August 1992.

40. Lyder, C.H., et al. "Validating the Braden Scale for the Prediction of Pressure Ulcer Risk in Blacks and Latino/Hispanic Elders: A Pilot Study," *Ostomy Wound Management* 44(suppl 3A):42S-49S, March 1998.

41. Lyder, C.H., et al. "The Braden Scale for Pressure Ulcer Risk: Evaluating the Predictive Validity in Black and Latino/Hispanic Elders," *Applied Nursing Research* 12(2):60-68, May 1999.

42. Maklebust, J., and Magnan, M.A. "A Quasi-experimental Study to Assess the Effect of Technology-assisted Training on Correct Endorsement of Pressure Ulcer Preventive Interventions," *Ostomy Wound Management* 55(2):32-42, 2009.

43. Maklebust, J., Sieggreen, M.Y., Sidor, D., Gerlach, M.A., Bauer, C. Anderson, C. "Computer-based Testing of the Braden Scale for Predicting Pressure Sore Risk," *Ostomy Wound Management* 51(4):40-52, 2005.

44. Bergstrom, N., et al. "Predicting Pressure Ulcer Risk: A Multisite Study of the Predictive Validity of the Braden Scale," *Nursing Research* 47(5):261-69, September-October 1998.

45. The Institute for Healthcare Improvement. "Medical-surgical Care Resources." Available at http://www.ihi.org/IHI/Topics/MedicalSurgicalCare/Medical-SurgicalCareGeneral/Resources. Accessed January 4, 2011.

46. World Union of Wound Healing Societies. "WoundPedia Pressure Ulcer Risk Assessment." Available at http://woundpedia.com/index.php?page=stream&topic=3&docID=369&docLocation=woundpedia. Accessed January 3, 2011.

47. Brem, H., and Lyder, C. "Protocol for the Successful Treatment of Pressure Ulcers," *American Journal of Surgery* 188:1A (Suppl to July), 9S-17S, 2004.

48. Baranoski, S. "Raising Awareness of Pressure Ulcer Prevention and Treatment," *Advances in Skin & Wound Care* 19(7):398-405, 2006.

49. Paralyzed Veterans of America. "Pressure Ulcer Prevention and Treatment Following Spinal Cord Injury: A Clinical Practice Guideline for Health-Care Professionals," Washington, DC, 2000. Available at http://www.pva.org/site/c.ajIRK9NJLcJ2E/b.6357755/apps/s/content.asp?ct=8825403. Accessed January 4, 2011.

50. Keast, D.H., Parslow, N., Hughton, P.E., Norton, L., Fraser, C. "Best Practice Recommendations for the Prevention and Treatment of Pressure Ulcers: Update 2006," *Wound Care Canada* 4(1):R19-R29, 2006.

51. Thompson, P., Langemo, D., Anderson, J., Hanson, D., Hunter, S. "Skin Care Protocols for Pressure Ulcers and Incontinence in Long-term Care: A Quasi-experimental Study," *Advances in Skin & Wound Care* 18(8):422-9, 2005.

52. Carr, D., Benoit, R. "The Role of Interventional Patient Hygiene in Improving Clinical and Economic Outcomes," *Advances in Skin & Wound Care* 22(2):74-8, 2009.

53. Brindle, C.T. "Outliers to the Braden Scale: Identifying High-risk ICU Patients and the Results of Prophylactic Dressing Use." *World Council of Enterostomal Therapists Journal* 30(1):11-18, 2010.

54. Duimel-Peeters, I.G.P., Halfens, R.J.G., Berger, M.P.F., Snoeckx, L.H. "The Effects of Massage as a Method to Prevent Pressure Ulcers: A Review of the Literature," *Ostomy Wound Management* 51(4):70-80, 2005.

55. Langemo, D., Thompson, P., Hunter, S., Hanson, D., Anderson, J. "Heel Pressure Ulcers: Stand Guard," *Advances in Skin & Wound Care* 21(6)282-92, quiz 293-5: 2008.

56. Campbell, K. E., Woodbury, M.G., Houghton, P.E. "Implementation of Best Practice in the Prevention of Heel Pressure Ulcers in the Acute Orthopedic Population," *International Wound Journal* 7(1):28-40,2010

57. Defloor, T., Grypdonck, M., De Bacquer, D. "The Effect of Various Combinations of Turning and Pressure Reducing Devices on the Incidence of Pressure Ulcers," *International Journal of Nursing Studies* 42(1):37-46, 2005.

58. Vanderwee, K., Grypdonck, M.H., De Bacquer, D., Defloor, T. "Effectiveness of Turning with Unequal Time Intervals on the Incidence of Pressure Ulcer Lesions," *Journal of Advanced Nursing* 57(1):59-68, 2007.

59. Rastinehad, D. "Effectiveness of a Pressure Ulcer Prevention Program in an At-risk Oncology Population," *World Council of Enterostomal Therapists Journal* 28(3):12-16, 2008.

60. Norton, L., Coutts, P., Sibbald, R.G. "A Model for Support Surface Selection as Part of Pressure Ulcer Prevention and Management: A Preliminary Study," *World Council of Enterostomal Therapists Journal* 28(3):25-29, 2008.

61. National Pressure Ulcer Advisory Panel. "Support Surface Standards Initiative (S3I)." Available at http://www.npuap.org. Accessed May 27, 2010.

62. Horn, S.D., Sharkey, S.S., Hudak, S., Gassaway, J., James, R., Spector, W. "Pressure Ulcer Prevention in Long Term Care Facilities: A Pilot Study Implementing Standardized Nurse Aide Documentation and Feedback Reports," *Advances in Skin & Wound Care* 23(3):120-31, 2010.

63. Milne, C.T., Trigilia, D., Houle, T.L., DeLong, S., Rosenblum, D. "Reducing PU Prevalence Rates in the LTC Setting," *Ostomy Wound Management* 55(4):50-59, 2009.

64. "Preventing Pressure Ulcers: A Patient's Guide," Volume 3 AHCPR PUB. NO.92-0048, May 1992. Available at http://www.ncbi.nlm.nih.gov/books/NBK12258/. Last accessed January 4, 2011.

65. National Pressure Ulcer Advisory Panel. "Pressure Ulcers Prevalence, Cost, and Risk Assessment: Consensus Development Conference Statement," *Decubitus* 2(2):24-28, May 1989.

66. Shea, J.D. "Pressure Sores: Classification and Management," *Clinical Orthopaedics and Related Research* 112:89-100, October 1975.

67. International Association of Enterostomal Therapy (IAET). "Dermal Wounds: Pressure Sores. Philosophy of the IAET," *Journal of Enterostomal Therapy* 15(1):9-15, January-February 1988.

68. National Pressure Ulcer Advisory Panel. "Pressure Ulcer Stages Revised by NPUAP." February 2007. Available at www.npuap.org/pr2.htm. Accessed January 5, 2011.

69. National Pressure Ulcer Advisory Panel. "Mucosal Pressure Ulcers. An NPUAP Position Statement." Available at http://www.npuap.org/Mucosal_Pressure_Ulcer_Position_Statement_final.pdf. Accessed January 5, 2011.

70. National Pressure Ulcer Advisory Panel. "National Pressure Ulcer Advisory Panel Position Paper on Staging Pressure Ulcers." Available at http://www.npuap.org/NPUAP_position_on_staging%20final%5B1%5D.pdf. Accessed January 5, 2011.

71. Lyder, C.H., Krasner, D.L., Ayello, E.A. "Clarification from the American Nurses Association on the Nurse's Role in Pressure Ulcer Staging," *Advances in Skin & Wound Care* 23(1):8-10, 2010.

72. Patton, R.M. "Is Diagnosis of Pressure Ulcers Within an RN's Scope of Practice?" *American Nurse Today* 5(1):20, 2010.

73. Ayello, E.A., and Lyder, C.H. "Pressure Ulcers in Persons of Color: Race and Ethnicity," in Cuddigan, J., et al., eds. *Pressure Ulcers in America: Prevalence, Incidence, and Implications for the Future.* Reston, VA: National Pressure Ulcer Advisory Panel, 2001.

74. Van Gilder, C., MacFarlane, G.D., Meyer, S. "Results of Nine International Pressure Ulcer Prevalence Surveys: 1989 to 2005," *Ostomy Wound Management* 54(2):40-54, 2008.

75. Sprigle, S., et al. "Clinical Skin Temperature Measurement to Predict Incipient Pressure Ulcers," *Advances in Skin & Wound Care* 14(3):133-37, May-June 2001.

76. Ayello, E.A., Baranoski, S., Salati, D.S. "Best Practices in Wound Care Prevention and Treatment," *Nursing Management* 37(9): 42-48, 2006.

77. Zulkowski, K. Ayello, E.A. "Urban and Rural Nurses' Knowledge of Pressure Ulcers in the USA," *World Council of Enterostomal Therapists Journal* 25(3):24-30, 2005.

78. Ayello, E.A., Baranoski, S., Salati, D.S. "A Survey of Nurses' Wound Care Knowledge," *Advances in Skin & Wound Care* 18(5):268-75, 2005.

79. Ayello, E.A., Baranoski, S., Salati, D.S. "Wound Care Survey Report," *Nursing2005* 35(6):36-45, 2005.

80. European Pressure Ulcer Advisory Panel. "ePUCLAS2. Pressure Ulcer Classification." Available at http://www.puclas.ugent.be/puclas/e/. Accessed January 5, 2011.

81. National Database of Nursing Quality Indicators. "Pressure Ulcer Training." Available at https://www.nursingquality.org/ndnqipressureulcertraining/default.aspx. Accessed January 5, 2011.

82. Maklebust, J. "Policy Implications of Using Reverse Staging to Monitor Pressure Ulcer Status," *Advances in Wound Care* 10(5):32-35, 1997.

83. Roberson, S., Ayello, E.A., Levine, J. "Clarification of Pressure Ulcer Staging in Long-term Care under MDS 2.0." *Advances in Skin & Wound Care* 23(5):206-10, 2010.

84. National Pressure Ulcer Advisory Panel. "NPUAP Statement on Reverse Staging of Pressure Ulcers." Available at http://www.npuap.org/archive/positn2.htm. Accessed January 5, 2011.

85. Aydin, A.K., Karadağ, A. "Assessment of Nurses' Knowledge and Practice in Prevention and Management of Deep Tissue Injury and Stage I Pressure Ulcer," *Journal of Wound, Ostomy and Continence Nursing* 37(5):487-94, 2010.

86. Stewart T.P., Magnano, S.J. "Burns or Pressure Ulcers in the Surgical Patient?" *Decubitus* 1(1):36-40, 1988.

87. Gefen, A. "Deep Tissue Injury from a Bioengineering Point of View," *Ostomy Wound Management* 55(4):26-36, 2009.

88. Black, J. "Deep Tissue Injury: An Evolving Science," *Ostomy Wound Management* 55(2):4, 2009.

89. Quintavalle, P.R., Lyder, C.H., Mertz, P.J., Phillips-Jones, C., Dyson, M. "Use of High-resolution, High-frequency Diagnostic Ultrasound to Investigate the Pathogenesis of Pressure Ulcer Development," *Advances in Skin & Wound Care* 19(9):498-505, 2006.

90. National Pressure Ulcer Advisory Panel. "Not All Pressure Ulcers Are Avoidable [Press Release]." Available at http://www.npuap.org/A_UA%20Press%20Release.pdf. Accessed January 5, 2011.

91. Langemo, D.K., Brown, G. "Skin Fails Too: Acute, Chronic, and End-stage Skin Failure," *Advances in Skin & Wound Care* 19(4):206-11, 2006.

92. CAWC Institute for Wound Management and Prevention. *Level 1 Workbook: Putting Knowledge into Practice – Knowledge Learning.* Toronto, Canada: Canadian Association of Wound Care, 2010.

93. Pieper, B., Langemo, D., Cuddigan, J. "Pressure Ulcer Pain: A Systematic Literature Review and National Pressure Ulcer Advisory Panel White Paper." *Ostomy Wound Management* 55(2):16-31, 2009.

94. Bates-Jensen, B.M. "The Pressure Sore Status Tool a Few Thousand Assessments Later," *Advances in Wound Care* 10(5):65-73, September-October 1997.

95. NPUAP PUSH Task Force. "Pressure Ulcer Scale for Healing: Derivation and Validation of the PUSH Tool," *Advances in Wound Care* 10(5):96, September-October 1997.

96. National Pressure Ulcer Advisory Panel. "Pressure Ulcer Scale for Healing (PUSH) Version 3.0." Available at http://www.npuap.org/PDF/push3.pdf. Accessed January 5, 2011.

97. Berlowitz, D.R., Ratliff, C., Cuddigan, J., Rodeheaver, G.T., and the National Pressure Ulcer Advisory Panel. "The PUSH Tool: A Survey to Determine Its Perceived Usefulness," *Advances in Skin & Wound Care* 18(9):480-83, 2005.

98. Wallenstein, S., and Brem, H. "Statistical Analysis of Wound-healing Rates for Pressure Ulcers," *The American Journal of Surgery* 188(1A)(Suppl):73S-78S, July 2004.

99. Jessup, R.L. "What Is the Best Method for Assessing the Rate of Wound Healing? A Comparison of 3 Mathematical Formulas," *Advances in Skin & Wound Care* 19(3):138, 140-142, 145-146, 2006.

100. Schubert, V., Zander, M. "Analysis of the Measurement of Four Wound Variables in Elderly Patients with Pressure Ulcers," *Advances in Wound Care* 9(4):29-36, 1996.

101. Xakellis, G., and Frantz, R.A. "Pressure Ulcer Healing: What Is It? What Influences It? How Is It Measured?" *Advances in Wound Care* 10(5):20-26, 1997.

102. Dyson, M., Lyder, C. "Wound Management Physical Modalities," in Morison, M, ed., *The Prevention and Treatment of Pressure Ulcers.* Edinburgh: Harcourt Brace/Mosby International, 2001.

103. Sibbald, R.G., Woo, K.Y., Ayello, E.A. "Healing Chronic Wounds: DIM Before DIME Can Help," *Ostomy Wound Management* 12(Suppl), April 2009.

104. Robson, M.C., and Heggers, J.P. "Bacterial Quantification of Open Wounds," *Military Medicine* 134(1):19-24, February 1969.

105. Barr, J.E. "Principles of Wound Cleansing," *Ostomy Wound Management* 41(Suppl 7A):15S-22S, August 1995.

106. Hellewell, T.B., et al. "A Cytotoxicity Evaluation of Antimicrobial Wound Cleansers," *Wounds* 9(1):15-20, 1997.

107. Wilson, J.R., Mills, J.G., Prather, I.D., Dimitrijevich, S.D. "A Toxicity Index of Skin and Wound Cleansers Used on in Vitro Fibroblasts and Keratinocytes," *Advances in Skin & Wound Care* 18(7):373-78, 2005.

108. Rodeheaver, G.T., et al. "Wound Cleansing by High Pressure Irrigation," *Surgery, Gynecology and Obstetrics* 141(3):357-62, September 1975.

109. Stevenson, T.R., et al. "Cleansing the Traumatic Wound by High Pressure Syringe Irrigation," *Journal of the American College of Emergency Physicians* 5(1):17-21, January 1976.

110. Bhaskar, S.N., et al. "Effect of Water Lavage on Infected Wounds in the Rat," *Journal of Periodontology* 40(11):671-72, November 1969.

111. Yarkony, G.M. "Pressure Ulcers: Medical Management," in *Spinal Cord Injury Medical Management and Rehabilitation*. Gaithersburg, MD: Aspen, 1994.

112. Dolychuck, K.N. "Debridement," in Krasner, D., et al., eds. *Chronic Wound Care: A Clinical Source Book for Health Care Professionals*, 3rd ed. Wayne, PA: HMP Communications, 2001.

113. Galpin, J.E., et al. "Sepsis Associated with Decubitus Ulcers," *American Journal of Medicine* 61(3):346-50, September 1976.

114. Kim, Y.C., et al. "Efficacy of Hydrocolloid Occlusive Dressing Technique in Decubitus Ulcer Treatment: A Comparative Study," *Yonsei Medical Journal* 37(3):181-85, June 1996.

115. Bolton, L.L., et al. "Quality Wound Care Equals Cost-effective Wound Care: A Clinical Model," *Advances in Wound Care* 10(4):33-38, July-August 1997.

116. Saydak, S. "A Pilot of Two Methods for the Treatment of Pressure Ulcers," *Journal of Enterostomal Therapy* 7(3):139-42, May-June 1990.

117. Lyder, C.H. "Examining the Cost-effectiveness of Two Methods for Healing Stage II Pressure Ulcers in Long-term Care." Unpublished data, 2010.

118. ter Riet, G., et al. "Randomized Clinical Trial of Ascorbic Acid in the Treatment of Pressure Ulcers," *Journal of Clinical Epidemiology* 48(12):1452-60, December 1995.

119. Rackett, S.C., et al. "The Role of Dietary Manipulation in the Prevention and Treatment of Cutaneous Disorders," *Journal of the American Academy of Dermatology* 29(3):447-53, September 1993.

120. Waldorf, H., Fewkes, J. "Wound Healing," *Advances in Dermatology* 10:77-81, 1995.

121. Erlich, H.P., Hunt, T.K. "Effects of Cortisone and Vitamin A on Wound Healing," *Annals of Surgery* 167(3):324-28, March 1968.

122. Kloth, L.C., McCulloch, J. "Promotion of Wound Healing with Electrical Stimulation," *Advances in Wound Care* 9(5):42-45, September-October 1996.

123. Gardner, S.E., et al. "Effect of Electrical Stimulation on Chronic Wound Healing: A Meta-analysis," *Wound Repair and Regeneration* 7(6):495-503, November-December 1999.

124. Courville, S. "Hyperbaric Oxygen Therapy: It's Role in Healing Problem Wounds," *Canadian Association of Enterostomal Journal* 17(4):7-11, 1998.

125. Gruber, R. P., et al. "Skin Permeability of Oxygen and Hyperbaric Oxygen," *Archives of Surgery* 101(1):69-70, July 1970.

126. Mustoe, T.A., et al. "A Phase II Study to Evaluate Recombinant Platelet-derived Growth Factor-BB in the Treatment of Stage 3 and 4 Pressure Ulcers," *Archives of Surgery* 129(2):213-19, February 1994.

127. Cuddigan, J., Ayello, E.A. and Sussman, C. (Eds.) *Pressure Ulcers in America: Prevalence, Incidence, and Implications for the Future*. Reston, VA: National Pressure Ulcer Advisory Panel, 2001.

128. Ayello, E.A., et al. "Methods for Determining Pressure Ulcer Prevalence and Incidence," in Cuddigan, J., et al., eds. *Pressure Ulcers in America: Prevalence, Incidence, and Implications for the Future*. Reston, VA: National Pressure Ulcer Advisory Panel, 2001.

129. VanGilder, C, MacFarlane, G.D. Harrison, P., Lachenbruch C., Meyer, S. "The Demographics of Suspected Deep Tissue Injury in the United States: An Analysis of the International Pressure Ulcer Prevalence Survey 2006-200," *Advances in Skin & Wound Care* 23(6):254-61, 2010.

130. National Pressure Ulcer Advisory Panel (NPUAP) Board of Directors. "An Executive Summary of the NPUAP Monograph Pressure Ulcers in America: Prevalence, Incidence and Implications for the Future," *Advances in Skin & Wound Care* 14(4):208-15, July-August 2001.

131. Armitage, P., and Berry, G. *Statistical Methods in Medical Research*. Cambridge, MA: Blackwell Scientific, 1987.

132. Springett, J., Cowell, J., Heanet, M. "Using Care Pathways in Pressure Area Management: A Pilot Study," *Journal of Wound Care* 8(5):227-30, 1999.

133. Odierna, E., and Zeleznik, J. "Pressure Ulcer Education: A Pilot Study of the Knowledge and Clinical Confidence of Geriatric Fellows," *Advances in Skin & Wound Care* 16:26-30, 2003.

134. Garcia, A.D., Perkins, C., Click, C., Bergstrom, N., Taffet, G. "Pressure Ulcer Education in Primary Care Residencies," in Ayello, E.A., Baranoski, S. (eds.), Research Forum: Examining the problem of pressure ulcers. *Advances in Skin & Wound Care* 18(4 Suppl):193-4, 2005.

135. Boxer, E., and Maynard, C. "The Management of Chronic Wounds: Factors That Affect Nurses' Decision Making," *Journal of Wound Care* 8(8):409-412, 1999.

136. Lamond, D., and Farnell, S. "The Treatment of Pressure Sores: A Comparison of Novice and Expert Nurses' Knowledge, Information Use and Decision Accuracy," *Journal of Advanced Nursing* 27:280-6, 1998.

137. Maylor, M., and Torrance, C. "Pressure Sore Survey Part 2: Nurses Knowledge," *Journal of Wound Care* 8(2):49-52, 1999.

138. Ayello, E.A., Zulkowski, K., Holmes, A.M., Edelstein, T. "A Collaborative Statewide Across Care Setting Initiative Reduces Pressure Ulcers," *Advances in Skin & Wound Care.* In review, 2011.

139. Agency for Healthcare Research and Quality. "Preventing Pressure Ulcers in Hospitals: A Toolkit for Improving of Quality Care." Developed by the Boston University Research Team. Available at http://www.ahrg.gov/research/etc/pressureulcertoolkit. Accessed April 22, 2011.

140. Zulkowski, K., Ayello, E.A., Wexler, S. "Certification and Education: Do They Affect Pressure Ulcer Knowledge in Nursing?" *Advances in Skin & Wound Care* 20(1):34-8, 2007.

141. Lyder, C.H., and Ayello, E.A. "An Annual Checkup—One Year after the Implementation of the CMS Present on Admission and Pressure Ulcers." *Advances in Skin & Wound Care* 22(10):476-84; quiz 485-6, 2009.

142. Armstrong, D.G., Ayello, E.A., Capitulo, K.L., et al. "New Opportunities to Improve Pressure Ulcer Prevention and Treatment: Implications of the CMS Inpatient Hospital Care Present on Admission Indicators/Hospital-Acquired Conditions Policy—A Consensus Paper from the International Expert Wound Care Advisory Panel," *Advances in Skin & Wound Care* 21(10):469-77, 2008.

143. Orsted, H.L., Rosenthal, S., Woodbury, M.G. "Pressure Ulcer Awareness and Prevention Program. A Quality Improvement Program Through the Canadian Association of Wound Care." *Journal of Wound Ostomy & Continence Nursing* 36(2):178-83, 2009.

144. Messer, M.S. "Pressure Ulcer Risk in Ancillary Services Patients," *Journal of Wound Ostomy & Continence Nursing* 37(2):153-58, 2010.

145. Pieper, B., and Ratliff, C. "National Pressure Ulcer Advisory Panel Registered Nurse Competency-based Curriculum: Pressure Ulcer Prevention." Available at http://www.npuap.org/NPUAP%20RN%20Curr%20landscape%5B1%5D.pdf. Accessed January 14, 2011.

146. Ayello, E.A., and Frantz, R.A. "A Competency-based Pressure Ucer Curriculum for Registered Nurses in America. Part I, Pressure Ulcer Prevention," *World Council of Enterostomal Therapists Journal* 25(1):8-12, 2005.

147. Ayello, E.A., and Frantz, R.A. "A Competency-based Pressure Ulcer Curriculum for Registered Nurses in America. Part 2, Pressure Ulcer Treatment," *World Council of Enterostomal Therapists Journal* 25(2):8-14, 2005.

148. Brandeis, G.H., Berlowitz, D.R., Katz, P. "Are Pressure Ulcers Preventable? A Survey of Experts," *Advances in Skin & Wound Care* 14:244, 2001.

149. Carasa, M., and Polycarpe, M. "Caring for the Chronically Critically Ill Patient: Establishing a Wound Healing Program in a Respiratory Care Unit," *The American Journal of Surgery* 188(1A Suppl):18S-21S, July 2004.

150. Ayello, E.A., for the Hartford Institute for Geriatric Nursing. "Try This Series: Predicting Pressure Ulcer Risk." Available at http://consultgerirn.org/uploads/File/trythis/try_this_5.pdf. Accessed January 5, 2011.

CHAPTER 14

Venous Disease and Lymphedema Management

Objectives

After completing this chapter, you will be able to:

- describe the anatomy and physiology of the venous system
- describe the pathophysiology of lower-extremity venous ulcers
- explain the physiology of edema formation
- describe systems for classifying venous disease
- state the signs and symptoms that comprise a venous assessment
- discuss vascular laboratory tests performed for patients with venous disease
- describe the components of local wound care for a patient with a venous ulcer
- describe surgical treatment for patients with venous ulcers
- identify education needs for patients with venous disease
- describe the epidemiology of lymphedema
- explain the physiology of edema formation
- describe prevention and proper management of lymphedema.

VENOUS DISEASE

Mary Y. Sieggreen, NP, CNS, APRN, CVN,
and Ronald A. Kline, MD, FACS, FAHA

"Peripheral vascular disease" is a term commonly used in reference to an arterial problem, even though it includes diseases and conditions of the venous and lymphatic systems as well as the arterial system. Patients with leg ulcers may present with a combination of arterial, venous, and lymphatic disease. This chapter presents information in two separate sections: (1) the pathogenesis and management of wounds resulting from venous insufficiency and (2) lymphatic disease.

VENOUS DISEASE: SCOPE OF THE PROBLEM

Approximately 10% to 35% of the population has some form of venous disease.[1] It is estimated that between 1% and 22% of the population over age 60 suffers from lower-extremity skin ulcers.[2-5] One study found the problem to be underestimated when a self-report survey indicated that high numbers of patients cared for their own ulcers without consulting a healthcare provider.[6] The principal leg ulcer etiology in most patients is some type of peripheral vascular disease. Chronic venous disease is the seventh most common chronic disease and is the underlying cause in 95% of leg ulcers[1, 7-9] In a U.S. community health survey, 5% of adults had skin changes in the leg and more than 500,000 suffered from venous ulcers. Over 2,000,000 work days are lost in the United States per year due to the associated morbidity of post-phlebitic syndrome.[9] Although it's understood that chronic wounds have physical, financial, and psychological effects, it's difficult to measure these effects on a patient's quality of life.[10] It's also difficult to obtain accurate etiological information about leg ulcers and, in about one-third of medical records, no ulcer etiology might be documented.

VENOUS ANATOMY AND PHYSIOLOGY

Venous system

The venous system begins at the postcapillary level. Venules begin to coalesce, forming small veins, which again coalesce into larger veins from the periphery to a more central location. The venous system mimics the arterial system in many respects but has greater anatomic variability than the arterial tree. In the leg, the veins that course with the tibial and peroneal arteries are usually paired with numerous cross-linking branches, resulting in a retia appearance in some patients. These branches ascend along the respective arteries to form the popliteal vein, which is the first vein of significant size in the lower leg. The popliteal vein proceeds toward the head and becomes the femoral vein, commonly called the superficial femoral vein—a name that causes confusion because the vein in question is actually a deep vein. The superficial femoral vein joins the deep femoral vein to form the common femoral vein. The deep femoral vein is the deep drainage system of the thigh. (See *Deep and superficial venous systems.*)

Dual venous system

The leg has a dual venous system—the deep system just described and the superficial system represented by the saphenous veins. The greater

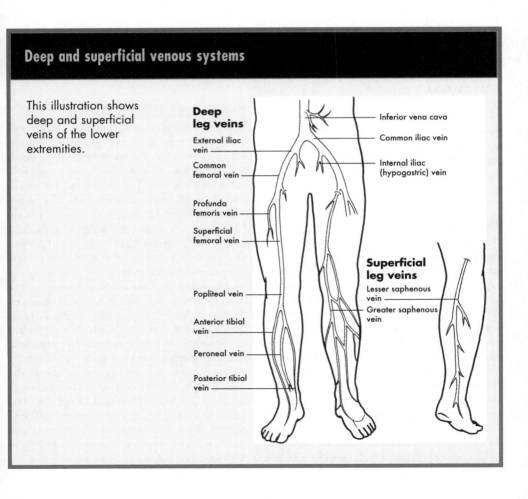

Deep and superficial venous systems

This illustration shows deep and superficial veins of the lower extremities.

Deep leg veins

External iliac vein

Common femoral vein

Profunda femoris vein

Superficial femoral vein

Popliteal vein

Anterior tibial vein

Peroneal vein

Posterior tibial vein

Inferior vena cava

Common iliac vein

Internal iliac (hypogastric) vein

Superficial leg veins

Lesser saphenous vein

Greater saphenous vein

saphenous vein courses along the medial aspect of the leg. The dorsal digital veins in the foot coalesce to form the greater saphenous vein, which is found medial and anterior to the medial malleolus. It ascends in the leg through a variable course and may be bifurcated or even trifurcated. At knee level, its course becomes deeper in relation to the skin. As it ascends the leg, it joins the common femoral vein at the fossa ovale. The lesser saphenous vein drains the posterior aspect of the calf. It perforates into the deep compartment of the calf at the level of the popliteal fossa to join the popliteal vein. As the common femoral vein ascends behind the inguinal ligament, it becomes the external iliac vein and joins the internal iliac vein to become the common iliac vein. The common iliac veins join at the level of the umbilicus and to the right of the aorta to become the inferior vena cava. The renal veins drain into the vena cava. More cephalad, the hepatic veins join the vena cava, which then empties into the right heart chamber.

The saphenous system is connected to the deep venous system through numerous perforator veins. Perforator veins shunt blood from the subcutaneous tissue and the greater saphenous system into the deep veins of the leg. They cross through the superficial fascia of the leg, hence their name. The location of perforator veins is somewhat variable, and some are ascribed proper names. The lowest perforator connecting the saphenous system with the deep venous system is just above the medial malleolus.

Valve anatomy

Unidirectional valves are present in the deep and superficial venous systems and in the perforator veins. These valves are located just before bifurcation points. The greater saphenous vein contains approximately six to eight valves. With rare exception, a valve is always present just below the insertion of the greater saphenous vein into the common femoral vein at the fossa ovale. The orientation of the valves allows venous blood to flow from distal to proximal. Perforator veins' valves are oriented to shunt blood from the lesser saphenous vein and the greater saphenous system into the deep veins of the leg.

Valve anatomy is that of a bileaflet with valve sinuses present on the lateral bases of each valve leaflet. These sinuses represent a dilation in the normal contour of the vein wall. Their function is to assist in valve closure, a passive act caused by the retrograde flow of venous blood into the sinus, thereby coapting (fitting together) the two valve leaflets. The valve leaflets are oriented parallel to the surface of the skin. It's the loss of valve function at various levels that results in varying degrees of venous insufficiency. Valve function is lost under a number of disease states. Inability of the valve to coapt can also occur with over-distention of the venous segment. This effectively stretches the valves apart so that they no longer come in direct contact, thereby allowing blood to reflux into the more dependent portion of the vein. Disease states that cause loss of valve function include:

* congenital valve absence
* deep vein thrombosis
* ectasia
* phlebitis
* valve atresia
* venous engorgement
* venous hypertension.

Venous wall architecture

Venous wall anatomy is similar to arterial wall anatomy except that the respective laminae are thinner. The outermost layer of a vein is the adventitia. The media varies most from the arterial media. The media within a vein contains both elastic and muscular fibers, but to a much lesser degree than the arterial media. Nonetheless, a vein can contract and adjust its size to correspond to the degree of venous blood flow. The intima layer is a delicate single layer of endothelial cells.

The relatively thin media accounts for the lack of venous compliance at increased pressures. At low pressures, the venous system is fairly compliant, but once arterial pressure is reached the venous wall becomes distended and rigid. Venoconstriction occurs in both the superficial and deep veins; the more peripheral the vein, the more readily it contracts. This reactivity is under sympathetic adrenergic control. Peripheral veins are more sensitive than central veins to this sympathetic drive. The ability of veins to relax and dilate enables the venous system to hold 75% of the total blood volume.

The upward flow of lower-extremity venous blood, although aided by unidirectional valves and arterial pressure, is mostly dependent upon the "muscular pump." Pedal dorsal vein pressure in the supine position should approximate that of central venous pressure. Upon assuming an erect posture, this pressure can approach 100 mm Hg. With active muscle contraction, intra-compartmental pressure markedly increases, thereby causing deep veins of the leg to compress and push venous blood upward. This pressure then approaches 200 mm Hg. This is possible because the muscular compartments of the leg are enclosed by relatively rigid fascial encasement. Back-flush of blood is reduced when valves are competent and reflux into the saphenous system is prevented by the unidirectional perforator valves.

ULCER PATHOPHYSIOLOGY

Venous ulcers

Venous ulcers are chronic skin and subcutaneous lesions usually found on the lower extremity at the pretibial and the medial supra-malleolar areas of the ankle, where the perforator veins are located. Venous ulcers were formerly known as "venous stasis" ulcers because their development was thought to be caused by blood pooled in the veins. More recent literature indicates that venous hypertension rather than venous stasis is both the cause of these ulcers and the reason they don't heal.[12] It's difficult to restore skin integrity in the presence of chronic venous hypertension because the underlying edema must be controlled in addition to healing the ulcer.

Venous ulceration may be precipitated by deep vein thrombosis (DVT), which can

Venogram

In this venogram, the patient's left venous valve (B) is intact. On the patient's right (A), collateral veins are present due to venous occlusion, possibly from an undiagnosed deep vein thrombosis.

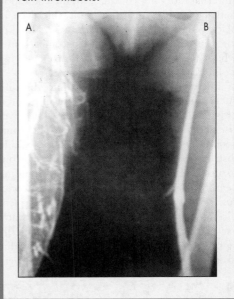

remain undiagnosed for years prior to the onset of the ulcer. (See *Venogram*.) It has long been thought that the natural course of lower-extremity DVT is the eventual development of leg ulcers.[13]

Symptomatic and asymptomatic thrombi may cause long-term complications by scarring the intima and creating valvular incompetence. When the valves are rendered incompetent, blood backs into the distal veins during diastole. With loss of perforator valve function, the high intracompartmental venous pressure, which can approach 200 mm Hg during active muscle contraction, results in distention of the saphenous system. This in turn causes a cascading effect with dilation of the greater saphenous vein and worsening of already compromised valvular function. The weight of the column of blood increases the pressure inside the capillaries.

CHARACTERISTICS OF VENOUS ULCERS

Venous hypertension distends the superficial veins, resulting in vein wall damage and exudation of fluid into the interstitial space, thereby causing edema of venous insufficiency. Over time, an actual leakage of red blood cells occurs through these compromised veins. As they break down, the red blood cells deposit hemosiderin into the tissues, causing a form of "internal tattooing" of the skin; the coloration is that of a brownish hue noticeable even in black skin. (See *Hemosiderin deposit*.) The skin loses its normal texture and becomes somewhat shiny and subsequently sclerotic, giving a taut skin appearance in these areas.

Edema and loss of red cells into the subcutaneous tissue occur at the point of greatest gravitational pressure, the ankle. This gives rise to the pathopneumonic features of chronic venous stasis, hyperpigmentation, and stocking distribution induration of the subcutaneous tissues,[14,15] the characteristics of long-standing venous insufficiency called lipodermatosclerosis. These areas are prone to subsequent ulceration or infection; extreme pruritus and excoriation are usually present, potentially aggravating the injured skin. Dermatitis due to endogenous or exogenous sources and severe

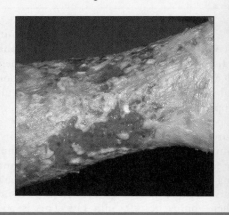

Venous ulcer with granulating base

The venous ulcer shown here has irregular borders and a granulating base with surrounding fibrotic tissue.

Hemosiderin deposit

Hemosiderin deposits caused the discoloration seen here in the patient's right leg.

allergic reactions may complicate the situation. The skin may present as itchy, erythematous, and weeping or dry and scaly. (See *Venous ulcer with granulating base*. See also *color section, Venous Ulcer*, page C22.) Chemical or mechanical factors may be responsible for contact dermatitis surrounding a leg ulcer.[16]

Another sequelae of venous hypertension is irritability of the musculature. Many patients with venous insufficiency—even those in whom the condition is mild—report nocturnal leg cramps. Depolarization may occur due to fluid distention of the muscular cells, causing tetanic-like contractions of various muscle groups. Distention of veins in the subdermal plexus results in the varicosities typically seen with venous insufficiency. (See *Varicose veins*.) The appearance of telangiectasias, more commonly called "spider veins," is the result of distention of the smaller subdermal capillary network. (See *Telangiectasias*.)

In some circumstances, venous aneurysms can occur due to massive dilation of the greater saphenous vein and its tributaries. Further stagnation of flow in these areas in the presence of an abnormal vessel wall can result in thrombophlebitis, which worsens the venous

Varicose veins

Note the presence of varicose veins in the patient's lower extremities, shown here.

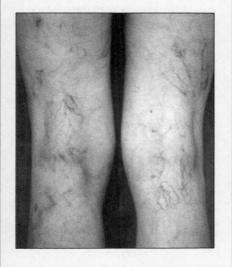

Telangiectasias

Telangiectasias, also known as "spider veins," are shown in the photograph below.

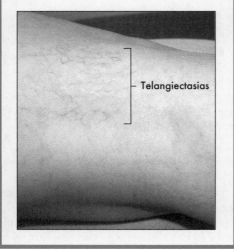

Telangiectasias

outflow of the leg and aggravates an already deleterious condition. Thrombosis adheres to the wall of the vein and although recanalization occurs eventually, the valves remain incompetent. In an attempt to compensate for the reduced venous return, the surrounding collateral veins dilate. Chronic edema occurs in the ankle. Increased venous pressure impedes capillary flow, decreasing oxygen available for transport from the capillaries to the tissues, and protein and red blood cells leak into the interstitial tissues. The effect is cumulative, eventually leading to tissue damage, scar formation and, ultimately, ulceration.

Endothelium in the normal saphenous vein facilitates contraction in response to noradrenaline. In varicose veins, the endothelial-enhanced noradrenaline vasoconstriction is decreased. Endothelial damage is thought to be a possible cause of venous dilatation and subsequent varicose veins.[17]

Venous leg ulcers are also correlated with increased ambulatory venous pressures. Nicolaides[21] obtained ambulatory venous pressure (AVP) from 220 patients admitted with venous problems. He found that no patients with an AVP less than 30 mm Hg had leg ulcers, while 100% of those with AVP greater than 90 mm Hg had ulcers. The incidence of ulceration wasn't preferentially associated with either superficial or deep venous disease.

Evidence-Based Practice

Nicolaides' study[18] suggests that AVP should be measured in patients with nonhealing venous ulcers to determine whether they may benefit from a procedure such as a venous valve transplant, which reduces the AVP to less than 30 mm Hg.

PATHOGENESIS OF VENOUS ULCERS

Several theories have been proposed to explain the mechanism of venous hypertension leading to ulceration. In 1917, Homans suggested that stasis of blood in dilated veins in the skin may cause anoxic cell death, leading to ulcers. In 1929,

CEAP classification system

The CEAP classification system for chronic venous disease consists of four elements:

- **c**linical classification
- **e**tiologic classification
- **a**natomic classification
- **p**athophysiological classification.

Clinical classification (C0-C6)

Class	Description
0	No signs of venous disease
1	Telangiectasias or reticular veins
2	Varicose veins
3	Edema
4	Skin changes
5	Healed ulcer
6	Active ulcer

Etiologic classification (E_C, E_P, E_S)

- Congenital (E_C)
- Primary (E_P)—with undetermined cause
- Secondary (E_S)—with known cause

Anatomic distribution classification (A_S, A_D, and A_P)

This element consists of classifications A_S, A_D, and A_P, and segments 1 through 18. See table below for a breakdown.

- Superficial veins (A_S)
- Deep veins (A_D)
- Perforating veins (A_P)

Segment	Classification
1	Superficial veins (A_S) Telangiectasias/reticular veins Greater (long) saphenous vein
2	• Above knee
3	• Below knee
4	• Lesser (short) saphenous
5	• Non-saphenous Deep veins (A_D)
6	Inferior vena cava Iliac
7	• Common
8	• Internal
9	• External
10	Pelvic-gonadal, broad ligament, other Femoral
11	• Common
12	• Deep
13	• Superficial
14	• Popliteal
15	Crural: Anterior tibial, posterior tibial, peroneal (all paired)
16	Muscular: Gastrocnemial, soleal, other Perforating veins (A_P)
17	Thigh
18	Calf

Pathophysiological classification (P_R, P_O)

- Reflux (P_R)
- Obstruction (P_O)
- Reflux and obstruction (P_R, P_O)

Adapted with permission from Kistner, R.L., and Eklof, B. "Clinical Presentation and Classification of Chronic Venous Disease," in Gloviczki, P., and Bergan, J.J., eds., *Atlas of Endoscopic Perforator Vein Surgery.* New York: Springer-Verlag, 1998.

Blalock[19] found blood oxygen content to be higher than normal in varicose veins, suggesting that arteriovenous communications may be responsible for venous hypertension. In 1972, however, a study using radioactive macro-aggregates refuted the arteriovenous shunting hypothesis.[20]

Two current hypotheses—the "fibrin cuff" and "white cell trapping" theories—are more recent attempts to explain venous ulcer formation. The fibrin cuff theory states that sustained venous hypertension causes distention of dermal capillary beds, which allows plasma exudate to leak into the surrounding tissue. Fibrin precipitation in the peripapillary space forms fibrin cuffs, which impair oxygen, nutrient, and growth factor transport. The tissues undergo inflammation and fibrosis.[21] A subsequent study suggests that peripapillary fibrin is present but doesn't influence healing of lower-extremity ulcers.[22]

The white cell trapping theory states that the neutrophil aggregation in the capillaries causes lipodermatosclerosis. Increasing venous pressure is thought to reduce capillary perfusion pressure and flow rate. Low capillary flow rate initiates white blood cell adherence to the cell wall. Endothelial cells and leukocytes interact and release proteolytic enzymes, oxygen-free radicals, and lipid products. The white cells are then activated, damaging the vessel walls, increasing capillary permeability, and allowing larger molecules such as fibrinogen to exit the capillaries.[23,24]

The trap hypothesis of venous ulceration was proposed by Falanga and Eaglstein.[25] This hypothesis proposes that fibrin and other macromolecules that leak out bind or trap growth factors and other substances necessary for maintaining normal tissues and healing.

CLASSIFYING VENOUS DISEASE

Chronic venous insufficiency has been defined as an abnormally functioning venous system caused by venous valvular incompetence with or without associated venous outflow obstruction, which may affect the superficial venous system, the deep venous system, or both.[26] Chronic venous insufficiency can result in post-phlebitic syndrome, which manifests as varicose veins and venous ulcers.

In 1994, the American Venous Forum developed a descriptive system based on clinical, etiologic, anatomic, and pathophysiologic (CEAP) data to categorize the key elements in chronic venous disease.[27] The CEAP system provides an objective classification method that clarifies relationships among contributing factors and improves communication regarding venous disease. (See *CEAP classification system*.) The system is subdivided into seven categories based on objective signs of chronic

venous disease.[28] In 2004,[29] this system was refined to add C_0 to the Clinical component to represent no visible or palpable signs of venous disease, and subclasses were also added.

C_4 was added to better define the differing severity of venous disease:

C_{4a}: Pigmentation or eczema
C_{4b}: Lipodermatosclerosis or atrophie blanche.

In 2000, The American Venous Forum developed an assessment tool called the Venous Clinical Severity Score (VCSS) to supplement the CEAP tool.[30] This assessment tool was revised and updated in 2010.[31] Designed to provide more information about severe chronic venous disease, the VCSS tool consists of six descriptors—pain, varicose veins, venous edema, skin pigmentation, inflammation, and induration—that are rated 0 (absent), 1 (mild), 2 (moderate), or 3 (severe). In addition, there are four descriptors for ulcers: number of active ulcers (0, 1, 2, or 3 or more), active ulcer duration (N/A, <3 months, >3 months but <1 year, not healed for 1 year), active ulcer size (N/A, <2 cm diameter, 2-6 cm diameter, >6 cm diameter), and compressive therapy (not used, intermittent use, wears most days, full compliance). This scoring system is an elaboration of the C or clinical component of the CEAP classification system. It is dynamic in that the numbers can change as the ulcers heal or the venous disease process is treated. Combining the two tools provides a method to communicate information about the ulcer in both objective and subjective terms. The VCSS and CEAP tools are expected to improve clinicians's ability to follow venous treatment outcomes.

DIAGNOSING VENOUS ULCERS

Venous disease and ulcer etiology can be determined by obtaining a thorough patient history and performing a physical examination. A focused vascular history includes a clear description of the presenting complaint, past medical history for vascular and related conditions, current and previously taken medications, and risk factors. Signs and symptoms of lower-extremity venous disease may include pain, tissue loss, or change in appearance or sensation. It is important to include assessment of the arterial system when evaluating venous and lymphatic disease. Adequate arterial perfusion is essential when using compression therapy for venous and lymphatic ulcers. It may be necessary to correct the arterial problem before the ulcer can be treated. Noninvasive vascular laboratory testing is used to identify the location of vascular pathology.

Physical examination

Physical examination provides direction for intervention, starting with skin inspection. Skin changes in venous disease include hyperpigmentation, dermatitis, lipodermatosclerosis, or atrophie blanche, a characteristic white patchy scarring at the site of previous ulcers. Because skin color may indicate venous congestion, the color of each toe should be noted and compared with the the color of other foot and toes. In venous insufficiency, the skin appears a dusky ruddy color. In chronic venous insufficiency, the skin may become atrophied with scarring from a previous ulcer or it may have weeping blisters or dry, scaly crusts.

Skin should be palpated for temperature changes. The skin over varicose veins is often warmer than the surrounding skin. Patients presenting with foot or leg ulcers should be tested for neuropathy, which is a common finding in the diabetic patient.

Edema is commonly found in lower-extremity venous disease. Early edema may be observed as a difference in calf circumference between legs and should be confirmed by measurement. After edema has been longstanding tissue fibrosis occurs. This makes the skin and subcutaneous tissues less resilient to palpation.

Venous signs and symptoms

Patients may report a gradual onset of discomfort associated with venous disease; however, often no symptoms are present initially. Most patients describe general nondescript aching rather than specific pain. Some terms used to describe sensations in the legs include fullness, swelling, tightness, aching, or heaviness. These symptoms can be reduced with leg elevation. Venous insufficiency accompanied by acute

deep vein thrombosis (DVT) may be described as sharp, severe, deep, aching pain.[32] Varicose veins occasionally produce a pulling, prickling, or tingling discomfort localized to the area of the varicose vein.[7] In severe cases of venous insufficiency, a form of claudication can occur. The patient may complain of foot edema that makes it difficult to wear shoes.

A venous ulcer is moist and may have a yellow fibrous film covering its surface. This fibrous tissue isn't a sign of infection and doesn't interfere with healing.[33] The ulcer edges may be irregular with firm fibrotic and indurated surrounding skin. The surrounding tissue may have a brownish rust color due to erythrocyte breakdown and deposition of hemosiderin. Scar tissue may indicate the site of a previous ulcer. Because of the subcutaneous scarring, there is no allowance for the tissue expansion that occurs with edema in skin of normal elasticity. Scar tissue also prevents blood vessels from transporting oxygen to the skin, further compromising healing.[34] Lipodermatosclerosis the term used for chronic inflammation and fibrosis of skin and subcutaneous tissues. It may be associated with diffuse inflammatory painful skin edema.

VASCULAR TESTING

Although an experienced vascular clinician can make a vascular diagnosis based on history and physical examination alone, vascular laboratory studies contribute to the accuracy of the diagnosis. The presence, location, and severity of arterial and venous disease are confirmed by vascular laboratory procedures. Information obtained by vascular studies can predict ulcer healing when the cause is arterial insufficiency.[7] Laboratory tests differentiate among conditions that contribute to a nonhealing ulcer.

Noninvasive vascular testing is divided into direct tests that image the vessel itself and indirect tests that demonstrate changes distal to the diseased vessel. These tests include Doppler ultrasound, venous duplex ultrasound, ankle-brachial index (ABI), transcutaneous pressure of oxygen ($TCPO_2$), segmental systolic pressures, and plethysmography.

Doppler ultrasound

In a Doppler ultrasound, a transmitting probe sends a signal which is reflected from an object to the receiving probe. If the signal strikes a moving object such as blood cells, a frequency shift is detected and reflected as sound. The audible signals of venous and arterial flow patterns can be distinguished.

Duplex ultrasound

The venous duplex allows one to evaluate various segments of the venous tree looking for more than 0.5 seconds reflux after either a muscle contraction or manual augmentation of cephalad flow. Another advantage of venous duplex imaging is that it can identify sites of thrombosis with high levels of accuracy. The disadvantage is that it's fairly time-consuming, taking 1 to 2 hours per evaluation for a full leg imaging.

Venous testing

It's possible to perform a crude venous assessment by physical exam using a Doppler ultrasound. By compressing the limb manually, the flow in the veins can be augmented and noted by the audible Doppler signal heard distal to the site of compression. This is a subjective test, and reliability is clinician dependent. The introduction of noninvasive vascular testing has provided much anatomical and physiological information to increase the accuracy of diagnosing venous diseases. Two tests are most commonly used to assess the severity of venous insufficiency. One is venous photoplethysmography (PPG), and the other is venous duplex imaging.[35]

PLETHYSMOGRAPHY

Plethysmography records volume changes in the limb. Several types of plethysmography are available:

- air plethysmography, which uses a pneumatic cuff as a segmental volume sensor
- strain-gauge plethysmography, which uses a fine-bore silicone rubber tube filled with mercury wrapped around the limb to be studied

- impedance plethysmography, which measures the relative change in resistive impedance of the passage of an electrical current through a segment of the body
- PPG, which measures the degree of light attenuation, which is proportional to the quantity of blood present and not actual volume change.[7,36]

Air plethysmography and PPG are the more common tests for chronic venous disease. A photoplethysmograph consists of an infrared light-emitting diode and a photo sensor mounted on a probe. The probe is applied to the skin over the area to be tested.[7] The advantage of venous PPG is that it's quick and gives assessment of overall venous refill time. On the other hand, it only evaluates the most dependent portion of the leg in the gator area.

TREATING VENOUS ULCERS

Treatment goals for all ulcers are to:

- provide an environment conducive to new tissue growth
- protect the wound
- prevent further tissue destruction.

Topical and systemic treatments are addressed simultaneously. It's imperative to consider the cause when deciding treatment because ulcers aren't all alike and treatment for one type may be inappropriate or harmful for another type. A vascular specialist consultation is appropriate for ulcers of mixed etiology.

Wound infection

Infected leg ulcers, soft-tissue cellulitis, and osteomyelitis are treated by administering systemic IV or oral antibiotics. Topical antibiotics are not indicated for all leg ulcers.[37] Chronic wounds are colonized with normal skin flora and shouldn't be treated with antibiotics. Rigorous and frequent ulcer cleansing assists in removing surface bacteria. Newer silver-impregnated dressings have been effective in managing bacteria and promoting healing by keeping the wound surface clean.[38]

Biopsy for a quantative culture of the inflamed tissue surrounding non-healing ulcers should be considered if true infection isn't responding to antibiotics. If carcinoma is suspected, biopsy of the lesion should be obtained. (See Chapter 7, Wound bioburden and infection.)

> ### ▶ PRACTICE POINT
>
> Because bone scans are expensive and may give false-positive results in the presence of inflammation, their use is indicated only when bone infection, abscess, or fluid collection is suspected.

Skin and wound care

A clean wound, free from dead tissue and wound debris, is necessary for healing to occur. Wound cleaning and debridement are the initial steps in wound care. Many commercial wound cleaners and disinfectants are cytotoxic. Povidone-iodine, hydrogen peroxide, and 0.25% acetic acid have shown evidence of interfering with fibroblast formation and epithelial growth.[39–42] There may be indications for using cidal agents in a wound; however, their use should be time-limited and each caregiver should have a clear understanding of what the goals are and when the goals have been reached.

> ### Evidence-Based Practice
>
> The advantage of cleaning the wound should be weighed against the risk of damaging new tissue growth.[43]

The safest wound cleanser is 0.9% saline solution. Wounds should be cleaned with a force strong enough to dislodge debris but gentle enough to prevent damage to newly growing tissue. The pressure to accomplish this goal ranges from 4 to 15 psi.[44] A 19-gauge needle or 19-gauge angiocatheter distributes approximately 8 psi when used with a 35-ml syringe. Using a Baxter cap on a saline irrigation bottle is a less expensive method to distribute an adequate amount of pressure (Fig. 14-1). Leg ulcers treated in the home are commonly irrigated with running tap water.

Hydrotherapy or whirlpool has been used to aid in cleaning and debridement of both arterial and venous leg ulcers.[45] A clinical pilot study found that whirlpool followed by vigorous rinsing reduced the bacterial load in venous ulcers more than the whirlpool alone.[46] This may suggest that the vigorous irrigation is the significant factor in cleaning the wound. Whirlpool may be contraindicated if the water and dependent position increase edema in the leg. There are no current studies to support or refute whirlpool as a standard recommendation for cleansing venous ulcers.

Dressings chosen for specific wounds depend on the condition of the wound bed and the goal for the wound. Many new dressings are designed to support moist wound healing. (See chapter 9, Wound treatment options.) Because the skin is fragile in patients with either arterial or venous disease and can be easily injured, tape and adhesive products should be used with extreme caution. Use other methods of securing dressings that

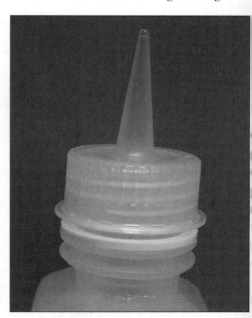

Figure 14-1. Baxter cap. (Photo courtesy M.J. Geyer.)

won't injure the skin. A *Cochrane* review on leg ulcer dressings found that the type of dressing material placed under compression had no influence on healing rates.[47,48] Other studies found no advantages with the use of either silver-impregnated[49] or honey-impregnated[50] dressings.

> ### PRACTICE POINT
>
> The preferred attachment device for dressings on vascular leg ulcers is roller gauze, or commercial devices (such as netting or tube gauze) that hold dressings in place without adhesive, which can damage fragile skin.

Compression

Venous hypertension and wounds are treated together. Wound care and edema management depend on whether or not the patient can be immobilized. Edema is controlled by conservative means, intermittent elevation, compression bandages, and intermittent pneumatic compression.[51] Studies have demonstrated that moist wound healing combined with compression improves wound-healing rate of venous ulcers.[52] Compression therapy is the mainstay of venous ulcer therapy.[53] Elevating the legs above the heart is recommended whenever the patient can be placed in this position. A compression dressing isn't required when the patient is immobilized with the leg elevated, such as during sleeping hours. Moist gauze dressings with frequent changes can be used instead.

Compression is the application of pressure to the limb. It is measured in millimeters of mercury (mm Hg) and is applied by bandages, elastic stockings, and/or intermittent pneumatic compression pumps. The amount of compression prescribed is determined by the diagnosis, comorbid conditions, and the patient's ability or willingness to accept the treatment. The following standard pressure classification[54] is suggested: mild (<20 mm Hg), moderate (21-40 mm Hg), strong (41-60 mm Hg), or very strong (≥61 mm Hg). Compression strength of 30 to 40 mm Hg is recommended to counteract the capillary filling pressures within the leg;

however, elderly or frail individuals or those who have difficulty donning the stockings may have compression ordered at 20 to 30 mm Hg. Many factors affect bandage pressure, including the bandage itself, the calf muscle and foot pump function, the shape of the leg, and the skill of the person applying the bandage.

The ambulatory venous patient is best served by semirigid dressings, such as the Unna boot, or by multi-component system compression wraps. Multi-component compression is more effective than single-component compression; both four-layer and short-stretch bandages have higher healing rates than paste plus an outer support (Unna boot). With the discovery of moist wound healing[55] and the advent of hydrocolloid and foam dressings, occlusive dressings may be used under compression wraps to promote growth of granulation tissue, reduce pain from the dressing rubbing against the ulcer, and promote autolytic debridement. One study found that ulcers treated with the foam dressing under the Unna boot healed twice as fast as ulcers treated without the foam.[56]

Bandages may be made of different materials, including elastic and inelastic materials or both. Stiff bandages are made of multiple layers of elastic or inelastic material. This type of bandage remains rigid and generates high pressure during exercise, which reduces venous hypertension.

Elastic bandages are considered long stretch and capable of stretching to double their size. Because these dressings can be stretched too tight, they are not recommended as a primary dressing for compression.[57]

Inelastic bandages are nonstretch bandages, short-stretch bandages, and zinc paste bandages. The resting pressure under inelastic bandages decreases over a 24-hour period, but the working pressure (with muscle movement) decreases less.

Compression wraps should be applied starting just below the toes and ending just below (two finger breadths) the popliteal fossa. A gauze roll or padded gauze dressing is typically placed over the wound area, and the dressing is covered with an elastic bandage. If the leg is misshapen, padding the leg to create symmetry facilitates a better bandage fit. Extra padding around bony prominences reduces the possibility of

Compression wrapping

This photograph shows a leg being wrapped with a four-layer compression therapy dressing.

creating a pressure ulcer. The concave area around the lateral and medial malleoli may need extra padding to ensure sufficient pressure is applied to those areas. Training should be ongoing to avoid complications associated with the application of compression wraps, such as ineffective pressure, pressure ulcers, bandage slippage, and limb distortion.[57] (See *Compression wrapping*.)

Complications from compression include pain, damage to skin and subcutaneous tissue from pressure, reduction of calf muscle, and skin problems. Interventions include carefully assessing to determine the cause of pain, avoiding excessive pressure under the dressing, encouraging exercise, and avoiding topical products that might cause allergies or irritations.[57]

Stockings reduce ambulatory venous pressure by decreasing venous reflux and improving calf muscle ejection capacity during use.[58] The benefit derived from stockings is in direct proportion to the fit.

In many cases, patients fail to wear the prescribed compression dressing or stocking because of difficulty donning the stockings or complaints of tightness. The importance of long-term external compression can't be overemphasized. Patients should be taught that the stockings must be replaced every 3 to 6 months. Two pairs should be purchased so that one can be worn while the other is laundered.

PRACTICE POINT

Long-term compression therapy is an essential part of the treatment of venous leg ulcers.

A pneumatic compression pump may be used to reduce lower-extremity edema. One study found improved venous ulcer healing when compression pumps were used; however, not all third-party payers agree with the use of these pumps for treatment.[59–62] Another study[63] found 4 hours of pump compression per day improved ulcer healing when used in conjunction with compression stockings. In yet another study,[64] an intermittent pneumatic compression device provided improved healing when used for 1 hour twice weekly in conjunction with conventional dressings. Patients who are immobile, are unable to tolerate bandages, have arterial insufficiency, or have problems with edema may benefit from intermittent pneumatic compression.[64]

Assessment of treatment

If a venous ulcer does not show signs of healing, the patient should be assessed for other comorbidities. Diabetes, heart failure, arterial insufficiency, venous reflux or history of venous thrombosis, fibrin on the wound surface, superficial colonization of bacteria, or infection all can slow healing.[65,66]

EXERCISE

A graded exercise program may be used to improve the calf muscle pump in those patients with abnormalities in pump function. One author[64] determined that a structured exercise program to improve muscle function may have a significant positive outcome in patients with venous disease.[67]

Effective edema removal from the leg reverses much of the associated comorbidity, particularly the skin changes. The achieved limb reduction must be maintained through the use of appropriately fitted compression hosiery or alternative compression product. The application and removal of such hosiery can be problematic in those with limited hand function or who are unable to see or reach their toes (obese, blind, arthritic, etc.). However, application aids are available and instruction in technique does help. Other strap-type leggings and boot-like devices[40] are available to decrease the functional burden. Therapists can be very creative in combining or layering different compressive products to achieve adequate levels of compression. Compliance is crucial to prevent recurrence of edema.

Surgical treatment for venous ulcers

Surgical treatment for venous ulcers is aimed at correcting the cause of the venous hypertension. Patients can have venous reflux without the symptoms of insufficiency. It is when reflux is severe enough that the insufficiency results in dermal venous hypertension and the eventual skin changes with which patients present. Procedures aimed at correcting insufficiency of the deep venous system include vein valve transplantation, direct valve repair, and veno-venous bypass. Outflow obstruction of a limb is addressed with veno-venous bypass, endovascular intervention, or a combination of the two. Varicose veins, the manifestation of superficial venous insufficiency, generally require ablation. Their treatment is usually by excision, ligation, injection, or the more recent method of endovenous ablation, depending on the size of the vein.

Surgical treatment for venous insufficiency remains far behind the more established treatment of arterial occlusive disease. Venous insufficiency can be grouped under two broad categories:

- venous reflux
- venous outflow obstruction.

The net result of both of these disease entities is venous hypertension and the sequelae resulting in dermal injury that ultimately ends with venous ulcerations. The mainstay for the treatment of venous insufficiency continues to be good external compression. In many patients, this is all that is required. Compression acts both as treatment for various states of venous insufficiency as well as prophylaxis for the development of the adverse sequelae. In some patients, the use of compression alone is inadequate; for these patients, surgical intervention is usually necessary.

Venous outflow obstruction is usually the result of DVT; however, other causes include obstruction from surgical excision of outflow vessels, tumor encasement of venous return, radiation-induced fibrosis, congenital atresia, injection-induced venous destruction (illicit or otherwise), obesity with immobility, and infection. When it involves isolated segments with normal segments proximal and distal, the obstruction can result in a cascading event resulting in venous insufficiency. In some patients, the outflow obstruction is the cause of the symptoms. In these patients it may be necessary to relieve the venous outflow obstruction and the corresponding venous hypertension by bypassing the obstructed segment, by balloon angioplasty of a sclerotic or stenotic segment with or without stent placement or, if the DVT is not chronic, by either open venous thrombectomy or mechanical thrombectomy.

Endovascular treatment of iliac vein obstruction is now possible on a routine basis. The morphology of this outflow obstruction and the measures to best treat it are ideally evaluated with the use of intravascular ultrasound (IVUS).[68] Although there is an early reocclusion rate of around 35% at 3 months, subsequent ulcer recurrence-free rates of almost 60% exist out to 5 years.[69] Early thrombosis and in-stent stenosis remain the most common causes of these early failures.

For years, obstruction from DVT has been approached in Europe with open venous thrombectomy, but this technique has never caught on in the United States. Mechanical thrombectomy via percutaneous routes is a focus of current interest. Two devices currently popular are Trellis drug dispersion and thrombectomy catheter (Bacchus, Santa Clara, CA),[70,71] and the AngioJet (Possis Medical, Minneapolis, MN).[72,73] Each uses a unique method of clot destruction and aspiration combined with lytic therapy. Trellis traps the thrombus between two balloons and emulsifies it with a rheolytic agent and oscillating wire. Once the clot is emulsified it is aspirated from between the two balloons. The AngioJet uses lytics and a high-velocity jet of liquid to fragment and then rapidly aspirate the thrombus fragments back into the catheter. Both methods are effective, with Trellis being quicker and AngioJet gentler on the vessel's intima. Whether these devices will have good long-term results is still in debate. Post-treatment patients need to be on warfarin.

Patients who require bypass are best served using an autogenous venous conduit. The proximal and distal anastomoses of the venous bypass are dictated by the obstruction site. For example, if a patient has an isolated iliofemoral thrombosis that has failed to recannulize or has only partially recannulized and the affected leg is symptomatic, a femoral-femoral bypass from the proximal portion of the symptomatic leg to the more distal portion of the contralateral leg can be performed. The saphenous vein is usually used for this, but in contrast to arterial bypasses the direction of the valve isn't reversed; rather the valve leaflets are oriented to prevent reflux. Similarly, a bypass from a more proximal vein within a symptomatic leg to the more cephalad iliac vein may be indicated.[74]

In patients with an outflow obstruction, but in whom insufficiency or hypertension is caused by occlusion of the greater saphenous vein, the venous hypertension may be alleviated by isolated partial saphenous vein ligation and stripping. This is usually done at the knee level with stripping of the affected saphenous segment. If, however, the reflux or hypertension is the result of the deep venous system, then stripping the greater saphenous vein wouldn't help and actually may be detrimental due to elimination of one of the venous outflow tracts of the extremity. This information must be known before a surgical procedure is performed to correct venous insufficiency. Three tests are available to evaluate reflux:

- ascending/descending venography
- duplex imaging
- venous PPG with sequential tourniquet placement.

These tests are all readily available through either an accredited vascular laboratory or a radiology department with experience in venous testing. Venous PPG can determine whether the deep or superficial system is involved with venous reflux. It is an excellent assessment of overall limb reflux and helps assess for perforator incompetence. Venous duplex, which interrogates specific segments of both the superficial and deep veins for reflux, gives a more detailed anatomic evaluation of the affected extremity. Both are needed to properly evaluate a patient with venous disease. Isolated valve segments of the more proximal venous system can be evaluated using descending venography looking for contrast reflux past the incompetent valve. Venography and venous duplex imaging can also determine sites of stenoses within the venous system. One of the problems associated with accurate duplex imaging is that it's dependent upon the competence of the technician performing the test.

Certain laboratories have more expertise in these areas than do others. This notwithstanding, duplex imaging has largely replaced venography in evaluating patients with venous disease. Venography is still used if surgical bypass and/or valvular surgery is planned.

When deep venous insufficiency is due to valvular incompetence, it isn't known how many competent valves are required and in what locations for the deep venous system to become competent again. Research in these areas is still ongoing as more attention is given to venous insufficiency.[75]

Three techniques are available for surgical correction of venous insufficiency due to valvular incompetence:

- artificial venous valve insertion
- autogenous vein valve transplantation using a segment of vein, usually from the upper extremities or axilla
- direct valvuloplasty.

Autogenous valve transplantation is a procedure in which a segment of vein with a competent valve, usually from the upper extremity or axilla, is identified. This section of vein is resected and an interposition graft placed at the harvest site. The vein is then transposed into the venous system of the affected extremity, maintaining the orientation of the valve to keep the leaflets open in a cephalic direction. Postoperative anticoagulation with heparin and subsequently warfarin is commonly used.

Approximately 75% of the stasis ulcers remain healed 12 months after valve transplantation.[76] However, considerable degradation occurred over the course of the second year in these patients, such that only 40% of limbs remain healed.[76] After the second year, results appear to stabilize without further deterioration although the reports on this are limited in both scope and number.[76]

Variations of this procedure using valve segments from other areas or even transposing a deep vein with a competent valve with another deep vein with an incompetent valve can be done. In Ko et al.'s study, the overall results with this method appeared to be similar to that of transposition of competent vein valve segments.[76]

Direct valvuloplasty is another technique for correcting valvular insufficiency. This is performed by suture approximation of two valve leaflets that don't fully close. It's done either with direct suturing within the areas of the cusps to obtain good apposition or by external buttressing of an incompetent vein valve sinus. Valve leaflets themselves are brought into apposition by placing the equivalent of a "girdle" around the dilated valve to reduce dilation and allow the valves to come in apposition in a more normal fashion. This sleeve technique is usually done with prosthetic material. Similarly, a transplanted valve that may deteriorate due to dilation can be made competent again by using this technique.[83]

An external valve repair known as the *Psathakis Silastic sling procedure* has been developed.[84] This procedure involves placing a Silastic sling around the popliteal vein and then attaching it to the two heads of the biceps femoris muscle. When these muscles contract, the sling is intended to occlude the popliteal vein during ambulation. The problem with this procedure is that the sling becomes intimately adherent to the vein and surrounding tissue and over time no longer functions in this fashion.

Two fairly recent publications on neovalve construction and valvular repair highlight the various techniques employed to restore venous competency of the deep system and their outcomes.[79,80] These are technically challenging operations that are not widely available. When successful, ulcer healing rates exceed 88%.

In patients in whom no suitable vein valve segment can be found or it's deemed an inadequate operation, the development and implantation of a prosthetic valve holds some promise. Currently, a prosthetic venous valve comprised of a complex titanium double-leaflet system is being developed and may hold promise.

The appropriate use of adequate compression is necessary in conjunction with all the surgical treatments. The application of compression hose and management of these patients are addressed elsewhere within this chapter.

Patients with recurrent leg ulcers due to incompetent perforators (Fig. 14-2) in the affected area were thought to benefit from a Linton flap. This august procedure requires

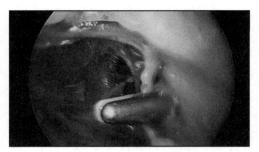

Figure 14-2. Incompetent vein.

elevation of the skin and fascia at the site of ulceration and transection with ligation of the incompetent perforator veins feeding the area. Proper application of compression is required afterward to reduce local venous hypertension. The morbidity associated with this procedure includes tissue slough along the area of incision and the overlying tissue, resulting in a prolonged healing period. This is thought to be due to the chronic disease state of the tissue at the ankle.

A subfascial ligation of incompetent perforator veins with an endoscope (SEPS) is a significant advancement in the Linton technique. Using equipment developed for laparoscopic cholecystectomies, the scope is passed from the medial infrageniculate area into the subfascial space. The fascia is raised, often with CO_2 insufflation. The perforator veins are ligated and transected through the endoscope. Advances in technology, such as smaller-diameter scopes (5 to 10 mm), high-resolution camera and LCD screens, and single-step electrocautery/transection, have made this procedure much easier to perform. The smaller-diameter endoscopes allow easy peri-malleolar inspection for perforators. This entire procedure routinely takes less than an hour to perform and in select patients can be done on an outpatient basis. The reason for ligating incompetent perforators is to eliminate the venous hypertension associated with the reflux of venous blood.[79] In a meta-analysis by Tenbrook et al., ulcers treated by SEPS with or without additional venous ablation healed in 88% of patients.[81,82]

There has been some interest in duplex ultrasound–guided foam sclerotherapy, which scleroses the perforator veins to achieve the same effect.[83,84] While this treatment is used extensively in Europe, it's not yet approved in the United States.[85] Further studies are needed to establish the overall effectiveness of this procedure for wound healing.

The use of endovenous ablation has really become widespread in the United States, supplanting traditional vein stripping. In most places, endovenous ablation is an outpatient office-based procedure. It involves ultrasound-guided cannulation of the distal saphenous vein, either lesser or greater, with a catheter whose tip is positioned 2 cm distal to the sapheno-femoral junction. The length of the vein is surrounded with tumescent anesthesia usually consisting of a dilute buffered lidocaine solution (usually 300 to 500 ml). This acts as a heat trap for the delivered energy, which destroys the vein wall and coagulates the blood within. The energy delivered is either in the form of a laser (endovenous laser therapy, EVLT) or radiofrequency (RF). Proponents of both forms claim superiority. The end result, if successful, is controlled thrombosis and destruction of the vein and thereby prevention of reflux through it. U.S. data show 99.6% successful occlusion initially,[86] falling to 86% to 89% at 4 years.[87] Devices of both types exist that can be used to directly ablate incompetent perforators under ultrasound guidance. However, neither of these devices is as easy to use as the main units.

RF and EVLT are quick procedures, routinely taking far less than 1 hour to perform. The patients generally do very well, and the procedures are well tolerated. The patient avoids a hospital stay and the need for a major anesthetic. Endovenous ablation has been widely accepted as a tool for the patient seeking removal of mostly asymptomatic varicosities but, when appropriately applied, the procedure can correct isolated saphenous reflux disease. While the procedure has a low complication rate, it has two major drawbacks that open vein stripping does not: usually leaves behind a distal segment of vein, and recannulation can occur. Some centers have combined endovenous ablation with a subsequent limited distal stripping or microphlebectomy, if needed. Depending on how extensive the condition, either of these procedures could be office based.

In some patients, the application of a split-thickness skin graft to an otherwise healthy stasis ulcer may be appropriate. This technique shouldn't be used in patients whose underlying venous problems haven't been addressed. The application of a split-thickness skin graft to an ulcer with persistent venous hypertension will fail, even if the patient is compliant with the use of a compression garment.

Options other than split-thickness grafting involve the use of bioengineered human dermal substitutes. These are intended to be used as carriers of human growth stimulants and to provide a scaffold upon which the patient's own dermis can regenerate, either spontaneously or with the use of a delayed thin skin graft. Dermal substitutes are not inexpensive however, and the underlying venous issue as well as the wound bed must still be addressed. Although skin substitutes appear to hasten wound closure, recurrence rates are high.[88]

Modern venous surgery now has in its armamentarium a wider array of treatment options for those patients with venous disease. As this area of vascular surgery matures, better paradigms for patient treatment are emerging.[89] No longer is it just an Unna boot and vein stripping.

SUMMARY

Chronic venous insufficiency is a permanent condition. Because of this, patients are given information about the disease process and rationale for intervention. The more information they have, the more likely they are to manage the condition effectively. Activities that promote venous return are encouraged. Extremity elevation should become a daily routine, and external compression is needed for life. Patients must understand the importance of this fact. Protection from skin trauma is essential. A small lesion may progress quickly to a large ulcer because of the edema. It may take years to heal, if at all. Small cuts or bruises should receive immediate medical attention. Leg exercises to increase muscle pump activity are taught to the patient. Patients are encouraged to use these exercises during long periods of standing or sitting. When sitting, the legs should be elevated.

Success in managing venous ulcers requires a total patient commitment. Risk factors and ulcer management are dependent upon the patient's activities; therefore, the patient must have as much information as possible to participate in therapy. An understanding of venous pathophysiology and its contribution to leg ulcers is critical in managing the ulcers. Venous reconstruction is in its infancy but shows promise to reduce the sequelae of postphlebitic syndrome. Venous ulcers always require external compression, ultimately in the form of compression stockings. Ulcers associated with lymphedema usually respond when the edema is reduced. A variety of wound care products are available for leg ulcers, but no research exists showing one product to be more effective than another. Economic concerns make it imperative to choose the appropriate dressings and treatment, but research demonstrates little increased benefit of the newer treatments over the old. Although surgical treatment for venous ulcer lags behind that for arterial occlusive disease, there are procedures that correct the insufficiency of the deep venous system. These are vein valve transplantation, direct valve repair, and veno-venous bypass.

PATIENT SCENARIO

Clinical Data

Mrs. MC is an 82-year-old woman who has had multiple recurrent superficial ulcers in the medial aspect of the left ankle region, presumably resulting from venous insufficiency. Some ulcers healed spontaneously, but more recently they required compression therapy at a wound center. The current episode was indolent for more than 8 months and has left Mrs. MC with macerated skin that cracks and weeps serous fluid (Fig. 14-3A). She recently moved in with her daughter but is quite independent. Although Mrs. MC is thin, her nutrition is adequate and she is compliant with leg elevation. She has worn proper compression hose in the past. She was referred to the Vascular Surgery Service for evaluation.

The left leg has no palpable pedal pulses, although Mrs. MC does not describe any claudication or rest pain. She has a remote history of limited smoking. Other than hypertension and the current left leg complaints, she is healthy. She underwent arterial and venous vascular lab evaluations consisting of arterial Doppler ultrasound, venous PPG, and venous duplex tests for reflux. Her ABIs were >0.95 bilaterally with triphasic waveforms. Venous refill times were markedly abnormal bilaterally, 12 seconds on the left and 15 seconds on the right. Tourniquet application indicated isolated greater saphenous vein (GSV) incompetence in both legs. Venous duplex testing revealed no DVTs, >0.5 seconds of reflux in the left proximal femoral vein and the entire left GSV. Reflux was also noted in the entire right GSV. Endovenous ablation of the left GSV was recommended.

Case Discussion

Mrs. MC's GSV incompetence on her symptomatic left side is most likely the cause of her recurrent venous ulcers and now chronic tissue and skin changes. Although there is reflux in the left proximal femoral vein, the GSV is the predominant source of her dermal venous hypertension. With ablation of this GSV and, once healed, wearing proper support hose, it is expected that her symptoms will improve and her ulcer heal. Because of her age and the desire to avoid both hospitalization and a major anesthetic, endovenous ablation with radiofrequency was the intervention of choice. This office-based procedure requires only local tumescent anesthesia.

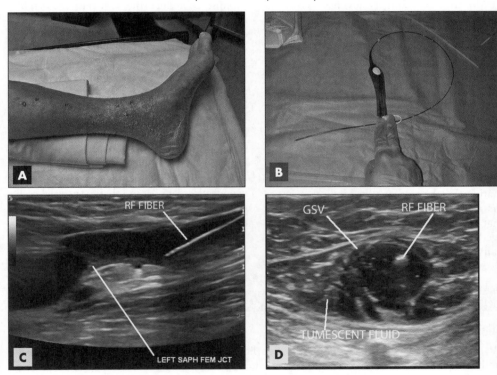

Figure 14-3. (A) Macerated skin due to multiple recurrent superficial ulcers in the medial aspect of the left ankle region. (B) Radiofrequency fiber. (C) Placement of the radiofrequency fiber approximately 2 cm distal to the junction of the common femoral vein. (D) Tumescent fluid infused around the GSV. (See *color section*, *Patient Scenarios*, page C44, for the color versions of A and B images.)

The radiofrequency fiber (Fig. 14-3B) was passed up the GSV after entry at the distal calf level via ultrasound guidance. After placement approximately 2 cm distal to the junction of the common femoral vein (Fig. 14-3C), tumescent infusion around the vein was performed (Fig. 14-3D). Several cycles of heat were applied as the fiber was sequentially pulled back. Once completed, the limb was compressed using thigh-high support hose of 30 to 40 mm Hg compression; support hose were worn for an initial 72 continuous hours followed by 7 additional days of non-sleep wear. The patient then returned for a series of duplex ultrasound tests to evaluate the ablation and to rule out DVT.

Mrs. MC is now doing well with well healed skin. This took an additional 2 months to achieve. She wears knee-high support hose of 30 to 40 mm Hg compression religiously on both limbs. The right leg remains asymptomatic.

LYMPHEDEMA

Caroline E. Fife, MD, CWS, Mary Y. Sieggreen, NP, CNS, APRN, CVN, and Ronald A. Kline, MD, FACS, FAHA

Edema (swelling) results when an increase in interstitial fluid volume occurs, representing an imbalance between capillary filtration and lymph drainage. *Lymphedema* represents a failure of lymphatic drainage.[1] This section examines the epidemiology of lymphedema as well as its mechanisms, manifestations, and management.

EPIDEMIOLOGY OF LYMPHEDEMA

As discussed by Logan[2] and Williams et al.,[3] the epidemiology of lymphedema has been difficult to ascertain due to a variety of issues in determining prevalence and incidence rates. Perhaps more importantly, lymphedema lacks a valid and consistent definition. This is due in part to the unavailability of a good diagnostic test and challenges in quantifying the severity of edema and the associated skin and tissue changes. For example, chronic lower-extremity edema (perhaps caused by heart failure or venous insufficiency) can mimic lymphedema. In this case, excess low-viscosity, protein-poor interstitial fluid resulting from increased capillary filtration accumulates in the subcutaneous tissue because a *normal* lymphatic system cannot handle the imposed load.

True "primary lymphedema" arises from congenital or developmental defects of the lymphatic system. Usually one limb is more severely affected, and the condition was once thought to be rare. "Secondary lymphedema," by contrast, is seen more frequently and is usually triggered in Western countries by lymph node dissection and perhaps irradiation treatment for cancer and in developing countries by parasitic infection. However, traumatic injury, chronic inflammation or infection, and other surgical interventions may also precipitate the condition. More recent evidence suggests that secondary lymphedema may be a subclinical form of primary lymphedema. Patients who develop lymphedema after surgery or trauma may have had marginal lymphatic function to begin with, which became dysfunctional due to injury or insult.

Left untreated, lymphedema in some patients can progress through several stages until it manifests as elephantiasis, a most disfiguring condition. Although lymphedema can be managed successfully with lifelong adherence to a maintenance protocol (manual lymph drainage, compression garments, skin care, and exercise) and psychosocial support, cure is not possible because the damaged lymphatic system cannot be repaired.

Globally, lymphedema resulting from filariasis (infection by the nematode *Wuchereria bancrofti*, which is carried by mosquitoes) affects nearly 119 million people or 2% of the world's population,[4] primarily in tropical areas of the world such as India, Africa, Haiti, and Malaysia. However, a discussion of filariatic lymphedema is beyond the scope of this chapter.

In Western countries, upper-extremity lymphedema due to complications resulting from breast cancer treatment is by far the most common presentation and is usually associated with surgery and/or irradiation of the lymph nodes. Risk factors identified for breast cancer–related lymphedema include irradiation, the extent of axillary node dissection, combined axillary dissection and irradiation, obesity, surgical wound infection, tumor stage, and extent of surgery.[3,5–7] Although surgical improvements have been made during the past few decades, the incidence of secondary lymphedema remains at about 30%, although the data may also reflect improved detection of the condition.[3,7] Cancer-related lymphedema in the lower extremity is less prevalent. Studies have demonstrated that the incidence of lower-extremity lymphedema is dependent on the location of the cancer; for example, the incidences are 40% and 55% following groin or ilioinguinal dissection, respectively, but 6% to 11% following combined pelvic and lymph node dissection for stage III melanoma.[8–10] Risk factors for development of this type of lymphedema include tumor location and factors similar to those identified for breast cancer–related lymphedema.

Although clinicians now understand the relationship between breast cancer treatment and lymphedema, they are less likely to be aware that chronic inflammation and ulceration have the potential to damage the lymphatic system.[11–14] Chronic venous disease, trauma, recurrent infection, and arthritis may contribute to lower-extremity lymphedema, yet many clinicians may not appreciate these conditions as causative agents.[2,11,15] Increasingly, obesity is a contributing factor; although the mechanism remains unclear, it is likely due in part to increasing venous insufficiency among the morbidly obese, exacerbated by immobility and volume overload. Clinicians may not be able to differentiate between lymphedema and lipedema, a condition involving abnormal fat distribution, typically around the legs or hips. Unfortunately, if lymphatic insufficiency is not recognized, ineffective treatment and increased morbidity are likely to ensue.

A UK study addressed some of the aforementioned epidemiological issues by using a broader operational definition of chronic edema/lymphedema and setting specific clinical criteria to identify cases.[12,16] These criteria included persistent edema lasting longer than 3 months, little

or no response to overnight elevation or diuretics, and the presence of skin changes (primarily thickened skin, hyperkeratosis, and papillomatosis). Individuals with congestive heart failure, hypoalbuminemia, or nephrotic syndrome were excluded from the study as these systemic disorders were likely the cause of the edema. The population included only those individuals known to, or being treated by, health professionals. While the study authors acknowledged that their broad definition of chronic edema/lymphedema made it likely that cases with mixed etiologies would be included, they argued that chronic edema thus identified represented some form of lymphatic insufficiency because a functional lymphatic system ought to be able to compensate for an increase in capillary filtration by increasing lymph drainage.[12,16]

A crude prevalence of 0.13% was reported in the study, with age-related increases reaching 0.54% for those older than 65 years and 1.0% for those over age 85.[17] Although these figures translate into some 100,000 cases of chronic edema/lymphedema in the United Kingdom or 395,000 in the United States based on current population estimates, it is doubtful that all patients were receiving treatment during the study period, and thus the prevalence estimates are likely to be on the conservative side. In a Norwegian study, Petlund reported a crude prevalence of 0.144% for chronic edema, which buttresses the UK figures.[18] Other important findings from the UK study illustrated the impact of the condition on patients' lives. For example, almost one-third of the study participants suffered an acute infection in the preceding year, and a quarter of these patients required hospitalization. The condition was also responsible for sick leave in 80% of individuals and a change in employment status in 9%. Moreover, while it is often reported in the literature that lymphedema is not painful, half of the patients indicated that they experienced pain or discomfort with the edema. These issues were also reflected by low scores in many domains of the well-validated SF-36 questionnaire, suggesting a poor quality of life.[17] In summary, chronic edema/lymphedema seems to be a frequently unrecognized complaint associated with significant morbidity and appears with a frequency equal to that of leg ulcers.

LYMPHATIC SYSTEM

Compared with the vascular systems in the leg, the lymphatic system is the least understood and its embryologic development remains relatively unknown. Lymphatic vessels are divided into three categories:

- Initial or terminal lymphatic capillaries
- Collecting vessels
- Lymph nodes.

Terminal lymphatic capillaries originate in the superficial layer of the dermis and have no valves. These lymphatic capillaries drain into the deep dermal and subdermal system, which is the level at which valved lymphatic vessels can be observed (pre-collectors), and vessels ascend the leg into lymph nodes at the popliteal fossa and the inguinal ligament. Generally, the lymphatic system parallels the larger veins of the proximal leg above the knee, with valves operating in much the same way as venous valves. The lymphatic system then drains though the iliac lymph nodes above the inguinal ligament level, eventually coalescing into the periaortic nodes, the cisterna chyli, and thoracic duct, which ascends along the thoracic aorta on the right side of the chest and empties into the left jugular vein slightly above the jugulo-subclavian junction. While the thoracic duct is considered the main terminus of the lymphatic system, some patients have an accessory right lymphatic duct that drains into the right jugular venous system.

Lymphatic vessels are much smaller than major arteries or veins—between one-seventh and one-tenth the size—because fluid flow is less. In terms of vessel anatomy, the outer adventitial layer is much thinner although the media contains some elastin fibers and smooth muscle striae, the latter being used to propel the lymphatic flow cephalad through contraction. The intimal layer consists of a single layer of endothelium.

Aspects of lymphatic flow

Lymphatic flow is a consequence of three factors: capillary blood pressure, osmotic pressure, and interstitial fluid pressure (hydrostatic). The intrinsic contractility of the lymphatic vessel wall, coupled with the action of muscular pumps such as the calf, which aids flow in the same way as for the venous system, creates a suction force distal to the major lymph vessels. In addition, the action of deep breathing, which creates a positive abdominal pressure and a negative thoracic pressure, also increases the cephalic lymph flow.

Because capillary cell walls are "leaky," acellular interstitial fluid containing protein and white blood cells accumulates, and thus the lymphatic system provides a means for drainage of this fluid as well as a mechanism for the return of white blood cells to the vasculature. A normal lymphatic system with intact functional architecture is required for unimpaired lymph circulation. Lymphedema results when disruption or injury occurs to the lymphatic system at a local level because interstitial fluid is no longer being drained adequately.

The lymphatic system can be considered a one-way transportation system that prevents the body from drowning in its own fluid. However, besides maintaining interstitial tissue fluid balance (volume and pressure), the lymphatic system also performs other key functions. Composed of a tree-like hierarchical network of vessels and organs, including the spleen, thymus, tonsils, bone marrow, and numerous lymph nodes, the lymphatic system biologically filters lymph at the nodes using macrophages and lymphocytes. The lymphatic organs and nodes also provide a means for lymphocyte maturation and transportation that is crucial to immune function; lymphocytes include natural killer cells involved in the innate immune system, whereas T-cells and B-cells are associated with the adaptive immune response.[12,19–21] In addition, the lymphatic system plays a role in certain kinds of fat absorption. Thus, when portions of the lymphatic system are injured, the local response to inflammation or infection likewise becomes disrupted by disturbing cytokine (growth factor) and cellular circulation in the affected area.[11] In other words, the lymphedematous extremities develop fatty deposits in response to chronic edema and the swollen limb really does become "fatter." For the purpose of this chapter, only the structures and mechanisms specific to lymphatic circulation of the lower limb are discussed.

While the anatomy of the lymphatic system mirrors that of the venous system in terms of general structure and function, there are distinct differences in that the lymphatic system has lymph nodes and the vessels are thinner and have more valves than their venous counterparts. Although little is known concerning the embryology of the lymphatic system, its development proceeds on a parallel with the venous system starting with origination in lymph sacs (for example, the jugular, iliac, retroperitoneal, and cisterna chyli sacs). Its venous origin has also been supported by recent work that demonstrates the presence of tyrosine kinase 4, a gene specific to both venous and lymphatic but not arterial endothelia early in the development process that ultimately becomes expressed solely within lymphatic endothelia.[11,22,23]

Lower limb lymphatic anatomy

The lymphatic system is comprised of the small, non-contractile initial lymphatic vessels, also known as lymphatic capillaries, whose function is to absorb interstitial fluid, linked to the progressively larger contractile collector vessels. Lymphatic capillaries begin as blind-ended tubes only a single cell in thickness, but the cells are arranged in a slightly overlapping pattern similar to the shingles on a roof and are connected to surrounding tissue through anchoring filaments. The interstitial pressure forces the cells to separate periodically, which allows lymph to enter but not escape as the cell walls then close to reestablish their overlapping pattern. This process resembles a one-way valve system.[20,24,25] Pre-collector vessels linked to the capillaries possess segments with capillary-like walls, as well as valves, and merge into larger contractile vessels termed collectors or trunks, which have valves and intervalve segments called lymphangions. The function of these entities is to propel lymph forward cephalically via vessel wall smooth muscle contractions initiated by pacemaker cells or modulated through sympathetic activation.[24,25]

Akin to the venous system, the deep fascia divides the lymphatic system into deep/subfascial and superficial/suprafascial networks connected by perforating vessels. Superficial capillaries originate in the dermis and drain into subcutaneous collectors, which are organized into progressively larger bundles. The superficial system drains both the dermis and subcutaneous tissue. While skin areas emptied of interstitial fluid by one collector form topographical strips known as *skin zones* in which the lymph vessels freely communicate, skin zones associated with all the collectors from a lymph vessel bundle form distinct territories that are separated by watersheds in which few vessels communicate.[26]

PRACTICE POINT

The communication ties or anastomoses between lymphatic capillaries in different areas provide an anatomical basis for "manual lymph drainage," an important component of the therapeutic intervention for lymphedema. MLD consists of specific manual techniques designed to increase lymph flow and remove excess tissue fluid from the congested area of one watershed via the lymphatic capillaries to another whose drainage is intact.

PRACTICE POINT

Smooth muscle contraction in the lymphangions is dependent on the influx of calcium ions. Therefore, calcium channel blocking agents commonly used to treat high blood pressure can have a negative effect on lymphatic contractility that contributes to peripheral edema.[12]

Muscles, bones, and joints are drained by the deep subfascial collectors. However, although subfascial collectors share the same perivascular sheath construction as their venous and arterial counterparts, lymph is directed from the deep to the superficial lymphatic system, which is the opposite of the venous system in which blood drains from superficial veins through the perforating veins into the deep veins.[27]

Lymph flow in the leg

Plasma that has escaped from the capillary vasculature mixes with other interstitial materials (forming pre-lymph) and enters the lymphatic capillaries and pre-collectors in a passive process aided by rhythmic contractions of the lymphangions upstream, nearby muscular contractions and arterial pulsation, suction pressure due to breathing, and manual lymph drainage. The lymph then flows into serially larger collectors of which the more proximal are known as *trunks*. Distention of the trunk wall is the stimulus for lymphangion contraction, which provides the primary propulsion necessary for lymph flow and which occurs at a rate of 6 to 10 beats per minute. In essence, the lymphangions function like miniature hearts in linear sequence[11] that are also capable of cardiac-like inotropic and chronotropic responses.[11,19,27] Under normal conditions, lymph flow can increase by an order of magnitude when an increased filtrate volume is present with higher pre-lymph uptake and a faster rate of lymphangion contraction,[16] ensuring a large margin of capacity. In other words, healthy lymphatics, like the heart, can work harder when more fluid is present.

PRACTICE POINT

Exercise or passive movement induces alternating changes in the interstitial fluid pressure, which translates to improved lymphatic capillary filling. This effect can partially compensate for damaged collectors whose contractility has failed. Applying a bandage or other form of external compression enhances the effect of movement (muscle contraction), thus increasing lymph flow.

Lymph is propelled by afferent collectors in the leg and funnels through some 7 to 15 trunks via an anteromedial route that follows the course of the great saphenous vein where it is filtered in the nodes of the popliteal fossa and the inguinal ligament.[11,12] From the inguinal nodes, lymph is moved cephalad

through several iliac nodes before coalescing into peri-aortic nodes and trunks, from there into the cisterna chyli, and finally into the thoracic duct. The thoracic duct is located on the right side of chest and follows the thoracic aorta before draining into the left jugular vein just above the jugulo-subclavian junction. In some individuals, an accessory right lymphatic duct, which drains into the right jugular venous system, may also be present.

Cephalic (towards the head) lymph flow in the central region of the body is particularly assisted by breathing and local arterial pulsation. Although the thoracic duct is traditionally considered to be chief drainage route for lymph back into the venous system, other drainage methods exist, for example, lymphovenous communications within muscle compartments and on the periphery of the body. However, it is thought these do not typically play a role in lymph drainage unless chronic obstruction of lymph vessels or nodes is present.[28]

PRACTICE POINT

Exercise, deep breathing, and manual lymph drainage are all considered essential components in the treatment of chronic edema/lymphedema because they all increase lymph flow.

TISSUE EDEMA

Pathophysiology of edema in venous disease

Regardless of the etiology of edema, the immediate cause is always an imbalance between capillary filtration and lymph drainage. Consequently, an understanding of the forces associated with interstitial fluid balance can be helpful. Capillary filtration is easily illustrated using the Starling equation, which describes flow across a semi-permeable membrane. The net movement of fluid from the inside of a capillary to the interstitium, often referred to as the capillary filtration rate, is governed by the difference between the capillary and interstitial hydrostatic pressures and the difference between the capillary and interstitial osmotic pressures. (Osmotic pressure is the force derived from the attraction of water to large-molecular-weight entities.)

Net filtration is also influenced by the permeability of the capillary wall to water, to small proteins that can exert an osmotic (or oncotic) effect, and to the surface area available for filtration. Under normal conditions, the Starling equation correctly predicts a net filtration rate, and the volume of interstitial fluid that is added over a period of time is also removed. In other words, the amount of fluid in the tissue remains stable. Otherwise, accumulation of fluid in the tissue spaces would result. For many years it was thought that reabsorption of the capillary filtrate was achieved primarily by venous capillaries, but more recent evidence from 12 types of tissue suggests that it is the lymphatic system that takes the major role of fluid uptake.[12,29,30] In other words, the lymphatics may be responsible for the majority of fluid returning to the heart. The lymphatic system returns 2 to 4 L of fluid containing approximately 240 g of protein back to the circulation, so it can be readily appreciated that without the lymphatic system, cardiovascular collapse would quickly occur, not to mention a life-threatening shortage of protein.

EDEMA DUE TO INCREASED FILTRATION

The most common form of edema, known as *high-volume lymphatic insufficiency*, develops when the capillary filtration rate exceeds lymph drainage capacity over a period of time. This is analogous to what happens when a municipal drainage system that, although it is still working, becomes overwhelmed by heavy rain, resulting in flooding. In this example, a high volume of fluid can overwhelm the capacity of the drainage system. Typically, increases in capillary filtration are the consequence of increased capillary pressure due to venous hypertension, heart failure, or fluid overload. However, reduced plasma osmotic pressure is another cause of increased capillary pressure.

In other words, fluid leaves the vasculature for the interstitium because osmolality in the interstitium is higher than in the blood vessels. This can be due to hypoalbuminemia, perhaps from nephrotic syndrome or liver failure. In addition, an increased capillary permeability to water and small proteins can occur. Inflammation may cause this increased capillary permeability; it may also increase blood flow, which further increases capillary pressure and capillary filtration rate. Thus, venous disease is associated with at least two potential causes of high-volume lymphatic insufficiency (increased capillary pressure and interstitial inflammation), and in cases in which the lymphatic system deteriorates, lymphedema may result.[21]

EDEMA DUE TO REDUCED LYMPHATIC TRANSPORT

The swelling present in lymphedema can also be caused by a gross mechanical failure of the lymphatic system to accommodate even a *normal* load of capillary filtrate.[26] This condition is also known as *low-volume lymphatic insufficiency*. This situation is analogous to the flooding that would occur from a small amount of rain if the municipal drains become blocked. The lymphatic failure can result from lymphatic capillaries and pre-collectors becoming unable to absorb capillary filtrate or from a dysfunction upstream that prevents conduction or filtering of a normal load.

MECHANISMS LIMITING EDEMA FORMATION

Because venous disease induces capillary hypertension and therefore increased capillary filtration, edema must result. Nevertheless, there are several mechanisms by which the edema can be limited. These mechanisms, which form the physiological basis for treatment, include:

- Increased interstitial pressure due to increased stiffness of the skin and soft tissues
- A reduction in the interstitial osmotic pressure
- Increased lymph flow
- Postural vasoconstriction in a dependent leg via the veni-arteriolar reflex
- Activation of the calf muscle pump.

INCREASED INTERSTITIAL FLUID PRESSURE

The ability of a tissue to resist swelling is directly related to its compliance—an inverse measure of its stiffness. Muscle or fibrotic tissue containing collagen or other extracellular matrix fibers resists swelling because a small increase in interstitial fluid volume results in a large increase in interstitial pressure, which opposes the capillary filtration force. Conversely, because compliant tissue (such as the skin of the eyelid) has elastic properties, it can accommodate a much higher volume of fluid before the interstitial pressure rises sufficiently to oppose filtration.

The venous-arteriolar reflex that generates vasoconstriction in a dependent leg also acts to oppose filtration by decreasing capillary pressure.

REDUCED INTERSTITIAL OSMOTIC PRESSURE

When the capillary filtration rate increases, the local interstitial protein concentration is reduced, particularly if the pre-lymph removal rate does not increase, and the plasma protein concentration is increased. The combined effects tend to decrease the interstitial osmotic pressure and increase the capillary osmotic pressure with the result that further increases in capillary filtration rate are resisted. This feedback mechanism is of major importance in protection against both pulmonary and peripheral edema.

> ### ▶ PRACTICE POINT
>
> Using a bandage or non-compliant compression stocking on the leg increases tissue stiffness, thereby increasing interstitial pressure, opposing filtration, and consequently reducing edema formation or preventing its re-accumulation. A short-stretch bandage will generate high interstitial pressure during muscle contraction, enhancing venous and lymphatic flow, but will conversely exert low pressure during muscle relaxation, allowing lymph vessels to refill.

INCREASED LYMPH FLOW

Increased capillary filtration is a consequence of the elevated venous pressure found in venous disease. In addition to the previously mentioned osmotic effects opposing filtration, the higher level of filtrate entering the lymphatic capillaries stimulates more forceful lymphangion contraction cephalad, and thus the lymph transportation rate is increased to match the load. The ability to dramatically increase transport capacity in response to increased lymphatic load is also known as the *lymphatic safety valve function* and is an important mechanism preventing edema formation. Other factors that limit edema formation include local pressure changes in tissues and capillaries induced by movement in active or passive exercise, manual lymph drainage, arterial pulsation and, in more central tissues, breathing. Activation of the calf muscle pump not only decreases venous pressure but also enhances lymph flow.

> ### ▶ PRACTICE POINT
>
> Bandaging and stockings enhance the pumping effect of exercise by providing a "shell" against which the foot and calf muscles can compress during contraction. Higher evacuation of venous blood leads to a decrease in venous capillary pressure and filtration. Intermittent changes in tissue pressure from walking and other rhythmic exercise increase lymphatic capillary filling and lymphangion contractility thereby increasing lymph flow.[30,31]

When venous disease is not attended by edema, this means that the previously mentioned mechanisms are compensating satisfactorily. On the other hand, the presence of edema with venous disease indicates that either the compensatory mechanisms are inadequate or that the capillary filtration rate greatly exceeds the forces that oppose it. The foremost contributory factor in the latter case is likely to be inflammation, which may advance along the perivascular perforating sheath or spread between divisions.[11,27,31]

LYMPHATIC FAILURE IN VENOUS DISEASE

Lymph flow increases during the early stages of venous disease but becomes compromised in later stages when lipodermatosclerosis and/or venous ulcers are present. Obese patients have many issues that contribute to lower-extremity lymphedema, including increased capillary filtration, decreased calf muscle pumping (due to decreased activity), and long periods of dependency (particularly in patients with sleep apnea who may be unable to sleep supine). There may be genetic factors that predispose to both obesity and lymphedema.

Many theories have been proposed to explain the generation of venous ulcers and, similarly, several ideas have been advanced to explain the development of lymphedema during chronic venous disease. One of the most intriguing concepts has been that patients who develop secondary lymphedema have already acquired subclinical manifestations of the condition from birth due to genetic defects; other patients may have fewer lymphatic vessels or vessels that have been damaged over a period of time from various causes. In one study of venous ulcers, light and electron microscopy demonstrated that superficial fibrin and inflammatory cell layers and the intermediate blood capillary layer of the ulcer bed did not contain lymphatics.[32] In addition, only a few lymphatic capillaries were present in the transition zone from granulation tissue to the deeper collagenous scar layer of the ulcer. These observations suggest greatly lowered fluid reabsorption and lymph flow in the affected area.[32] Fluorescent microlymphography studies have also observed a greatly diminished superficial lymphatic network with accompanying dilation of other lymphatics, as well as increases in permeability.[33–36] In post-thrombotic syndrome, lymphoscintigraphy showed that subfascial lymphatic drainage was substantially impaired,[37] and the same technique demonstrated that lymphatic function was reduced in legs exhibiting venous ulcers compared with legs that had no ulcers.[38,39] It is theorized that obliteration of lymphatic vessels that results is loss of function probably develops through lymphangiothrombosis or lymphangitis in a similar fashion to that which occurs in veins, although it is likely to be a much slower process. In addition, lymphangions may become dysfunctional by losing their contractile ability, although whether this might be linked to valvular incompetence and therefore lymph reflux is not known. One technique still under development that may help to validate these theories is near-infrared fluorescent imaging, which employs fluorophores such as indocyanine green and is much more sensitive than radiotracers. The technique has recently been used in humans for lymph mapping in breast cancer patients, intraoperative guidance, and real-time functional imaging.[40]

In the later stages of venous disease, which involve tissue fibrosis, the stiffness of the tissues may mitigate edema or prevent edema from being detected easily; some controversy exists regarding whether this stage should be termed chronic lymphatic insufficiency rather than lymphedema.[41,42] However, the 2003 consensus document from the International Society of Lymphology defines lymphedema as an external (or internal) manifestation of lymphatic insufficiency and deranged lymph transport,[21] and thus lymphatic failure in later stages of venous disease would be included under this definition.

The broadest classification of lymphedema pathology defines whether it is obstructive or nonobliterative. Obstructive pathology results from any perilymphangitis etiology, whereas nonobliterative pathology can result from endolymphangitis proliferans, primary thoracic duct pathology, lymph node obstruction, congenital defects, or lymphatic thrombosis.

In the United States, tumors are the most common cause of lymph node obstruction, but primary thoracic duct disease can be congenital or surgically acquired. Endolymphangitis is typically a result of repeated intraluminal injury from many types of noxious agents that cause repeated injury. Whereas lymphangiectasis is a true atrophy of the lymphatic channel rather than a developmental problem, congenital factors, which usually cause a nonobliterative disorder, result in either agenesis or hypoplasia. One of the most common phenotypes of the nonobliterative disorder is Meige's disease, representing approximately 3% of all cases of lymphedema. Meige's disease primarily affects females; the age of onset is variable, although it typically occurs near puberty.[43]

Lymphatic thrombosis is another form of the nonobliterative disease sometimes encountered. Although anticoagulants are ineffective, the administration of benzopyrones such as coumarin (not to be confused with Coumadin) may be able to reduce the edema by stimulating macrophage activity, which increases degradation of protein in lymph fluid.[44,45]

CLASSIFYING LYMPHEDEMA

The oldest classification of lymphedema divided the condition into three categories: congenital, lymphedema precox, and lymphedema tarda. Congenital lymphedema is diagnosed at birth or shortly thereafter, while lymphedema precox is diagnosed between birth and the age of 35 years, although the majority of cases are found around puberty. The term lymphedema tarda is simply applied to a case in which onset occurs after the age of 35. The classification system in use today is based on whether the lymphedema is primary or secondary.

Primary lymphedema can be described as either hyperplastic/hypoplastic/aplastic or obstructive/nonobstructive. Obstructive pathologies are usually described according to anatomical location and divided into distal obliterative or pelvic obliterative. For example, about 10% of patients have primary hyperplastic lymphedema, which is classified as bilateral hyperplasia, sometimes with megalymphatics (large valveless lymphatic ducts similar to varicosities); bilateral hyperplasia is characterized by capillary angiomata on both the sides of the feet. An obstructive process is usually present at the level of the cisterna chyli or thoracic duct, and valves can be observed when examined. The patient may exhibit little or no leg edema, but chylous reflux is present.

Secondary lymphatic obstructions result from of a variety of causes, including tumors, surgical intervention, trauma, or infection. Infections can be bacterial or filarial. In developing countries, the most common cause of lymphatic obstruction is filarial infection by *W. bancrofti*. As discussed above, our understanding of secondary lymphedema is changing with the advent of better imaging techniques.

One of the most common dilemmas facing wound care clinicians is differentiating between venous disease/other types of edema and lymphatic disorders, although it has been noted that venous disease may cause lymphedema. Differentiating between these conditions is important because treatment profiles differ considerably. Many pathological processes can mimic lymphedema and need to be excluded in order to make a diagnosis. These include arteriovenous malformations, lipedema (an abnormal accumulation of fat in the tissues of the leg), erythrocyanosis frigid (bluish discoloration of extremities secondary to cold exposure), factitious edema, and gigantism.

Differential diagnosis of edema
CHARACTERISTIC FEATURES OF LYMPHEDEMA

It is important to differentiate lymphedema from other forms of peripheral edema so that appropriate treatment can be provided. (See *color section, Lymphedema*, page C23.) Clinical history, physical examination, and simple tests often make this distinction possible, although imaging procedures may be needed to confirm diagnoses in some cases. For example, diuretics increase the excretion of water and salt, thereby reducing plasma volume, venous capillary pressure, and filtration. Thus, diuretics improve filtration edema but have no effect on lymph drainage over the long term.[11] Similarly, overnight elevation of the legs will improve 90% of a filtration-based edema because higher venous pressure is coupled with higher capillary filtration rates, but only a 10% to 20% improvement in edema will be observed, if there is any improvement at all, in lymphedema.[12] Thus, relative unresponsiveness in both these situations likely indicates lymphedema.

Onset of symptoms may also provide further clues, with lymphedema having a much slower duration of onset compared with edema from other causes. The distinctive skin thickening with fissures and other soft tissue changes (such as hyperkeratosis or papillomatosis) that occur in response to chronic lymphatic system congestion also point to lymphedema. While pitting is often present in the early stages of lymphedema and then disappears as the disease progresses, it can still be made to occur with prolonged compression to accommodate for the increase in fibrosis and skin thickness. Another maneuver, the Kaposi-Stemmer sign, tests the inability to pinch and pick up a fold of skin at the base of the second toe and is predictive of lymphatic insufficiency,[26] although it is not infallible. (The test is "positive" if the clinician is *not* able to pinch a fold of skin at the base of the second toe, indicating lymphedema.) Finally, an increase in swelling of more proximal segments of the affected limb, the contralateral limb, and/or the adjacent trunk quadrant in response to compression (bandaging, garments, or intermittent pneumatic compression) is an indication of lymphatic insufficiency proximal to the limb segment undergoing compression. Regrettably, not all clinicians make this observation if it occurs. Along with continuing inappropriate compression therapy, this missed observation can lead to a situation in which a patient incurs further congestion of the more proximal segment with associated damage to the lymphatic system. This problem is not uncommon in patients with late-stage venous disease in whom the leg has been decongested but lymphedema has developed in the region of the thigh, buttock, or genital area. Individuals with this response should be referred to a certified lymphedema therapist because appropriate treatment will require complex decongestive therapy, including manual lymph drainage, and may require treatment of the trunk and/or contralateral limb. (See *Complex decongestive therapy*. Also, in the United States, refer to www.lymphnet.org for a list of Lymphology Association of North America–certified therapists by state.)

Lymphatic failure in venous disease: Implications for management

Improving lymph drainage is a goal in all edema therapy because edema is caused by either the

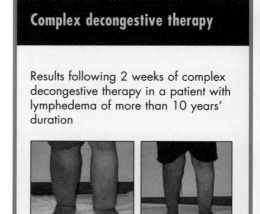

Complex decongestive therapy

Results following 2 weeks of complex decongestive therapy in a patient with lymphedema of more than 10 years' duration

increased capillary filtration rate overwhelming the intact lymphatic system or primary failure of the lymphatic system to transport lymph. While similarities do exist between venous disease and lymphedema in terms of treatment, it is important to detect lymphatic insufficiency in the later stages of venous disease; otherwise, improper treatment and further damage to the lymphatics could follow. Besides treatment, measures to prevent worsening of the condition are also crucial, and these include meticulous skin and wound care, interventions to reduce capillary filtration edema, and interventions to increase lymph flow using compression therapy, exercise, and/or manual lymph drainage.

SKIN AND WOUND CARE

In lymphatic insufficiency, a diminished immune response coupled with the high protein content of the interstitial fluid creates ideal conditions for bacterial growth and an increased risk for infection, particularly cellulitis. Such infections may be recurrent and can occur without skin ulcers being present.[17] In particular, fibrotic skin changes, such as fissures, together with hyperkeratosis, papillomatosis, and increased surface debris and scale, elevate the possibility of bacterial or fungal colonization or invasion. Furthermore, increased edema is associated with higher rates of wound drainage, which means clinicians need to be cognizant about the risk of skin maceration, more frequent dressing changes, selection of more absorptive dressings, and appropriate bandaging. The toes and forefoot are especially vulnerable, as compression wrapping of the toes and foot is often necessary to accomplish graduated compression all the way to the knee. The use of multiple layers of short-stretch bandages and padding is generally advisable because the altered size and shape of the leg make bandaging a complex effort; in obese patients, other techniques, such as the use of Velcro strapping devices (e.g., FarrowWrap, Farrow Medical Innovations, Bryan, TX, or CircAid T3, CircAid Medical Products, San Diego, CA), may be more suitable. Patients will also need to be educated about functional ambulation, a key component of treatment, and may require assistive devices as compression bandages often limit mobility. Adjunct treatments, such as deep breathing exercises and manual lymph drainage, will benefit venous ulcer patients with lymphedema, and the latter is also an important component of pure lymphedema therapy.

DECREASING FILTRATION EDEMA

During the day, leg elevation is frequently prescribed for patients who depend on wheelchairs for mobility. To do any good, however, the patient must lie supine with his or her legs at least at the level of the heart, if not above; "in-between" times, resting positions with the patient's torso in an upright condition and the legs raised are only partially effective. Moreover, the effective resting posture does not encourage ambulation, which might be more effective in the long term if performed regularly. Diuretics should only be prescribed in cases of sodium and fluid retention associated with heart failure or nephrotic syndrome; while they decrease venous volume and ultimately filtration rate, they do not enhance lymph flow and their long-term use in lymphedema is ineffective and may be harmful.

SUMMARY

Lymphedema results when there is an imbalance between capillary filtration and lymphatic drainage. In the United States, lymphedema occurs most commonly due to injury or obstruction, such as from cancer treatment, or associated with severe venous insufficiency and/or obesity. There is no cure, but treatment with compression can effect significant improvement and control of symptoms, which may include skin changes, limb distortion, and cellulitis.

PATIENT SCENARIO

Clinical Data

Mrs. A is a 56-year-old white woman with morbid obesity and longstanding venous insufficiency who developed lymphedema 10 years ago after recurrent episodes of cellulitis, particularly in the left leg. The recurrent episodes of infection have led to worsening lymphedema and dramatic leg enlargement. She now has diffuse areas of skin breakdown circumferentially on the left leg that drain copiously (Fig. 14-4A). She is able to wear a compression stocking on the right leg but not the left due to its deformity and girth. Her husband is also morbidly obese, and his legs, which contact hers in bed, have had cellulitis with similar organisms (Fig. 14-4B).

Case Discussion

The patient and her husband were treated simultaneously with intravenous antibiotics followed by oral antibiotics. Topical antimicrobial products and highly absorbent dressings were used underneath short-stretch lymphedema bandages, which were changed daily until the ulcerations closed (Fig. 14-4C). Eventually the patient was placed in a semi-rigid Velcro strap device (Fig. 14-4D). The patient was also provided with a pneumatic compression device ("lymphedema pump"), which she was to use for 1 hour daily in hopes of achieving long-term control of her lymphedema, and was placed on an oral antibiotic prophylaxis regimen for 1 year.

(continued)

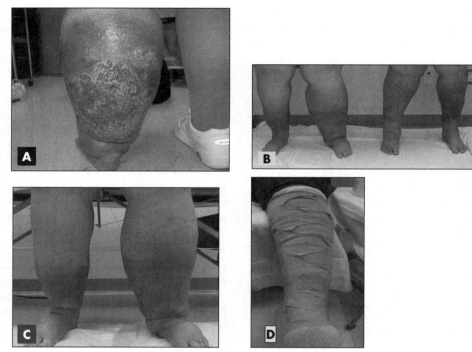

Figure 14-4. (A) Diffuse areas of skin breakdown in an obese patient with lymphedema in the left leg. (B) Skin breakdown due to cellulitis also seen in the patient's husband. (C) Resolution of ulcerations in the patient following antibiotic treatment. (D) Semirigid Velcro strap device used to control lymphedema. (Photos courtesy of C.Fife, MD.) (See *color section*, *Patient Scenarios*, page C45, for the color versions of these images.)

SHOW WHAT YOU KNOW: VENOUS DISEASE

1. The cause of venous ulcers is:
   A. venous stasis.
   B. venous hypertension.
   C. embolic phenomenon.
   D. varicose veins.

   ANSWER: B. *Venous stasis was thought to cause venous ulcers because of pooled blood in the veins. However, current literature reports that venous hypertension is responsible for increased pressure along the vein wall and in the subcutaneous tissue.*

2. The ankle-brachial index (ABI) is an indicator of loss of perfusion in the lower extremity.
   A. True
   B. False

   ANSWER: A. *Perfusion of the lower extremity is indirectly measured by the ABI.*

3. The most important treatment component for venous ulcers is:
   A. moist wound healing.

(continued)

B. antibiotics.
C. compression.
D. revascularization.

ANSWER: C. *Compression is the most important component—the edema must be managed in order for venous and lymphatic ulcers to heal.*

4. The most detrimental activity a patient with any vascular disease can do is:
A. walk into the pain.
B. sleep with legs dependent.
C. use nicotine.
D. fail to monitor pulses.

ANSWER: C. *Nicotine shouldn't be used in any form. It constricts vessels and contributes to atherosclerosis and venous disease.*

SHOW WHAT YOU KNOW: LYMPHEDEMA

1. Which of the following statements about the epidemiology and course of lymphedema in the developed world is <u>false?</u>
A. It is most commonly the result of cancer treatment.
B. Overnight elevation and aggressive diuresis are likely to improve it.
C. While treatment improves symptoms, lymphedema is not curable.
D. Lymphedema may be confused with lipedema, a genetically mediated fatty deposition syndrome.

ANSWER: B. *A broad definition of lymphedema is persistent edema lasting longer than 3 months, little or no response to overnight elevation or diuretics, and the presence of skin changes (primarily thickened skin, hyperkeratosis, and papillomatosis). In the Third World, the most common cause is infection by the nematode* W. bancrofti, *which is carried by mosquitoes. In the developed world, damage to lymphatics—usually from cancer treatment—is the most common cause. There is no cure. The differential diagnosis of leg enlargement can be challenging because lipedema, a pathological deposition of fat, usually below the waist, may be confused with lymphedema. Although there may be orthostatic edema, the feet are spared. However, lipedema can develop into lymphedema.*

2. Which of the following scenarios is likely to contribute to edema in the lower limb?
A. A decrease in capillary filtration rate
B. A decrease in interstitial fluid pressure
C. A decrease in intravascular oncotic pressure
D. A decrease in capillary ultrafiltrate

ANSWER: C. *Lymphatic flow is determined by several factors, including capillary blood pressure, osmotic pressure, and interstitial fluid pressure (hydrostatic pressure). Anything that increases capillary filtration means that more fluid is in the interstitial space (because of an increase in either the rate of filtration or the total amount of ultrafiltrate, perhaps due to an increase in blood pressure or volume overload). This will cause the interstitial fluid pressure to increase. If the oncotic pressure inside the blood vessels decreases (due, for example, to decreased albumin), then more fluid will leave the blood vessels for the interstitial space, and edema will increase.*

(continued)

SHOW WHAT YOU KNOW: LYMPHEDEMA *(continued)*

3. Optimal care of lower-extremity lymphedema includes all of the following except:
   A. Compression with short-stretch bandages and fitting of appropriate compression garments
   B. Manual lymphatic drainage
   C. Routine use of diuretics
   D. Exercise and ambulation

   ANSWER: C. *Diuretics may cause dehydration and thus increase interstitial oncotic pressure, thereby increasing edema. The lynchpin of therapy is compression with short-stretch garments, which have a low resting pressure (and thus cannot cause ischemia) but a high working pressure, able to work with the muscle pump as the patient ambulates.*

REFERENCES

Venous Disease

1. Young, J.R. "Differential Diagnosis of Leg Ulcers," *Cardiovascular Clinics* 13(2):171-93, 1983.
2. Cornwall, J.V., et al. "Leg Ulcers: Epidemiology and Aetiology," *British Journal of Surgery* 73(9):693, September 1986.
3. Coon, W.W., et al. "Venous Thromboembolism and Other Venous Disease in the Tecumseh Community Health Study," *Circulation* 48(4):839-46, October 1973.
4. Dewolfe, V.G. "The Prevention and Management of Chronic Venous Insufficiency," *Practical Cardiology* 6:197-202, 1980.
5. Callam, M.J., et al. "Chronic Ulcers of the Leg: Clinical History," *British Medical Journal* (Clinical Research Edition) 294(6584):1389-91, May 30, 1987.
6. Nelzen, O., et al. "The Prevalence of Chronic Lower-limb Ulceration has been Underestimated: Results of a Validated Population Questionnaire," *British Journal of Surgery* 83(2):255-58, February 1996.
7. Rutherford, R.B. "The Vascular Consultation" in *Vascular Surgery*, Vol. 1, 4th ed. Philadelphia: WB Saunders, 1995.
8. Moore, W.S. (ed). *Vascular Surgery: A Comprehensive Review*, Philadelphia: WB Saunders, 1991.
9. Browse, N.L., et al. *Diseases of the Veins: Pathology, Diagnosis, and Treatment.* London: Edward Arnold, 1988.
10. Phillips, T.J., and Dover, J.S. "Leg Ulcers," *Journal of the American Academy of Dermatology* 25(6 Pt 1):965-89, December 1991.
11. Levick, J. "Revision of the Starling Principle: New Views of Tissue Fluid Balance," *Journal of Physiology* 557(3):704, 2004.
12. Browse, N.L., and Burnand, K.G. "The Cause of Venous Ulceration," *Lancet* 2(8292):243-45, July 31, 1982.
13. Dodd, H., and Cockett, F. "The Postthrombotic Syndrome and Venous Ulceration," in Dodd, H., and Cockett, F. (eds.), *The Pathology and Surgery of the Veins of the Lower Limbs.* New York: Churchill Livingstone, 1976.
14. Burnand, K., et al. "Venous Lipodermatosclerosis: Treatment with Fibrinolytic Enhancement and Elastic Compression," *British Medical Journal* 280(6206):7-11, January 5, 1980.
15. Nicolaides, A., et al. "Chronic Deep Venous Insufficiency," in Haimovici, H., et al. eds., *Haimovici's Vascular Surgery*, 4th ed. Oxford: Blackwell Science, 1996.
16. Powell, S. "Contact Dermatitis in Patients with Chronic Leg Ulcers," *Journal of Tissue Viability* 6(4):103-106, October 1996.
17. Owens, J.C. "Management of Postphlebitic Syndrome," *British Journal of Surgery* 68:807-96, 1981.
18. Nicolaides, A.N., et al. "The Relation of Venous Ulceration with Ambulatory Venous Pressure Measurements," *Journal of Vascular Surgery* 17(2):414-19, February 1993.
19. Blalock, A. "Oxygen Content of Blood in Patients with Varicose Veins," *Archives of Surgery* 19:898-905, 1929.
20. Lindemayr, W., et al. "Arteriovenous Shunts in Primary Varicosis? A Critical Essay," *Vascular Surgery* 6(1):9-13, January-February 1972.
21. Burnand, K.G., et al. "Peripapillary Fibrin in the Ulcer-bearing Skin of the Leg: The Cause of Lipodermatosclerosis and Venous Ulceration," *British Medical Journal* (Clinical Research Edition) 285(6):1071-72, November-December 1982.
22. Falanga, V., et al. "Pericapillary Fibrin Cuffs in Venous Ulceration: Persistence with Treatment and During Ulcer Healing," *Journal of Dermatology, Surgery, & Oncology* 18(5):409-14, May 1992.
23. Coleridge Smith, P.D., et al. "Causes of Venous Ulceration," *British Journal of Hospital Medicine*

(Clinical Research Edition) 296(6638):1726-27, June 18, 1988.

24. Sarin, S., et al. "Disease Mechanisms in Venous Ulceration," *British Journal of Hospital Medicine* 45(5):303-5, May 1991.

25. Falanga, V., and Eaglstein, W.H. "The 'Trap' Hypothesis of Venous Ulceration," *Lancet* 341(8851):1006-08, April 17, 1993.

26. Porter, J.M., et al. "Reporting Standards in Venous Disease," *Journal of Vascular Surgery* 8(2):172-81, August 1988.

27. Ad Hoc Committee of the American Venous Forum. "Classification and Grading of Chronic Venous Disease in the Lower Limbs: A Consensus Statement," in Gloviczki, P. and Yao, J.S.T. (eds.), *Handbook of Venous Disorders: Guidelines of the American Venous Forum*. London: Chapman & Hall, 1996.

28. Kistner, R.L., et al. "Diagnosis of Chronic Venous Disease of the Lower Extremities: The CEAP Classification," *Mayo Clinic Proceedings* 71(4): 338-45, April 1996.

29. Eklof, B., Rutherford, R.B., Bergan, J.J., et al. "Revision of the CEAP Classification for Chronic Venous Disorders: Consensus Statement." Presented at the Sixteenth Annual Meeting of the American Venous Forum, Orlando, Florida, February 26-29, 2004.

30. Rutherford, R.B., Padberg, F.T., Jr., Comerota, A.J., Kissner, R.I., Meissner, M.H., Moneta, G.I., American Venous Forum's Ad Hoc Committee on Venous Outcomes Assessment. "Venous Severity Scoring: An Adjunct to Venous Outcome Assessment," *Journal of Vascular Surgery* 31: 1307-12, 2000.

31. Vasquez, M.A., Rabe, E., McLafferty, R.B., Shortell, C.K., Marston, W.A., Gillespie, D., Meissner, M.H., Rutherford, R.B. "Revision of the Venous Clinical Severity Score: Venous Outcomes Consensus Statement: Special Communication of the American Venous Forum Ad Hoc Outcomes Working Group," *Journal of Vascular Surgery* 52(5):1387-96, 2010.

32. Fahey, V.A., and White, S.A. "Physical Assessment of the Vascular System," in Fahey, V.A. (eds.), *Vascular Nursing*. Philadelphia: WB Saunders, 1994.

33. Douglas, W.S., and Simpson, N.B. "Guidelines for the Management of Chronic Venous Leg Ulceration: Report of a Multidisciplinary Workshop," *British Journal of Dermatology* 132(3):446-52, March 1995.

34. Lane, K., Worsley, D., McKenzie, D. "Exercise and the Lymphatic System: Implications for Breast-Cancer Survivors," *Sports Medicine* 35(6):461-471, 2005.

35. Belcaro, G., et al. "Noninvasive Tests in Venous Insufficiency," *Journal of Cardiovascular Surgery* 34(1):3-11, February 1993.

36. Nicolaides, A.N., and Miles, C. "Photoplethysmography in the Assessment of Venous Insufficiency," *Journal of Vascular Surgery* 5(3):405-12, March 1987.

37. Burton, C., "Venous Ulcers," *American Journal of Surgery* 167(1A Suppl):S37-S41, January 1994.

38. Jones, S.A., Bowler, P.G., Walker, M., Parsons, D. "Controlling Wound Bioburden with a Novel Silver Containing Hydrofiber Dressing," *Wound Repair and Regeneration* 12:288-94, 2004.

39. Lineaweaver, W., et al. "Topical Antimicrobial Toxicity," *Archives of Surgery* 120(3):267-70, March 1985.

40. Lineaweaver, W., et al. "Cellular and Bacteriologic Toxicities of Topical Antimicrobials," *Plastic & Reconstructive Surgery* 75(3):94-96, March 1985.

41. Cooper, M., et al. "The Cytotoxic Effects of Commonly Used Topical Antimicrobial Agents on Human Fibroblasts and Keratinocytes," *Journal of Trauma* 31(6):775-84, June 1991.

42. McCauley, R.L., et al. "In Vitro Toxicity of Topical Antimicrobial Agents to Human Fibroblasts," *Journal of Surgical Research* 46(3):267-74, March 1989.

43. Maklebust, J. "Using Wound Care Products to Promote a Healing Environment," *Critical Care Nursing Clinics of North America* 8(2):141-58, June 1996.

44. Maklebust, J., and Sieggreen, M. *Pressure Ulcers: Guidelines for Prevention and Management*, 3rd ed., Springhouse, PA: Springhouse Corp., 2001.

45. Niederhuber, S.S., et al. "Reduction of Skin Bacterial Load with Use of Therapeutic Whirlpool," *Physical Therapy* 55(5):482-86, May 1975.

46. Bohannon, R.W. "Whirlpool versus Whirlpool and Rinse for Removal of Bacteria from a Venous Stasis Ulcer," *Physical Therapy* 62(3):304-308, March 1982.

47. O'Meara, S., Cullum, N.A., Nelson, F.A. "Compression for Venous Leg Ulcers," *Cochrane Database of Systematic Reviews* 1:CD000265, 2009.

48. Palfryman, S.S.J., Nelson, E.A., Lochiel, R., Michaels, J.A. "Dressings for Healing Venous Leg Ulcers," *Cochrane Database of Systematic Reviews* 3:CD001103, 2006.

49. Michaels, J., Palfreyman, S., Shackley, P. "Randomized Controlled Trial and Cost Effectiveness Analysis of Silver-donating Antimicrobial Dressings for Venous Leg Ulcers (VULCAN Trial)," *British Journal of Surgery* 96:1147 -56, 2009.

50. Jull, A., Walker, N., Parag, V., Molan, P., Rogers, A. "Randomized Clinical Trial of Honey-

impregnated Dressings for Venous Leg Ulcers," *British Journal of Surgery* 95:175-82, 2008.

51. Goldman, M.P., et al. "Diagnosis and Treatment of Varicose Veins: A Review," *Journal of the American Academy of Dermatology* 31(3 PH): 393-416, September 1994.

52. Cordts, P.R., et al. "A Prospective, Randomized Trial of Unna's Boot versus Duoderm CGF Hydroactive Dressing plus Compression in the Management of Venous Leg Ulcers," *Journal of Vascular Surgery* 15(3):480-86, March 1992.

53. Mayberry, J.C., et al. "Nonoperative Treatment of Venous Stasis Ulcer," in Bergan, J.J., and Yao, J.S.T. (eds.), *Venous Disorders*. Philadelphia: WB Saunders, 1991.

54. Partsch, H. Clark, M., Mosti, G., et al. "Classification of Compression Bandages: Practical Aspects," *Dermatology Surgery* 34:600-9., 2008.

55. Winter, G.D. "Formation of a Scab and the Rate of Epithelialization of Superficial Wounds in the Skin of a Pig," *Nature* 193:293-94, 1962.

56. Loiterman, D.A., and Byers, P.H. "Effect of a Hydrocellular Polyurethane Dressing on Chronic Venous Ulcer Healing," *Wounds* 3(5):178-81, September-October 1991.

57. World Union of Wound Healing societies (WUWHS). *Principles of Best Practice: Compression in Venous Leg Ulcers. A Consensus Document.* London: MEP Ltd, 2008.

58. Noyes, L.D., et al. "Hemodynamic Assessment of High Compression Hosiery in Chronic Venous Disease," *Surgery* 102(5):813-15, November 1987.

59. Pekanmaki, K., et al. "Intermittent Pneumatic Compression Treatment for Postthrombotic Leg Ulcers," *Clinical & Experimental Dermatology* 12(5):350-53, September 1987.

60. Scurr, J.H., et al. "Regimen for Improved Effectiveness of Intermittent Pneumatic Compression in Deep Venous Thrombosis Prophylaxis," *Surgery* 102(5):816-20, November 1987.

61. Mulder, G., et al. "Study of Sequential Compression Therapy in the Treatment of Nonhealing Chronic Venous Ulcers," *Wounds* 2:111-15, 1990.

62. Allsup, D.J. "Use of the Intermittent Pneumatic Compression Device in Venous Ulcer Disease," *Journal of Vascular Nursing* 12(4):106-11, December 1994.

63. Smith, P.C., et al. "Sequential Gradient Pneumatic Compression Enhances Venous Ulcer Healing: A Randomized Trial," *Surgery* 108(5):871-75, November 1990.

64. Mirand, F., Perez, M., Castigloni, M., et al. "Effect of Sequential Intermittent Pneumatic Compression on Both Leg Lymphedema Volume and on Lymph Transport as Semi-quantitatively Evaluated by Lymphoscintigraphy," *Lymphology* 34:135-41, 2001.

65. Margolis, D.J., Berlin, J.A., Strom, B.L. "Risk Factors Associated with the Failure of a Venous Leg Ulcer to Heal," *Archives of Dermatology* 135(8):920-26, 1999.

66. Chaby, G., Viseux, V., Ramelet, A.A., et al. "Refractory Venous Leg Ulcers: A Study of Risk Factors," *Dermatologic Surgery* 32(4): 512-19, 2006.

67. Szuba, A., Cooke, J., Yousuf, S., Rockson, S. "Decongestive Lymphatic Therapy for Patients with Cancer-Related or Primary Lymphedema," *The American Journal of Medicine* 109(4):296-300, September 2000.

68. Neglén, P., Raju, S. "Intravascular Ultrasound Scan Evaluation of the Obstructed Vein," *Journal of Vascular Surgery* 35:694-700, 2002.

69. Neglén, P., Hollis, K.C., Olivier, J., Raju, S. "Stenting of the Venous Outflow in Chronic Venous Disease: Long-term Stent-related Outcome, Clinical, and Hemodynamic Result," *Journal of Vascular Surgery* 46:979-90, 2007.

70. Kasirajan, K., Ramaiah, V.G., Diethrich, E.B. "The Trellis Thrombectomy System in the Treatment of Acute Limb Ischemia," *Journal of Endovascular Therapy* 10:317-21, 2003.

71. Tsetis, D.K., Katsamouris, A.N., Androulakakis, Z., et al: "Use of the Trellis Peripheral Infusion System for Enhancement of rt-PA Thrombolysis in Acute Lower Limb Ischemia," *Cardiovascular and Interventional Radiology* 26:572-75, 2003.

72. Kasirajan, K., et al. "Percutaneous AngioJet thrombectomy in the Management of Extensive Deep Venous Thrombosis," *Journal of Vascular and Interventional Radiology* 12:179-85, 2001.

73. Kim, H.S., et al. "Adjunctive Percutaneous Mechanical Thrombectomy for Lower-extremity Deep Vein Thrombosis: Clinical and Economic Outcomes," *Journal of Vascular and Interventional Radiology* 17:1099-110, 2006.

74. Gloviczki, P., Pairolero, P.C., Toomey, B.J., Bower, T.C., Rooke, T.W., Stanson, A.W., Hallett, J.W., Jr., Cherry, K.J., Jr. "Reconstruction of Large Veins for Nonmalignant Venous Occlusive Disease," *Journal of Vascular Surgery* 16:750-61, 1992.

75. Kistner, R.L. "Valve Reconstruction for Primary Valve Insufficiency," in Bergan, J.J., and Kistner, R.L. (eds.), *Atlas of Venous Surgery*. Philadelphia: WB Saunders, 1992.

76. Ko, D., Lerner, R., Klose, G., Cosimi, A. "Effective Treatment of Lymphedema of the Extremities," *Archives of Surgery* 133:452-458, April 1998.

77. Raju, S. "Axillary Vein Transfer for Postphlebitic Syndrome," in Bergan, J.J., and Kistner, R.L.

(eds.), *Atlas of Venous Surgery*. Philadelphia: WB Saunders, 1992.

78. Kistner, R.L. "Transposition Techniques," in Bergan, J.J., and Kistner, R.L. (eds.), *Atlas of Venous Surgery*. Philadelphia: WB Saunders, 1992.

79. Maleti, O., Lugli, M. "Neovalve Construction in Postthrombotic Syndrome," *Journal of Vascular Surgery* 43:794-99, 2006.

80. Tripathi, R., Sienarine, K., Abbas, M., Durrani, N. "Deep Venous Valve Reconstruction for Non-healing Leg Ulcers: Techniques and Results," *Australian and New Zealand Journal of Surgery* 74:34-9, 2004.

81. Gloviczki, P., Bergan, J., (eds.). *Atlas of Endoscopic Perforator Vein Surgery*. London: Springer-Verlag, 1998.

82. Tenbrook, J.A., Jr., Iafrati, M.D., O'Donnell, T.F., Jr., et al: "Systematic Review of Outcomes after Surgical Management of Venous Disease Incorporating Subfascial Endoscopic Perforator Surgery," *Journal of Vascular Surgery* 39:583-89, 2004.

83. Breu, F.X., and Guggenbichler, S. "European Consensus Meeting on Foam Sclerotherapy," *Dermatologic Surgery* 30(5):709-17, May 2003.

84. Frullini, A., Cavezzi, A. "Sclerosing Foam in the Treatment of Varicose Veins and Telangiectasia: History and Analysis of Safety and Complications," *Dermatologic Surgery* 28:11-15, 2002.

85. Scurr, J.H. "Alternative Procedures in Deep Venous Insufficiency," in Bergan, J.J., and Kistner, R.L. (eds.), *Atlas of Venous Surgery*. Philadelphia: WB Saunders, 1992.

86. Proebstle, T.M., Vago, B., Alm, J., Göckeritz, O., Lebard, C., Pichot, O. "Treatment of the Incompetent Great Saphenous Vein by Endovenous Radiofrequency Powered Segmental Thermal Ablation: First Clinical Experience," *Journal of Vascular Surgery* 47:151-56, 2008.

87. Proebstle, T.M., Lehr, H.A., Kargl, A., Espinola-Klein, C., Rother, W., Bethge, S., Knop, J. "Endovenous Treatment of the Greater Saphenous Vein with a 940 nm Diode Laser: Thrombotic Occlusion after Endoluminal Thermal Damage by Laser Generated Steam Bubbles," *Journal of Vascular Surgery* 35:729-36, 2002.

88. Falanga, V., Sabolinski, M. "A Bilayered Living Skin Construct (APLIGRAF) Accelerates Complete Closure of Hard-to-heal Venous Ulcers," *Wound Repair and Regeneration* 7:201-17, 1999.

89. Lawrence, P.F., Chandra, A., Wu, M., Rigberg, D., DeRubertis, B., Gelabert, H., Jimenez, J.C., Carter, V. "Classification of Proximal Endovenous Closure Levels and Treatment Algorithm," *Journal of Vascular Surgery* 52:388-93, 2010.

Lymphedema

1. Mortimer, P. "The Pathophysiology of Lymphedema," American Cancer Society Lymphedema Workshop. *Cancer* 83(12 Suppl American): 2798-802,1998.

2. Logan, V. "Incidence and Prevalence of Lymphoedema: A Literature Review," *Journal of Clinical Nursing* 4:213-19, 1995.

3. Williams, A., Franks, P., Moffat, C. "Lymphoedema: Estimating the Size of the Problem," *Palliative Medicine* 19:300-13, 2005.

4. Bundy, M., Grenfell, B. "Reassessing the Global Prevalence and Distribution of Lymphatic Filariasis," *Parasitology* 112(Pt 4):409-28, 1996.

5. Armer, J. "The Problem of Post-Breast Cancer Lymphedema: Impact and Measurement Issues," *Cancer Investigation* 23(1):76-83, 2005.

6. Petrek, J., Senie, R., Peters, M., Rosen, P. "Lymphedema in a Cohort of Breast Carcinoma Survivors 20 Years after Diagnosis," *Cancer* 92(6):1368-77, 2001.

7. Geller, B., Vacek, P., O'Brien, P., Secker-Walker, R. "Factors Associated with Arm Swelling After Breast Cancer Surgery," *Journal of Women's Health (Larchmt)* 12:921-930, 2003.

8. Okeke, A., Bates, D., Gillatt, D. "Lymphoedema in Urological Cancer," *European Urology* 45(1):18-25, 2004.

9. Shaw, J., Rumball, E. "Complications and Local Recurrence Following Lymphadenectomy," *British Journal of Surgery* 77:760-64, 1990.

10. James, J. "Lymphedema Following Ilio-Inguinal Lymph Node Dissection," *Scandinavian Journal of Plastic and Reconstructive Surgery* 16:167-71, 1982.

11. Mortimer, P. "Implications of the Lymphatic System in CVI-Associated Edema," *Angiology* 51(1):3-7, 2000.

12. Mortimer, P., Levick, R. "Chronic Peripheral Oedema: The Critical Role of the Lymphatic System," *Clinical Medicine* 4(5):448-53, 2004.

13. Duran, W., Pappas, P., Schmid-Schonbein, G. "Microcirculatory Inflammation in Chronic Venous Insufficiency: Current Status and Future Directions," *Microcirculation* 7(6 [Pt 2]):S49-58, 2000.

14. Tiwari, A., Cheng, K., Button, M., Myint, F., Hamilton, G. "Differential Diagnosis, Investigation, and Current Treatment of Lower Limb Lymphedema," *Archives of Surgery* 138(2): 152-61, 2003.

15. Olszewski, W., Pazdur, J., Kubasiewicz, E., Zaleska, M., Cooke, C., Miller, N. "Lymph Draining From Foot Joints in Rheumatoid Arthritis Provides Insight into Local Cytokine and Chemokine Production and Transport to

Lymph Nodes," *Arthritis & Rheumatism* 44(3): 541-49, 2001.

16. Topham, E., Mortimer, P. "Chronic Lower Limb Oedema," *Clinical Medicine* 2(1):28-31, 2002.

17. Moffat, C., Franks, P., Doherty, D., Williams, A., Badger, C. "Lymphoedema: An Underestimated Health Problem," *Quarterly Journal of Medicine* 96:731-738, 2003.

18. Petlund, C. *Prevalence and Incidence of Chronic Lymphoedema in a Western European Country, in* Nishi, M., Uchina, S., Yabuki, S. (eds.), *Progress in Lymphology,* Vol XII. Amsterdam: Elsevier Science Publishers BV, 1990, pp 391–94.

19. Lane, K., Worsley, D., McKenzie, D. "Exercise and the Lymphatic System: Implications for Breast-Cancer Survivors," *Sports Medicine* 35(6): 461-71, 2005.

20. Guyton, A., Hall, T. *Textbook of Medical Physiology.* Philadelphia: WB Saunders, 1999.

21. International Society of Lymphology. "The Diagnosis and Treatment of Peripheral Lymphoedema. Consensus Document of the International Society of Lymphology Executive Committee," *Lymphology* 36:84-91, 2003.

22. Kaipainen, A., Korhonen, J., Mustonen, T., et al. "Expression of the FMS-like Tyrosine Kinase 4 Gene Becomes Restricted to Lymphatic Endothelium During Development," *Proceeding of the National Academy of Science USA* 92(8): 3566-70, 1995.

23. Saharinen, P., Tammela, T., Karkkainen, M., Alitalo, K. "Lymphatic Vasculature: Development, Molecular Regulation and Role in Tumor Metastasis and Inflammation," *Trends in Immunology* 25(7):387-95, 2004.

24. Schmid-Schonbein, G. "Microlymphatics and Lymph Flow," *Physiological Reviews* 70(4): 987-1028, 1990.

25. Schmid-Schonbein, G. "Mechanisms Causing Initial Lymphatics to Expand and Compress to Promote Lymph Flow," *Archives of Histology and Cytology* 53(Suppl):107-14, 1990.

26. Foeldi, M., Foeldi, E., Kubik, S. *Textbook of Lymphology: for Physicians and Lymphedema Therapists,* 5th ed. Munich: Urban & Fischer Verlag, 2003.

27. Foldi, E., Foldi, M., Clodius, L. "The Lymphedema Chaos: A Lancet," *Annals of Plastic Surgery* 22(6):505-15, 1989.

28. Threefoot, S. "The Clinical Significance of Lymphaticovenous Communications," *Annals of Internal Medicine* 72(6):957-58, 1970.

29. Adamson, R., et al. "Oncotic Pressures Opposing Filtration Across Non-fenestrated Rat Microvessels." *Journal of Physiology* 557:889-907, 2004.

30. Levick, J. "Revision of the Starling Principle: New Views of Tissue Fluid Balance," *Journal of Physiology* 557(3):704, 2004.

31. Macdonald, J. "Wound Healing and Lymphedema: A New Look At an Old Problem," *Ostomy Wound Management* 47(4):52-7, 2001.

32. Eliska, O., Eliskova, M. "Morphology of Lymphatics in Human Venous Crural Ulcers with Lipodermatosclerosis," *Lymphology* 34:111-23, 2001.

33. Bollinger, A., Isenring, G., Franzeck, U. "Lymphatic Microangiopathy: A Complication of Severe Chronic Venous Incompetence," *Lymphology* 15:60-65, 1982.

34. Bollinger, A., Leu, A., Hoffmann, U., Franzeck, U. "Microvascular Changes in Venous Disease: An Update," *Angiology* 48(1):27-31, 1997.

35. Leu, A., Leu, H-J., Franzeck, U., Bollinger, A. "Microvascular Changes in Chronic Venous Insufficiency — A Review," *Cardiovascular Surgery* 3(3):237-45, 1995.

36. Junger, M., Steins, A., Hahn, M., Hafner, H.M. "Microcirculatory Dysfunction in Chronic Venous Insufficiency (CVI)," *Microcirculation* 7(6 Pt 2): S3-12, 2000.

37. Franzeck, U., Haselbach, P., Speiser, D., Bollinger, A. "Microangiopathy of Cutaneous Blood and Lymphatic Capillaries in Chronic Venous Insufficiency (CVI)," *Yale Journal of Biology and Medicine* 66:37-46, 1993.

38. Brautigam, P. "The Importance of the Subfascial Lymphatics in the Diagnosis of Lower Limb Edema: Investigations with Semiquantitative Lymphoscintigraphy," *Angiology* 44:464-70, 1993.

39. Bull, R., Ansell, G., Stanton, A.W., Levick, J.R., Mortimer, P.S. "Normal Cutaneous Microcirculation in Gaiter Zone (Ulcer-susceptible Skin) Versus Nearby Regions in Healthy Young Adults," *International Journal of Microcirculation, Clinical and Experimental* 15(2):65-74, 1995.

40. Rasmussen, J.C., Tan, I.C., Marshall, M.V., Fife, C.E., Sevick-Muraca, E.M. "Lymphatic Imaging in Humans with Near-infrared Fluorescence," *Current Opinion in Biotechnology* 20(1):74-82, 2009.

41. Bernas, M., Witte, M. "Consensus and Dissent on the ISL Consensus Document on the Diagnosis and Treatment of Peripheral Lymphedema," *Lymphology* 37:165-67, 2004.

42. Foldi, M. "Remarks Concerning the Consensus Document of the ISL 'The Diagnosis and Treatment of Peripheral Lymphedema,'" *Lymphology* 37: 168-73, 2004.

43. Fahey, V.A., White, S.A. "Physical Assessment of the Vascular System," in Fahey, V.A. (ed.), *Vascular Nursing*. Philadelphia: WB Saunders, 1994.

44. Douglas, W.S., and Simpson, N.B. "Guidelines for the Management of Chronic Venous Leg Ulceration: Report of a Multidisciplinary Workshop," *British Journal of Dermatology* 132(3):446-52, 1995.

45. Belcaro, G., Labropoulos, N., Christopoulos, D., et al. "Noninvasive Tests in Venous Insufficiency," *Journal of Cardiovascular Surgery (Torino)* 34(1): 3-11, 1993.

46. Fife, C.E., Maus, E.A., Carter, M.J. "Lipedema: A Frequently Misdiagnosed & Misunderstood Fatty Deposition Syndrome," *Advances in Skin & Wound Care* 23(2):81-92, Quiz 93-94, 2010.

47. Macdonald, J.M., Ryan, T.J. *Lymphoedema and the Chronic Wound: The Role of Compression and Other Interventions.* Geneva, Switzerland: World Health Organization, 2010, pp. 63-83.

CHAPTER 15

Arterial Ulcers

Mary Y. Sieggreen, NP, CNS, APRN, CVN
Ronald A. Kline, MD, FACS, FAHA
R. Gary Sibbald, BSc, MD, MEd, FRCPC (Med Derm), MACP, MAPWCA
Gregory Ralph Weir, MBChB, MMed (Surg), CVS

> ## Objectives
> After completing this chapter, you'll be able to:
> - identify the structure and explain the function of the lower-extremity arterial system
> - assess the signs and symptoms of lower-extremity arterial disease and ulcers
> - select appropriate vascular laboratory diagnostic testing for lower-extremity arterial disease
> - evaluate medical and surgical treatment options for lower-extremity arterial disease
> - design appropriate patient education for prevention and appropriate lifestyle change.

SCOPE OF THE PROBLEM

Peripheral vascular disease is commonly used to refer to arterial problems in the legs. Some authors also include diseases of the venous and lymphatic systems in their definition of peripheral vascular disease, so the reader should be aware that there may be discrepancies in how this condition is discussed.

Leg and foot ulcers may have several different etiologies, including arterial, venous, and lymphatic disease along with trauma, infections, inflammatory diseases, and malignancy. This chapter describes the arterial component, including anatomy and physiology, and examines the treatment of lower-extremity arterial ulcers.

Approximately 8% to 10% of patients with leg and foot ulcers have pure arterial insufficiency.[1] It's estimated that between 1% and 22% of the population over age 60 suffers from lower-extremity skin ulcers.[2–5] One self-report survey study found the problem to be underestimated when high numbers of patients indicated that they cared for their own ulcers without consulting a healthcare provider.[6] The principal etiology of leg ulcers is chronic venous disease, whereas foot ulcers are much more commonly caused by arterial disease.[1,7–9] Although it's understood that chronic wounds have physical, financial, and psychological effects, it's difficult to measure those effects on a patient's quality of life.[10] It's also difficult to obtain accurate etiological information about leg ulcers because no ulcer etiology documentation exists in about one-third of medical records.

VASCULAR ANATOMY AND PHYSIOLOGY

Vascular anatomy includes the arterial, venous, and lymphatic systems. Vascular ulcers may develop in any of these systems from a variety of causes. For the purposes of this chapter, we will confine our discussion to the arterial system.

Arterial system

Lower-extremity arterial perfusion begins with adequate cardiac performance. As blood exits the left ventricle, it begins its downward course through the descending thoracic aorta. The intercostal arteries, which arise from the descending thoracic aorta, are the first important collaterals to perfusion in the legs. These become important when they are the sole collaterals in distal aortic occlusive disease. As the aorta exits the thorax and enters the true abdominal cavity, its caliber begins to decrease after every major arterial branch. Its greatest reduction in size occurs distal to the renal arteries.

Lumbar arteries usually arise as paired vessels at each vertebral level in the abdomen. The lumbar arteries become important collateral pathways to the lower extremities in distal aortic occlusions or severe aortoiliac occlusive disease. At the level of the umbilicus, the abdominal aorta bifurcates into the common iliac arteries, which in turn branch into internal and external iliac arteries. The internal iliac arteries perfuse the lower sigmoid colon and rectum. They also, by way of the gluteal and pudendal branches, provide another collateral pathway to perfusion of the legs. The external iliac artery becomes the common femoral artery at the level of the inguinal ligament. It's at this level that one can first appreciate the quality of the pulse wave by palpating the femoral artery.

ASPECTS OF THE FEMORAL ARTERY

The common femoral artery bifurcates into the superficial femoral artery and the deep femoral artery. The deep femoral artery is the single most important collateral pathway for perfusion of the lower portion of the leg. Its muscular perforators allow reconstitution of the popliteal artery in superficial femoral artery occlusions. The superficial femoral artery becomes the popliteal artery after it exits the adductor hiatus, also known as *Hunter's canal*. (See *Arterial system*.)

Arterial system

This illustration shows the major arteries of the lower extremities.

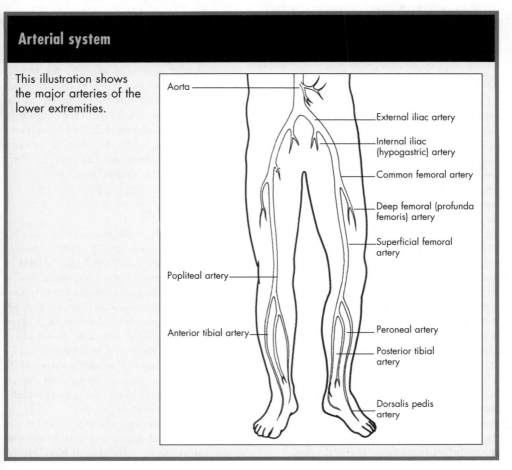

Aorta

External iliac artery

Internal iliac (hypogastric) artery

Common femoral artery

Deep femoral (profunda femoris) artery

Superficial femoral artery

Popliteal artery

Anterior tibial artery

Peroneal artery

Posterior tibial artery

Dorsalis pedis artery

The superficial femoral artery is the most commonly occluded artery in the legs of patients with peripheral vascular occlusive disease. Its occlusion infrequently results in significant ischemia to the lower leg. Below the knee, the popliteal artery bifurcates into the tibioperoneal trunk and the anterior tibial artery. The anterior tibial artery proceeds from the popliteal fossa through the interosseous membrane, which connects the tibia and fibula; it then courses down the anterior muscle compartment into the foot. The tibioperoneal trunk (also known as the tibiofibular trunk) at a variable distance then bifurcates into the peroneal (also known as the fibular) artery and the posterior tibial artery.

The peroneal artery courses down toward the ankle in the deep muscular compartment, whereas the posterior tibial artery descends into the foot in a more superficial fashion. The peroneal artery provides important muscular profusion branches. It's commonly patent even in the presence of severe lower-extremity peripheral vascular occlusive disease.

ASPECTS OF THE TIBIAL ARTERIES

The anterior and posterior tibial arteries proceed into the foot with the anterior tibial artery becoming palpable as it becomes the dorsalis pedis artery. The posterior tibial artery then courses behind the medial malleolus and at this level also becomes palpable. The posterior tibial artery provides both deep and superficial components to the plantar arch. Perforators from the plantar arch provide arterial perfusion to the heel, sole, and branches to the digits.

The anterior tibial artery, which becomes the dorsal pedal artery and is palpable on the dorsum of the foot, eventually communicates with the plantar arch, forming a complete circuit in the foot. The peroneal artery, although it stops above the level of the ankle joint, does provide medial and lateral tarsal branches that communicate with the distal-most portions of the anterior and posterior tibial arteries. This is another important collateral pathway for revascularization of the plantar arch in patients with occlusive disease. Vascular surgeons can perform bypass operations to any of these named vessels, with modern procedures successfully bypassing more distal vessels.

ARTERIAL WALL ARCHITECTURE

The arterial wall typically consists of three laminae. The outer lamina, the adventitia, is a layer of loose connective tissue that provides moderate strength to the arterial wall. The media, or middle layer, contains both elastic and muscular fibers and is responsible for arterial strength, elasticity, and contractility. The intima, the innermost layer, is the endothelial lining of an artery and a few cell layers thick. As the arterial tree descends from the center to the periphery, muscular functions become more evident. Vessels below the common femoral artery have a greater propensity for rapid vasoconstriction or vasodilation in direct relationship to perfusion. The tibioperoneal vessels can quickly accommodate changes in perfusion by relaxation or dilation.

Arteries are capable of increasing in size to maintain constant shear stress when atherosclerotic accumulation decreases luminal surface area. However, once a stenosis reaches 50% of the vessel diameter, the artery loses its ability to relax any further and any increase in atherosclerotic accumulation impedes arterial perfusion. Further restriction in flow through this stenotic area results in a decrease in the diameter of the artery distal to the stenosis in order to accommodate diminished blood flow. Compliance of an artery decreases as the arterial wall becomes more rigid as seen in calcific atherosclerosis. (See *Arterial wall*.)

ARTERIAL PERFUSION

As blood descends through successively smaller arterial conduits, it eventually reaches the arteriolar level. Blood flow (rheologic factors) in this precapillary bed plays an important role in perfusion. Blood is a non-Newtonian thixotropic fluid; that is, its viscosity is inversely proportional to its shear rate. Shear rate can be equated to the velocity of blood flow. The slower blood is propulsed, the more viscous it becomes. The primary determinant of whole blood viscosity at any given shear rate is the hematocrit. As red cell mass increases, blood viscosity markedly increases and the flow decreases.

Dehydration or polycythemia, two of many disease states that increase whole blood viscosity, can result in a sludging of blood in the

Arterial wall

In the layers of the arterial wall shown here, the plaque formation and thrombus significantly reduce blood flow through the vessel.

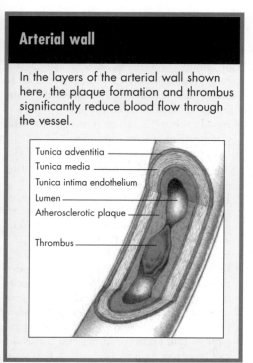

Tunica adventitia
Tunica media
Tunica intima endothelium
Lumen
Atherosclerotic plaque
Thrombus

precapillary bed and a decrease arterial tissue perfusion. In many elderly patients with arterial occlusive disease, even mild dehydration can result in poor extremity perfusion. Simple rehydration can reduce the red cell mass and allow for better perfusion. In other cases of increased blood viscosity, such as multiple myeloma, plasmapheresis may be necessary to remove the abnormal concentrations of proteins. Nonetheless, in the "normal" atherosclerotic patient, it's the red cell mass, measured by hematocrit, which is the primary determinant of viscosity.

As blood proceeds into the capillary bed, the diameter of the vessel approaches that of the red cell—approximately 8 μ (microns) in diameter. Red cells pass through capillaries sequentially. Red cell deformability plays a role in perfusion at this level. In conditions in which the red cell membrane is relatively rigid, tissue perfusion decreases because of increased transit time for a red cell to pass from the precapillary to postcapillary level. Although nutrient and oxygen extraction are increased by this increase in transit time, the per-unit perfusion of the tissues is decreased overall. Medications such as pentoxifylline reportedly facilitate red

cell deformability, thereby increasing the per-unit perfusion of tissues.[7,8]

In normal states, arterial tissue perfusion is well above minimal requirements. Certain tissues, such as muscle, can change their metabolic requirements. Muscle becomes more efficient under anaerobic conditions (this is called the Cori cycle)—for example, in a trained person who engages in long-distance running. The process is gradual, but it's useful in patients with claudication. A regular exercise program can increase the distance walked before claudication occurs. The skin does not have the same kind of compensatory mechanism where exercise can gradually increase blood flow.

ARTERIAL ULCER PATHOPHYSIOLOGY

The pathophysiology of vascular ulcers varies according to the type of ulcer. Arterial ulcers are wounds that will not heal due to compromised or inadequate arterial blood flow or ischemia. Hypoxia due to anemia might exacerbate ischemia. Precipitating events for arterial ulcers vary. Limbs with arterial compromise may have minimal but adequate blood flow to maintain tissue viability. Ischemic lower-extremity ulcers are often precipitated by trauma or infection.

The location of traumatic ulcers varies depending on the cause, but these wounds are commonly found on the foot or on the anterior tibial area of the lower leg. Traumatic ulcers may be caused by an acute physical injury, such as blunt trauma (for example, bumping into a piece of furniture or dropping a heavy object on the foot), or by acute or chronic pressure (such as the continual pressure from ill-fitting footwear). Several other conditions may be responsible for tissue breakdown, including thermal extremes, chemicals, or a localized clot or embolus, which can also lead to decreased cellular nutrition from impaired arterial flow. *Regardless of the cause, when ischemia is present, wound healing is inhibited.* Although some wounds heal in the presence of ischemia, arterial inflow must usually be improved for healing to occur. Injury repair requires more than baseline oxygen consumption and increased tissue nutritional need because diminished arterial flow causes tissue hypoxia in arterial insufficiency and can

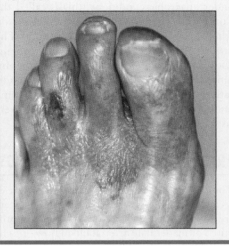

Ischemic forefoot

This photograph shows an ischemic forefoot.

eventually lead to gangrene or tissue necrosis. (See *Ischemic forefoot.*)

DIAGNOSING VASCULAR ULCERS

Vascular disease and ulcer etiology can be determined by obtaining a thorough patient history and performing a physical examination. A focused vascular history includes a clear description of the presenting complaint, past medical history for vascular and related conditions, current and previous medications, and risk factors. Signs and symptoms of lower-extremity vascular disease may include pain, tissue loss, or change in appearance or sensation. Noninvasive vascular laboratory testing is required to identify the location of vascular pathology.

The first question to ask every patient is about his or her history of allergies. This question is important if there is a known sensitivity to medications that may be ordered or to dyes used for angiography. The next question should be about the patient's medications and then about his or her occupation.[11]

The important points to remember about a patient's history include remembering the ABCDEs,[11] all of which are increased risk factors for arterial disease. They are:

- **A**$_{1C}$: Hemoglobin A$_{1C}$ refers to the personal or family history of diabetes or arterial disease. Arterial disease often manifests at an earlier age in males and in individuals who smoke or have other risk factors.
- **B**lood pressure: Find out if it is elevated and if the patient is on medications.
- **C**holesterol: Elevated cholesterol is a risk factor, and the use of statin cholesterol-lowering agents may reduce this risk.
- **D**iet and obesity: Increased weight, especially a body mass index above 25, indicates an increased risk for heart and peripheral vascular disease as well as diabetes.
- **E**xercise: Individuals who exercise regularly have a lower risk of peripheral vascular disease and can build up a greater tolerance to overcome compromised circulation. In general, individuals with leg pain at rest or when in bed have severe ischemia, those who have pain or claudication (aching and throbbing calf muscles) with walking up a few stairs or less than 50 yards have moderate disease, and individuals with symptoms after walking one or two blocks have mild disease.
- **S**moking: One cigarette decreases circulation by 30% for 1 hour and the more pack-years of accumulated smoking history, the greater the risk. Ask patients how many cigarettes they smoke a day and how many years they have been smoking. (For example, 30 years of smoking a half a pack a day is 15 pack-years [30 × 0.5 = 15.])

Other risk factors include increased levels of homocysteine and hypothyroidism.[12] If peripheral vascular disease is present, it is also more common to have a history of coronary artery disease and previous stroke.[12]

Physical examination

Skin inspection is an important part of the physical examination. It includes examining the distal extremities for taut or shiny, atrophic skin that's present with arterial disease. Because skin color may indicate arterial perfusion, each toe should be noted and compared with the other foot and toes. Arterial insufficiency causes ischemic tissue to first become pale, progressing to a mottled netlike appearance (livedo reticularis) and subsequently to a dark purple hue, and finally black. (See *color section, Arterial ulcer*, page C22.) Elevating the foot at a 45-degree angle causes the ischemic limb to become pale. Immediately after positioning the ischemic foot in a dependent position, it becomes dark red or ruddy. This finding is the reactive hyperemia of ischemic tissue. There may be a loss of hair distally, and the nails may lose their luster and become thickened. Make sure to distinguish nail changes from changes that occur with a fungal infection or psoriasis.

Palpate the skin for temperature changes. The skin of the distal part of an ischemic limb feels cool or cold, with temperature demarcation that correlates to the diseased artery. Capillary refill time is determined by compressing the skin (dorsum of the foot or toe pad) with the thumb to remove the local profusion leading to a local blanching of color. Then release the thumb to observe the capillary refill and return of color as a good indicator of arterial skin perfusion. Perform this test with the foot slightly elevated. Normal capillary refill time is less than 3 seconds from pallor to normal skin color.

Palpate pulses for presence, rate, regularity, strength, and equality. The most common objective physical finding is the presence or absence of pulses. Care must be taken when palpating pedal pulses. *It's common to mistake a contracting tendon for the presence of a pulse.* No universal consensus exists regarding a pulse grading system. According to the Inter-Society Consensus for the Management of Peripheral Arterial Disease (TASC II),[13] pulses are graded as 0 (absent), 1 (diminished), or 2 (normal). The American Heart Association's guideline adds a grade of 3 for bounding pulses. To ensure consistency, adhere to local policy. A high degree of observer variability exists in determining the presence or absence of pulses. It can be confusing if clinicians report 2+ or 3+ pulse examinations. Communication is better facilitated if pulses are recorded simply as present or absent. However, even this seemingly obvious assessment parameter may not always be accurate. One study found only a 50% chance that two observers would agree with a third observer about the presence or absence of dorsalis pedis or posterior tibial pulses.[14] This same study found the dorsalis

pedis pulse congenitally absent in 4% to 12% of subjects and the posterior tibial pulse absent in 0.24% to 12.8%.[14] Additional descriptors of pulse, such as "weak" or "bounding," can be added to clarify your findings.

> ### PRACTICE POINT
>
> The best way to document pulses is to use descriptor terms, such as present or absent, rather than numerical ratings, such as 2+ or 3+. Use modifier words, such as weak or bounding, to further describe and clarify the pulse findings.

Although pulses in the foot may be present at rest, they may disappear with exercise. A patient who presents with claudication but has clearly discernable pulses should have an exercise test done in the vascular laboratory. Clinicians are often tempted to skip the assessment of the elusive popliteal pulse, particularly when the dorsalis pedis and posterior tibial pulses are strong. While good pedal pulses indicate foot perfusion, finding bounding popliteal pulses may indicate a popliteal aneurysm. Popliteal aneurysms can be a source of emboli to the lower leg with resulting tissue or limb loss.

Test patients with foot or leg ulcers for neuropathy. This is a common finding in persons with diabetes, but there are several other causes associated with a loss of protective sensation. For example, neuropathy commonly obscures a traumatic or pressure-induced wound in an ischemic limb. Lack of pain sensation and injury awareness prevents the patient with diabetes from seeking appropriate care early. Evaluate neuropathy by testing light touch with monofilaments for the sensory component, examining for dry skin as part of the autonomic component, and eliciting reflexes for the motor component. You can remember to assess for neuropathy with the mnemonic SAM (**S**ensory, **A**utonomic, and **M**otor). An objective assessment of significant neuropathy is best done by using the 5.07 Semmes-Weinstein monofilament.[15] To perform this assessment, ask the patient to close their eyes and indicate when he or she feels the monofilament. Test the areas over the plantar aspect of the first, third, and fifth toe; the first, third, and fifth metatarsal head; both sides of the plantar aspect of the midfoot; the plantar heel; and, lastly, the dorsum of the foot. Place the monofilament on the test position until it bends slightly, and then move it to the next position. Record the number of negative sites the patient reports; if there are four or more negative sites, then neuropathy is present, which indicates a loss of protective sensation. (See chapter 16, Diabetic foot ulcers, page 423, *Practice Point: Assessing Protective Sensation with a Monofilament.*)

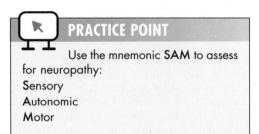

PRACTICE POINT

Use the mnemonic **SAM** to assess for neuropathy:
Sensory
Autonomic
Motor

ARTERIAL SIGNS AND SYMPTOMS

Arterial insufficiency is commonly associated with complaints of pain[16] resulting from atherosclerotic arterial changes interrupting blood flow to tissues.[17] Claudication pain is pain that occurs with exercise and is relieved by rest; it occurs in the muscle group distal to the stenosed or occluded artery. While the calf is the most common location for claudication, it can also occur in the buttocks, thighs, or feet and is predictable and reproducible. Claudication is described by patients as muscle cramping, aching, or weakness. The distance the patient is able to walk until the claudication first develops is referred to as the *initial claudication distance*. The distance the patient is able to walk before

PRACTICE POINT

When taking a history, it's important to find out exactly how far the patient can walk before he or she needs to stop; a shorter distance indicates more severe atherosclerosis. Reported changes in ambulatory distance may indicate progressive atherosclerotic disease.

he or she has to stop is called the *absoluteclaudication distance*. The period of time the patient needs for the pain to subside after he or she is forced to stop is referred to as the *recovery time*.

The patient with leg ulcers and poorly perfused tissue commonly seeks care because of sharp, severe, and possibly constant pain at the ulcer site and the distal extremity. Pain that occurs at rest represents inadequate perfusion and is a sign of threatened limb viability or critical limb ischemia. This pain is referred to as *rest pain*. The patient may describe waking at night with pain across the distal metatarsal area of the foot. In an attempt to relieve the pain, the patient will get out of bed and lower the foot, which has increased blood flow due to increased hydrostatic pressure, to improve tissue perfusion. The patient may even ambulate. The ischemic pain may be relieved by the small contribution of blood flow from collateral vessels if the limb is placed in a dependent position. The patient with pain at rest may begin sleeping with the legs dependent, and leg edema may develop due to the chronic dependent position. Elevation of this edematous limb will further exacerbate rest pain, distinguishing it from venous insufficiency and other causes of edema.

PRACTICE POINT

Rest pain represents end-stage arterial insufficiency and commonly requires revascularization.[18,19]

Patients with extensive sensory neuropathy—for example, those with diabetes—may not experience pain even with severely ischemic ulcers. On the other hand, these patients may experience such intense hyperesthesia associated with the neuropathy that they cannot bear the light touch of stockings. Ulcers in patients with neuropathy are typically found on the plantar side of the foot and are surrounded by calluses from long-term local pressure. These patients may describe the sensations of burning, stinging, shooting, and stabbing pain (neuropathic pain) rather than the more characteristic gnawing, aching, throbbing, and tender pain (nociceptive pain) associated with an acute injury of peripheral vascular disease.

When obtaining a history, note previous arterial surgery for vascular disease, including coronary artery disease and cerebrovascular disease. Vascular disease isn't limited to any one organ but can occur in all body systems: 60% of patients with peripheral arterial disease will have coronary artery disease, and 40% will have cerebrovascular disease. Document all medications, especially vasoconstrictor drugs. Ischemic symptoms are exacerbated by nicotine. Patients with symptomatic vascular disease may aggravate their symptoms by using tobacco, nicotine gum, or nicotine patches for smoking cessation.

Another arterial finding upon examination is gangrene. In ischemic tissue, gangrene initially appears pale, then blue-gray, followed by purple and, finally, black. Gangrenous tissue eventually becomes black, hard, and mummified. The hardened tissue isn't painful, but significant pain may be present at the line of demarcation between the gangrene and the live but ischemic tissue. Gangrene may be a small skin lesion or extend to an entire limb depending on the location of the arterial lesion. If a small patch of skin is affected, the skin will dry and fall off, producing a skin ulcer. Large areas of gangrene may require debridement, skin graft, or potential amputation. *Do not attempt this prior to revascularization.*

Other findings upon examination are ulcers that may appear as small black or dark purple dots, circular areas found on the distal toes, or localized infarcts around the toe nail beds. (See *Blue toe syndrome.*) Ulcers found in these areas are caused by tissue ischemia from arteriosclerosis or by atheromatous debris embolizing from a proximal artery. Arterial ulcers may also be found between the toes, starting as a small, moist, macerated spot on the skin surface extending deep into the bony structure of the foot. This may also be caused by pressure due to ill-fitting footwear.

Arterial ulcers typically have distinct borders with a pale-gray or yellow-dry base. They may contain exposed tendons, fascia, fat, muscle, bone, or joint structures in their base. The surrounding tissue may appear pale compared with skin elsewhere on the body, or it may be reddened if the leg is dependent. Chronic ischemic skin may appear thin and shiny. Foot elevation will produce skin pallor. The red or ruddy color of a dependent ischemic limb is called *dependent rubor* or *reactive hyperemia.*

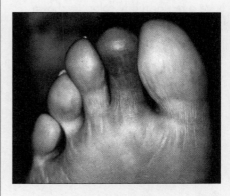

Blue toe syndrome

This photograph shows "blue toe syndrome" in the second toe caused by tissue ischemia from arteriosclerosis.

(See *Dependent rubor,* page 406.) Even in a person of color, the difference in hue is discernible when the ischemic limb is compared with the contralateral well-perfused limb.

Arterial pressure is one of the most reliable physical findings in peripheral arterial disease.[20] However, lower-extremity blood pressures aren't obtained as a part of the routine physical examination. Bilateral brachial pressures should always be obtained on the initial examination to identify whether a discrepancy exists between them. The correct pressure is always the higher of the two pressures. This pressure is used to determine the ankle-brachial index when assessing lower-extremity perfusion.

VASCULAR TESTING

Although an experienced vascular clinician can make a vascular diagnosis based on history and physical examination alone, vascular laboratory studies help pinpoint the diagnosis. The presence, location, and severity of arterial disease are confirmed by vascular laboratory procedures. Information obtained by vascular studies can predict potential ulcer healing (healable ulcer) when the cause is arterial insufficiency.[7] Laboratory tests differentiate among conditions contributing to a nonhealing ulcer.

Dependent rubor

Foot elevation produces skin pallor in patients with ischemic skin (Beurger sign). When dependent, the ischemic limb will have a red or ruddy color, as shown here in the patient's right leg. This is called dependent rubor or reactive hyperemia (Goldflam sign).

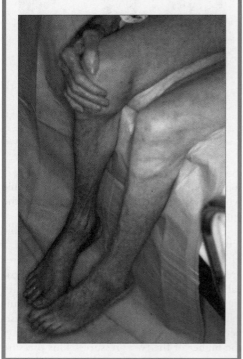

Noninvasive vascular testing is divided into direct tests that image the vessel itself and indirect tests that demonstrate changes distal to the diseased vessel. These tests include segmental arterial Doppler ultrasound with pressures, arteriogram, ankle-brachial index (ABI), transcutaneous pressure of oxygen (TcPO$_2$), and toe pressures.

Handheld Doppler ultrasound

A Doppler ultrasound transmitting probe sends a signal, which is reflected from an object to the receiving probe. If the signal strikes a moving object such as blood cells, a frequency shift is detected and reflected as sound (Doppler principle). The audible signals of arterial flow patterns can then be determined. The handheld Doppler is used to detect an audible signal on the dorsum of the foot or ankle (dorsalis pedis artery and posterior tibial artery). A blood pressure cuff is then placed around the lower calf and inflated until the audible signal disappears. The cuff is then slowly deflated, and when the signal returns the systolic pressure is determined from the reading on the cuff gauge.

Arteriogram

An arteriogram is an invasive test used to identify an operative lesion in the arterial system by outlining the patent arterial lumen. (See *Arteriogram*.) Indications for a surgical procedure include incapacitating claudication, rest pain, nonhealing ulcers, and gangrene. An arteriogram is not indicated unless a bypass or dilation procedure is required. It's also not indicated when the patient is too ill for surgery or is refusing surgical intervention.

Arterial testing

Propagation of a pulse wave originating in the heart is easily measured by auscultation of a peripheral artery with Doppler ultrasound.

Arteriogram

The arteriogram below shows iliac stenosis.

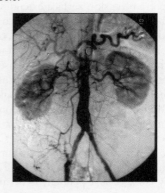

Arterial waveform changes

The arterial changes corresponding to occluded arteries are illustrated here.

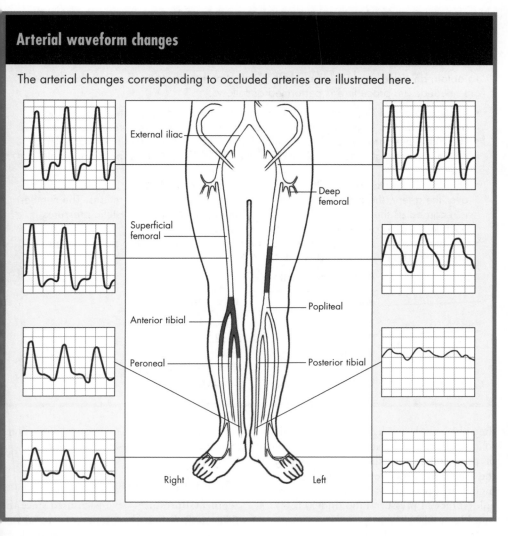

Recording the Doppler shift demonstrates the normal triphasic signal representing the three phases of the pulsation in a normal peripheral artery. The first wave represents forward flow of blood and arterial distention. The second phase represents the arterial relaxation and subsequent retrograde flow of blood. The third phase or portion of the triphasic Doppler signal is believed to represent the bulging of the aortic valve, which occurs during diastole. Some authors suspect that the third phase represents the rebound of the compliant, elastic arterial wall.

The third phase of the triphasic arterial signal is first lost as an artery becomes less compliant and is followed by loss of the second phase of the triphasic Doppler signal. With worsening occlusive disease proximal to the area of auscultation, the normally sharp first wave becomes flattened and broader. In severely diseased arteries, the Doppler signal can be a monophasic, low-amplitude wave. The minimum systolic pressure that can result in forward Doppler flow is used in the calculation of the ABI, a measurement of arterial perfusion in the leg. (See *Arterial waveform changes*.)

Ankle-brachial index

Additional tests for arterial disease include ABI, segmental pressures and waveforms, duplex ultrasound, and exercise treadmill for claudication. Perfusion is indirectly measured by the ABI—the Doppler systolic pressure of

Obtaining an ankle-brachial index

To obtain an ankle-brachial index (ABI), a sphygmomanometer and a Doppler device are needed. The procedure is performed as follows:

- Bilateral brachial Doppler pressures are obtained while the patient is supine. The higher of the two Doppler pressures is used as the brachial pressure in the ratio.
- The blood pressure cuff is placed on the leg just above the malleoli. The Doppler probe is placed at a 45-degree angle to the dorsalis pedis or the posterior tibial artery.
- The cuff is inflated until the Doppler signal is obliterated. With the Doppler probe over the artery, the cuff is slowly deflated until the Doppler signal returns. The number is recorded as the ankle systolic pressure. The higher of the two systolic pressures in each leg is used as the ankle pressure for that leg.
- The higher of the ankle pressures is divided by the higher of the systolic brachial pressures. The ratio obtained is the ABI.

ABI interpretation

ABI	Interpretation
1.0-1.2	Normal
0.75-0.90	Moderate disease
0.50-0.75	Severe disease
<0.5	Rest pain or gangrene
Unreliable	Diabetes

the ankle artery divided into the brachial systolic pressure. ABI ratios reflect the degree of perfusion loss in the lower extremity. If the higher leg pressure is 80 mm Hg and the higher arm pressure is 100 mm Hg, then the ankle-brachial pressure ratio (index) is 80/100 mm Hg or 0.80.

In most individuals, the resting ankle pressure in a supine position is equal to or greater than the brachial pressure, with an ABI value of 1 or more. An individual with claudication may have a normal ABI in this position and have it drop during and after exercise. Patients with pain even in the resting state will have an abnormally low ABI (< 0.5). With exercise, the ABI in the patient with rest pain usually doesn't fall because the arteries are already maximally dilated. Inadequate perfusion creates local tissue factors that result in vasodilation. Collateral pathways can't provide the additional tissue perfusion required, resulting in rest pain. A patient with ischemic tissue loss usually has a perfusion picture that is more consistent with rest pain than claudication.[7] (See *Obtaining an ankle-brachial index*.)

Segmental pressures

Segmental pressures have been used since the 1950s to determine the location of arterial vascular lesions.[21] Pressures obtained at the level of the thigh, above the knee, calf, and ankle are compared with each other and with pressures in the other leg. An arterial lesion can be isolated with a 20 mm Hg gradient between cuff pressures. If no pressure gradient exists on a limb that claudicates, the patient is asked to exercise and repeat pressures are obtained.

A palpable pulse indicates an arterial flow pressure of approximately 80 mm Hg or more in the foot. With calcification of the intima, the arterial pressures derived in the larger vessels of the leg can be falsely elevated. If an ABI is over 1.2, the results are not reliable. The vascular laboratory will then have to rely on accessory tests, such as the toe pressure procedure or $TcPO_2$ test.

TOE PRESSURES

In patients with severe atherosclerosis (diabetes, chronic renal failure, advanced age), the tibial vessels become circumferentially calcified, which renders them incompressible. Toe pressure tests measure the flow through the large toe where the vessel is small enough that calcium deposits don't circle the entire vessel and compressibility is usually present. A toe pressure of 50 mm Hg or higher, even in a person with diabetes, is usually adequate for healing. Toe pressures of 20 to 30 mm Hg usually indicate some vascular compromise, and the wound healing will be more difficult. Pressures below 30 mm Hg may be adequate if the skin is intact, but as soon as injury results and disrupts the cutaneous barrier, the vascular supply is often inadequate for the repair process.

Evidence-Based Practice

A falsely high pressure reading is commonly seen in patients with diabetes due to incompressible artery walls caused by medial sclerosis of the arteries.[19] When the vessels are incompressible, toe pressures are obtained because they're reported to be more accurate.

TREATING VASCULAR ULCERS

When treating vascular ulcers, follow the "preparing the wound bed" paradigm below:[22, 23]

- Treat the cause: bypass, stents, or dilation with a consult to a vascular specialist
- Patient-centered concerns: pain, quality of life, and activities of daily living
- Local wound care:

    — Healable wound: debridement, moisture balance, and bacterial balance
    — Maintenance wound: procedures may be more conservative because of patient or system factors causing the wound to not heal
    — Nonhealable wound: requires conservative debridement, moisture reduction, and bacterial reduction.

With a healable wound, debridement of slough or nonviable tissue is actively promoted to create a clean wound. This may include careful sharp surgical debridement (with bleeding after debridement) or the use of mechanical, enzymatic, or autolytic debridement methods with dressings (usually alginates, hydrogels, or hydrocolloids).

A maintenance wound—one that could heal but patient factors such as smoking, inconsistent treatment, excessive obesity, or uncontrolled diabetes may make sustained healing less likely—requires conservative, superficial debridement (with no bleeding after debridement), accompanied by local wound care for bacterial and moisture balance. If a wound doesn't have enough blood supply to heal, the surface of the wound or necrotic gangrenous tissue should be allowed to dry and demarcate. This can be done by removing the soft slough around the proximal intersection of the necrotic and viable tissue but leaving the necrotic cap intact. Moisture and bacterial reduction may best be served with antiseptic agents, such as povidone-iodine or chlorhexidine, which may reduce bacterial counts with acceptable tissue toxicity.[23] Both of these agents have a broad spectrum of action, a sustained residual effect, and acceptable tissue toxicity for this indication. Agents such as sodium hypochlorite, quaternary ammonium agents, and various aniline dyes (crystal violet) have higher cellular toxicities and more limited antibacterial effects.[23]

Wound infection

It's important to remember that all chronic ulcers contain bacteria (contamination). When bacteria are attached to tissue and multiply, they become colonized and can lead to damage that delays healing (such as with critical colonization, increased bacterial burden, covert infection, and superficial infection). Patients with critical colonization don't have all the classic signs and symptoms of a deep tissue infection. Infection can be diagnosed with a bacterial swab that helps identify resistant organisms or serves as a guide to antimicrobial therapy. The superficial compartment of the wound bed should be examined for more than one sign of bacterial damage. The key features of a wound bed can be remembered by the NERDS mnemonic.[24] (See NERDS© and STONES© in chapter 7,

Wound bioburden and infection. Also see *color section, NERDS,*© page C7.)

Topical treatment for critically colonized wounds could include the various new silver dressings or cadexomer iodine in healable wounds. Povidone-iodine or chlorhexidine may be considered for wounds with inadequate blood supply to support healing.

Deep tissue infection requires systemic antimicrobial agents. The classic signs of warmth, tenderness, swelling, and erythema can be supplemented for persons with chronic wounds by the mnemonic STONES.[24] (See NERDS© and STONES© in chapter 7, Wound bioburden and infection. Also see *color section, STONES©*, pages C8–C9.) If exudate and odor are present, other criteria are needed to determine whether the infection is superficial or deep.

PRACTICE POINT

- The diagnosis of superficial or deep tissue infection can be made clinically with a bacterial swab to help with treatment decisions.
- Persons with diabetes, neuropathy, and foot ulcers often have a false-negative X-ray of the foot for osteomyelitis, and other criteria, such as probing bone, should be used to make a diagnosis.[25]
- The use of a bone scan is limited because it is expensive and may give false-positive results in the presence of inflammation. Magnetic resonance imaging may be more helpful diagnostically.

Wound cleaning

A clean wound, free from dead tissue and wound debris, is necessary for healing to occur. Many commercial wound cleaners have some cytotoxicity, but they have surfactant properties that are often useful. Povidone-iodine, chlorhexidine, hydrogen peroxide, and 0.25% acetic acid have been shown to interfere with fibroblast formation and epithelial growth.[26–29] The selective use of these agents, particularly povidone-

Evidence-Based Practice

The advantage of wound cleansing should be weighed against damaging new tissue growth.[30]

iodine and chlorhexidine, should be reserved for wounds that don't have the ability to heal or for time-limited use in wounds in which bacterial burden is more important than cellular toxicity.

The safest wound cleanser is 0.9% saline solution or water. Wounds should be cleaned with a force strong enough to dislodge debris but gentle enough to prevent damage to newly growing tissue. The pressure to accomplish this goal ranges from 4 to 15 pounds per square inch (psi).[31] A 19-gauge needle or 19-gauge angiocatheter distributes approximately 8 psi when used with a 35-ml syringe. A Baxter cap on a saline irrigation bottle is a less expensive method to distribute adequate pressure. Hydrotherapy or whirlpool debridement has been used to aid in cleaning and debridement of arterial ulcers.[32] This may suggest that vigorous irrigation is the significant factor in cleaning the wound. (For more information about wound cleaning, see chapter 7, Wound bioburden and infection.)

Dressings chosen for specific wounds depend on the wound bed condition and the goal for the wound. Many new dressings are designed to support moist wound healing (see chapter 9, Wound treatment options). Because skin is fragile in patients with either arterial or venous disease and can be easily injured, tape and adhesive products should be used with extreme caution. The use of methods to secure dressings that won't injure the skin are recommended. Of the available adhesive products, soft silicones are less likely to cause

PRACTICE POINT

The preferred attachment device for dressings on vascular leg ulcers is a gauze roll or commercial devices (such as netting or tube gauze) that hold dressings in place without adhesive, which can damage fragile skin.

local trauma during dressing changes. Products without adhesives that secure dressings are the first choice when they are available.

Arterial ulcer treatment

Treatment of arterial ulcers includes increasing the blood supply to the area. Positioning the extremity in a dependent position may facilitate blood flow by gravity through collateral vessels. Use caution if devices such as a foot cradle are used for protection because an insensate foot is subject to trauma from the cradle's hard wood or metal. Debridement of nonviable tissue should not be performed in the presence of ischemia because the blood flow is insufficient to heal the new surgical wound. Ulcers without adequate arterial inflow must be kept dry—in contrast to the principle of moist wound healing for ulcers with adequate blood supply. Moisture provides a bed for bacterial growth if eschar, slough, or gangrenous tissue is present. This tissue, if kept dry, can be left in place until demarcation or debridement is indicated.

Ulcers with adequate blood supply that are expected to heal should be dressed with products that support moist wound healing principles. These dressings include hydrocolloids, thin films, foams and, if nothing else is available, moist saline gauze. The surrounding intact tissue should be protected from fluid accumulation, which can macerate the healthy skin at the ulcer border.

Arterial reconstruction is the treatment of choice to improve the circulation for most patients.[33] Treatment for arterial leg ulcers requires reinstating arterial inflow before any other treatment is established. This is usually preceded by a noninvasive vascular test, an arteriogram (computerized tomography angiogram, magnetic resonance angiogram, digital subtraction angiogram) followed by angioplasty and/or surgery. Simultaneously, local ulcer treatment can be determined. Usually the arterial ulcer has a dry ulcer bed. The patient may have several punctate ulcers with regular borders as well as dry eschar or gangrene distal to the most perfused tissue—usually the tips of the toes or an entire toe. This tissue must be kept dry until adequate arterial perfusion occurs. Moistened gangrenous tissue can provide a medium for bacterial growth. (See *Keeping gangrene dry*.)

Keeping gangrene dry

Gangrenous tissue must be kept dry until adequate arterial perfusion is restored to the area. In the photograph below, the necrotic toes are left open to the air with alcohol wipes placed between them to promote drying.

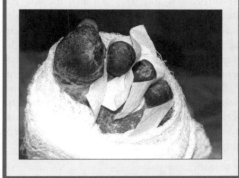

SURGICAL TREATMENT FOR ARTERIAL ULCERS

Surgical treatment should be considered when patients have incapacitating claudication, rest pain, nonhealing ulcers, or progressive gangrene and infection that cannot be controlled. For arterial ulcers, surgical treatment is aimed at restoring tissue perfusion. Bypass grafting may be performed using autologous veins or, when autologous veins are not available, prosthetic grafts, either reversed or in situ. Despite the fact that endovascular techniques are not superior to surgical techniques with regard to vessel patency, wound healing and limb salvage can be attained by using endovascular techniques for patients previously considered ineligible for revascularization. There are poor long-term results from percutaneous balloon angioplasty and stent insertions, atherectomy (percutaneous endoluminal removal of atherosclerotic plaque),[34] and laser ablation of atherosclerotic lesions,[35] except in the common iliac arteries. However, these minimally invasive procedures are very useful in the high-risk patient and expand treatment options.

Ulcers with large skin loss may require skin grafting to close the defect. The recently published BASIL (Bypass versus Angioplasty in

Severe Ischemia of the Leg) trial,[36] which compared bypass surgery and angioplasty, clearly showed that bypass surgery was superior in achieving amputation-free survival. Also, those patients who underwent bypass surgery first fared better than those who underwent angioplasty first. However, this superiority was not significant until after 2 years. The BASIL trial[36] also showed that autologous veins were superior to prosthetic conduits for these bypasses. Unfortunately, the trial did not include the much more common practice of hybrid procedures, combined bypass surgery, and endovascular intervention. Nevertheless, it reinforces the long-held concept in limb salvage surgery that being aggressive is usually better for the patient.

The treatment of ulceration due to arterial insufficiency depends on the level that the occlusive disease occurs. Surgeries for arterial insufficiency are generally grouped into three major areas:

- aortoiliac bypass
- femoropopliteal bypass
- distal bypass.

Restoring tissue perfusion

Occlusive disease in many patients is multileveled. The rule of thumb is to improve inflow first in these patients and then, if necessary, perform an outflow procedure. Inflow usually involves the aortoiliac segments. The exact surgery is tailored to the individual patient's physiologic status and need. For example, an elderly, frail patient with severe aortoiliac occlusive disease may not be a candidate for an aortobifemoral bypass graft. In this type of patient, an extra-anatomic axillobifemoral bypass graft is considered. By avoiding intra-abdominal surgery and clamping of the abdominal aorta, the overall morbidity for these surgeries can be reduced. However, the trade-off for this is that an axillobifemoral bypass graft generally doesn't have the long-term patency rates that an aortobifemoral bypass graft does.

Percutaneous balloon angioplasty

The development of percutaneous balloon angioplasty, with or without stent placement, has significantly reduced the need for routine aortobifemoral bypass surgery in patients with aortoiliac occlusive disease.[37] Isolated short-segment stenoses can be treated successfully with balloon angioplasty. Short-segment stenoses are gener-

ally defined as those less than 10 cm in length, commonly less than 5 cm. With more recent advances in stent development, acute occlusions occurring as a result of atherosclerotic plaque rebound have decreased. The long-term patency rate for stents approaches that for arterial bypass, but only in the aortoiliac segments.[38] Good long-term outcomes with bare metal stents are still haunted by the occurrence of in-stent restenosis. The development of covered stents, with graft material (usually polytetrafluoroethylene [PTFE]) either on one side of the stent metal or enclosing it completely, may hold the answer.[39] Infra-inguinal balloon angioplasty with or without stent placement is still inferior to surgical intervention. However, this procedure still holds a place in the treatment of high-risk patients.

According to the TASC II Guidelines,[13] arterial reconstruction by means of endovascular techniques should be considered before more invasive surgical techniques when possible. Percutaneous intraluminal balloon angioplasty and/or stenting are considerations for arterial stenoses and occlusions classified as TASC A or B lesions. TASC C and D lesions are usually longer and more extensive and often require bypass operations. Newer hybrid procedures include a combination of open surgical and endovascular techniques.[13]

Femoropopliteal bypass graft

A femoropopliteal bypass graft is the standard treatment for femoral popliteal disease. In contrast to an aortoiliac bypass, where the bypass conduit is that of a synthetic material, the femoropopliteal segment may have either a prosthetic conduit or an autogenous venous conduit. The patency rate for a bypass of the femoral popliteal segment depends upon the choice of conduit and the distal level of the bypass. In an above-knee femoropopliteal surgery, the patency rate between autogenous vein and prosthetic material has no significant difference, although long-term patency rates are better when an autogenous venous conduit is used. In a below-knee femoropopliteal bypass, prosthetic material is far inferior to that of autogenous venous conduits.[40] An autogenous venous conduit should be used in the below-knee position whenever possible. (See *Graft patency rates.*)

Below-knee femoropopliteal bypasses using veins have a higher patency rate than above-knee

Graft patency rates

This chart shows the percentage of grafts that remain patent after 1, 2, 3, and 4 years.

Type of graft	1 year	2 years	3 years	4 years
ABOVE-KNEE FEMOROPOPLITEAL GRAFTS				
Reverse saphenous vein	84%	82%	73%	69%
Polytetrafluoroethylene (PTFE)	79%	74%	66%	60%
BELOW-KNEE FEMOROPOPLITEAL GRAFTS				
Reverse saphenous vein	84%	79%	78%	77%
PTFE	68%	61%	44%	40%
Limb salvage				
Reverse saphenous vein	90%	88%	86%	75%
Reverse saphenous vein	94%	84%	83%	
INFRAPOPLITEAL GRAFTS				
Reverse saphenous vein	84%	80%	78%	76%
PTFE	46%	32%	21%	
Limb salvage				
Reverse saphenous vein	85%	83%	82%	82%
PTFE	68%	60%	56%	48%
AT OR BELOW-ANKLE GRAFTS				
Reverse bypass vein	85%	81%	76%	
In-situ vein bypass	92%	82%	72%	
Foot salvage	93%	87%	84%	

femoropopliteal bypasses because a certain amount of atherosclerotic disease at the level of the knee joint can be missed if only anterior-posterior arteriography views are obtained. For this reason, many vascular surgeons require oblique views of the popliteal artery so as to preclude this as a source of decreased long-term patency rates.

Distal bypass

A distal bypass, below the tibial peroneal trunk, requires an autogenous venous conduit. It's reserved for patients with tissue loss when pulsatile arterial perfusion to an ischemic area is desired. Although somewhat controversial, either a reversed venous bypass or an in situ bypass can be performed. Patency rates were equivalent in large series comparing these two techniques.[40] The in situ technique is generally reserved for patients with considerable size disparity between the proximal and distal venous conduit, such as the greater saphenous

vein. An in situ bypass is technically more demanding and requires more operative time than a reversed venous bypass. Some vascular surgeons advocate the creation of a controlled arteriovenous fistula in order to promote long-term patency rates of the prosthetic conduit, when these are used for distal bypasses. The BASIL trial would disagree with this. (See Surgical treatment for arterial ulcers section.)

A patient with calf claudication requires improved perfusion to the posterior calf muscles. Claudication can occur in the buttocks, thighs, or isolated compartments of the lower legs. The perfusion of the respective symptomatic musculature is what determines the level of the outflow portion of the bypass. In patients with combined aortoiliac superficial femoral popliteal disease, 90% of the claudication can be improved by merely improving the inflow to the profundal system by some form of aortoiliac bypass. It is for this reason that routine combined aortofemoral and femoropopliteal bypasses should be avoided. In patients with lifestyle-limiting claudication with isolated superficial femoral artery disease, a femoropopliteal bypass is usually all that is needed.

Patients with ischemic tissue loss usually require pulsatile arterial flow to heal their lesions. If these lesions are in the foot, then whatever bypass is necessary to restore pulsatile arterial flow to the affected area should be performed. Combined with the appropriate vascular bypass procedure, an area of ischemic tissue loss with gangrenous edges should be debrided to create viable tissue. In some patients, however, if there is dry gangrene, autoamputation can be anticipated once adequate perfusion is restored. Some clinicians allow the gangrenous eschar to autoamputate to enable normal epithelial coverage of the underlying eschar before eschar separation. If, however, the area of tissue loss involves a digit, amputation with primary closure may be recommended if no infection is present. This can be done in conjunction with the vascular bypass procedure, or the procedures can be separated by several days if deemed appropriate.

Arterial reconstruction with an in situ graft may be used to revascularize the lower extremity well below the knee. An in situ graft is a vein left in its natural location, anastomosed to the arterial system above and below the arterial stenoses, after the valves are lysed. This procedure allows the surgeon to reconstruct the smaller distal arteries in the lower extremity near the foot. These reconstructed vessels are close to the skin surface. The surgeon must use extreme care not to cause injury to underlying vessels when using sharp debridement for the necrotic ulcers. Autolytic debridement is a safer debriding alternative.

Medical treatment

Medical treatment of arterial disease may include antiplatelet drugs, such as aspirin or clopidogrel, which inhibit the binding of adenosine triphosphate (ATP). Clopidogrel was shown to be slightly better than aspirin in a comparative study.[41] In addition, cilostazol[42–44] has been used not only to decrease platelet aggregation but also to act as a vasodilator that may facilitate an increase in exercise capacity. However, it cannot be used in patients with heart failure. In addition, building up exercise tolerance with a conditioning program may also be important.

Measuring healing

Calculating healing rates is problematic when no standard measurement for wound healing parameters exists. Following wounds to complete healing is one method, but this method is not satisfactory if changes in therapy are needed. Healing rates can be expressed as percent of ulcer area, measurement of change in ulcer perimeter, or percent of ulcer area healed. However, the perimeter and surface area are much greater in large ulcers. Using these measurements will give erroneously high healing rates for larger ulcers compared with smaller ulcers. For example, if the percent of ulcer healed is used as a measurement, smaller ulcers will appear to heal faster than large ulcers by comparison.

Another method traces ulcers on a celluloid screen then measures them over time. The area and circumference of the tracing are calculated by a computer program. In general, a healing trajectory will be established if a wound is 20% to 40% smaller by week 4 and that wound should heal by week 12 provided that the same healing rate is maintained.[45–47]

There are some patients whose ulcers do not heal at the expected rate. If tissue damage has progressed beyond salvage, surgery is too risky, or the limitations of the ischemic limb are interfering with quality of life, amputation may be considered.

PATIENT EDUCATION

The patient may inadvertently neglect the ulcer or fail to use prevention measures if the nature of the condition is not understood. Patient education includes the reason for the ulcer and the treatment rationale. Patient-centered concerns should be central to the treatment process, and active patient involvement includes the recognition and reporting of changes that indicate problems with healing. Patient and family education includes assessment of patient and family needs and level of comprehension about the arterial ulcer and its etiology. Teaching methods vary and are chosen specifically to facilitate the most appropriate method for each patient and family.

Risk factors

Factors that increase risk for arteriosclerosis include smoking, diabetes, hyperlipemia, and hypertension.[48] Smoking is a risk factor in 73% to 90% of patients with atherosclerotic arterial disease. Up to 30% of patients with arterial disease are reported to have diabetes,[49] and 16% to 58% of patients with diabetes have arterial disease.[50–52] Hypertension is present in 29% to 39% of patients with atherosclerosis, and 31% to 57% of patients with atherosclerosis have hyperlipidemia.[48] Risk factor modification is part of the treatment for vascular ulcers to reduce the possibility of further breakdown.

Patients can help themselves by positioning and reducing activities that impair blood flow. After a surgical or percutaneous intervention to restore arterial flow, the patient should continue behaviors that promote vascular health and reduce risk factors. (See *Patient Teaching: Teaching about arterial ulcers.*)

Smoking cessation

Smoking cessation is critical for patients with arterial insufficiency. The direct relationship between tobacco use and ischemia is well known. Smokers are nine times more likely to develop claudication than nonsmokers.[53] However, the link between smoking and vascular disease isn't well recognized by many patients; in one study, only 37% of smokers with peripheral vascular disease understood the strong association between smoking and vascular disease.[43] Patients must be informed of the negative effects of smoking on the vascular system. They should be referred to smoking cessation specialists if needed. Teach the patient the ABCDE mnemonic to remember the risk factors of arterial disease.[11]

SUMMARY

Success in managing arterial ulcers requires a total patient commitment. Risk factors and ulcer management are so dependent upon the patient's activities that the patient must have as much information as possible to participate in the treatment process. An understanding of the peripheral vascular blood supply and the need for adequate tissue oxygenation is critical to the management of arterial ulcers in the legs and feet.

Arterial reconstruction is the hallmark of treatment for arterial disease. In general, dry arterial ulcers or those with fixed, stable, dry eschar should be kept dry until the tissue is revascularized. Economic concerns make it imperative to choose the appropriate dressings and treatment. Research demonstrates little increased benefit of the newer treatments over the old in healing rates; however, some modern wound dressings often improve quality-of-life and pain issues.

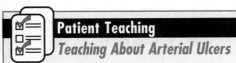
Patient Teaching
Teaching About Arterial Ulcers

Teach the patient with an arterial ulcer to:

- monitor arterial or graft patency by palpating pulses
- recognize signs and symptoms of graft failure and what to report
- avoid nicotine in any form, including second-hand smoke
- begin or maintain a regular exercise program
- manage blood glucose, if diabetes is present
- control hyperlipidemia
- manage hypertension
- reduce weight, if indicated
- perform meticulous foot care
- manage ulcer care.

PATIENT SCENARIO

Clinical Data

Mrs. DA is a 59-year-old black woman who presented in the emergency room with pain in her right foot and dark purple-blue coloring on the skin of both great toes. Her medical history includes diabetes mellitus, tobacco smoking, stroke, peripheral vascular disease, dyslipidemia, and hypertension. Her surgical history is significant for cardiac catheterization performed 1 year

(continued)

ago. Current medications include Plavix 75 mg daily, Crestor 10 mg nightly, aspirin 81 mg daily, Percocet as needed for pain, Colace 100 mg twice daily, Neurontin 300 mg three times daily, Pantoloc 40 mg daily, and enalapril 10 mg daily. She has no known drug allergies.

Mrs. DA smokes a half pack of cigarettes per day and does not drink alcohol or use illicit drugs. She lives in an assisted living complex because of a mild residual left hemiparesis from her stroke.

On physical examination, Mrs. DA appears older than her stated age. She is thin and favors a contracted position in bed with her hips and knees bent, although she is able to extend her legs when asked. She is 5'5" (165.1 cm) tall and weighs 46.5 kg (102.3 lb). Her temperature is 37.6° C (99.7°F), blood pressure 170 to 190/50 to 88 mm Hg, and heart rate 86 bpm. Her feet are painful on palpation and cool to the touch.

Case Discussion

A noninvasive study in the Vascular Lab showed an ABI of 0.2 in the right lower extremity. Mrs. DA was admitted to the hospital, where a vascular surgery consult was obtained.

An arteriogram revealed severe vascular disease. Mrs. DA underwent a combined open aorto-bifemoral bypass and selective balloon angioplasty of the popliteal and peroneal arteries with stent placement to the right popliteal artery (Fig. 15-1). Results were good: She did not have palpable pulses in the foot, but the foot was warm and Doppler signals were present. She then underwent a right transmetatarsal amputation. The wound was left open because of a soft tissue infection in the foot. Mrs. DA's ABI increased to 0.96 on the right side, but this was thought to be falsely elevated because of her diabetes. Negative pressure wound therapy was started on the open foot wound postoperatively with a porous sponge in the wound. The dressing was changed every 3 days.

The pain in the right foot decreased postoperatively, but the left foot became more painful. The gangrene on the left began to extend to the plantar surface of the foot, and an X-ray demonstrated bone changes consistent with osteomyelitis. The ABI on the left was 0.43, with the following absolute pressures: brachial, 191 mm Hg, posterior tibial, 83 mm Hg, dorsalis pedis, 62 mm Hg, and digital, 23 mm Hg. The waveforms in the ankle were monophasic and severely diminished in the digits. The diagnosis was severe left femorotibial occlusive disease.

Mrs. DA was then scheduled for a femorotibial balloon angioplasty and stent placement. A completion arteriogram showed that the vessels were patent. The foot was debrided of necrotic tissue. Again, this wound was left open and treated with negative pressure wound therapy.

Two months after her hospitalization, Mrs. DA was free from pain. The wounds eventually healed by contraction and did not require skin grafting. During her hospitalization, the nursing and pulmonary staffs were able to work with Mrs. DA on a smoking cessation program, and she remained tobacco-free after discharge.

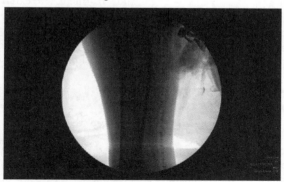

Figure 15-1. Balloon angioplasty of the popliteal artery.

1. Risk factors for the development of arterial ulcers include all of the following <u>except</u>:
   A. smoking.
   B. hypercholesterolemia.
   C. diabetes mellitus.
   D. varicose veins.
   E. hypertension.

   ANSWER: D. *Varicose veins of the lower legs are an early sign of venous insufficiency, and the presence of venous disease is not a known risk factor for the development of arterial disease. Smoking, hypercholesterolemia, diabetes mellitus, and hypertension are risk factors for arterial disease.*

2. Patients with arterial ulcers that do not have adequate blood supply to heal should have local wound care that includes:
   A. aggressive local debridement to bleeding tissue.
   B. silver dressings that promote moisture balance.
   C. local antiseptics such as povidone-iodine and chlorhexidine.
   D. moisture balance dressings such as a hydrogel.

   ANSWER: C. *In patients without the ability to heal, antimicrobials that will work with moisture reduction, such as povidone-iodine or chlorhexidine, are a necessary treatment. Other treatments include conservative debridement of the slough, moisture reduction, and antibacterials that work in a dry environment. For silver to be effective in a wound bed, it requires moisture to be converted to the ionized form, and this is contraindicated in ulcers without the ability to heal.*

3. Which of the following is most likely to be associated with an arterial ulcer?
   A. Lipodermatosclerosis
   B. Reduced blood flow
   C. Edema
   D. Systemic hypertension
   E. Diabetes mellitus

   ANSWER: B. *An arterial ulcer by definition is always associated with arterial insufficiency or reduced blood flow (100%). Lipodermatosclerosis and edema are associated with venous ulcers. There is a less common but significant association of arterial ulcers with diabetes (30%) and hypertension in 29% to 39% of patients.*

4. The ankle-brachial index (ABI) is an indicator of loss of perfusion in the lower extremity.
   A. True
   B. False

   ANSWER: A. *Perfusion of the lower extremity is indirectly measured by the ABI.*

5. Surgical treatment for arterial ulcers most commonly includes:
   A. a graft.
   B. valvoplasty.
   C. a bypass graft.
   D. phlebectomy.

   ANSWER: C. *Arterial ulcers are associated with arterial insufficiency, and a bypass graft is meant to restore the arterial circulation to the ischemic tissues. The other options are incorrect.*

REFERENCES

1. Young, J.R. "Differential Diagnosis of Leg Ulcers," *Cardiovascular Clinics* 13(2):171-93, 1983.

2. Cornwall, J.V., et al. "Leg Ulcers: Epidemiology and Aetiology," *British Journal of Surgery* 73(9):693, September 1986.

3. Coon, W.W., et al. "Venous Thromboembolism and Other Venous Disease in the Tecumseh Community Health Study," *Circulation* 48(4): 839-46, October 1973.

4. Dewolfe, V.G. "The Prevention and Management of Chronic Venous Insufficiency," *Practical Cardiology* 6:197-202, 1980.

5. Callam, M.J., et al. "Chronic Ulcers of the Leg: Clinical History," *British Medical Journal* (Clinical Research Edition) 294(6584):1389-91, May 30, 1987.

6. Nelzen, O., et al. "The Prevalence of Chronic Lower-limb Ulceration Has Been Underestimated: Results of a Validated Population Questionnaire," *British Journal of Surgery* 83(2):255-58, February 1996.

7. Rutherford, R.B. "The Vascular Consultation," in *Vascular Surgery,* Vol. 1, 4th ed. Philadelphia: WB Saunders, 1995.

8. Moore, W.S. (ed.). *Vascular Surgery: A Comprehensive Review.* Philadelphia: WB Saunders, 1991.

9. Browse, N.L., et al. *Diseases of the Veins: Pathology, Diagnosis, and Treatment.* London: Edward Arnold, 1988.

10. Phillips, T.J., and Dover, J.S. "Leg Ulcers," *Journal of the American Academy of Dermatology* 25(6 Pt 1): 965-87, December 1991.

11. Sibbald, R.G, and Ayello, E.A. "Assessing Arterial Disease History Using ABCDE's Mnemonic," Presented at School of Nursing, Wenzhou University Wound Care Symposium, Wenzhou, China, November 2009.

12. Aronow, W.S. "Management of Peripheral Arterial Disease," *Cardiology in Review* 13(2):61-68, March-April 2005.

13. Norgren, L., Hiatt, W.R., Dormandy, J.A., Nehler, M.R., Harris, K.A., Fowkes, F.G. "Inter-Society Consensus for the Management of Peripheral Arterial Disease (TASC II)," *Journal of Vascular Surgery* 45(Suppl S):S5-67, 2007.

14. Lubdbrook, J., et al. "Significance of Absent Ankle Pulse," *British Medical Journal* 1:1724, 1962.

15. Mayfield, J.A., Sugarman, J.R. "The Use of the Semmes-Weinstein Monofilament and Other Threshold Tests for Preventing Foot Ulceration and Amputation in Persons with Diabetes," *Journal of Family Practice* 49(11 Suppl):S17-S29, November 2000.

16. Taylor, L.M., and Porter, J.M. "Natural History and Nonoperative Treatment of Chronic Lower Extremity Ischemia," in Moore, W.S., ed. *Vascular Surgery: A Comprehensive Review.* Philadelphia: WB Saunders, 1993.

17. Blank, C.A., and Irwin, G.H. "Peripheral Vascular Disorders: Assessment and Intervention," *Nursing Clinics of North America* 25(4):777-94, December 1990.

18. Fahey, V.A., and White, S.A. "Physical Assessment of the Vascular System," in Fahey, V.A., ed. *Vascular Nursing.* Philadelphia: WB Saunders, 1994.

19. Baker, J.D. "Assessment of Peripheral Arterial Occlusive Disease," *Critical Care Nursing Clinics of North America* 3(3):493-98, September 1991.

20. Brantigan, C.O. "Peripheral Vascular Disease: A Comparison between the Vascular Laboratory and the Arteriogram in Diagnosis and Management," *Colorado Medicine* 77(9): 320-27, September 1980.

21. Winsor, T. "Influence of Arterial Disease on the Systolic Blood Pressure Gradients of the Extremity," *American Journal of Medical Science* 220, 1950.

22. Sibbald, R.G, et al. "Preparing the Wound Bed 2003: Focus on Infection and Inflammation," *Ostomy Wound Management* 49(11): 24-51, November 2003.

23. Sibbald, R.G, et al. "Best Practice Recommendations for Preparing the Wound Bed: Update 2006," *Wound Care Canada* 4(1):R6-R18, 2006.

24. Sibbald, R.G., et al. "Increased Bacterial Burden and Infection: The Story of NERDS and STONES," *Advances in Skin & Wound Care* 19(8): 462-63, October 2006.

25. Grayson, M.L., et al. "Probing to Bone in Infected Pedal Ulcers. A Clinical Sign of Underlying Osteomyelitis in Diabetic Patients," *Journal of the American Medical Association* 273(9):721-23, March 1, 1995.

26. Lineaweaver, W., et al. "Topical Antimicrobial Toxicity," *Archives of Surgery* 120(3): 267-70, March 1985.

27. Lineaweaver, W., et al. "Cellular and Bacteriologic Toxicities of Topical Antimicrobials," *Plastic & Reconstructive Surgery* 75(3):94-96, March 1985.

28. Cooper, M., et al. "The Cytotoxic Effects of Commonly Used Topical Antimicrobial Agents on Human Fibroblasts and Keratinocytes," *Journal of Trauma* 31(6):775-84, June 1991.

29. McCauley, R.L., et al. "In Vitro Toxicity of Topical Antimicrobial Agents to Human Fibroblasts," *Journal of Surgical Research* 46(3):267-74, March 1989.

30. Maklebust, J. "Using Wound Care Products to Promote a Healing Environment," *Critical Care Nursing Clinics of North America* 8(2):141-58, June 1996.

31. Maklebust, J., and Sieggreen, M. *Pressure Ulcers: Guidelines for Prevention and Management*, 3rd ed., Springhouse, PA: Springhouse Corp., 2001.

32. Niederhuber, S.S., et al. "Reduction of Skin Bacterial Load with Use of Therapeutic Whirlpool," *Physical Therapy* 55(5):482-86, May 1975.

33. Husni, E.A. "Skin Ulcers Secondary to Arterial and Venous Disease," in Lee, B.Y., ed. *Chronic Ulcers of the Skin*. New York: McGraw Hill, 1985.

34. Ramaiah, V., Gammon, R., Kiesz, S., et al: "Midterm Outcomes from the TALON Registry: Treating Peripherals with SilverHawk: Outcomes Collection," *Journal of Endovascular Therapy* 13:592-602, 2006.

35. Laird, J.R., Zeller, T., Gray, B.H., et al: "Limb Salvage Following Laser-assisted Angioplasty for Critical Limb Ischemia: Results of the LACI Multicenter Trial," *Journal of Endovascular Therapy* 13:1-11, 2006.

36. Bradbury, A., et al. "Final Results of the BASIL Trial (Bypass Verses Angioplasty in Severe Ischaemia of the Leg)," *Journal of Vascular Surgery* 51(10S), May 2010.

37. Mousa, A.Y., Beauford, R.B., Flores, L., Faries, P.L., Patel, P., Fogler, R. "Endovascular Treatment of Iliac Occlusive Disease: Review and Update," *Vascular* 15(1):5-11, 2007.

38. Schurmann, K., Mahnken, A., Meyer, J., et al: "Long-term Results 10 Years After Iliac Arterial Stent Placement," *Radiology* 224:731-38, 2002.

39. Kedora, J., Hohmann, S., Garrett, W., et al: "Randomized Comparison of Percutaneous Viabahn Stent Grafts vs Prosthetic Femoral-popliteal Bypass in the Treatment of Superficial Femoral Arterial Occlusive Disease," *Journal of Vascular Surgery* 45:10-16, 2007.

40. Dalman, R.L. "Long-term Results of Bypass Procedures," in Porter, J.M. and Taylor, L.M. (eds.), *Basic Data Underlying Clinical Decision Making in Vascular Surgery. Annals of Vascular Surgery* 141-43, 1995.

41. CAPRIE Steering Committee. "A Randomised, Blinded, Trial of Clopidogrel versus Aspirin in Patients at Risk of Ischaemic Events," *Lancet* 348:1329-39, 1996.

42. Hughson, W.G., et al. "Intermittent Claudication: Prevalence and Risk Factors," *British Medical Journal* 1(6124):1377-79, May 27, 1978.

43. Clyne, C.A., et al. "Smoking, Ignorance, and Peripheral Vascular Disease," *Archives of Surgery* 117(8):1062, August 1982.

44. Cavezzi-Marconi, P. "Manual Lymphatic Drainage," in Cavezzi, A., and Michelini, S. (eds.), *Phlebolymphoedema: From Diagnosis to Therapy*. Bologna, Italy: Edizioni PR, PR Communications, 1998.

45. Falanga, V., et al. "Initial Rate of Healing Predicts Complete Healing of Venous Ulcers," *Archives of Dermatology* 133(10):1231-34, October 1997.

46. Margolis, D.J., et al. "The Accuracy of Venous Leg Ulcer Prognostic Models in a Wound Care System," *Wound Repair and Regeneration* 12(2):163-68, March-April 2004.

47. Margolis, D.J., and Kantor, J. "A Multicentre Study of Percentage Change in Venous Leg Ulcer Area as a Prognostic Index of Healing at 24 Weeks," *British Journal of Dermatology* 142(5):960-64, May 2000.

48. Barnes, R.W. "The Arterial System," in Sabiston, D.C., ed. *Essentials of Surgery*. Philadelphia: WB Saunders, 1987.

49. Coffman, J.D. "Principles of Conservative Treatment of Occlusive Arterial Disease," in Spittell, J.A., ed. *Clinical Vascular Disease*. Philadelphia: FA Davis, 1983.

50. Kilo, C. "Vascular Complications of Diabetes," *Cardiovascular Reviews & Reports* 8(6):18-23, June 1987.

51. Levin, M.E., and Sicard, G.A. "Evaluating and Treating Diabetic Peripheral Vascular Disease: Part 1," *Clinical Diabetes* 62-70, May-June 1987.

52. Dowdell, H.R. "Diabetes and Vascular Disease: A Common Association," *AACN Clinical Issues* 6(4):526-35, November 1995.

53. Hughson, W.G., et al. "Intermittent Claudication: Prevalence and Risk Factors," *British Medical Journal* 1(6124):1377-79, May 27, 1978.

CHAPTER 16

Diabetic Foot Ulcers

Lawrence A. Lavery, DPM, MPH

James B. McGuire, DPM, PT, CPed, CWS, FAPWCA

Sharon Baranoski, MSN, RN, CWCN, APN-CCRN, DAPWCA, FAAN

Elizabeth A. Ayello, PhD, RN, ACNS-BC, CWON, MAPWCA, FAAN

Steven R. Kravitz, DPM, FACFAS, FAPWCA

Objectives

After completing this chapter, you'll be able to:

- state the significance of foot ulcers in patients who have diabetes mellitus
- list strategies for preventing foot ulcers in patients with diabetes
- describe wound characteristics and assessment parameters for a patient with diabetes
- list options for reducing pressure for a patient with diabetes who has a foot ulcer
- discuss the rationale for use of diagnostic imaging in patients with diabetes.

DIABETES: A GROWING PROBLEM

Diabetes mellitus is a significant healthcare problem worldwide. The American Diabetes Association (ADA) defines diabetes as "a disease in which the body doesn't produce or properly use insulin." The incidence of diabetes has increased 48% over the past 10 years, with a 70% increase in patients in their 30s. However, of the 20.8 million Americans (7% of the population) who have diabetes, only 14.6 million are diagnosed, leaving more than one-third, or 6.2 million people, unaware they have the disease. Blacks, Hispanics, Native Americans, and Asian-Americans have the highest prevalence of diabetes mellitus.[1]

Between 5% and 10% of people with diabetes have type 1 diabetes—the autoimmune form of the disorder that causes destruction of pancreatic beta-cells and requires insulin therapy to prevent life-threatening complications. Type 1 diabetes is characterized by a sudden onset of clinical signs and symptoms associated with hyperglycemia, with a strong propensity for the development of ketoacidosis. However, although the clinical onset may be abrupt, the pathophysiologic insult is a slow, progressive phenomenon.[1]

Between 90% and 95% of Americans (19.7 million) have type 2 diabetes, making it the most common form of the disease in the United States[2]; it's also severely underdiagnosed.[3] Indeed, almost 30% of patients with type 2 diabetes don't know they have it.[3] The failure to diagnose this patient population results in progressive morbidity and mortality, with severe insulin resistance existing for years before the onset of hyperglycemia. Patients with type 2 diabetes have this relative insulin deficiency because their bodies either fail to make enough insulin or are unable to use insulin properly. Additionally, type 2 diabetes is a heterogeneous disorder for which specific secondary genetic causes of the metabolic syndrome are being rapidly identified. Type 2 diabetes, which is usually seen in older adults, is now being identified in a much younger population.[1]

Diabetes is the single most common underlying cause of lower-extremity amputation in the United States. Foot problems are one of the most common complications of diabetes that lead to hospitalization.[4-7] Indeed, admissions for foot complications account for 20% to 25% of all hospital days for patients with diabetes.[4,8,9] In the United States, approximately 120,000 nontraumatic lower-extremity amputations are performed each year, with 45% to 83% of these amputations involving patients with diabetes.[7,10,11] The risk of lower-extremity amputation in diabetics is 15 to 46 times higher than in nondiabetic patients.[4,5,7,10]

After the initial amputation, the risk of reamputation or amputation of the contralateral extremity is also high: 9% to 17% of patients will experience a second amputation within the same year,[4,12] and 25% to 68% will have an amputation of the contralateral extremity within 3 to 5 years.[4,13,14] The 5-year survival rate after a lower-extremity amputation ranges from 41% to 70%.[10,14]

Diabetes is a contributing factor in 75% to 83% of all amputations among blacks, Hispanics, and Native Americans.[4,7,15] The incidence of lower-extremity amputation is 1.5 times higher in Hispanics and 2.1 times higher in blacks compared with non-Hispanic whites. (See *ADA contact information*.)

ADA contact information

The American Diabetes Association (ADA)[1] offers much information for diabetic patients and their families as well as for health care professionals. General information about diabetes is available, along with advice on exercise, nutrition, and daily meal planning. To contact the ADA:

1701 N. Beauregard Street
Alexandria, VA 22311
1-800-DIABETES
www.diabetes.org

ETIOLOGY OF AND RISK FACTORS FOR FOOT ULCERS

A number of local and systemic risk factors for foot ulceration and amputations should be considered in the prevention and treatment of the diabetic foot. Perhaps the strongest and easiest risk factor to identify is the presence of a previous ulceration or amputation, which indicates the potential for recurrence due to scar formation or biomechanical abnormalities. The underlying pathology usually is not reversible, and most disease processes affecting the diabetic foot will continue to worsen over time. Three primary pathways or mechanisms of injury have been identified in the development of foot ulcers. These include wounds that result from ill-fitting shoes (low-pressure injuries that are associated with prolonged or constant pressure), ulcers on weight-bearing areas (repetitive moderate pressure and shear forces on the sole), and penetrating injuries from puncture wounds or other traumatic events (high-pressure injuries with a single exposure of direct pressure).[16] (See *color section*, *Diabetic Foot Ulcers*, page C24.)

In recent years, some studies have suggested that the incidence of amputations is declining in both the general population and in patients with diabetes. Rayman et al.[17] conducted a prospective study over a 3-year period in a large district general hospital population. This study was performed to show that diabetic foot interventions were having a positive result. Rayman et al. reported that amputation rates declined from 9.6 to 7.1 per 100,000 of the general population and from 3.48 to 2.61 per 1,000 people in their diabetic population.[17]

Neuropathy

Diabetes affects sensory, motor, and autonomic nerve function. In patients with sensory neuropathy, pain—the primary natural warning system that alerts the body to take action and seek medical care—is defective. Sensory neuropathy contributes to an inability to perceive injury to the foot due to what is commonly referred to as loss of protective sensation (LOPS).[18] LOPS represents a level of sensory loss where patients can injure themselves without recognizing the injury.

Motor neuropathy contributes to wasting of the intrinsic muscles of the foot; muscle imbalance; structural foot deformity, such as claw toes and subluxated metatarsophalangeal joints; and limited joint mobility. Autonomic neuropathy causes shunting of blood[19] and loss of sweat and oil gland function, which leads to dry, scaly skin that can easily develop cracks and fissures. The combined effect of these neuropathies results in a foot with structural deformity and biomechanical faults; dry, poorly hydrated integument; and an inability to respond to pain and repetitive injury.

Neuropathy is one of the most common risk factors for lower-extremity complications.[7, 18] It is unusual to see a patient with a foot ulceration who does not have sensory neuropathy.[20] Several screening methods can be used to identify sensory neuropathy, including a systematic clinical examination, vibration perception threshold (VPT) testing with a VPT Meter, and pressure assessment with Semmes-Weinstein monofilaments.[18, 21, 22] Although these methods are noninvasive and have good sensitivity and specificity to identify patients with loss of protective sensation,[23] Semmes-Weinstein monofilaments in particular may present several problems, which should be considered before using the device. Semmes-Weinstein monofilaments should be purchased from a vendor that sells *calibrated* instruments because considerable variability exists among different brands of monofilament.[24] Booth and Young found that some brands of monofilaments buckled at 8 g of force rather than at the 10 g for which they were designated.[24] In addition, the material properties of the monofilament wear out after repetitive testing. Young and colleagues[25] found that after 500 cycles of testing (or the equivalent of testing 10 sites on each foot for 25 patients), there was an average reduction of 1.2 g of testing force. A worn-out monofilament may result in patients being diagnosed as having sensory neuropathy with loss of protective sensation when they are not at risk. (See *Practice Point: Assessing protective sensation with a monofilament*.)

A systematic clinical examination can be an effective way to diagnose neuropathy and identify high-risk patients.[26] Abbott et al. used a modification of the neuropathy disability score to evaluate a large cohort of patients ($n = 9,710$) with diabetes.[26] The neuropathy disability score evaluates vibration with a 128-Hz tuning fork (Fig. 16-1), pin-prick, hot-cold perception, and Achilles deep tendon reflex. The deep tendon reflex is scored 0 if it is normal, 1 if reinforcement is required, and 2 if it is absent. The other tests are scored 0 for normal and 1 for abnormal. Each foot is scored, for a possible high score of 10. Abbott showed that high neuropathy disability scores (> 6) were associated with a higher ulcer incidence.

VPT testing is a quantitative evaluation that measures large myelinated nerve function. It is less prone to inter-operator variation than are monofilaments, and it does not need to be replaced to continue providing accurate results. The VPT Meter is a handheld device with a rubber head that is applied to a bony prominence, such as the medial aspect of the first metatarsal head or the tip of the great toe. The unit contains a linear scale that displays the applied voltage, ranging from 0 to 100 V. The amplitude is then slowly increased until the patient can feel the vibration. The inability

---

PRACTICE POINT

Not all monofilaments are of the same quality or last forever; be sure to use a calibrated instrument in your patient assessments.

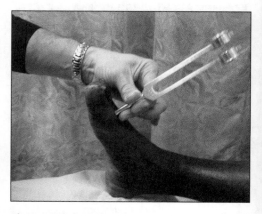

Figure 16-1. Vibration testing using a 128-Hz tuning fork.

PRACTICE POINT

Assessing Protective Sensation with a Monofilament

A Semmes-Weinstein 10-g (5.07 log) monofilament is commonly used to assess protective sensation in the feet of patients with diabetes. You can order the Semmes-Weinstein monofilament from the following companies:

- Center for Specialized Diabetic Foot Care: 1-800-543-9055
- North Coast Medical, Inc.: 408-283-1900
- Sensory Testing Systems: 1-888-289-9293
- Smith & Nephew Rehabilitation Division: 1-800-558-8633.

Use the 10-g (5.07 log) monofilament wire on each foot at the following 10 sites:

- plantar aspect of the first, third, and fifth digits
- plantar aspect of the first, third, and fifth metatarsal heads
- plantar midfoot medially and laterally
- plantar heel
- dorsal aspect of the midfoot.

Performing the test

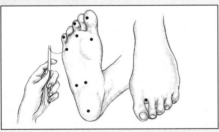

Place the patient in a supine or sitting position. Remove his socks and shoes and provide support for his legs. Touch the monofilament to the patient's arm or hand to demonstrate what it feels like. Then ask him to respond "yes" each time he feels the monofilament on his foot.

Place the patient's foot in a neutral position with his toes pointing straight up, and tell him to close his eyes. Remind him to say "yes" when he feels the monofilament on his foot. Hold the monofilament perpendicular to the patient's foot and press it against the first site, increasing the pressure until the monofilament wire bends into a C shape. Make sure it doesn't slide over the skin. Hold the monofilament in place for about 1 second. Record the patient's response on a foot-screening form. Use a "φφ" for a positive response and a "−" for a negative response. Then move to the next site.

Test all 10 sites at random and vary the time between applications so that the patient won't be able to guess the correct response. If he has a scar, callus, or necrotic tissue at a test site, apply the monofilament along the perimeter of the abnormality, not directly on it.

Loss of protective sensation is indicated if the patient can't feel the monofilament at any site on his foot. It's essential to teach a patient who has lost protective sensation to inspect and protect his feet.

Adapted with permission from Sloan, H.L., and Abel, R.J. "Getting in Touch with Impaired Foot Sensitivity," *Nursing* 28(11):50-51, November 1998; and Armstrong, D.G., et al. "Choosing a Practical Screening Instrument to Identify Patients at Risk for Diabetic Foot Ulceration," *Archives of Internal Medicine* 158(3):289-92, February 9, 1998.

to feel greater than 25 V is indicative of LOPS and puts the patient at risk for ulceration and amputation.

Peripheral arterial disease (PAD) in patients with diabetes is characterized by multiple occlusive plaques of small- and medium-sized arteries of the infrapopliteal vessels.[19] PAD puts the patient with diabetes at greater risk for foot ulcers, infections, and amputations.[7,27] Several theories attempt to explain the microvascular changes that occur in diabetes. One theory proposes that increased microvascular pressure and flow results in direct injury to the vascular endothelium, which in turn causes the release of extravascular matrix proteins. This leads to microvascular sclerosis and thickening of the capillary basement membrane. Capillary fragility also leads to microhemorrhage, which could be the reason that infection spreads through the tissue planes in patients with diabetes.[19,28] In addition to the direct effect on the vessels, an additional indirect effect on the microvasculature is mediated by the autonomic nervous system. LoGerfo and colleagues[29,30] believe that there is no microcirculatory occlusive process; rather, they suggest that some other indirect physiologic abnormality occurs. Altered microvascular blood flow is a complication of diabetic autonomic neuropathy that causes a shunting of blood away from the skin, making it prone to ulceration and impairing the healing process.[31]

It is likely that any theory of microvascular involvement in the process of diabetic ulceration and healing must include both the direct effects of glycosylation and local inflammation and the indirect effect of alteration of microvascular hemodynamics associated with autonomic dysfunction.

Evaluating vascular status should include a thorough history of symptoms of intermittent claudication, ischemic rest pain, and peripheral vascular surgery; clinical signs of ischemia, such as skin temperature, dependent rubor, pallor, hair loss, and shiny skin; and a clinical assessment of lower-extremity pulses.[32] According to the American College of Cardiology (ACC)/American Hospital Association (AHA) guidelines[33] for the management of patients with peripheral arterial disease, physicians should screen their patients for a diagnosis of PAD by determining bilateral resting ankle-brachial indices (ABIs). Patients 70 years or older suspected of having lower-extremity PAD are those with exertional leg pain or a nonhealing wound. The disease should also be suspected if the patient is 50 or older and has a history of smoking or diabetes. In addition, a toe-brachial index should be used when the ABI is not reliable because of excessively high systolic pressures in the ankle. When the ABI is greater than 1.3, the arteries are considered to be noncompressible. Segmental pressure measurements are useful to localize the site of lower-extremity PAD when planning a vascular intervention.

Laser Doppler assessment of skin perfusion pressure has been used in recent years as an objective method to assess the severity of PAD and to predict wound healing.[34] Castronuovo et al.[35] evaluated whether skin perfusion pressure could be used to distinguish foot ulcer patients with critical limb ischemia who would require vascular reconstruction or amputation from patients whose wounds would heal with local wound care or a minor amputation. They concluded that skin perfusion pressure measurement was approximately 80% accurate in diagnosing which patients with critical limb ischemia would not respond to less invasive care.

SKIN AND NAIL EXAMINATION

Evaluation of the skin and nails is critical to identify the subtle signs of impending injury, including high-pressure areas, cracks, maceration, or fissures in the skin. Patient education is an important aspect of care. All patients should be instructed on how to perform skin self-examinations as a preventive measure. (See *Patient Teaching: Skin-care teaching tips.*) Discoloration of a callus or bleeding under a callus is a sign of a preulcerative lesion. Likewise, deformed and thickened nails are commonly the source of abnormal pressure on the nail bed that can cause subungual ulcerations. Common nail disorders seen in patients with diabetes mellitus include onychomycosis (tinea unguium) and onychocryptosis (ingrown toenail).[32] While these are usually minor problems in persons without diabetes,

Patient Teaching
Skin-Care Teaching Tips

Teach your diabetic patient the following self-care points:

- Keep your diabetes well controlled. People with high sugar levels tend to have dry skin and less ability to fend off harmful bacteria. Both conditions increase the risk of infection.
- Keep skin clean and dry. Use talcum powder in areas where skin touches skin, such as armpits and groin.
- Avoid very hot baths and showers. If your skin is dry, don't use bubble baths. Moisturizing soaps, such as Dove or Basis, may help. Afterward, use an oil-in-water skin cream, such as Lubriderm or Alpha-Keri. Don't put lotions between your toes—the extra moisture there can encourage fungus to grow.
- Prevent dry skin. Moisturize your skin to prevent chapping.
- Don't scratch dry or itchy skin because doing so can tear the skin, allowing infection to occur.
- Treat cuts right away. Wash minor cuts with soap and water. Don't use mercurochrome antiseptic, alcohol, or iodine to clean skin because these agents are too harsh. Use an antibiotic cream or ointment only if your doctor says it's okay. Cover minor cuts with sterile gauze. See a doctor right away if you get a major cut, burn, or infection.
- During cold, dry months, keep your home more humid. Bathe less during this weather if possible.
- Use mild shampoos and unscented soaps. Don't use feminine hygiene sprays.
- See a dermatologist about skin problems if you aren't able to solve them yourself.
- Take good care of your feet. Check them every day for sores and cuts. Wear broad, flat shoes that fit well. Check your shoes for foreign objects before putting them on.

they can result in cellulitis, osteomyelitis, neuropathy, and vascular impairment in patients with diabetes.

MUSCULOSKELETAL EXAMINATION

In patients with neuropathy, ulcerations typically develop as a result of repetitive pressure and shear on the sole of the foot or from shoe pressure on the top or sides of the foot; however, no specific level of pressure has been determined to be abnormal or pathologic.[7,36–38] Diabetes alters biomechanics in patients with preexisting structural and functional foot deformities. Motor neuropathy is thought to contribute to atrophy and weakness of the intrinsic muscles of the foot. This leads to what has been called the "intrinsic minus foot," which describes wasting of the small (intrinsic) muscles that originate in the foot (flexor digitorum brevis, flexor hallucis brevis, extensor digitorum brevis, extensor hallucis brevis, lumbricales, interossei, and abductor hallucis).

Metatarsal ulcers can develop when digital deformities are irritated by the toe-box of a shoe or because of loss of fat pad and increased pressure under the metatarsal head (Fig. 16-2). The lesser digits contract and sublux dorsally, resulting in a claw toe deformity and a strong plantar flexor force at the metatarsophalangeal joints.[19,36,39] As the toes deform and the metatarsophalangeal joints dislocate, the metatarsal heads are literally driven through the bottom of the foot. The tips and dorsal aspects of the toes and the area beneath the metatarsophalangeal heads are subjected to increased pressure and friction, which, in the presence of loss of protective sensation, can lead to ulceration (Fig. 16-3).[19,36,40] Limited mobility of the ankle and metatarsophalangeal joints has been associated with soft tissue glycosylation

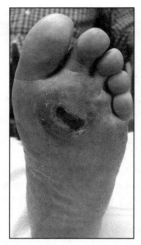

Figure 16-2. Metatarsal ulcer.

involving the gastro-soleus-Achilles complex and periarticular tissues. Limited motion of the ankle, subtalar, and metatarsophalangeal joints has been associated with high pressures in the forefoot. Often patients with an intrinsic minus foot will appear to have a high arch; however, this is not a congenital deformity but rather is due to atrophy of the abductor hallucis muscle belly on the medial side of the foot.

Infection

Soft tissue and bone infections are very common in persons with diabetic foot ulcerations. The majority of patients with diabetic foot ulcers (56%) will be treated for soft tissue

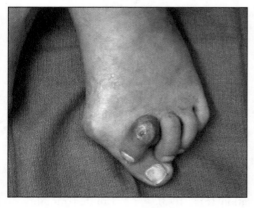

Figure 16-3. Ulcer on digital deformity. (Photo courtesy of J. McGuire. Used with permission.)

infection during the course of their ulceration. Approximately 20% of these patients will develop infection of the underlying bone.[41]

Identification of foot infections in patients with diabetes requires vigilance because the normal signs of infection may be blunted or absent.[2] Hyperglycemia impairs leukocyte functioning, including phagocytosis and intracellular killing function.[19] Patients with diabetes may also demonstrate a diminished inflammatory response, even when severe soft tissue and bone infections are present. However, frequent wound culture and the use of superficial swab cultures in wounds without clinical signs of infection are not helpful and should be discouraged. All open wounds have a normal bacterial flora, and routine swab culture will reveal several types of bacteria colonizing the wound.[42,43] Instead, wounds should be thoroughly débrided and cleansed before any cultures are taken. Tissue samples from the base of the wound should be sent for culture. Aerobic and anaerobic cultures should also be ordered when signs and symptoms of infection are present. (See chapter 7, Wound bioburden and infection.)

Wound depth is the strongest predictor of both soft tissue and bone infections. Compared with superficial wounds, the risk of infection for wounds that extend to the bone is 23.08 times higher for soft tissue and 6.71 times higher for bone (see Table 16-1).

Risk stratification

Evaluation of risk factors and risk stratification is important to prioritize the patient's treatment according to his or her individual needs.[44-46] Many healthcare providers either never evaluate the feet or generally consider everyone with diabetes to be "at-risk" for foot problems. This usually leads to no preventive care, but it can also contribute to unnecessary services for low-risk patients. To help evaluate individual risk factors, a risk classification system endorsed by the International Working Group on the Diabetic Foot[46,47] provides a validated scheme to stratify subjects based on their risk of ulceration and amputation. Key elements of the lower-extremity examination should help to risk-stratify subjects in order to

TABLE 16-1	Risk Factors for Soft Tissue and Bone Infections		
	Relative risk	**95% Confidence intervals**	**P value**
Risk factors for soft tissue infection			
Wound penetrates to bone	23.08	8.47-62.92	.0001
Previous history of ulceration prior to enrollment	2.15	1.07-4.32	.03
Recurrent/multiple wounds during study period	1.92	1.20-3.06	.007
Risk factors for bone infection			
Ulcer depth to bone	6.71	2.27-19.85	.001
Ulcer duration >30 days	4.66	1.62-13.37	.004
Recurrent foot ulceration	2.41	1.28-4.53	.006
Traumatic etiology to ulcer	2.36	1.12-4.98	.02
Peripheral vascular disease	1.93	1.04-3.56	.04

Adapted from Lavery, L.A., Armstrong, D.G., Wunderlich, R.P., Mohler, M.J., Wendel, C.S., Lipsky, B.A. "Risk Factors for Foot Infections in Individuals with Diabetes," *Diabetes Care* 29(6):1288, June 2006; and Lavery, L.A., Peters, E.J., Armstrong, D.G., Wendel, C.S., Murdoch, D.P., Lipsky, B.A. "Risk Factors for Developing Osteomyelitis in Patients with Diabetic Foot Wounds," *Diabetes Research in Clinical Practice* 83(3):347-52, March 2009.

identify the frequency and level of preventive care required. (See Table 16-2.)

MULTIDISCIPLINARY STRATEGIES

Many strategies can be used to help prevent foot complications in diabetic patients. Although the specific elements of a multispecialty approach to prevention haven't been studied, both systemic disease factors and local treatment are believed to be pivotal elements of long-term prevention.[47]

Careful management of systemic disease processes, including heart failure, renal insufficiency, and diabetes, is essential in order to minimize complications. Control of glucose level is critical to slow the multiple disease processes involved in diabetes-related foot complications. Indeed, hyperglycemia has been associated with a higher risk of ulceration and a poor healing response in patients with diabetes.[7] Effective glycemic control can be achieved through a comprehensive team effort that addresses dietary management, self-glucose monitoring, proper exercise, appropriate medication, and early recognition and treatment of hyperglycemia.[19] Several clinical studies have reported a 48% to 78%[48,49] reduction in amputations and a 47% to 49%[50,51] reduction in lower-extremity–related hospitalizations when high-risk diabetic patients are treated in specialty clinics. These clinics often include multiple specialties that focus on both prevention and care of acute complications in patients with diabetes. Further, consensus documents for prevention measures related to the "diabetic foot" have been developed by the American Orthopaedic Foot and Ankle Society,[52] the American College of Foot and Ankle Surgery,[53] the Registered Nurses' Association of Ontario, and the International Working Group on the Diabetic Foot.[47]

Foot care

Regular foot evaluation is essential to identify new risk factors and prevent impending complications. Podiatric physicians provide for debridement of callus and nails as well as

TABLE 16-2 Lavery-Peters Diabetic Foot Risk Classification

Category	Risk factors	Ulcer incidence	Amputation incidence	Prevention and treatment
1	No neuropathy No peripheral arterial disease (PAD) No history of ulcer	2%	0.04%	• Reevaluation once a year
2	Neuropathy ± deformity No PAD No history of ulcer or amputation	3.4%	0.05%	• Podiatry every 6 months • Over-the-counter shoes and insoles; evaluate appropriate fit
3	PAD No history of ulcer or amputation	13.8%	3.7%	• Podiatry every 2 to 3 months • Professionally fit therapeutic shoes and insoles • Patient education
4	Previous ulcer or amputation	31.5%	8.1%	• Podiatry every 1 to 2 months • Professionally fit therapeutic shoes and insoles • Patient education

Adapted from Lavery, L.A., Peters, E.J., Williams, J.R., Murdoch, D.P., Hudson, A., Lavery, D.C. "Reevaluating the Way We Classify the Diabetic Foot: Restructuring the Diabetic Foot Risk Classification System of the International Working Group on the Diabetic Foot," *Diabetes Care* 31(1):154-6, January 2008.

regular evaluation of shoes and insoles. These routine encounters offer an additional opportunity to reinforce key educational elements, such as the need to avoid going barefoot, hydrate the skin, and inspect the feet daily. Protective footwear and insoles can be prescribed for the patient and then evaluated and monitored for their effectiveness.

Protective footwear and pressure redistribution

The primary role of therapeutic footwear is to protect the foot from repetitive injuries and eliminate the shoe as a source of pathology. Extra-depth shoes have a high toe-box with

enough depth throughout the shoe to accommodate a total contact molded insole or orthotic. These are often recommended for patients with structural foot deformities, such as claw toes or dislocated metatarsophalangeal joints. These types of shoes usually allow for up to a ⅜"-thick accommodative insole to fit without irritating the top or sides of the foot. (See *Wide-toe shoe with insert*.) The combination of a correctly sized shoe and a protective insole can reduce pressure on the sole, top, and sides of the foot by as much as 20%.[54, 55]

Custom-molded shoes are individually made from a mold of the patient's foot. Because custom-molded shoes can be expensive and require several weeks or months to make, however,

Wide-toe shoe with insert

Shoes with a deep toe-box and that are "extra depth" throughout the shoe are the mainstay of diabetic wound preventive care. The shoes typically come with laces, as shown here, or with Velcro closures.

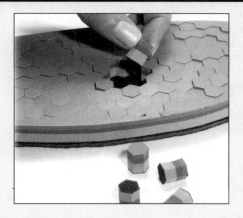

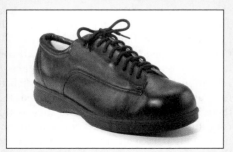

The combination of a correctly sized shoe and an accommodative insole can reduce pressure on the sole, top, and sides of the foot. The insert is customized to relieve pressure, according to the patient's needs, and then placed inside the shoe.

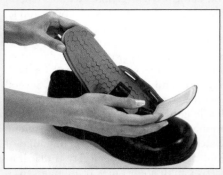

Photographs courtesy of Royce Medical Co.

they are only necessary in a small percentage of high-risk patients with severe foot deformities that cannot be accommodated by off-the-shelf shoes. For most patients with less severe deformities, there are a number of more affordable athletic, comfort, and therapeutic shoes with multiple sizes and extra depth to accommodate a wide variety of foot deformities.

THE DIABETIC SHOE BILL

Patients with diabetes who are "at risk" for foot disease and who have Medicare Part B are eligible for Medicare's Therapeutic Shoe Bill.[56] In order to qualify, a patient must have diabetes and one or more of the following: previous amputation of part or all of either foot; a history of previous foot ulceration or preulcerative calluses; peripheral neuropathy with evidence of callus formation; foot deformity; or poor circulation.

The bill covers one of the following annually: one pair of off-the-shelf extra-depth shoes and three additional pairs of multi-density inserts or custom-molded orthoses; one pair of off-the-shelf extra-depth shoes, including a modification and two additional pairs of multi-density inserts; or one pair of custom-molded shoes and two additional pairs of multi-density inserts.

Elective and prophylactic surgery

Is there good evidence that elective or prophylactic foot surgery in patients who have diabetes will prevent ulceration in the future? Armstrong and colleagues validated a four-tier surgery classification that consists of elective, prophylactic, curative, and emergent surgery.[57] Elective surgery is planned reconstructive surgery in a patient with foot deformity to eliminate pain or to enhance function. Prophylactic surgery is intended to prevent ulcer recurrence. Curative surgery is intended to facilitate wound healing in a patient with an existing foot wound. Emergent surgery is intended to remove infection or devitalized tissue.[57]

There is no evidence that elective surgery reduces the risk of future ulceration. Patients with diabetes should undergo elective foot surgery only if they have severe deformity, pain, or functional limitations that warrant surgery rather than an expectation that surgery will prevent a foot ulcer in the future.

Prophylactic surgery includes toe and bunion deformity correction, Achilles tendon lengthening, and exostectomy. For example, percutaneous lengthening of the Achilles tendon[58] has been shown to reduce plantar foot pressures in subjects with prior ulceration. This type of surgery has been used for both prophylactic and curative treatment. Several authors have reported on the use of Achilles tendon lengthening in patients with forefoot ulcerations due to a tight Achilles tendon associated with limited ankle joint range of motion. The rationale for surgery is that limited active ankle joint range of motion causes more pressure and shear stresses on the ball of the foot, leading to ulceration. Armstrong and colleagues demonstrated a reduction of about 27% reduction in forefoot loading after lengthening the Achilles.[59]

Several clinical studies have described the procedure and clinical results of Achilles tendon lengthening to prevent ulcer recurrence. Lin et al.[60] reported on a cohort of patients with diabetic foot ulcers that failed to heal after a period of immobilization via a total contact cast (TCC). Using the Achilles lengthening procedure, 93% of patients (14/15) healed in an average of 39 days with no ulcer recurrence in the subsequent 17 months.[60] In a randomized clinical trial, Mueller compared neuropathic ulcer healing in patients using the same procedure versus TCC immobilization.[61] Ulcers healed in all of the patients who underwent surgery ($n = 31$) as compared with 88% ($n = 33$) of patients in the TCC group. Patients with Achilles lengthening had less than half the incidence of ulcer recurrence (31% vs. 81%) compared with patients in the TCC group.[61]

Preventive education

Education has long been assumed to be an essential component of any program designed to reduce the incidence of diabetic foot ulcers. Preventive education usually takes the form of an intensive introduction to the disease and includes practical steps to cope with the manifestations of diabetes over time. In a 2004 *Cochrane Review*[62] of nine randomized, controlled trials to determine the effectiveness of educational programs in preventing diabetic foot ulceration, the authors concluded that there was only weak evidence to suggest that education reduces foot ulceration and amputations in high-risk patients. On the other hand, the studies reinforced the idea that increased knowledge of foot care had a positive effect on patient behavior in the short term. While this initial approach is good, continual education and reinforcement may be necessary, especially among high-risk patients, in order to have a continued effect on patient outcomes. The data from this review suggest not only that more study is needed in this area but also that the educational programs we currently employ need to be revamped to improve their effectiveness over the long term.

To complicate matters, many diabetics have severe limitations to classical education methods. A large proportion of patients both with and without foot ulcers lacked the visual acuity, manual dexterity, or joint flexibility to perform the self-examination necessary to care for their feet.[7] Among ulcer patients, 49% could not position or see their feet, and 15% were legally blind in at least one eye. When patients are obese or have limited joint mobility or impaired vision, education and self-assessment skills should be directed to both the patient and his or her spouse or caregiver.[7] Repetition and regular reinforcement should be practiced by every member of the healthcare team to help the patient and family maintain an understanding of the disease process and continue to practice protective behaviors to avoid some of the serious complications of diabetes.

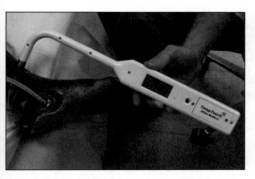

Figure 16-4. TempTouch infrared temperature monitoring device. (Diabetica Solutions, San Antonio, TX.)

Temperature monitoring

At-home temperature monitoring is a new concept for high-risk patients to identify early warning signs of tissue injury before a foot ulcer actually develops (Fig. 16-4). Because neuropathy inhibits the natural warning system, local inflammation and pain as a result of tissue trauma go unnoticed. Several studies have used temperature assessment as a surrogate to identify tissue injury in patients at risk for diabetic foot ulcers and pressure ulcers. Indeed, two randomized clinical trials demonstrated a 3- to 10-fold reduction in foot complications among high-risk patients using at-home temperature assessment as compared with standard prevention therapy, consisting of therapeutic shoes and insoles, regular podiatry evaluation, and foot-specific education.[63,64]

Two main barriers contribute to poor results with "standard" prevention practices. First, patients often cannot visualize their feet in order to evaluate them.[7] Second, the visual signs of tissue injury are probably too subtle for even the most motivated patient or family member to accurately identify. In a randomized study by Lavery and colleagues,[63] for example, by the time the majority of patients identified "areas of concern," an ulcer had already developed. Therefore, self-monitoring with an infrared temperature device provides a mechanism to identify the precursor to ulcer and gives the high-risk patient enough time to reduce his or her activity in order to avoid ulcer development.

> **PRACTICE POINT**
>
> At-home temperature monitoring can provide objective feedback to warn patients with neuropathy that their feet are injured before an ulcer develops.

WOUND CHARACTERISTICS AND ASSESSMENT

Several classification systems can be used to classify diabetic ulcers. The University of Texas ulcer classification system (Table 16-3) is a validated system that includes a mechanism to document wound depth as well as the presence of infection and vascular impairment—two pivotal factors in predicting clinical outcomes.[6,65] Using this system, the risk of amputation has been shown to be predictive of amputation as wounds increase in depth (grade 0 to III) and progress from no infection (class A), to infection (class B), to PAD (class C), and to infection and PAD (class D).

A classification scheme first described by Meggitt[66] and popularized by Wagner[67] has also been used extensively but has the disadvantage of not consistently including wound depth or the presence of infection (Table 16-4). Osteomyelitis is the only type of infection included, and end-stage disease events of gangrene are the only vascular parameters included. Furthermore, the system is difficult to use for more subtle disease processes that are critical for clinical decision making.

The ADA Consensus report[2] recommends that a systematic wound assessment include the following questions in the evaluation:

- Has the patient experienced trauma? Is the ulcer a result of penetrating trauma, blunt trauma, or burn?
- What is the duration of the wound? Is the ulcer acute or chronic?
- What is the progression of local or systemic signs and symptoms? Is the wound getting better, is it stable, or is it deteriorating?
- Has the patient had any prior treatment of the wound or previous wounds? What treatments worked? What failed?

TABLE 16-3 University of Texas Diabetic Wound Classification System

Class	Grade 0	I	II	III
A	Preulcerative or postulcerative lesion, completely epithelialized	Superficial wound, not involving tendon, capsule, or bone	Wound penetrating to tendon or capsule	Wound penetrating to bone or joint
B	Preulcerative or postulcerative lesion, completely epithelialized with infection	Superficial wound, not involving tendon, capsule, or bone, with infection	Wound penetrating to tendon or capsule with infection	Wound penetrating to bone or joint with infection
C	Preulcerative or postulcerative lesion, completely epithelialized with ischemia	Superficial wound, not involving tendon, capsule, or bone, with ischemia	Wound penetrating to tendon or capsule with ischemia	Wound penetrating to bone or joint with ischemia
D	Preulcerative or postulcerative lesion, completely epithelialized with infection and ischemia	Superficial wound, not involving tendon, capsule, or bone, with infection and ischemia	Wound penetrating to tendon or capsule with infection and ischemia	Wound penetrating to bone or joint with infection and ischemia

Reprinted with permission from Armstrong, D.G., et al. "Validation of a Diabetic Wound Classification System: The Contribution of Depth, Infection, and Ischemia to Risk of Amputation," *Diabetes Care* 21(5):855-69, May 1998.

TABLE 16-4 Meggitt-Wagner Ulcer Classification

Grade	Wound characteristics
0	Preulceration lesions, healed ulcers, presence of bony deformity
1	Superficial ulcer without subcutaneous tissue involvement
2	Penetration through the subcutaneous tissue; may expose bone, tendon, ligament, or joint capsule
3	Osteitis, abscess, or osteomyelitis
4	Gangrene of digit
5	Gangrene of foot

Reprinted with permission from Wagner, F.W. "The Dysvascular Foot: A System for Diagnosis and Treatment," *Foot & Ankle* 2(2):64-122, September 1981; and Meggitt, B. "Surgical Management of the Diabetic Foot," *British Journal of Hospital Medicine* 16:227-32, 1976.

In addition, blood glucose control and comorbidities should be evaluated. Clinical assessment should identify:

- signs of ischemia—adequate blood flow to heal the wound
- signs of soft tissue or bone infection—unpleasant odor, cellulitis, abscess, or osteomyelitis
- wound depth—undermining or exposed tendon, joint capsule, or bone
- appearance—surrounding callus, devitalized tissue, granulation tissue, drainage, eschar, or necrosis.

PRACTICE POINT

Six essentials of the ADA treatment algorithm[68]

- debridement, early and often
- reducing pressure
- moist-wound healing
- treating infection
- correcting ischemia (below the knee disease)
- preventing amputation.

Debridement

Sharp debridement of the ulcer removes devitalized tissue, reduces the bacterial load of the wound, eliminates proteases from the wound bed, and provides a bleeding wound bed. A diabetic ulcer typically has a thick rim of keratinized tissue surrounding it. Debridement must remove all of the callus and devitalized tissue, so that a clean wound edge is created and all edge pressure from the callus is removed. Enzymatic or autolytic debridement may be an option if sharp debridement is not possible or if the patient has PAD.[32] Ongoing debridement may be needed throughout the healing process.[19,69] Indeed, higher healing rates have been observed in patients who have had more frequent debridement.[69] In addition, in a post-hoc evaluation from the becaplermin gel pivotal trial, Steed reported a higher proportion of healed wounds in both the treatment and placebo study groups when wound debridement was performed more frequently.[70]

STRATEGIES TO REDUCE PRESSURE

Reduction of pressure and shear forces on the foot may be the single most important yet most often neglected aspect of neuropathic ulcer treatment. Off-loading therapy is a key part of the treatment plan for diabetic foot ulcers. The goal is to reduce the pressure at the ulcer site and keep the patient ambulatory.[19,54,71, 72] Several methods are available to protect the foot from abnormal pressures (see Table 16–5). Off-loading strategies must be tailored to the age, strength, activity, and home environment of the patient. In general, however, more restrictive off-loading approaches will result in less activity and better wound healing. Education is critical to improve compliance with off-loading. The patient must understand that the wound is a result of repetitive pressure and that every unprotected step is literally tearing the wound apart.

PRACTICE POINT

Methods to off-load the diabetic foot include:

- bed rest
- wheelchair
- ambulatory aids (crutches, walker)
- felted foam padding
- half-shoes
- therapeutic shoes
- custom shoes
- custom total contact foot orthoses
- custom splints or braces
- prefabricated cast walkers
- total contact casting.

Total contact cast

Use of a TCC is considered the gold standard for off-loading the foot. TCCs reduce pressure at the ulcer site while still allowing the patient to be ambulatory.[19,71] A skilled clinician or technician is required to apply the molded plaster cast to ensure a proper fit. A TCC is a modification of a traditional fracture cast that uses minimal cast padding and includes a covering to protect the toes. The cast is molded to the

TABLE 16-5	Off-Loading Modalities and Wound Healing		
Off-loading modality	**Mean healing time**	**Percent healed**	**Source**
Total contact cast	• Forefoot ulcers: 30 days • Midfoot and hindfoot ulcers: 63 days	90%	Myerson, M., et al.[99]
Total contact cast	• 38 days	73%	Helm, P.A., et al.[75]
Total contact cast	• 44 days	82%	Sinacore, D.R., et al.[76]
Total contact cast	• Forefoot ulcers: 31 days • Nonforefoot ulcers: 42.1 days	Not reported	Walker, S.C., et al.[73]
Total contact cast	• Midfoot ulcers: 28 days	100%	Lavery, L.A., et al.[77]
Total contact cast Cast boot Half-shoe	• 34 days • 50 days • 61 days	90% 65% 58%	Armstrong, D.G., et al.[78]
Total contact cast Shoe insole	• 42 days • 65 days	90% 32%	Mueller, M.J., et al.[79]
Scotch cast boot	• 112 days • 181 days	80%	Knowles, E.A., et al.[86]
Half-shoe	• 70 days	96%	Chantelau, E., et al.[87]
Custom splint	• 300 days	Not reported	Boninger, M.L., and Leonard, J.A.[88]

contour of the foot and leg so that no movement is possible within the cast (Fig. 16-5). TCCs are generally changed every 1 to 2 weeks but may need to be replaced more frequently in patients with edema or other concerns.

A TCC is one of the most effective ways of treating plantar neuropathic foot ulcers.[71,73,74] Numerous studies[73–76,78–81] have shown that TCCs can heal ulcers in 6 to 8 weeks. In descriptive and randomized clinical trials, the proportion of wounds that heal with TCCs is consistently much higher than those using topical growth factors, bioengineered tissue, or special dressings.[82–85]

One of the main advantages of using a TCC is that it forces patient compliance with off-loading. The ulcer is protected with every step the patient takes. Using a TCC to facilitate wound healing is analogous to using a cast to heal a fracture—in both cases, healing is facilitated by rest

and immobilization. The TCC reduces the patient's activity level,[78] decreases stride length and cadence, and significantly reduces pressure at the ulcer site.[71,74] The main disadvantages for patients are the same as their complaints with a fracture cast—a cast is heavy and hot and makes bathing, walking, and sleeping difficult.

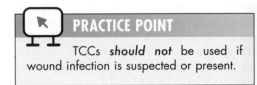

PRACTICE POINT

TCCs *should not* be used if wound infection is suspected or present.

Removable cast walkers

The effectiveness of removable cast walkers to reduce pressure at ulcer sites has been shown in several studies to be comparable to that

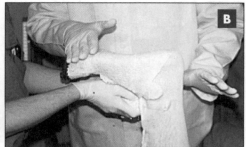
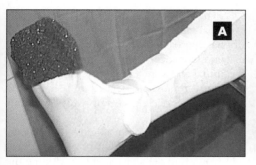
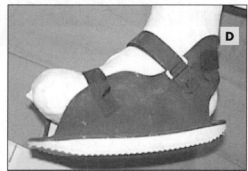
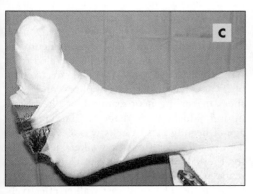

Figure 16-5. Applying a total contact cast (TCC). (A) A foam layer covers the toes for protection, and padding is applied over bony prominences before the first layer of casting material is applied. (B) Application of the TCC. (C) Completed TCC. (D) A cast boot covers the TCC.

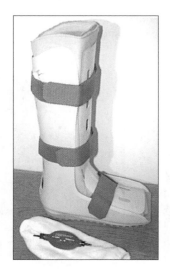

Figure 16-6. Removable walking boot. This prefabricated boot is used as an off-loading device.

of TCCs (Fig. 16-6).[71,74] Many practitioners consider removable cast walkers to be their preferred off-loading device because they are less time-consuming and easier to apply than TCCs and they are more readily accepted by patients. In addition, the TCC has several precautions and contraindications that aren't issues with removable walkers. Edema can be overcome with constant adjustments to the fit of the device, and compression dressings can be applied in conjunction with the removable cast boot. Wounds can be inspected regularly and treated with advanced wound care products such as growth factors, electrical stimulation, and other biologically active dressings. Because the wound and limb can be inspected frequently, the vascular concerns inherent in the occlusive irremovable TCC aren't an issue.

Additional advantages of removable walking boots (as compared with TCCs) are that

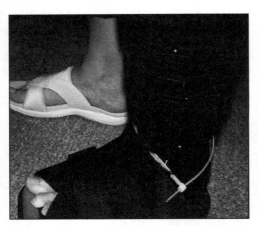

Figure 16-7. Instant total contact cast (ITCC) (irremovable cast walker) with a cable tie to prevent removal of the device.

they're relatively inexpensive, the protective insole can be easily replaced if it shows signs of wear, no special training is required for correct and safe application, and they can be easily removed to assess and débride the wound as appropriate.[74,78,79,86–88] It's also possible to modify removable walkers into non-removable devices by securing the walker with cast material or a non-removable cable tie; this is known as an instant TCC (ITCC; Fig. 16-7). If patients can't remove the walker, the element of forced compliance that makes the TCC attractive is maintained and the outcomes for healing improve to the levels seen with the TCC.[72,89–91]

No one off-loading device is appropriate for every patient. McGuire[92] has suggested a transitional approach to healing and maturing the diabetic foot ulcer that uses the instant TCC for initial pressure management and transitioning to removable devices and shoe-based platforms before the patient is ready for definitive footwear.

A number of removable walking boots have been designed to help protect and heal foot wounds in diabetic patients, including the Royce Medical Active Hex Walker (formerly known as the DH Pressure Relief Walker), the Bledsoe Diabetic Conformer Boot, the DonJoy Diabetic Walker, and the Aircast Pneumatic Walker.[90,93] In a randomized controlled trial, Armstrong et al.[94] compared the effectiveness of TCCs, removable cast walkers, and half-shoes in healing neuropathic foot ulcerations in individuals with diabetes. The percentage of healing at 12 weeks was 89.5% for the TCC, 65.0% for the cast walker, and 58.3% for the half-shoe.[94] When the cast walker is made non-removable (ITCC), the difference between the TCC and cast walker effectively disappears.[95]

ROYCE ACTIVE HEX WALKER

The Royce Active Hex Walker has been shown to be identical to TCCs in pressure reduction at the site of ulcerations on the sole (Fig. 16-8).[74] The walker is a low-profile boot with a fixed ankle rocker sole. The interior holds a patented insole

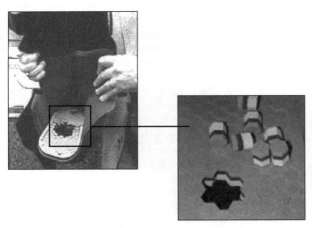
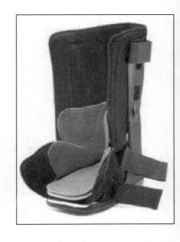

Figure 16-8. Royce Medical Active Hex Walker.

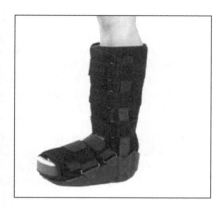

Figure 16-9. Donjoy High-Tide Diabetic Walker.

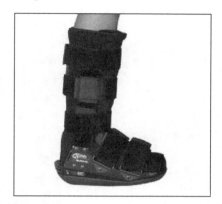

Figure 16-10. Bledsoe Diabetic Conformer Boot.

comprised of a series of hexagonal plugs attached to its base by Velcro. The plugs are made of layers of firm-density urethane, medium-density ethylene vinyl acetate, and soft urethane. The insole can absorb shock, conform to the shape of the foot and, because of the independent motion of the hex plugs, reduce shear forces during ambulation. The hex plugs can be removed in areas of high pressure to aid in ulcer healing. In a study by Lavery et al., the off-loading capacity of the Royce walker was the best of several other cast walkers and comparable to that of the TCC.[71,74]

DONJOY DIABETIC WALKER

A similar system is used in the DonJoy Diabetic Walker, which incorporates removable diamond-shaped sections in a Plastazote contact layer, thus eliminating the need to cover the removed sections to prevent loosening (Fig. 16-9).

BLEDSOE CONFORMER DIABETIC BOOT

The Bledsoe Conformer Diabetic Boot also incorporates a fixed ankle, rigid rocker design with a "memory foam" insole. In a study by Pollo et al., the Bledsoe walker was shown to be superior to the TCC in off-loading all areas of the foot tested (Fig. 16-10).[96]

AIRCAST DIABETIC WALKER

The Aircast Diabetic Walker has a wide-profile rocker sole and a multi-density Plastazote insole that can be heated or dynamically

molded to create a total contact footbed for the walker (Fig. 16-11).

Healing sandals and half-shoes

A number of healing sandals and half-shoes or wedged shoes are available to reduce pressure on the forefoot (Fig. 16-12). These sandals and shoes are useful for patients who can't tolerate a TCC or for those who need a transitional device after removal of a TCC while they're awaiting custom-made therapeutic shoes and insoles. A modification of the Carville healing sandal can be made from a standard surgical shoe with a total contact direct-molded Plastazote insole (Fig. 16-13).[97]

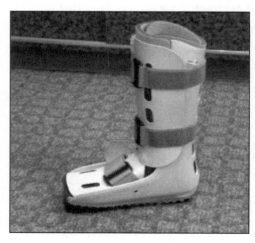

Figure 16-11. Aircast Diabetic Walker.

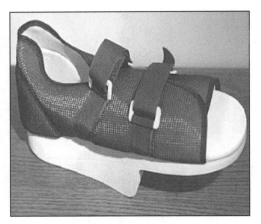

Figure 16-12. Wedged forefront-relief shoe.

Surgical shoes with a rocker sole design are preferable to the flat design for postoperative use. Royce Medical has a healing sandal that utilizes the Active Hex insole, described above, and can be used as a transitional device after closing the wound.

The OrthoWedge shoe by Darco products was originally designed to protect the forefoot after elective surgery. This shoe has a sole that's wedged at a 10-degree dorsiflexion angle, effectively removing pressure from the forefoot area. Studies by Needleman[27] and Lair[98] provide support for its role in postoperative patients following surgery on the forefoot. However, these types of shoes aren't well accepted by patients because they're difficult to walk in, they typically cause pain of the contralateral extremity, and they are not safe for

use in patients with postural instability. Also, most diabetics have equinus and can't tolerate the negative heel position created by the shoe. Further, suspension of the heel during ambulation increases pressure on the forefoot and stresses the midfoot, a common site for collapse in the diabetic Charcot foot. In a randomized clinical trial that compared TCCs with healing sandals and removable cast boots, patients in the healing sandal group were less compliant and used the device during walking significantly less than did subjects in the TCC group.[36,77,78]

Ankle-foot orthoses

Custom-made ankle-foot orthoses can be used for lower-extremity pathology, including Charcot fractures, tendon injuries, and neuropathic ulcers (Fig. 16-14). The Charcot Restraint Orthotic Walker (Fig. 16-15), for example, initially was used to treat patients with neuropathic fractures. It provides protection to the neuropathic foot and aids in controlling lower-extremity edema. This device looks like a ski boot; it has a rigid polypropylene shell with a rocker bottom sole.[36]

The primary drawback to custom-made devices is that they typically cost more than $1,000. If the structure of the foot changes or local edema resolves, the device can no longer be used. Since a number of less expensive, off-the-shelf products are now available to treat neuropathic wounds, custom ankle-foot orthoses are used less commonly. Off-the-shelf devices should be replaced at regular intervals

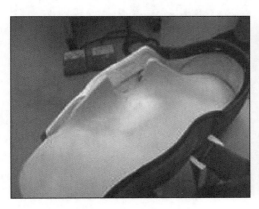

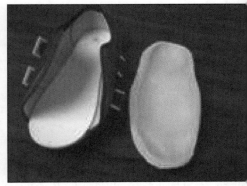

Figure 16-13. Carville healing sandal.

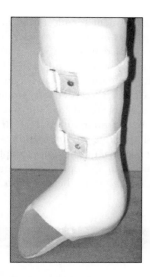

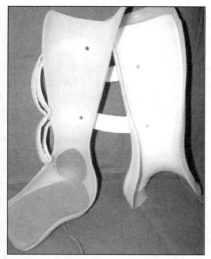

Figure 16-14. Custom-made ankle-foot orthoses.

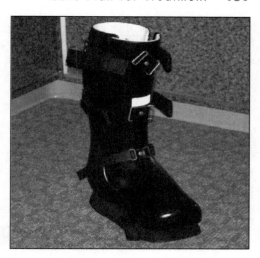

Figure 16-15. Charcot Restraint Orthotic Walker.

because the materials in the insoles will lose their effectiveness over time.[55]

DIAGNOSTIC IMAGING

Whenever there's an open wound on the foot it's always wise to order an X-ray initially to check for the presence of osteomyelitis. If the wound has been open for several weeks or if bone can be palpated with a sterile probe, further investigation is warranted even if standard X-rays are negative.[9]

After radiography, most clinicians would agree that the magnetic resonance imaging is the next diagnostic modality of choice to detect the presence of osteomyelitis. If X-ray reveals bone destruction and magnetic resonance imaging reveals osteomyelitis, a bone biopsy should be obtained prior to considering an ablative procedure such as an amputation.

Technetium bone scans are often ordered for patients with expected infection. These scans show increased uptake in the area of infection, but they're nonspecific and also show increased uptake in any area of osseous activity, such as with arthritis or a Charcot fracture. White blood cell–labeled bone scans, such as an indium–technetium scan or a hexamethyl propylene amine oxime scan, can also be compared with standard technetium scan. In the presence of Charcot fracture, the bone will exhibit increased uptake in the techneium scan but not in the labeled scan.

CARE PLAN FOR TREATMENT

A comprehensive care plan is vital to treating foot ulcers in persons with neuropathy. Glycemic control as measured by hemoglobin A1c may influence selection of some advanced therapies. Assessment of vascular supply and adequate circulation is also essential for wound healing.

SUMMARY

Diabetic foot ulcer care is a challenge for both the patient and the healthcare provider. As the population continues to age, the incidence of diabetes will continue to increase, which will in turn lead to more diabetic wounds. A team approach—with total involvement of the healthcare system and the necessary partnership with the patient—will be the infrastructure for achieving better outcomes of care.

Early assessment for ulceration in persons with diabetes is essential. A variety of methods must be used to identify at-risk persons. Appropriate skin care and properly fitting shoes are mandatory for any person with diabetes. Clinicians can choose among many products available to off-load the diabetic foot. Infection is an important concern in diabetic ulcers and warrants prompt identification and treatment. Adjuvant therapies coupled with debridement and appropriate dressings can be critical in salvaging the diabetic limb.

PATIENT SCENARIO

Clinical Data

Mr. JS is a 55-year-old white man who came to our clinic 4 months ago with an open wound on the plantar surface of the right foot under the first metatarsal head (Fig. 16-16A). According to Mr. JS, the wound had been open for 4 months but did not concern him because he was completely pain-free. He discovered the wound one evening after noticing an area of drainage on his sock. Beyond covering the wound with an adhesive bandage, Mr. JS ignored it initially; however, persistent drainage from the wound forced him to seek care from his local podiatrist. The patient could not recall any single precipitating event for the wound and had been trying to maintain a full work schedule as a salesman while allowing the wound to heal.

Mr. JS has had type II diabetes for the past 15 years. He has been hypertensive (135/90 controlled) for the past 10 years and already has a mildly elevated creatinine level (1.8). His medications include valsartan and metformin.

Initial treatment consisted of debridement, topical mupirocin ointment, becaplermin gel, and dry sterile dressings. The only off-loading device prescribed was an unmodified wedge-style surgical shoe (Fig. 16-16B). Mr. JS frequently wears dress shoes for long periods of time for work rather than the surgical shoe prescribed for him as an off-loading device. The ulcer has not improved over the past 4 months.

During the current visit, Mr. JS's feet are warm, dry, and scaling bilaterally. Both feet have thick callus under the first metatarsal head but no other significant keratotic lesions. The right foot has an ulcer under the head of the first metatarsal; the ulcer is red and measures 3.0 × 2.5 × 0.4 cm. The wound is assigned a grade of 2A on the University of Texas classification system after X-rays reveal that no osteomyelitis is present.

A Semmes-Weinstein 5.07 nylon monofilament is used to check for neuropathy. The patient is unable to feel the monofilament at any site tested, revealing significant bilateral neuropathy. He also has no pain or temperature sensation in either foot.

He has good pulses bilaterally with a 2/4 grade on the dorsalis pedis and posterior tibial arteries. The capillary refill time is less than 2 seconds on all digits.

Biomechanical evaluation reveals a plantar-flexed, non-weight-bearing first metatarsal with significant equinus bilaterally (0-degree ankle dorsiflexion with the knee straight). When not in dress shoes, Mr. JS wears comfortable shoes with a flexible sole, such as sneakers. He has depth shoes but doesn't like to wear them in public.

(continued)

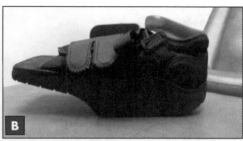
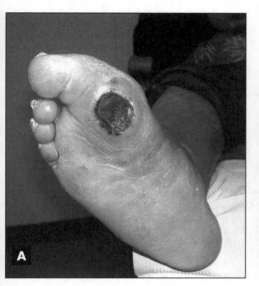
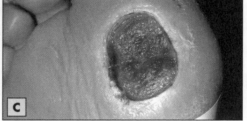

Figure 16-16. Neuropathic diabetic ulcer sub–first metatarsal. (A) The wound on initial presentation. (B) The off-loading device prescribed initially. (C) The wound following debridement and cleansing. (Photos courtesy of J. Mc Guire, DPM, PT.) (See *color section, Patient Scenarios*, page C46, for the color versions of these images.)

Case Discussion

Sharp debridement was employed to remove callus from the wound edges and fibrous tissue from the wound base, and the wound was cleansed with a superoxygenated water solution (Fig. 16-16C). Because of the age of the wound, a sample of tissue from the wound base was sent for culture. No predominant microorganism was identified. No bone could be palpated when the wound was examined with a sterile probe. The wound was dressed with oxidized regenerated cellulose with silver and covered with a non-adherent silver alginate dressing. Similar dressings were ordered for the patient for home application every other day. He was placed in a cast walker with removable segments in the insole that could be removed during a subsequent visit if further pressure relief became necessary. The cast walker was made non-removable by securing the boot to the leg with a single plastic cable tie. The patient was told to leave the boot in place until he returned in 5 days. He was given a pair of crutches and instructed by the physical therapy department on how to use them safely.

The wound healed steadily for 9 weeks and had just closed when the patient was transitioned to a removable cast walker so that he could exercise the foot and ankle and begin bathing and hydrating the skin. At 12 weeks, he was transitioned to a modified healing sandal and measured for depth shoes with custom-molded insoles and rigid rocker soles. He began wearing his new shoes 2 weeks later. He returns every 8 weeks for callus debridement and assessment of his feet.

SHOW WHAT YOU KNOW

1. According to the ADA, how many people are unaware that they have diabetes mellitus?
   A. 50%
   B. 30%
   C. 75%
   D. 25%

   ANSWER: B. *One-third of people with diabetes are unaware of their condition.*

2. The single leading cause of lower-extremity amputation is:
   A. diabetes mellitus.
   B. lymphedema.
   C. arterial occlusion.
   D. venous disease.

   ANSWER: A. *Diabetes mellitus is the single leading cause of lower-extremity amputation. While B, C, D are conditions that can contribute to complications in the diabetic patient, they aren't listed as the leading cause for amputation.*

3. According to the ADA, good skin care for patients with diabetes includes all of the following except:
   A. keeping skin clean and dry.
   B. applying moisturizers between toes.
   C. avoiding very hot showers and tub baths.
   D. checking feet daily for cracks or fissures.

   ANSWER: B. *Moisturizers shouldn't be applied between the toes—fungal infections can occur. All others are ADA recommendations for good skin care.*

4. Off-loading strategies must be tailored to the age, strength, activity, and home environment of the patient.
   A. True
   B. False

   ANSWER: A. *Off-loading must be tailored to the individual.*

5. For which of the following treatment strategies have healing rates for diabetic foot ulcers been found to be comparable to those with TCCs?
   A. Wedged shoe
   B. Half shoe
   C. Wide-toe shoe
   D. Walker boot rendered irremovable (ITCC)

   ANSWER: D. *Studies have found that making walking boots irremovable (ITCC) offers patients the same level of healing as with the gold standard of off-loading, the TCC. The other options are all removable shoes, but research has not demonstrated healing rates comparable to TCC.*

REFERENCES

1. American Diabetes Association. www.diabetes.org. Accessed November 7, 2010.
2. "American Diabetes Association: Clinical Practice Recommendations." *Diabetes Care* 21(Suppl 1):1999.
3. Centers for Disease Control and Prevention. *The Public Health of Diabetes Mellitus in the United States*. Atlanta, GA: Department of Health and Human Services, 1997.
4. Reiber, G.E., et al. "Lower Extremity Foot Ulcers and Amputations in Diabetes," in Mi, H., ed.

Diabetes in America, 2nd ed. Washington, DC: National Institutes of Health, 1995.

5. Lavery, L.A., et al. "Increased Foot Pressures After Great Toe Amputation in Diabetes," *Diabetes Care* 18(11):1460-62, November 1995.

6. Lavery, L.A., et al. "Classification of Diabetic Foot Wounds," *Journal of Foot and Ankle Surgery* 35(6):528-31, November-December 1996.

7. Lavery, L.A., et al. "Practical Criteria for Screening Patients at High Risk for Diabetic Foot Ulceration," *Archives of Internal Medicine* 158(2):157-62, January 26, 1998.

8. Miller, A.D., et al. "Diabetes Related Lower-extremity amputation in New Jersey 1979 to 1981," *Journal of the Medical Society of New Jersey* 82(9):723-26, September 1985.

9. Pecoraro, R.E. "Chronology and Determinants of Tissue Repair in Diabetic Lower Extremity Ulcers," *Diabetes* 40(10):1305-13, October 1991.

10. Lavery, L.A., et al. "In-hospital Mortality and Disposition of Diabetic Amputees in the Netherlands," *Diabetic Medicine* 13(2):192-97, February 1996.

11. van Houtum, W.H., et al. "The Impact of Diabetes-Related Lower-Extremity Amputations in the Netherlands," *Journal of Diabetes and Its Complications* 10(6):325-30, November-December 1996.

12. Lavery, L.A., et al. "Diabetes-related Lower-extremity Amputations Disproportionately Affect Blacks and Mexican Americans," *Southern Medical Journal* 92(6):593-99, June 1999.

13. Edmonds, M.E., et al. "Improved Survival of the Diabetic Foot: The Role of a Specialized Foot Clinic," *Quarterly Journal of Medicine* 60(232): 763-71, August 1986.

14. Most, R.S., and Sinnock, P. "The Epidemiology of Lower-Extremity Amputations in Diabetic Individuals," *Diabetes Care* 6(1):87-91, January-February 1983.

15. Lavery, L.A., et al. "Variation in the Incidence and Proportion of Diabetes-Related Amputations in Minorities," *Diabetes Care* 19(1):48-52, January 1996.

16. Lavery, L.A., Peters, E.J., Armstrong, D.G. "What Are the Most Effective Interventions in Preventing Diabetic Foot Ulcers?" *International Wound Journal* 5(3):425-33, June 2008.

17. Rayman, G., Krishnan, S.T., Baker, N.R., Wareham, A.M., and Rayman, A. "Are We Underestimating Diabetes-Related Lower-Extremity Amputation Rates? Results and Benefits of the First Prospective Study," *Diabetes Care* 27(8):1892-96, August 2004.

18. Armstrong, D.G., et al. "Choosing a Practical Screening Instrument to Identify Patients at Risk for Diabetic Foot Ulceration," *Archives of Internal Medicine* 158(3):289-92, February 1998.

19. Calhoun, J.H., et al. "Diabetic Foot Ulcers and Infections: Current Concepts," *Advances in Skin & Wound Care* 15(1):31-42, January-February 2002.

20. Lavery, L.A., Peters, E.J., Williams, J.R., Murdoch, D.P., Hudson, A., Lavery, D.C. "Reevaluating the Way We Classify the Diabetic Foot: Restructuring the Diabetic Foot Risk Classification System of the International Working Group on the Diabetic Foot," *Diabetes Care* 31(1):154-6, January 2008.

21. Levin, M. "Diabetic Foot Wounds: Pathogenesis and Management," *Advances in Wound Care* 10(2):24-30, March-April 1997.

22. Rith-Najarian, S.J. et al. "Identifying Diabetic Patients at High-Risk for Lower-Extremity Amputation in a Primary Health Care Setting. A Prospective Evaluation of Simple Screening Criteria," *Diabetes Care* 15(10):1386-95, October 1992.

23. Wunderlich, R.P., et al. "Defining Loss of Protective Sensation in the Diabetic Foot," *Advances in Wound Care* 11(3):123-28, May-June 1998.

24. Booth, J., and Young, M.J. "Differences in the Performance of Commercially Available 10-g Monofilaments," *Diabetes Care* 23(7):984-87, July 2000.

25. Young, R., et al. "The Durability of the Semmes-Weinstein 5.07 Monofilament," *Journal of Foot and Ankle Surgery* 39(1):34-38, January-February 2000.

26. Abbott, C.A., Carrington, A.L., Ashe, B.H., et al. "The North-West Diabetes Foot Care Study: Incidence of and Risk Factors for New Diabetic Foot Ulceration in a Community-based Patient Cohort," *Diabetes Medicine* 19(5):377-84, May 2002.

27. Needleman, R.L. "Successes and Pitfalls in the Healing of Neuropathic Forefoot Ulcerations with the IPOS Postoperative Shoe," *Foot & Ankle International* 18(7):412-17, July 1997.

28. Tooke, J.E., and Brash, P.D. "Microvascular Aspects of Diabetic Foot Disease," *Diabetic Medicine* 13(Suppl 1):S26-S29, 1996.

29. LoGerfo, F.W., and Coffman, J.D. "Current Concepts, Vascular and Microvascular Disease of the Foot in Diabetes. Implications for Foot Care," *New England Journal of Medicine* 311(25):1615-19, December 20, 1984.

30. LoGerfo, F.W., and Misare, F.D. "Current Management of the Diabetic Foot," *Advances in Surgery* 30:417-26, 1997.

31. Chao, C.Y.L., Cheing, G.L.Y. "Microvascular Dysfunction in Diabetic Foot Disease and Ulceration," *Diabetes/Metabolism Research and Reviews* 25:604-614, 2009.

32. Mulder, G.D. "Evaluating and Managing the Diabetic Foot: An Overview," *Advances in Skin & Wound Care* 13(1):33- 36, January-February 2000.

33. Hirsch, A.T., et al. "ACC/AHA Guidelines for the Management of Patients with Peripheral Arterial Disease (Lower Extremity, Renal, Mesenteric, and Abdominal Aortic): A Collaborative Report from the American Association for Vascular Surgery/Society for Vascular Surgery, Society for Cardiovascular Angiography and Interventions, Society of Interventional Radiology, Society for Vascular Medicine and Biology, and the American College of Cardiology/American Heart Association Task Force on Practice Guidelines (Writing Committee to Develop Guidelines for the Management of Patients With Peripheral Arterial Disease)," Available at http://www.sirweb.org/clinical/cpg/PAD_Full_Text.pdf. Accessed December 29, 2010.

34. Yamada, T., Ohata T., Ishibashi, H., Sugimoto, J., Iwata, H., Takahashi, M., Kawanishi, J. "Clinical Reliability and Utility of Skin Perfusion Pressure Measurement in Ischemic Limbs—Comparison with Other Noninvasive Diagnostic Methods," *Journal of Vascular Surgery* 47(2):318-23, February 2008.

35. Castronuovo Jr., J.J., Adera, H.M., Smiell, J.M., Price, R.M. "Skin Perfusion Pressure Measurement Is Valuable in the Diagnosis of Critical Limb Ischemia," *Journal of Vascular Surgery* 25(4):629-37, October 1997.

36. Catanzariti, A.R., et al. "Off-loading Techniques in the Treatment of Diabetic Plantar Neuropathic Foot Ulceration," *Advances in Wound Care* 12(9):452-58, November-December 1999.

37. Gibbons, G.W., and Habershaw, G.M. "Diabetic Foot Infections: Anatomy and Surgery," *Infectious Diseases Clinics of North America* 9(1):131-42, March 1995.

38. Frykberg, R.G. "The Team Approach in Diabetic Foot Management," *Advances in Wound Care* 11(2):71-77, March-April 1998.

39. Lavery, L.A., and Gazewood, J.D. "Assessing the Feet of Patients with Diabetes," *Journal of Family Practice* 49(11 Suppl):S9-S16, November 2000.

40. Lavery, L.A., et al. "Ankle Equinus Deformity and Its Relationship to High Plantar Pressure in a Large Population with Diabetes Mellitus," *Journal of the American Podiatric Medical Association* 92(9):479-82, October 2002.

41. Lavery, L.A., Armstrong, D.G., Wunderlich, R.P., Tredwell, J., Boulton, A.J.M. "Diabetic Foot Syndrome: Evaluating the Prevalence and Incidence of Foot Pathology in Mexican Americans and Non-Hispanic Whites From a Diabetes Disease Management Cohort," *Diabetes Care* 26:5, 2003.

42. Lipsky, B.A., et al. "The Diabetic Foot: Soft Tissue and Bone Infection," *Infectious Diseases Clinics of North America* 4(3):409-32, September 1990.

43. Lipsky, B.A. "Infections of the Foot in Patients with Diabetes," in Pfeifer, M.A., and Bowker, J.H., eds., *The Diabetic Foot*, 6th ed. St. Louis: Mosby–Year Book, Inc., 2001.

44. Lavery, L.A., Armstrong, D.G., Wunderlich, R.P., Mohler, M.J., Wendel, C.S., Lipsky, B.A. "Risk Factors for Foot Infections in Individuals with Diabetes," *Diabetes Care* 29(6):1288, June 2006.

45. Lavery, L.A., Peters, E.J., Armstrong, D.G., Wendel, C.S., Murdoch, D.P., Lipsky, B.A. "Risk Factors for Developing Osteomyelitis in Patients with Diabetic Foot Wounds," *Diabetes Research in Clinical Practice* 83(3):347-52, March 2009.

46. Peters, E.J., and Lavery, L.A. "Effectiveness of the Diabetic Foot Risk Classification System of the International Working Group on the Diabetic Foot," *Diabetes Care* 24(8):1442-47, August 2001.

47. Lavery, L.A., Peters, E.J., Williams, J.R., Murdoch, D.P., Hudson, A., Lavery, D.C. "Reevaluating the Way We Classify the Diabetic Foot: Restructuring the Diabetic Foot Risk Classification System of the International Working Group on the Diabetic Foot," *Diabetes Care* 31(1):154-6, January 2008.

48. Holstein, P., et al. "Decreasing Incidence of Major Amputations in People with Diabetes," *Diabetologia* 43(7):844-47, July 2000.

49. Larsson, J., et al. "Decreasing Incidence of Major Amputation in Diabetic Patients: A Consequence of a Multidisciplinary Foot Care Team Approach?" *Diabetic Medicine* 12(9):770-76, September 1995.

50. Patout, C.A., et al. "Effectiveness of a Comprehensive Diabetes Lower-Extremity Amputation Prevention Program in a Predominantly Low-Income African-American Population," *Diabetes Care* 23(9):1339-42, September 2000.

51. Runyan, J.W. Jr., et al. "The Memphis Diabetes Continuing Care Program," *Diabetes Care* 3(2):382-86, March-April 1980.

52. Pinzur, M.S., et al. "Guidelines for Diabetic Foot Care," *Foot & Ankle International* 29(11):695-702, November 1999.

53. Frykberg, R.G., et al. "Role of Neuropathy and High Foot Pressures in Diabetic Foot Ulceration," *Diabetes Care* 21(10):1714-19, October 1998.

54. Lavery, L.A., et al. "Reducing Plantar Pressure in the Neuropathic Foot: A Comparison of Footwear," *Diabetes Care* 20(11):1706-10, November 1997.

55. Lavery, L.A., et al. "A Novel Methodology to Obtain Salient Biomechanical Characteristics of Insole Materials," *Journal of the American Podiatric Medical Association* 87(6):260-65, June 1997.

56. Sugaman, J.R., et al. "Use of the Therapeutic Footwear Benefit among Diabetic Medicare Beneficiaries in Three States," *Diabetes Care* 21(5):777-81, May 1998.

57. Armstrong DG, Nguyen HC, Lavery LA, et al. "Off-loading the Diabetic Foot Wound: A Randomized Clinical Trial," *Diabetes Care* 24(6):1019-22, June 2001.

58. Armstrong D.G., et al. "Lengthening of the Achilles Tendon in Diabetic Patients Who Are at High Risk for Ulceration of the Foot," *Journal of Bone & Joint Surgery [Am]* 81(4):535-38, April 1999.

59. Armstrong, D.G., Stacpoole-Shea, S., Nguyen, H., Harkless, L.B. "Lengthening of the Achilles Tendon in Diabetic Patients," *Journal of Bone & Joint Surgery [Am]* 82A(10):1510, October 2000.

60. Lin, S.S., Lee, T.H., Wapner, K.L. "Plantar Forefoot Ulceration with Equinus Deformity of the Ankle in Diabetic Patients: the Effect of Tendo-Achilles Lengthening and Total Contact Casting," *Orthopaedics* 5:465-75, May 1996.

61. Mueller, M., Sinacore, D.R. "Effect of Achilles Tendon Lengthening on Neuropathic Plantar Ulcers: a Randomized Clinical Trial," *Journal of Bone & Joint Surgery* 8:1436-45, August 2003.

62. Dorresteijn, J.A., Kriegsman, D.M, Assendelft, W.J.J., Valk, G.D. "Patient Education for Preventing Diabetic Foot Ulceration," *The Cochrane Database of Systematic Reviews* 12(5):CD001488, 2010.

63. Lavery, L.A., Higgins, K.R., Lanctot, D.R., et al. "Preventing Diabetic Foot Ulcer Recurrence in High-Risk Patients: Use of Temperature Monitoring as a Self-Assessment Tool," *Diabetes Care* 30(1):14-20 January 2007.

64. Armstrong, D.G., Holtz-Neiderer, K., Wendel, C., Mohler, M.J., Kimbriel, H.R., Lavery, L.A. "Skin Temperature Monitoring Reduces the Risk for Diabetic Foot Ulceration in High-risk Patients," *American Journal of Medicine* 120(12):1042-6; December 2010. Erratum in *American Journal of Medicine* 121(12), December 2008.

65. Armstrong, D.G., et al. "Validation of a Diabetic Wound Classification System: The Contribution of Depth, Infection and Ischemia to Risk of Amputation," *Diabetes Care* 21(5):855-59, May 1998.

66. Meggitt, B. "Surgical Management of the Diabetic Foot," *British Journal of Hospital Medicine* 227-32, 1976.

67. Wagner, F.W., Jr. "The Dysvascular Foot: A System for Diagnosis and Treatment," *Foot & Ankle* 2(2):64-122, September 1981.

68. Sheehan, P. "American Diabetes Association (ADA): Presentation of Consensus Development Conference on Diabetic Foot Wound Care," *Wounds* 13(5 Suppl E):6E-8E, 2001.

69. Steed, D.L., et al. and the Diabetic Ulcer Study Group. "Effect of Extensive Debridement and Treatment on the Healing of Diabetic Foot Ulcers," *Journal of the American College of Surgery* 183(1):61-64, July 1996.

70. Steed, D.L. "The Wound Healing Society (WHS) Evaluation of the Science to Arrive at Guidelines," *Wounds* 13(5 Suppl E):15E-16E, 2001.

71. Lavery, L.A., et al. "Total Contact Casts: Pressure Reduction at Ulcer Sites and the Effects on the Contralateral Foot," *Archives of Physical Medicine & Rehabilitation* 78(11):1268-71, November 1997.

72. Frykberg, R.G. "A Summary of Guidelines for Managing the Diabetic Foot," *Advances in Skin & Wound Care* 18(4):209-14, May 2005.

73. Walker, S.C., et al. "Total Contact Casting and Chronic Diabetic Neuropathic Foot Ulcerations: Healing Rates by Wound Location," *Archives of Physical Medicine & Rehabilitation* 68(4):217-21, April 1987.

74. Lavery, L.A., et al. "Reducing Dynamic Foot Pressures in High-Risk Diabetic Subjects with Foot Ulcers: A Comparison of Treatments," *Diabetes Care* 19(8):818-21, August 1996.

75. Helm, P.A., et al. "Total Contact Casting in Diabetic Patients with Neuropathic Foot Ulcerations," *Archives of Physical Medicine & Rehabilitation* 65(11):691-93, November 1984.

76. Sinacore, D.R., et al. "Diabetic Plantar Ulcers Treated by Total Contact Casting: A Clinical Report," *Physical Therapy* 67(10):1543-49, October 1987.

77. Lavery, L.A., et al. "Healing Rates of Diabetic Foot Ulcers Associated with Midfoot Fracture Due to Charcot's Arthropathy," *Diabetic Medicine* 14(1):46-49, January 1997.

78. Armstrong, D.G., et al. "Off-loading the Diabetic Foot Wound: A Randomized Clinical Trial," *Diabetes Care* 24(8):1509, August 2001.

79. Mueller, M.J., et al. "Total Contact Casting in Treatment of Diabetic Plantar Ulcers. Controlled Clinical Trial," *Diabetes Care* 12(6):384-88, June 1989.

80. Sinacore, D.R. "Total Contact Casting for Diabetic Neuropathic Ulcers," *Physical Therapy* 76(3):296-301, March 1996.

81. Caputo, G.M., et al. "The Total Contact Cast: A Method for Treating Neuropathic Diabetic Ulcers," *American Family Physician* 55(2):605-11, February 1, 1997.

82. Veves, A., et al. "Graftskin, A Human Skin Equivalent, Is Effective in the Management of Noninfected Neuropathic Diabetic Foot Ulcers: A Prospective Randomized Multicenter Clinical Trial," *Diabetes Care* 24(2):290-95, February 2001.

83. Veves, A., et al. "A Randomized, Controlled Trial of Promogran (A Collagen/Oxidized

Regenerated Cellulose Dressing) Versus Standard Treatment in the Management of Diabetic Foot Ulcers," *Archives of Surgery* 137(7):822-27, July 2002.

84. Gentzkow, G.D., et al. "Use of Dermagraft, A Cultured Human Dermis, to Treat Diabetic Foot Ulcers," *Diabetes Care* 19(4):350-54, April 1996.

85. Wieman, T.J., et al. "Efficacy and Safety of a Topical Gel Formulation of Recombinant Human Platelet-Derived Growth Factor-BB (Becaplermin) in Patients with Chronic Neuropathic Diabetic Ulcers. A Phase III Randomized Placebo-Controlled Double-Blind Study," *Diabetes Care* 21(5):822-27, May 1998.

86. Knowles, E.A., et al. "Off-loading Diabetic Foot Wounds Using the Scotchcast Boot: A Retrospective Study," *Ostomy/Wound Management* 48(9):50-53, September 2002.

87. Chantelau, E., et al. "Outpatient Treatment of Unilateral Diabetic Foot Ulcers with 'Half Shoes,'" *Diabetic Medicine* 10(3):267-70, April 1993.

88. Boninger, M.L., and Leonard, J.A. Jr. "Use of Bivalved Ankle-foot Orthosis in Neuropathic Foot and Ankle Lesions," *Journal of Rehabilitation Research & Development* 33(1):16-22, February 1996.

89. Armstrong, D.G., Lavery, L.A., Wu, S., et al. "Evaluation of Removable and Irremovable Cast Walkers in the Healing of Diabetic Foot Wounds; a Randomized Controlled Trial," *Diabetes Care* 28(3):551-54, March 2005.

90. McQuire, J.B. "Pressure Redistribution Strategies for the Diabetic or At-risk Foot: Part II," *Advances in Skin & Wound Care* 19(5):270-77, June 2006.

91. Sibbald, R.G., Woo, K., Ayello, E.A. "Increased Bacterial Burden and Infection: The Story of NERDS and STONES," *Advances in Skin & Wound Care* 19(8):447-61, October 2006.

92. McGuire, J. "Transitional Off-loading: An Evidence-Based Approach to Pressure Redistribution in the Diabetic Foot." *Advances in Skin & Wound Care* 23(4):175-88, April 2010.

93. Frykberg, R.G. "Diabetic Foot Ulcers: Pathogenesis and Management," *American Family Physician* 66:1655-62, November 2002.

94. Armstrong, D.G., Lavery, L.A., Frykberg, R.G. "Validation of a Diabetic Foot Surgery Classification," *International Wound Journal* 3: 240-246, September 2006.

95. Katz, I.A., Harlan, A., Miranda-Palma, B., et al. "A Randomized Trial of Two Irremovable Off-loading Devices in the Management of Plantar Neuropathic Diabetic Foot Ulcerations," *Diabetes Care* 28(3):555-59, March 2005.

96. Pollo, F.E., Crenshaw, M.S., Brodsky, M.D., Kirksey, B.S. "Plantar Pressures in Total Contact Casting Verses a Diabetic Walking Boot," Paper presented at the Annual Meeting of the Orthopedic Research Society, San Francisco, February 25-28, 2001.

97. Department of Health and Human Services, Health Resources and Services Administration. "Sandals." Available at http://www.hrsa.gov/hansens/clinical/footcare/sandals_PT.htm. Accessed December 29, 2010.

98. Lair, G. *Use of the Ipos Shoe in the Management of Patients with Diabetes Mellitus*. Cleveland, OH: Cleveland Clinic Foundation, 1992.

99. Myerson, M., et al. "The Total-Contact Cast for Management of Neuropathic Plantar Ulceration of the Foot," *Journal of Bone & Joint Surgery [Am]* 74(2):261-69, February 1992.

CHAPTER 17

Sickle Cell Ulcers

Terry Treadwell, MD, FACS

The contributions of Harold Brem, MD, FACS, and Angela Collette Willis, RN, CWS, CDE, to the previous editions of this chapter are greatly appreciated.

Objectives

After completing this chapter, you'll be able to:

- understand the pathogenesis of sickle cell anemia (or sickle cell disease)
- discuss the pathogenesis of sickle cell ulcers
- differentiate sickle cell ulcers from arterial and venous ulcers
- implement protocols for prevention and treatment of complications of sickle cell ulcers.

SICKLE CELL ANEMIA

Sickle cell ulcers are a complication of sickle cell anemia, an inherited, genetic disorder of the oxygen carrying hemoglobin in red blood cells. Sickle cell anemia (or sickle cell disease) was first reported in 1910 by Dr. J.B. Herrick.[1] It is a disease primarily seen in black individuals and is more prevalent in the United States and Africa. The disease is seen in two main forms: when the individual receives a gene for the abnormal hemoglobin (hemoglobin S) from both the mother and the father, the person has homozygous sickle cell disease, which is the most severe form; when the individual receives only one gene for the abnormal hemoglobin from either the mother or father and the other gene is for normal hemoglobin, the person has heterozygous sickle cell disease, which is the less severe form.

Prevalence and incidence

The patient with the homozygous form of sickle cell disease is most likely to develop a sickle cell ulcer. Studies have shown that males are more likely to develop leg ulcers due to sickle cell disease than females.[2] The same study found that 5% of males with sickle cell disease who were over 10 years of age had sickle cell ulcers,[2] and 75% of patients over age 30 had a sickle cell ulcer at some time during the course of their disease.[3] According to the National Heart, Lung and Blood Institute of the National Institutes of Health, sickle cell anemia affects 70,000 to 100,000 Americans.[4] The disease occurs mainly in blacks (1 in every 500 black births and 1 in 36,000 Hispanic births).[4] Approximately 2 million Americans have the sickle cell trait, or 1 in 12 blacks.[4] This makes the number of patients with sickle cell ulcers a significant health concern.

> ### PRACTICE POINT
>
> Lower extremity ulcers in young black patients, especially males, could be due to undiagnosed sickle cell disease.

ULCER PATHOGENESIS

The abnormal hemoglobin molecule in the red blood cell in the patient with sickle cell disease does not affect the amount of oxygen the red blood cell can carry. After the red blood cell

447

Sickled cell

The illustration below show a normal red blood cell and a sickled cell

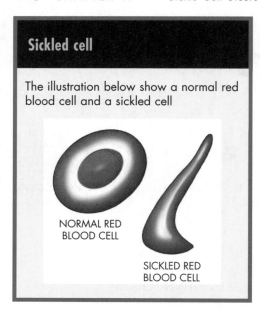

NORMAL RED
BLOOD CELL

SICKLED RED
BLOOD CELL

and its hemoglobin give up the oxygen to the tissue, the abnormal hemoglobin causes the red blood cell to distort and become rigid. This results in the cell becoming deformed into a sickle shape (See *Sickled cell*.)

When the red blood cell is reoxygenated, the cell resumes its normal shape. Unfortunately, while the cells are in the sickled shape, they tend to increase blood viscosity and become "sticky." This causes slowing of the blood flow in small vessels and subsequently clotting of the vessels, which results in ischemia of tissue and organs. Over time the patient suffers repeated episodes of pain, tissue damage and, eventually, organ failure. Many times the cells become damaged while they are in the sickled shape and have a shortened lifespan. Anemia results because these cells are removed from the circulation faster than normal. (See *Conditions associated with sickle cell anemia*.[5])

Conditions associated with sickle cell anemia

Complication	Cause
"Crisis" with fever and pain	Sickling of cells due to abnormal hemoglobin
Pain in bones, joints, and back	Sickling of cells and ischemia of tissues
Severe abdominal pain	Sickling of cells and ischemia of tissues
Pregnancy problems Fertility problems	Uncontrolled sickling of cells
Increased infections Pneumonia Urinary tract	Deficient immune response
Salmonella osteomyelitis	Ischemia of bones, bone infarcts, sepsis
Chronic leg ulcers	Sickling of cells and ischemia of tissues
"Hand-foot" syndrome	Sickling of cells and ischemia of bones
Avascular necrosis of femoral or humeral head	Ischemic necrosis of bones due to sickling
Visual problems	Ischemia of retina due to sickling
Pulmonary infarction	Ischemia of lung due to sickle cell emboli

Conditions associated with sickle cell anemia (continued)

Complication	Cause

Congestive heart failure
  Cardiac murmurs
  EKG abnormalities
	Myocardial ischemia

Jaundice	Hemolytic anemia Gallstone production and obstructive jaundice
Cirrhosis of liver	Ischemia of liver and cell necrosis
Hepatitis	Multiple blood transfusions
Enlarged spleen (infancy only)	Increased blood production
Splenic infarction (late teens, adult)	Ischemia of tissue due to sickling of cells

Renal dysfunction
  Hematuria
  Infections
	Ischemia of kidney with infarction of tissue

Renal vein thrombosis	Sickling of cells
Priapism (especially in children)	Sickling of cells
Impotence	Damage of penis by priapism and ischemia
Anemia	Hemolysis of abnormal cells
"Aplastic crisis"	Failure of bone marrow to produce cells due to infarction of marrow
Folate deficiency	High folate requirement of hemolytic anemia

Adapted from Conley, C. Lockard, "The Hemoglobinopathies and Thalassemias" in *Textbook of Medicine*, eds. Beeson, PB, McDermott, W, 13th Edition, W.B. Saunders Co., Philadelphia, pp.1501-1503, 1971.

Although the exact cause of sickle cell ulcers is not clear, they have been associated with trauma, infection, severe anemia, warm temperatures,[6] and venous insufficiency,[7,8] and they are most likely to occur in the malleolar area of the lower extremities. Laboratory evaluation has shown that sickle cell ulcer patients have lower hemoglobin levels and higher levels of lactate dehydrogenase, bilirubin, aspartate transaminase, and reticulocytes than do patients with sickle cell disease who do not have ulcers.[9] When cells become sickled and rigid, they occlude small vessels in the microcirculation, resulting in ischemia and tissue necrosis.[10] The sickle cells can cause chronic damage to the microcirculation in the skin at the ankle, including injury to the capillary walls, thickening of the intimal lining of the capillary, and increased permeability of the vessel wall, allowing macromolecules to escape into the tissue.[11] These changes can also result in the skin having a reduced blood supply, making it more susceptible to minor trauma and less likely to heal.[12] As a result, these areas of involvement are more likely to be the sites of skin breakdown and ulceration. It has also been suggested that a reduction in the amount of the smooth muscle relaxant (nitric oxide) in the microcirculation can result in unrestrained vasoconstriction of the small vessels, ischemia of the skin, and skin necrosis.[12]

Diagnosis
MEDICAL HISTORY

Evaluation of the patient with a suspected sickle cell ulcer is of utmost importance so that the correct diagnosis can be made and appropriate treatment planned. The patient's medical history should be recorded, and the events surrounding the ulcer development should be investigated. Is this the first ulcer the patient has had? How long has the ulcer been present? How did the ulcer first develop? Was there trauma to the area? How did the area first look? Any history of lower extremity edema; unexplained swelling of the hands, feet, or knees; osteomyelitis; episodes of abdominal or joint pain; episodes of severe unexplained pain; recurrent urinary tract infections or pneumonia; or anemia should be noted. Sickle cell patients are prone to develop unexplained episodes of fever that tend to resolve without therapy. These patients may carry a diagnosis of fever of unknown origin.

Physical examination

A complete physical examination should be part of the patient evaluation. Vital signs, especially temperature, should be taken because, as mentioned above, unexplained fever may be a sign of sickle cell disease. Abdominal examination can detect enlargement of the liver. The spleen may be enlarged in early childhood as it is a primary blood-forming organ but is usually small in later life due to ischemic infarction.

Scars on the extremity suggest that the patient may have had a sickle cell ulcer in the past. The location of the ulcer or ulcers is important as most sickle cell ulcers are found on the lower third of the leg and usually over the medial or lateral malleoli (or both) of the ankle.[6] The size of each ulcer should be measured by determining the length and width or by using one of the more advanced measuring modalities described elsewhere in this book. (See chapter 6, Wound assessment.)

The presence of an ulcer in a patient with varicose veins, venous insufficiency, and sickle cell disease can be especially troublesome as it may lead to misdiagnosis. (See *Undiagnosed sickle cell ulcer treated initially as a "venous ulcer."*) In addition, venous incompetence in the patient with sickle cell disease may predispose him to develop an ulcer and is correlated with the development of a recurrent sickle cell ulcer.[8] Noninvasive venous studies can be helpful in establishing the correct therapeutic approach in these patients.

> **PRACTICE POINT**
>
> Misdiagnosis—and thus mistreatment—of sickle cell ulcer as a venous "stasis" ulcer makes it imperative to get the differential diagnosis correct.

Undiagnosed sickle cell ulcer treated initially as a "venous ulcer"

Ulcer assessment

Examination of the wound bed is essential to determine the presence of granulation tissue or fibrinous material ("slough"). (See *color section, Slough* and *Differentiating tendon from slough,* page C10.) In addition, the presence of peri-ulcer erythema or cellulitis should also be documented. The presence and character of any drainage should be noted. Tenderness of the lower extremity to palpation or the presence of pain in the ulcer or surrounding area should be also recorded. A brief vascular examination should always be performed to be sure the patient has adequate blood flow to the area. The presence of dorsalis pedis and posterior tibial pulses should be noted. If there is a question about the adequacy of the circulation, the patient will need to be referred for noninvasive vascular studies or arteriography. The microcirculation in the periwound area can be evaluated with the laser Doppler and transcutaneous oxygen pressure ($TcPO_2$) measurements, if available.

> **▶ PRACTICE POINT**
>
> A complete history and physical examination are vital when evaluating a patient with a sickle cell ulcer.

Laboratory assessment

Laboratory evaluation depends on the condition of the patient. If the patient does not have a diagnosis of sickle cell disease, but it is suspected, the clinician should order blood tests that check for anemia, sickle cells, and abnormal hemoglobin. This usually involves a complete blood count (CBC), sickle "prep," and hemoglobin electrophoresis. Although hemoglobin electrophoresis is considered the diagnostic tool of choice, it has its limitations, especially if the patient has had recent blood transfusions.[5] In such a case, referral to a hematologist may be necessary. If the patient with known sickle cell disease has an ulcer, the laboratory workup should consist of a CBC with differential white blood cell count and reticulocyte count.

Patients with sickle cell disease are especially prone to develop infections; therefore, it is important to obtain a wound culture using appropriate technique if the wound bioburden appears elevated. We have found that a significant number of patients with sickle cell ulcers have wounds covered by biofilm, which must be removed before the ulcer can heal. The most frequent way to remove a biofilm is with sharp debridement, but recently we have turned to ultrasonic debridement techniques, which are less painful for the patient. (See *color section, Sickle cell ulcer,* page C25.) Dressings that enhance autolytic debridement can also be helpful. Following initial debridement, an enzymatic agent can be used for maintenance debridement.[13] Other methods for removing biofilms will be available in the near future. (See chapter 7, Wound bioburden and infection.)

Infection and osteomyelitis

Patients with sickle cell disease and a deep, painful ulcer should be evaluated radiologically for the presence of osteomyelitis, especially if the patient has fever or leukocytosis. Patients with sickle cell disease are prone to developing salmonella osteomyelitis.[5] Radiologic evaluation can be done by several methods. Plain film X-rays are the least sensitive method and usually don't show any evidence of osteomyelitis until late in the course of the infection. In addition, they can be especially confusing in the patient with sickle cell disease because the disease can result in periosteal elevation and other bone changes that mimic osteomyelitis.[5] Nuclear medicine bone scans are slightly more helpful, but it must be remembered that routine bone scans only detect areas of inflammation. Also, if the patient has an ulcer overlying the bone in question, the bone scan is virtually useless.

Magnetic resonance imaging appears to be the imaging modality of choice in terms of sensitivity and specificity. It has been suggested that bone biopsy and culture may be the only definitive way to determine whether osteomyelitis is present,[6] but it should be done with great care so as not to cause an infection in the bone. Biopsy of the wound bed and wound margin may be advisable if the ulcer has been present for longer than 3 months, does not respond to therapy, or just doesn't "look right." This should be done to rule out the possibility of malignancy and can help with the diagnosis.[14]

PAIN

Because of the painful nature of sickle cell ulcers and the need to do biopsy cultures, the practitioner must be aware of recent studies about the use of topical and local anesthetics. Berg et al.[15] have shown that EMLA cream, a topical anesthetic agent commonly used before wound biopsies, is highly antibacterial. Within 1 hour of exposure to EMLA cream, most common bacteria were killed. This included strains of *Staphylococcus aureus* (both methicillin-resistant and methicillin-sensitive strains), *Streptococcus pyogenes*, *Escherichia coli*, and *Pseudomonas aeruginosa*. Injected solutions of 1% lidocaine were also found to be antibacterial for the same organisms but at greater than 2 hours after local injection. Berg and colleagues recommend that EMLA cream not be used for anesthesia when biopsy cultures are being done. Local injection of preservative-free 1% lidocaine would be satisfactory to use if the biopsy culture is done within 2 hours of the injection.[15]

Although sickle cell ulcers tend to be extremely painful, pain assessment is an area that can be easily overlooked because the patient is often fearful of experiencing even more pain and may not want you to look at the ulcer much less touch it. This makes debridement and treatment of these ulcers very difficult. (A useful pain assessment tool for evaluating a patient's pain is outlined elsewhere in this book [see chapter 12, Pain management and wounds]). It has been the author's experience that if the provider does not address the pain problem, many of the patients will not return for follow-up care. Indeed, most patients would rather keep their ulcer than deal with potentially being in more pain than they already are. For this reason, significant debridements must be done with some type of anesthesia, such as topical anesthesia (xylocaine ointment or EMLA cream), injectable local anesthesia, regional anesthesia, or general anesthesia. Some of these techniques will require hospitalization of the patient.

Pain control can be managed with topical anesthetic agents. Topical xylocaine ointment or EMLA cream can be used on a regular basis for pain control. Applied every 4 to 6 hours, these agents can make the patient's daily activities much more manageable. They also make dressing changes more comfortable. Other therapies, including opioid analgesics and regional medications (xylocaine patches), are useful but many times have to be managed by a pain specialist. (See chapter 12, Pain management and wounds.)

> ▶ **PRACTICE POINT**
>
> Sickle cell ulcers are extremely painful. Evaluation and treatment of the patient's pain should be a top priority and should be the first step in instituting therapy.

Treatment

Treatment of sickle cell ulcers can be challenging and frustrating. Even in this day of evidence-based therapies, it is noteworthy that there are no published trials of treatments of sickle cell ulcers.[6] One of the more interesting findings about the treatment of sickle cell ulcers is that most ulcers will heal with prolonged bed rest.[6] Obviously, this is not a practical therapy as extended hospitalization is no longer possible and complete bed rest at home is not realistic. However, any therapy that results in a long period of immobilization, such as surgical intervention, must take into account that it is the bed rest and not the treatment that is healing the ulcer. With this in mind, one must begin with the basics of what we know constitutes good wound care.

The basics of good wound care include debridement of devitalized tissue, control of infection, assurance of adequate circulation, and maintenance of a moist wound environment. The major addition in the treatment of sickle cell ulcers is control of wound pain. Many times the ulcers are so painful that manipulation of the wound is impossible. Treatment of the wound with topical anesthetics has been addressed previously and must not be overlooked. If the therapy for the wound is painful, most people will forgo your advice and treat the ulcer themselves in ways that do not cause more pain. It is unfortunate that many of these patients are labeled as "noncompliant" when it is a poor choice of therapy by the clinician and not the compliance of the patient that should be in question. Once the pain is controlled, the wound can be debrided and treated, as indicated. Use of dressings that enhance autolytic debridement should be strongly considered, as previously mentioned. Debridement with sterile maggots can be a consideration and is less painful, but convincing the patient may be difficult!

The evaluation of sickle cell ulcers for infection and the evaluation of the patient for circulation problems have been covered previously. The importance of moist wound care has been known since Winter's 1962 publication on the topic.[16] It is now known that wounds treated with wet-to-dry dressings do not heal well and that removing a dry dressing that adheres to the wound causes pain and wound reinjury.[17] Wounds treated with moist dressings heal faster, are less painful, and have less scarring. Numerous wound dressings currently available will maintain a moist wound environment. (See chapter 9, Wound treatment options.)

If the wound is believed to be infected, topical antimicrobials should be considered. Oral or IV antibiotics are indicated only if the patient has a leukocytosis, cellulitis, or fever. Silver dressings have become popular in the treatment of the wound with a clinically significant bacterial burden (critical colonization) or with frank infection. Numerous silver dressings are available for use on these wounds. At this time, I believe one should pick the silver dressing that best meets the patient's needs instead of debating the amount of silver in the dressing. If excess drainage is present, a silver alginate, hydrocolloid, or foam might be indicated. If there is significant odor, then a silver dressing with odor control properties might be most beneficial. If only a bandage delivering silver ions is needed, those are also available. It is suggested that once the bacterial burden is under control, the silver dressing should be discontinued and other moisture control dressings used. This is because of the potential for toxicity of the silver to the growing tissue.[18,19] Dressings containing Cadexomer iodine are useful in treating wounds that are critically colonized with bacteria or infected wounds.[20,21]

Other therapies that may be helpful include oral zinc sulfate (200 mg three times/day)[22] and zinc oxide–impregnated Unna boot. An Unna boot applied to the lower extremity and covered with an elastic wrap has been especially beneficial for patients with edema. The bandages are changed weekly until the ulcer heals.[6] In a recent series, the topical growth factor molgramostim (granulocyte macrophage–colony-stimulating factor) had some degree of success in the treatment of these very difficult wounds.[23]

Based on the work of Aslan and Freeman[12] suggesting that sickle cell ulcers may result from a decrease in microcirculatory smooth muscle nitric oxide with resultant vasoconstriction, in my practice patients with sickle cell ulcers are treated with a combination of L-methyl folate, pyridoxal-5'-phosphate, and methylcobalamin (Metanx). This oral combination and formulation of vitamins has been shown to reduce endothelial cell homocysteine levels and raise nitric oxide levels, resulting in improved wound healing.[24] It has also helped reduce the pain associated with sickle cell ulcers and increased the blood flow in the microcirculation at the wound margin. (See *Treatment of sickle cell ulcer with nitric oxide–producing medication,* page 454.) It is my impression that healing is improved in these patients, but further analysis is pending. Whether this treatment will reduce the incidence of sickle cells ulcers or their recurrence is yet to be determined.

The revival of the use of natural honey, a therapeutic product that dates back to ancient Egypt, for treatment of sickle cell ulcers has been tried and has met with mixed results.[26] Because natural honey is unsterile, some important implications must be considered for treatment of wounds, the most serious of which is the presence of clostridial spores that could cause wound botulism. However, the

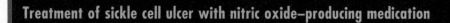

Treatment of sickle cell ulcer with nitric oxide–producing medication

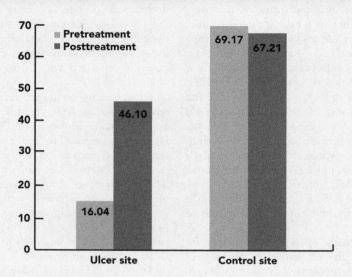

Before treatment, $TcPO_2$ levels at the ulcer site and control site were 16.04 and 69.17, respectively. The periwound $TcPO_2$ level is below what would be expected for healing to occur. After 1 week of oral therapy with the nitric oxide–producing medication Metanx, there was marked improvement in the periwound $TcPO_2$ while the control site stayed essentially the same.[25] With this improvement, the wound began to heal. Based on this, we treat all of our sickle cell ulcer patients with this medication.

introduction of the sterilized honey product, Manuka honey from New Zealand, opens new opportunities for the treatment of sickle cell ulcers.[27]

The use of tissue-engineered skin in the treatment of sickle cell ulcers has met with some degree of success.[28] Prior to applying any advanced therapeutic product the wound bed must be well prepared, which means ensuring that the wound bed has been debrided to remove all necrotic tissue, that infection has been controlled, and that the wound environment has been optimized.[29] To achieve the goal of wound environment optimization, Treadwell et al.[30] recommend pretreating the wound with a protease-modulating agent for 2 to 3 weeks to reduce the abnormal protease levels. These agents include oral or topical doxy-

cycline or an oxidized, regenerated cellulose product.[31,32] Early data show that pretreatment of any chronic wound with these protease-modulating agents prior to application of a human skin equivalent improves the healing rate.[30] Once treated with the tissue-engineered skin product, patients experience significant relief of their pain as well as healing of their ulcer. (See *color section, Recurrent sickle cell ulcer,* page C26.) One patient's ulcer healed within 8 weeks following a single application of the human tissue–engineered skin. Over 80% of patients treated with human skin equivalent will heal with only one application.[30] It is also of note that sickle cell ulcers treated with tissue-engineered skin seem to have a more normal-appearing and stable scar. One of the treatments of sickle cell disease is hydroxyurea, which is known to improve symptoms associated with sickle cell disease. Unfortunately, hydroxyurea is known to cause leg ulcers in patients taking this medication.[33,34] The medication must be stopped before the ulcer will heal.[35] Fortunately, it has been found that ulcers related to hydroxyurea therapy respond promptly to treatment with tissue-engineered skin.[35]

The use of split-thickness skin grafts or pinch grafts to treat patients with sickle cell ulcers may be a reasonable therapeutic alternative. However, the procedures require hospitalization and anesthesia, making them less cost-effective. It has also been reported that split-thickness skin grafting has a very low success rate in healing sickle cell ulcers and that the recurrence rate is very high in those that do heal.[36] Success has been noted with the use of muscle flaps, myocutaneous flaps, and free flaps to cover large lower extremity sickle cell ulcers,[37,38] although success has not been uniform.[39]

Transfusion therapy has been attempted in the treatment of patients with sickle cell ulcers who have been resistant to all other therapies. The goals of transfusion therapy are to keep the hematocrit between 30 and 35 volume percent and to keep the level of normal hemoglobin (hemoglobin A) greater than 70% of the total.[36] The transfusions are continued until the ulcer heals or for 6 months, at which time they are discontinued. Unfortunately, 20% to 30% of patients treated with multiple blood transfusions can develop antibodies to blood products, minimizing their use when anemia is profound.[40] The possibility of iron overload with this therapy must be considered.[10]

Another interesting approach to treating sickle cell ulcers has been the use of IV arginine butyrate. The concept is that the arginine butyrate will change the concentration of abnormal hemoglobin, thus allowing the wounds to heal. Two studies have shown reasonable success with this method,[41,42] but no randomized controlled trials have been done as of this time.

Other therapies for sickle cell ulcers include medications, such as pentoxifylline (Trental), negative pressure wound therapy, hyperbaric oxygen therapy, and electromagnetic stimulation. Others therapies are still considered experimental, and their utility in treating these patients with difficult wound problems will be determined by future studies.

Sickle cell ulcers will respond better to any therapy if the sickle cell disease is under control. If the patient's anemia is profound (<5 g Hg/100 mL) or if the abnormal hemoglobin-containing cells represent more than 50% of the total volume of red blood cells, then the success of any therapy is problematic. This has recently been supported by work reported by Eckman and Platt.[36]

PREVENTING ULCERS

Prevention of sickle cell ulcers is paramount. Use the patient teaching points listed below to educate patients with sickle cell disease.

Patient Teaching
Key Teaching Points for Preventing Sickle Cell Ulcers

Instruct the patient with sickle cell disease about the following:

- Good skin care, including keeping the skin moisturized, is very important.
- Prevent trauma to the lower legs and ankles, for example, by using insect repellants to avoid insect bites.
- Watch for signs of swelling in the lower extremities. Edema is the single most common occurrence prior to recurrence of an ulcer.[36]
- Wear support hose or elastic wraps.
- Seek medical care promptly for any minor injury to the extremities.

SUMMARY

Sickle cell ulcers are a potential reality for any person with the inherited disease sickle cell anemia. Treatment of these ulcers can be frustrating and require multiple modalities. Unfortunately, recurrence is common. With modalities to treat the underlying disease on the horizon, these problems eventually may be of historical interest only. In the meantime, persistent treatment and understanding will aid the patient and you with the best available therapy.

PATIENT SCENARIO

Clinical Data

A 28-year-old black woman with a history of anemia was referred to the wound center because of an extremely painful ulcer of the right lower extremity that has been present for 3 months. The patient has a history of ulceration of the right lower extremity with episodes of healing followed by recurrence. The ulceration usually occurs over and proximal to the medial malleolus. She has no history of thrombophlebitis, trauma to the leg, or total joint replacement. She was diagnosed with homozygous sickle cell anemia as a child and has had multiple hospital admissions for abdominal pain, pneumonia, and profound anemia requiring transfusion. Three years prior to this visit, the patient suffered a miscarriage. She has complained of pain in her left hip, but no X-ray evidence of bone problems has been detected. The patient was taking hydroxyurea for her sickle cell disease.

Examination showed a 6 cm × 4 cm, painful, full-thickness ulcer of the right lower extremity involving the medial malleolus. The ulcer was covered with a fibrotic tissue. There was no evidence of surrounding infection, but 3+ pitting edema was present from the knee to the foot. She had palpable dorsalis pedis and posterior tibial pulses at the ankle. Her $TcPO_2$ at the wound margin was 16, with a reference value of 69. Screening blood tests confirmed the presence of homozygous sickle cell disease, a hemoglobin level of 4 gm%, and a hematocrit of 12%.

Case Discussion

Because of the biofilm and severe pain, the wound was treated with a combination of xylocaine ointment 5% and Santyl (collagenase). Because of the edema, she was also treated with a compression bandage. Systemic therapy was started by giving the patient a combination medication of L-methyl folate, pyridoxal-5'-phosphate, and methylcobalamin (Metanx). A narcotic was also prescribed for pain. Arrangements for blood transfusion were made. Hydroxyurea was discontinued because of the possible association between the medication and the occurrence of sickle cell ulcers.

The patient's pain was markedly improved by the topical pain medication and the Metanx. After 5 days, no further narcotic pain medications were needed. The periwound $TcPO_2$ had risen to 46, with the reference value of 67. The fibrotic wound tissue was slowly removed until a clean, granulating wound bed was present, after which the patient's wound was dressed twice weekly with an oxidized, regenerated cellulose/collagen/silver wound dressing (Prisma). After receiving a multi-unit blood transfusion to bring her hemoglobin to 10.6 gm% and hematocrit to 31%, the ulcer began to heal. The wound slowly improved until healing was complete. Metanx has been continued, and she has had no recurrence to date.

1. Which of the following is <u>not</u> correct?
   A. Sickle cell disease is an inherited disease of the blood's hemoglobin molecule.
   B. Sickle cell disease is seen primarily in black individuals.
   C. Individuals with heterozygous sickle cell disease are at higher risk for developing an ulcer.
   D. The most severe form of sickle cell disease is seen when an individual inherits an abnormal hemoglobin gene from both parents.

   ANSWER: C. *Persons with heterozygous sickle cell disease receive only one gene for abnormal hemoglobin from one of their parents and are at less risk of ulceration than persons who have abnormal hemoglobin genes from both parents (homozygous). A, B, and D are true statements.*

2. Sickle cell ulcers are more likely to develop in males with sickle cell disease than in females.
   A. True
   B. False

   ANSWER: A.

3. Which one of the following can signal that a patient with sickle cell disease might ulcerate?
   A. Edema
   B. Hemoglobin A1c of 7
   C. Absence of fever
   D. Resolution of pain in the leg

   ANSWER: A. *Edema is a key indicator that a person with sickle cell disease may get an ulcer. B is incorrect as hemoglobin A1c is not related to sickle cell disease but to diabetes mellitus. C is incorrect as patients with sickle cell disease often have fever of unknown origin. D is incorrect because pain is frequently part of sickle cell ulcers.*

4. Which one of the following is not part of the evaluation of the patient with a sickle cell ulcer?
   A. History, including a family history
   B. General physical examination
   C. Assessment of wound bed and pulses
   D. A bone scan

   ANSWER: D. *A bone scan is virtually useless in diagnosing osteomyelitis; magnetic resonance imaging is preferred. A, B, and C are all correct and should be part of the assessment of a patient with a sickle cell ulcer.*

5. Comprehensive treatment of the patient with sickle cell ulcer could include all of the following <u>except</u>:
   A. Restriction of dietary iron intake
   B. Debridement of the ulcer
   C. Wound pain management
   D. Compression modalities

   ANSWER: A. *There is no reason to restrict iron in the diet of persons with sickle cell disease. B, C, and D are all important parts of the holistic plan of care of patients with a sickle cell ulcer.*

REFERENCES

1. Herrick JB. "Peculiarly Elongated and Sickle-Shaped Red Blood Corpuscles in a Case of Severe Anemia," *Trans Assoc Am Physicians* 25:553, 1910.

2. Powars DR, Chan LS, Hiti A, Ramicone E, Johnson C. "Outcome of sickle cell anemia: a 4-decade observational study of 1056 patients," *Medicine (Baltimore)* 84:363-76, 2005.

3. Charache S. "One view of the pathogenesis of sickle cell diseases," *Bull Eur Physiopathol Respir* 19:361-66, 1983.

4. National Heart, Lung and Blood Institute. "Who is at risk for sickle cell anemia?" Retrieved May 25, 2010 from http://www.nhlbi.nih.gov/health/dci/Diseases/Sca/SCA_WhoIsAtRisk.html.

5. Conley, C. Lockard, "The Hemoglobinopathies and Thalassemias" in *Textbook of Medicine,* eds. Beeson, PB, McDermott, W, 13th Edition, W.B. Saunders Co., Philadelphia, pp. 1501-1503, 1971.

6. The Sickle Cell Information Center: *The Management of Sickle Cell Disease*, 4th ed. Retrieved August 15, 2010 from http://scinfo.org/index.php?option=com_content&view=category&id=15:the-management-of-sickle-cell-disease-4th-ed&Itemid=27&layout=default.

7. Cumming V, King L, Fraser R, Sergeant G, Reid M. "Venous Incompetence, Poverty, and Lactic Dehydrogenase in Jamaica are Important Predictors of Leg Ulceration in Sickle Cell Anemia," *Br J Haematol* 142:119-125, 2008.

8. Clare A, FitzHenley M, Harris J, Hambleton I, Serjeant GR. "Chronic leg ulceration in homozygous sickle cell disease: the role of venous incompetence," *Br J Haematol*. 119(2):567-571, 2002.

9. Nolan VG, Adewoye A, Baldwin C, et.al. "Sickle cell ulcers: association with haemolysis and SNPs in Klotho, TEK and genes of the TGF-Beta/BMP pathway," *Br J Haematol*. 133(5):570-578, 2006.

10. Trent JT, Kirsner RS. "Leg Ulcers in Sickle Cells Disease," *Adv Skin Wound Care* 17(8):410-416, 2004.

11. Morris CR, Kuypers FA, Larkin S, Sweeters N, Simon J, Vichinsky EP, Styles LA. "Arginine therapy: a novel strategy to induce nitric oxide production in sickle cell disease," *Br J Haematol* 111:498-500, 2000.

12. Aslan M, Freeman BA. "Oxidant-mediated impairment of nitric oxide signaling in sickle cell disease—mechanisms and consequences," *Cell Mol Biol* 50:95-105, 2004.

13. Falanga V. "Wound Bed Preparation and the Role of Enzymes: A Case for Multiple Actions of Therapeutic Agents," *Wounds* 2002;14(2):47-57

14. Ackroyd JS, Young AE. "Leg ulcers that do not heal," *Br Med J* 286:207-208, 1983.

15. Berg JO, Mossner BK, Skov MN, et al. "Antibacterial Properties of EMLA and Lidocaine in Wound Tissue Biopsies for Culturing," *Wound Rep Reg* 14:581-585, 2006

16. Winter, G.D. "Formation of the Scab and the Rate of Epithelialization of Superficial Wounds in the Skin of Young Domestic Pigs," *Nature* 193:293-94, 1962.

17. Ovington LG. "Hanging wet-to-dry dressings out to dry," *Home Healthcare Nurse* 19:477-83, 2001.

18. Leaper DJ. "Silver dressings: their role in wound management," *Int Wound J* 3:282-294, 2006.

19. Alvarez OM, Mertz PM, Eaglstein WH. "The effect of occlusive dressings on collagen synthesis and re-epithelialization in superficial wounds," *J Surg Res* 35:142-8, 1983.

20. Lamme EN, Gustafsson TO, Middelkoop E. "Cadexomer-iodine ointment shows stimulation of epidermal regeneration in experimental full-thickness wounds," *Arch Dermatol Res* 290:18-24, 1998.

21. Holloway GA, Jr., Johansen KH, Barnes RW, Pierce GE. "Multicenter trial of cadexomer iodine to treat venous stasis ulcer," *West J Med* 151:35-38, 1989.

22. Serjeant GR, Gallaway RE, Gueri MC. "Oral zinc sulphate in sickle cell ulcers," *Lancet* 2:891-892, 1970

23. Mery L, Girot R, Aractingi S. "Topical effectiveness of molgramostim (GM-CSF) in sickle cell leg ulcers," *Dermatology* 208:135-37, 2004.

24. Boykin JV, Baylis C. Homocysteine—A Stealth Mediator of Impaired Wound Healing: A Preliminary Study. *Wounds* 18(4):101-114, 2006.

25. Treadwell TA. Unpublished data. Institute for Advanced Wound Care, October, 2009.

26. Okany CC, Atimomo CE, Akinyanju OO. "Efficacy of natural honey in the healing of leg ulcers in sickle cell anemia," *Niger Postgrad Med J* 11(3): 179-181, 2004.

27. White R, Cooper R, Molan P, eds. *Honey: A Modern Wound Management Product*. Aberdeen, UK: Wounds UK Publishing, 2005.

28. Gordon S, Bui A. "Human skin equivalent in the treatment of chronic leg ulcers in sickle cell disease patients," *J Am Podiatr Med Assoc* 93(3):240-241, May-June 2003.

29. Schultz GS, Falanga V, et al. "Wound bed preparation: A systematic approach to wound management," *Wound Rep Reg* 11(Suppl):1-28, 2003.

30. Treadwell TA, Fuentes ML, Walker D. "Wound Bed Preparation Prior to the Use of Bi-layered Tissue Engineered Skin: The Role of Protease Modulation." *Wound Rep Reg.* 16:A19, 2008.

31. Chin GA, Schultz GS. "Treatment of chronic ulcer in diabetic patients with a topical metalloproteinase inhibitor, doxycycline," *Wounds* 15(10): 315-323, 2003.

32. Cullen, B., et al. "Mechanism of action of Promogran, a protease-modulating matrix, for the treatment of diabetic foot ulcers," *Wound Rep Reg* 10:16-25, 2002.

33. Best JP, Daoud MS, Pittelkow MR, Petit RM. "Hydroxyurea-induced leg ulceration in 14 patients," *Ann Int Med* 128: 29-32, 1998.

34. Weinlich G, Schuler G, Greil R, Kofler H, Fritsch P. "Leg ulcers associated with long-term hydroxyurea therapy," *J Am Acad Dermatol.* 39: 372-374, 1998.

35. Flores F, Eaglstein WA, Kirsner RS. "Hydroxyurea-induced leg ulcers treated with Apligraf," *Ann Intern Med* 132(5): 417-418, March 2000.

36. Eckman J, Platt A. *Leg Ulcers. Sickle Cell Information Center Guidelines*. Retrieved June 21, 2010 from www.scinfo.org/legulcr.htm.

37. Heckler FR, Dibbell DG, McCraw JB. "Successful use of muscle flaps or myocutaneous flaps in patients with sickle cell disease," *Plast Reconst Surg* 59:902-908, 1997.

38. Khouri RK, Upton J. "Bilateral lower limb salvage with free flaps in a patient with sickle cell ulcers," *Ann Plast Surg* 27:574-6, 1991.

39. Richards RS, Bowen CVA, Glynn MFX. "Microsurgical free flap transfer in sickle cell disease," *Ann Plastic Surg* 29:278-281, 1992.

40. Steinberg MH. "Management of Sickle Cell Disease." *NEJM* 340:1021-1030, 1999.

41. Sher GD, Olivieri NF. "Rapid healing of chronic leg ulcers during arginine butyrate therapy in patients with sickle cell disease and thalassemia," *Blood* 84:2378-2380, 1994.

42. Atweh GF, Sutton M, Nassif I, et al. "Sustained induction of fetal hemoglobin by pulse butyrate therapy in sickle cell disease," *Blood* 93:1790-97, 1999.

CHAPTER 18

Surgical Reconstruction of Wounds

Joyce M. Black, PhD, RN, CPSN, CWCN, FAAN
Steven B. Black, MD, FACS

Objectives

After completing this chapter, you'll be able to:

- explain the intrinsic and extrinsic causes of surgical wounds that have failed to heal
- describe the reconstructive ladder
- describe how the reconstructive ladder is used to achieve wound closure
- explain the surgical principles that guide care of patients who require skin, tissue, or bone transplantation for wound closure.

Surgical wounds are common in hospitalized patients; however, due to the body's amazing ability to heal acute wounds, hospitalized patients are seldom seen by wound care specialists unless their wounds have failed to heal. This chapter addresses common surgical wounds, complex wounds healed via surgical procedures, and surgical wounds that have failed to heal in a timely manner.

ASSESSMENT

When examining a patient with a nonhealing surgical wound, it's imperative that the initial reason for surgery and the operation performed be fully understood. The answers to the following questions must be clear in the examiner's mind: What was the preoperative condition that required surgery? For example, did the patient have gastric bypass or repair of abdominal lacerations? What was the patient's condition before surgery? Was the patient healthy or was the patient chronically ill due to diabetes or cancer? What was the intended operation? Were organs or tissue removed? Was the operation clean or contaminated (for example, penetrating trauma, perforated diverticulum)? Were

foreign materials implanted? Was the operation carried out as planned? For example, has the wound been closed with permanent sutures or mesh? Has healing been occurring along a normal trajectory until now? If so, what has happened to alter the course of healing? What medications is the patient taking that might impact healing? Has the nutritional status of the patient been normal since surgery? Was it normal prior to surgery?

From this initial assessment, a comprehensive understanding of the patient who has the wound, not just the wound itself, will be obtained. And, although treating the wound is of utmost importance, treating the patient, whose body will heal the wound, is equally imperative.

EXTRINSIC AND INTRINSIC CAUSES OF NONHEALING WOUNDS

Causes of nonhealing wounds can be grouped into two large categories: extrinsic and intrinsic. Extrinsic causes are those factors that exist outside of the wound itself, such as pressure or tension, smoking, and malnutrition. Intrinsic factors exist within the wound, such as infection, tension, and arterial insufficiency.

Determining which of these factors is present in a wound is an important initial step in wound care. Removing any obstacles to healing is also important; local treatments won't be effective in healing the wound if the underlying cause of the disruption in healing is not addressed.

Early wound care focuses on removing the obstacles to healing. Although wound care has seen technological advances, the great 16th century surgeon Ambrose Paré is still correct in that we as healthcare providers don't heal wounds, we create them and nature heals them.[1] Indeed, our role is to support the body so that the wound can heal. Wound care practitioners must exercise caution when moving too quickly into treatments for wounds until the underlying causes of the delay in wound healing are fully understood.

GOALS OF CARE

For acute wounds, wound closure with the return of form and function is the usual goal of care. Left alone to close via contraction and scar formation, wounds seldom have either form or function and will often recur and look unpleasant. The ability to reach ideal and complete healing without unsightly scarring, such as seen in fetal wounds is impossible. Therefore, the return of acceptable healing with sustained function and anatomic continuity becomes the ideal end point.

Reconstructive ladder and planning reconstruction

A decision-making process in choosing the appropriate method to achieve wound closure is based on the following information and the "rungs" of the reconstructive ladder. (See *Reconstructive ladder*.) Following are some important questions to consider.

IS THE WOUND MISSING TISSUE?

If the wound hasn't lost any tissue, it may be possible to close it primarily. Wounds are capable of healing by primary intention, which occurs when the wound edges are approximated (pulled together) and retained by sutures, staples, or glue. The dynamics of healing begin, and new tissue is synthesized.

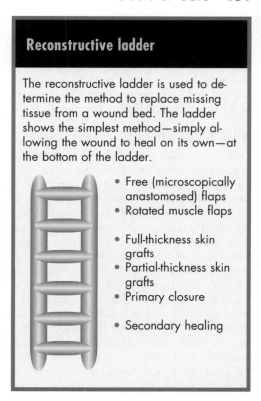

Reconstructive ladder

The reconstructive ladder is used to determine the method to replace missing tissue from a wound bed. The ladder shows the simplest method—simply allowing the wound to heal on its own—at the bottom of the ladder.

- Free (microscopically anastomosed) flaps
- Rotated muscle flaps

- Full-thickness skin grafts
- Partial-thickness skin grafts
- Primary closure

- Secondary healing

A healing ridge (an induration beneath the skin, extending to approximately 1 cm) forms directly under the suture line between 5 and 9 days after surgery. All forms of wound healing lead to scar, and primary wound closure is no different. If the scar is over tissue that is very mobile, it is prone to exaggerated scar formation, such as hypertrophic scar.

WHAT KIND OF TISSUE, IF ANY, IS MISSING?

Wounds that only lack portions of skin may be allowed to granulate closed if they're small, or skin may be grafted to speed the healing process. Wounds that have lost tendon, muscle, or bone may require transplantation of this tissue to provide form and function. Such operations require flaps of skin, muscle, fascia, or bone. Such flaps are named for their composition, such as an osteocutaneous flap, which is a bone and skin flap. Another type of flap is the free flap, which employs the surgical technique of freely removing tissue from one area, detaching the nutrient artery and vein from their supply vessels, and moving the tissue to the recipient site where these vessels are reattached to new supply vessels. For example, a radial free-arm flap contains radius bone, overlying muscle, and skin. It is commonly used to reconstruct the face and jaw after wide excision of cancer of the mandible and floor of the mouth.

WHAT DONOR-SITE MORBIDITY MAY OCCUR?

Donor sites have some form of scarring and may exhibit some loss of function, depending on the tissue removed. Split skin graft donor sites should heal with minimal effort; there is no loss of function but a scar remains. When the breast is reconstructed using the latissimus dorsi muscle from the back, the woman may lose some functions of the shoulder. Although some patients perceive the loss of function as tolerable, other patients—for example, a tennis player—may undoubtedly perceive it differently. If a thumb is lost, a patient may opt to transplant the great toe to provide opposition for hand function; however, most people wouldn't want to sacrifice a thumb to replace the great toe. In other words, the degree of loss a patient is willing to experience is proportional to his or her need for the sacrificed tissue.

WHAT'S THE SIMPLEST METHOD TO ACHIEVE WOUND CLOSURE?

The easiest method available to close the wound is often used first. Wounds that can heal quickly on their own via granulation and epithelialization are allowed to do so. Skin grafting is the next simplest method and is used to treat wounds that are missing only skin. Skin grafting can be full or partial-thickness, depending on the kinds of tissue missing in the recipient site and the condition of the site. Wounds that could close on their own, but with accompanying contracture and loss of function, may also be grafted. If muscle is missing, muscle flaps may be used to fill the wound defect or cavity, but the muscle isn't made functional (that is, an insertion, origin, and nerve aren't restored to create a functional muscle). The blood supply to the muscle is restored so that it remains viable. The ample blood flow into muscle is commonly used to treat complex wound problems such as osteomyelitis. Restored blood flow may also transport antibiotics and immune cells to the wound.

Muscle has been shown to supply overlying islands of skin through a series of vessels that perforate the muscle body. Surgeons can simultaneously transplant a muscle and the island of skin to both fill a wound cavity and provide skin coverage. Such a flap is called a musculocutaneous flap. Often the specific muscle is noted, as in the case of the tensor fascia lata flap, which is used to close a trochanteric pressure ulcer. If a large amount of skin is missing, the muscle may be transplanted and then covered with skin grafting to achieve the same effect. Such an operation is called a muscle-flap and split-thickness skin graft, with the specific muscle being grafted added to the name.

Muscle is brought to the recipient site in one of two ways:

- it's rotated along an arc with its original blood supply left intact
- it's freed from its blood supply and the artery and vein are reattached via a microscope at the recipient site.

Freeing the muscle, skin, and other parts of a flap allows the flap to be used for reconstruction in areas that the muscle normally couldn't reach, such as the lower third of the leg.

It's important to note that, as often as possible, tissue should be replaced with similar tissue. Similar hair bearing, appearance, and thickness improve aesthetic appearance on the reconstructed wound. This process of choosing a method to close a wound has been called a reconstructive ladder. (See *Reconstructive ladder.*) The easiest method, secondary healing, is at the bottom of the ladder.

Wounds without missing tissue

Some wounds don't require grafts because they aren't missing tissue, or local tissue can be undermined and lifted to close the original wound.

SIMPLE LACERATIONS

Traumatic wounds are often missing little or no tissue and can be closed primarily; however, the full extent of the injury must be known before any closure is attempted. Laceration of arteries and veins is usually obvious by the amount of bleeding present. Facial lacerations are especially bloody due to the robust blood supply in the face. The patient with a facial laceration is assessed for function of motor and sensory nerves, muscle, and parotid and other salivary glands in the area prior to injection with lidocaine, which would obscure the findings. Repair of vessels, tendons, ligaments, and nerves is commonly completed in the operating room because it is a sterile environment and sometimes has the added benefit of an operating microscope. Wounds are irrigated copiously to remove any debris. Skin closure is accomplished by undermining surrounding tissue to facilitate its movement and suturing layers of tissue with minimal tension. Drains may be placed in wounds with contamination or large amounts of dead space. The appearance of the wound should ideally mimic the ipsilateral appearance. However, traumatic amputation or extensive debridement may leave an appearance that's less than acceptable.

Removing all forms of tension on the wound reduces the scar. Wounds that must be mobilized to gain function, such as incisions over joints, heal with wider scars and this may be disturbing to the patient's self-image. Stented dressings, immobility (for example, limited chewing or talking with facial lacerations), and thin applications of topical antibiotics may help to minimize scars. Moist wound-healing techniques, used throughout the healing process, will minimize healing time and potentially the amount of scarring. However, it's important for the patient, the patient's family, and members of the healthcare team to realize that scarring is inevitable and only after the scar has matured, which can take more than 1 year, will scar revision be attempted. Silicone-based dressings may be used over some healed wounds to help minimize scar buildup during the maturation phase.

EXTENSIVE LACERATIONS

Extensive lacerations, while unsightly, are seldom life-threatening. Life-saving care of the heart, lungs, and brain precedes definitive wound care. Initial wound care includes debridement of obvious dirt, glass, grass, or other foreign bodies. Massive lacerations are packed with moist dressings to prevent tissue desiccation and, when the patient is stable, the wounds are debrided and surgically closed, if possible.

Extensive wounds may require multiple debridements until viable tissue is present; these wounds may also require more complex forms of delayed closure, such as flaps.

Wounds that are not closed within the first 6 hours after injury are considered contaminated and cannot be closed primarily after that time. Some clean facial wounds are an exception to this rule, and their closure may be delayed longer in healthy patients who are on antibiotics.

PENETRATING ABDOMINAL WOUNDS

Penetrating abdominal wounds include stab wounds, impalements, gun shots, and so forth. These are serious wounds due to direct tissue injury, risk of contamination and sepsis, and the potential for excessive bleeding. Depending on the degree of contamination from environmental agents (e.g., dirt) or penetration of the bowel or bladder, the wound may not be closed completely. Frequently in traumatic injuries, these wounds are not closed external to the fascia. If the fascia cannot be closed, leaving the abdomen open is also a challenge. These patients require multiple re-explorations while simultaneously reducing or controlling abdominal fluid secretion and preserving the fascia for closure. Currently, no protocols exist for the management of the open abdomen and care is based on clinical judgment.

ABDOMINAL COMPARTMENT SYNDROME

Abdominal compartment syndrome (ACS) is similar to compartment syndrome of the extremity. ACS can occur during elective abdominal operations, following abdominal trauma or pelvic fracture, and with pancreatitis. Normal intra-abdominal pressure in surgical patients is 2 to 10 mm Hg; a value above 12 mm Hg indicates intra-abdominal hypertension, and a value above 20 mm Hg is considered an indicator of abdominal compartment syndrome. Intra-abdominal pressure can be determined using simple water-column manometry with a bladder catheter. When pressure is mildly increased to 10 to 15 mm Hg, the cardiac index rises due to compression of the vena cava. With further elevations, there is progressive organ dysfunction due to intra-abdominal pressure on the abdominal organs and vena cava. Direct compression on the hollow intestine and portal-caval system causes these structures to collapse. When the bowel is compressed it becomes ischemic, allowing bacteria to thrive. Vasoactive substances such as histamine and serotonin increase endothelial permeability, further capillary leakage impairs red cell transport, and ischemia worsens. As pressure rises, ACS not only impairs visceral organs but also damages the cardiovascular and the pulmonary systems; it may also cause a decrease in cerebral perfusion pressure. Therefore, ACS should be recognized as a possible cause of decompensation in any critically injured patient.[2-5]

It is important to include ACS in a wound healing chapter because the treatment of ACS is not closure of the abdomen. If the abdomen is at all difficult to close, this procedure should be abandoned and alternative techniques applied. A good rule of thumb is as follows: when looking at the abdomen horizontally, if you can see the gut above the level of the wound, consider leaving the abdomen open and using temporary closure.

The easiest way to control the open abdomen is to use a silo-bag closure.[5] This short-term therapy has increasingly been replaced by negative pressure wound therapy (NPWT). The use of NPWT has been shown to allow successful fascial closure in patients who in the past would have required mesh grafting for closure. While NPWT increases the use of primary closure, it also shortens time to recovery.[6]

Wounds requiring tissue transplantation for closure

Tissue transplantation is a phrase used to describe closure techniques for a group of wounds that have missing tissue. In order to achieve closure, various tissue (skin, muscle, fascia, bone) can be grafted or flapped into the wound. These wounds can be quite complex to manage.

BURNS

Surgical management of burn wounds includes escharotomy, excision of eschar, skin grafting, and scar revision. Because many burned patients must undergo multiple operations, it is beneficial to have a dedicated team for these patients to reduce some of the anxiety associated

with surgery, anesthesia, and pain management. It is wise to have burned patients go directly from their inpatient room to surgery, not stopping in preoperative areas.

Escharotomy

Escharotomy is a decompressive operation to reduce compartment syndrome in the extremities, respiratory compromise, abdominal compartment syndrome, and even orbital compression. Full-thickness burned skin cannot stretch; therefore, during fluid resuscitation the fluid that moves into the interstitial spaces places pressure on vessels and nerves. Indications for escharotomy include compartment syndrome of the extremities (pallor, pain, pulselessness, paresthesia, and paralysis), falling oximetry with respiratory difficulty, increased abdominal pressure, and changes in vision. Escharotomy is completed by incising the burned tissue along the longitudinal axis of the extremities or across the chest and/or abdomen. The surgical site is left open to allow for both edema and chest wall movement with respiration. Once the capillary bed has stabilized and fluid leaves the interstitial spaces, the escharotomy incisions will approximate. The incisions are not closed, but rather are allowed to heal secondarily; therefore, they should be packed with saline-moistened gauze.

Excision of eschar

Years ago, eschar was removed slowly with weeks of daily submersion in tanks and debridement with scissors. This process is still used for some burns, but many burns today are debrided with pressurized water knives and some burns are completely excised and grafted early to promote rehabilitation. Burns of the hand are typically managed in this fashion in order to quickly mobilize the hand and restore function.

Skin grafting

The only way to permanently heal a burn wound is to graft the wound. Skin grafts are portions of the patient's skin removed from a donor site of unburned skin or healed burned skin that are moved to cover an open burn wound. They are often referred to as split-thickness skin grafts. Skin grafts are harvested in the operating room and placed on the freshly debrided burn wound. The skin graft lives off of the serum in the wound bed; it does not have a blood supply (unlike a flap). As the capillary beds in the wound bed grow into the skin graft, it becomes pink in color. This pink color is called a "take" and often expressed as a percentage (e.g., 50% take of the split-thickness skin graft).

A crucial aspect of skin graft healing is immobilization of the graft onto the wound bed. Most surgeons use fibrin glue, stent the graft in place, or suture it to the edges of the wound. Because edema in the space between the wound bed and the skin graft can separate the graft from capillary ingrowth, NPWT is often used to promote attachment. If NPWT is used, the suction should be continuous and not interrupted.

The dressings are usually removed at 72 hours to inspect the graft. Dressings after that point vary, but many surgeons continue to dress the newly grafted site with an antimicrobial dressing.

Skin grafts fail for several reasons. The primary reason is edema in the wound bed that lifts the grafted skin off the bed. It is imperative that all precautions to keep the grafted area elevated be followed. Too many well-meaning patients have convinced nurses that during a quick trip to the bathroom, rather than the bedside commode, the leg will remain elevated. Unfortunately, those short periods of time with the leg down may be all that is required to allow edema to lift the graft off of the wound bed!

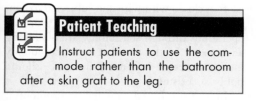

Patient Teaching

Instruct patients to use the commode rather than the bathroom after a skin graft to the leg.

Skin grafts can also fail due to infection in the wound. If infection is suspected it should be ruled out with quantitative cultures of the wound bed prior to grafting.

Pruritus is a common and distressing problem in healed burn wounds. Skin grafts do not carry sweat or oil glands with them, making the transplanted skin prone to dryness and pruritus from heat retention. In addition, burn scars are not elastic, making them prone to injury. Persistent pruritus is estimated to occur in about 87% of burned patients.[7] Methods to treat pruritus have not been compared systematically and the use of histamine-receptor agonists is commonly based on the belief that pruritus is mediated by mast cells. Newer thoughts on the etiology of pruritus following skin grafting are that it is a variant of pain; and newer treatments for pruritus have examined eutectic mixture of local anesthetic (EMLA) cream, transcutaneous electrical nerve stimulation (TENS), colloidal oatmeal, massage, and sedatives. The problem of pruritus is in great need of ongoing study.

Scar revision

Scars continue to mature over 6 to 12 months following a burn. Burned areas that were allowed to heal without grafting have the most robust scars. When the scars reach across joints, the joints can be pulled into contracture. Z-plasty is a procedure that can be performed if there is adequate tissue in one dimension and not the other, for example, adequate tissue in length but not width. Z-plasty transfers the excess tissue to the area in need of tissue, thereby releasing the contracture. Many times, however, there is not enough tissue in either direction, and so skin grafting is needed.

NONHEALING SURGICAL WOUNDS

Surgical wounds can be slow to heal because of underlying disease states, such as infection, poorly controlled diabetes, protein-calorie malnutrition, and compromised immunity. By convention, any surgical wound of 3 to 4 weeks' duration that is not responding to conventional therapy is considered nonhealing. From the surgical perspective, only debridement can be offered as treatment.

Infection, including the development of biofilms, is a common culprit of nonhealing. Biofilms promote inflammation, and inflammation delays healing. Common bacterial causes include *Staphylococcus*, *Pseudomonas*, and *Enterobacter*. Debridement, performed either traditionally or using low-frequency ultrasound, destroys the biofilm and is an important component of wound care.[8]

ABDOMINAL WOUND DEHISCENCE AND EVISCERATION

Wound dehiscence is the separation of the edges of a surgical wound. The strength of a wound lies in the musculo-aponeurotic layer of the abdomen. In the early postoperative period, wounds stay closed as a result of the strength of the sutures used or through normal healing processes as muscles regain their strength. However, some wounds are susceptible to dehiscence, thus requiring tissue transplantation.

Risk factors for wound dehiscence may be technical or related to patient factors. Technical factors are due to the type of closure used. Indeed, wound dehiscence may occur because sutures break, sutures stretch or cut through the tissue, knots slip, the suture is too thin, or an insufficient number of sutures is used. Closure is best achieved when long-lasting, absorbable, or permanent sutures are used, with secure knots that do not slip or invite bacteria to harbor in them. Sutures should be placed about 1 cm from the abdominal wound and 1 cm apart from each other. This closure places the suture in healthy fascia that will not be cut by suture material. In wounds that are healing securely, a healing ridge of palpable thick tissue about 0.5 cm appears along the incision. This ridge is almost always absent in wounds that rupture.

Patient factors that precipitated wound dehiscence were reported in a large retrospective study.[9] The most significant patient-related factors for dehiscence were age over 65 years, emergency operation, cancer, hemodynamic instability, intra-abdominal sepsis, wound infection, hypoalbuminemia, obesity, and use of steroids. Factors that were not significant included gender, anemia, and the presence of diabetes mellitus or pulmonary disease. Overall morbidity and mortality in the patients studied were 30% and 16%, respectively, correlating directly with the number of risk factors present.[9]

Obesity, heavy coughing or retching, and ascites, all of which strain the wound during healing, predispose to dehiscence. However, many surgeons believe that if a wound is closed securely, these complications will not occur. Usually the first sign of an impending problem is the sudden discharge of serosanguineous fluid

from the wound, but some patients present with sudden evisceration following an episode of coughing or retching. When the edges of the wound separate and internal organs such as the gut are protruding from the wound, this is known as evisceration.

Evisceration is a frightening experience for the patient. Immediate treatment includes helping the patient to remain calm, medicating for pain, and holding the abdominal contents in the abdomen by keeping the viscera moist with a sterile moist towel. Exposed intestines should not be forced back into the abdomen. The patient should be kept NPO and prepared for immediate surgery. Lower the head of the bed so it is flat or no more than 20 degrees.[5] Monitor the patient's vital signs and assess for signs and symptoms of shock.[5] The wound is explored urgently in surgery, devitalized tissue is excised, and the abdomen is closed with nonabsorbable interrupted suture taking secure bites into healthy tissue. Hernia formation is relatively common, reaching 30% in wounds that eviscerated and reclosed. If the wound has dehisced and the patient cannot tolerate another anesthetic, the wound can be packed with dressings, an abdominal binder used or a vacuum-assisted closure applied to obtain secondary healing. These wounds will inevitably develop hernia.

MEDIAN STERNOTOMY WOUNDS

Median sternotomy incisions are extremely complex wounds to close following surgery. Bone stabilization is usually done by rigid fixation and immobilization, but the sternum is often closed with wire and subjected to constant movement with respiration. Further, operations through sternotomy are often long and bloody, so the fact that some sternotomy incisions become infected and dehisce should not be surprising.

Indeed, infected medial sternotomy[10] wounds following cardiac surgery are a dreaded complication. High-risk patients include those who are obese (body mass index over 30) and those with diabetes, heart failure, previous myocardial infarction, urgent operative status, and hypertension. Perfusion time over 200 minutes, use of an intra-aortic balloon pump, and three or more distal anastomoses are risk factors for very serious infections, but these conditions rarely occur. Control of blood glucose and improvement of heart failure prior to surgery are helpful interventions. Sternal incision contamination from intranasal organisms can be reduced by using intranasal mupirocin (Bactroban) ointment.[9] Additionally, the use of transparent adhesive dressings is also helpful to prevent environmental exposure while the wound closes.[11,12]

Early wound infection, such as the aforementioned suppurative mediastinitis, appears as cellulitis, purulent wound drainage, and obvious tracking between the skin, sternum, and mediastinum. Left untreated, these infections smolder down into the mediastinum and may even extend into aortic suture lines, prosthetic grafts, and intracardiac prostheses. Local wound care is based on the condition of the wound and the condition of the patient. Wound-bed preparation may include packing, debridement, or the use of NPWT, which may be used as a first line of treatment to drain the superficial infection down to the sternum because it splints the chest wall. NPWT can be used as a bridge to allow the patient to recover or stabilize. Preliminary data show improved survival rates of patients with mediastinitis who were treated with NPWT.[6]

Caution is required when treating deep wounds that are packed. One continuous piece of rolled gauze is the preferred method for packing to avoid losing single dressings in the chest cavity. Further, if wounds require topical application of solutions, the large amount of open tissue will quickly absorb the fluids. Use of such products as povidone-iodine solution in these large wounds has resulted in iodine toxicity due to the large absorptive surface. Wounds that extend to or around the myocardium should be gently packed between heartbeats. Packing the wound tightly can constrict myocardial filling during relaxation; therefore, the wound must be tucked loosely with gauze.

CHEST WALL RECONSTRUCTION

Reconstruction of the chest wall can range from skin closure to chest wall stabilization. Defects following excision of a tumor, tissue loss from infection of the pleural space, and dehiscence of sternal wounds after coronary bypass grafting are examples of chest wall wounds that usually require reconstruction. Failure to stabilize the chest wall can lead to paradoxical chest motion with breathing, which results in compromised respiratory function. Prior to surgery, the patient's cardiac and pulmonary function, nutritional status, and wound bed should be maximized.

When a defect is limited to skin and subcutaneous tissue, local skin flaps can frequently be used to close the wound. A skin flap can be rotated or advanced to cover the wound. The deltopectoral skin flap can also be used to cover chest wounds, although its blood supply is stretched to do so. The principal blood supply to the flap is from two large perforating arteries arising from the second or third intercostal space lateral to the sternal border. Therefore, any tension of the flap or chest can interfere with blood supply to the flap. The weight and torsion of the breast tissue or an obese chest can place tension on the flap, so a loose-fitting bra or binder should be used to support the tissue.

Loss of the sternum is especially complex because without the sternum, ribs are pulled inward with inspiration (for example, flail chest). Patients can usually tolerate the loss of four ribs if the wound is closed with a muscle flap, such as the latissimus dorsi flap. Massive chest injuries or defects will require bony reconstruction; if bone is not used, acrylics or synthetic mesh can be used. However, the risks of infection and rejection are ever-present when synthetic materials are used.[11-13]

> ### ⬛ PRACTICE POINT
> Immediately report to the surgeon any signs of flap ischemia, such as pale, dusky, mottled, or cool tissue.

When the chest wall defect is large, several muscles may be needed for reconstruction, depending on the location of the wound. The latissimus dorsi, pectoralis major, rectus abdominis, and trapezius are the most common muscles used for chest wall reconstruction.[1] The pectoralis muscle is commonly used because it is near the defect. Its blood supply is through the thoraco-acromial artery, located in the axilla. The muscle is also supplied with perforating arteries from the internal mammary artery. If the pectoralis muscle is used, the patient will lose some ability to adduct and rotate the arm and may have some weakness with lifting. Due to the severity of the defect, this loss of donor site mobility is usually justified.

Following surgery, vascular inflow and outflow must be closely monitored. Arterial insufficiency in the flap is a major hazard, and problems can occur from too much tension on the artery, hematoma in the underlying tissue, extravasated blood, increased blood viscosity, spasm of the artery, or injury or disease of the arterial vessels. Venous outflow problems occur from edema in the flap or compression of the veins. A flap with arterial inflow problems will appear pale and feel cool. Flaps with venous congestion will look engorged and purple and feel tense or full.[14]

PRESSURE ULCER REPAIR

Repairing a pressure ulcer for surgical closure is a process that involves multiple steps that begin well before surgery. After the pressure ulcer bed is clean, it can be closed surgically. However, before any decisions are made for surgery, such plans must be considered in light of the patient's situation, condition, and goals. While various surgical options may be technically possible, performing these operations for the right reasons is an essential first step. Surgery shouldn't be entered into lightly. For some patients, not closing the wound surgically may be the best decision. With proper nutrition, pressure redistribution, and local wound care, deep pressure ulcers may remain stable for the duration of the patient's life. Adjunctive therapies, such as NPWT, electrical stimulation, and the use of bioengineered tissue products, may be considered to help with closure of these chronic wounds.[15]

Preparing the patient for surgery

Prior to any surgery, the patient's nutritional status and comorbidities must be controlled.

Although operative blood loss is usually modest with this type of surgery, general anesthesia is commonly used and the patient must be able to tolerate the stress. General anesthesia is also used in paralyzed patients. The need for general anesthesia for repairs in these patients is often an area of question, with the patient and/or family asking "why do I need anesthesia if I can't feel below my waist?" This question should be answered in the following way: "Even though you may not feel pain, reflex arcs are frequently intact and the stress of the surgery and blood loss make blood pressure erratic." Many pressure ulcers are repaired with the patient in a prone position, and general anesthesia is necessary to maintain a patent airway and oxygenation.

If malnutrition is the primary cause of non-healing, surgery should be delayed until the patient has achieved positive nitrogen balance. Calorie counts provide clear data on actual intake of protein and calories, and adjustments can be made to reach ideal intake levels of 25 to 35 cal/kg of calories and 1.5 to 3.0 g/kg of protein. Monitoring albumin is a reasonable marker, although the half-life of albumin is 20 to 21 days, which seldom reflects current nutritional status. Further, albumin is also lowered by inflammatory processes. With a half-life of 3 days, serum prealbumin is now accepted as a better marker for assessing visceral protein status. In patients with impaired renal function, prealbumin is artificially high because it is not removed with dialysis. Therefore, patients on dialysis should be classified as malnourished if the prealbumin level is less than 30 mg/dl, whereas the usual normal range is 16 to 35 mg/dl. More accurate nutritional information on protein status can benefit the healing potential for the patient. Indirect calorimetry is helpful to obtain more exact information on nutritional expenditure. It's important to recognize that patients who are malnourished are often deficient in vitamins (especially vitamin C) and minerals (especially zinc and iron); these supplements should be given throughout the course of care. The recent guidelines on pressure ulcer treatment[16] do not advise the routine use of vitamins and minerals for healing; they are recommended here only if the patient is deficient in them.

Again, the need for aggressive nutritional support is a common area for clinical questions. Families and patients may view tube feeding as "artificial life support" and resist its use. The healthcare team needs to explain that unless the patient is eating adequately, there will be no reserve to heal. Acute wounds need more calories and protein to heal, and tube feeding (or hyperalimentation) should be considered as a short-term method to increase the likelihood of healing. (See chapter 10, Nutrition and wound care, for additional information.)

If the ulcer is due primarily to pressure (such as ischial ulcers in a paraplegic patient), pressure must be redistributed both before and after surgery. Long-term plans for continued pressure redistribution must be included in the operative plan, such as fitting the patient for a wheelchair and appropriate off-loading device, and teaching the patient pressure-relief techniques to avoid high rates of recidivism.[15]

If the ulcer is due to a combination of erosion, shear, and pressure (such as ulcers on the sacrum in a patient with dyspnea and incontinence), all contributing factors need to be addressed. Similarly, long-term pressure reduction and proper skin care management must be included in the care plan. There is a finite number of available flaps; therefore, all efforts must be directed to prevent recurrent ulcers, especially through education of the patient. The social network of the patient with a spinal cord injury has been shown to be very crucial in maintaining a healed wound.[17]

Wound infection may not be evident from the surface appearance of the wound. The presence of osteomyelitis should be considered and ruled out in all stage III and IV ulcers. The workup for suspected osteomyelitis includes a complete blood count, erythrocyte sedimentation rate, and X-rays. This combination of studies has a sensitivity of 73% and specificity of 96%.[15] CT bone scans can be used to diagnose, as needed. Biopsy after adequate debridement can also be used if osteomyelitis is still suspected and the above studies are negative.

Other infections must also be controlled prior to surgery. Urinary tract infections are common in people with diabetes, elderly women, patients with catheters, and those with sacral wounds. Urosepsis is a serious complication and should be considered as the cause of malnutrition and changes in mental status or vital signs malnutrition. Chronic urinary antibiotics may be needed for persistent urinary tract infections. Wound infection can also lead to sepsis. (See chapter 7, Wound bioburden and infection.)

Spasms are often a contributing factor to both shear and friction injuries and may also complicate a postoperative course by putting undo tension on wound closure sites. Spasms are common after spinal cord injury due to loss of supraspinal inhibitory pathways. The higher the level of spinal cord injury, the more likely spasms will occur. People with cervical injury have almost a 100% chance of spasm compared with those with injury in the lower thoracic or lumbar spine, who have a 50% chance of spasm. Spasm must be controlled prior to surgery with medications such as baclofen (Lioresal) or dantrolene (Dantrium). Botulinum toxin (Botox) can also be injected into the muscle to attempt to reduce spasm; however, the efficacy of this treatment is unrecorded. Spastic limbs may lead to wound dehiscence and postoperative wound complications and therefore must also be controlled.

Contracture develops in patients with long-standing denervation caused by tightening of the muscle and joint capsules. Because hip flexors are so strong, hip contraction is common and can make positioning difficult, with bony prominences resting on each other and leading to ulcers. Contractures can be minimized with proper, persistent positioning, splinting, and a program of aggressive (often passive) range-of-motion exercises. Patients with significant contracture can't be placed in a supine position; if surgery is performed on one hip, only one side will be available as a turning surface, which will require a sophisticated pressure redistribution system to prevent complications or undue pressure at the other hip. A defined turning schedule is essential in these cases. If contractures can be released via tenotomy, the wound may heal. However, leaving a limb flaccid after tenotomy may leave the patient bedridden if he or she relies on the spastic limb for postural support while moving.

Preparing the wound for surgery

Debridement of nonviable tissue is an important first step in the treatment of full-thickness necrotic pressure ulcers or infected, dehisced surgical wounds. Debridement of adherent eschar in pressure ulcers is advised to reduce the wound bioburden and risk of sepsis. The true stage of a pressure ulcer can't be determined until adequate debridement has been performed because the true depth of the wound is obscured. Debridement can result in extensive wounds. For example, pelvic pressure ulcers can extend to the scapula and to the vagina or trochanters. Removal of necrotic tissue may enhance the wound healing cascade and diminishes the risk of infection. (See chapter 8, Wound debridement.) Dry and stable gangrene should usually not be removed from foot ulcers in patients with impaired arterial supply. Changing a closed and stable wound to an open and ischemic wound creates a greater problem.

Wound debridement is most thoroughly completed in the operating room. Bedside debridement may be used to unroof hard eschar but can seldom be completed to the level of a clean wound bed. Enzymatic debridement will often provide reasonable wound debridement but may take many weeks. However, in the patient who is a poor surgical risk, enzymatic agents are a good alternative.

Determining which wounds would benefit from debridement is the first step. Necrotic tissue is generally understood to be a healing deterrent because it allows infection. Necrotic tissue has no blood supply, so antibiotics and antibodies are not present in it. The wound and surrounding tissue should be examined fully to assess for fluid collection, abscess formation, and extensions into surrounding tissue.

Whether or not heels should be débrided remains controversial. Most clinicians feel that stable, dry, adherent eschar on ischemic heels should not be debrided.[16] The foot, especially the posterior heel, has very limited blood flow

and only a small amount of subcutaneous fat. Once the underlying fatty tissue is exposed to the environment, it may become infected quickly due to desiccation and its limited blood flow. If bone is exposed during debridement, osteomyelitis may be an inevitable occurrence.[15] Stable, dry eschar that has no openings should be left intact, assessed often, and off-loaded completely by placing pillows under the calves or floating the heel in orthotic splints/boots. The phrase "float the heels" is an appropriate order to convey the idea that no pressure is to be applied to the heels. If the eschar softens or breaks or the tissue around the ulcer becomes fluctuant or inflamed, the tissue should be excised to prevent deeper bacterial invasion and sepsis. Chemical debridement may be needed to continue the process of wound bed preparation. Moist wound-healing techniques should be instituted at this time. Off-loading should continue throughout the course of treatment.

FLAPS FOR PRESSURE ULCER REPAIR

Large areas of skin or skin and muscle may be missing from a pressure ulcer. Surgical repair options depend on what kind of tissue needs replacement. If skin is missing on a sacral wound, for example, rotational flaps of skin or skin and fascia can be rotated to close the wound. If muscle is missing, such as in a deep stage IV ulcer, the gluteus may be used to provide padding and protection of the bony structures. The muscle moved into the wound doesn't function as muscle; it atrophies over time due to denervation. Muscle tissue provides padding and robust blood supply to combat osteomyelitis. Muscle also carries more skin with its named blood vessels, so more skin can be moved without ischemia developing. (See *Flaps for pressure ulcer repair*. See also *color section*, *Surgical closure of a pressure ulcer*, page C27.)

Postoperative care

The transplanted muscle flap requires adequate perfusion of arterial blood and drainage of venous blood to survive. Because a limited number of flaps are available to reconstruct any wound, the consequence of flap failure is great. Early flap failure is most commonly due to arterial spasm or clots in the venous drainage. Flaps

Flaps for pressure ulcer repair

This chart presents common closure options for pressure ulcers at common sites.

Pressure ulcer site	Muscle flap options	Skin or fasciocutaneous flap options
Sacral ulcer	• Gluteus maximus (superiorly or inferiorly based) or V-Y advancement	Tensor fascia lata (may retain sensation)
Ischial ulcer	• Gluteus maximus (superiorly based) • Biceps femoris • Semimembranosus • Semitendinosus • Gracilis	• Transverse or vertical lumbosacral • Posterior thigh advancement flap with skin graft of donor site • Posterior V-Y advancement flap • Medial thigh rotation flap
Trochanteric ulcer	• Tensor fascia lata (may retain sensation)	

that have impaired arterial flow appear pale, have poor to absent capillary refill, and show sluggish bleeding when lanced. These wounds require quick restoration of their arterial supply by opening the wound and examining the arterial inflow. Occasionally, arterial spasm is the culprit. Spasm can be treated by positioning the flap dependently and warming the area.

PRACTICE POINT

Early signs of arterial flap failure are:

- pale color
- poor or absent capillary refill
- sluggish bleeding when lanced
- loss of audible pulses by Doppler.

Flaps that have impaired venous drainage appear dark blue and swollen. The problem is seldom a faulty anastomosis site; usually, it results from the sluggish exit of venous blood. Venous congestion can be treated by elevation and application of leeches to drain excess blood from the flap. NPWT may also be recommended to decrease fluid collection. Drains are commonly used to empty fluid

accumulation in dead space and can be left in place for a week or longer until drainage has subsided.

Tension on the incision line can lead to dehiscence. Bolster dressings are typically used to close the wound with little tension. Suture lines are slow to heal, especially in the denervated patient, and sutures are left in place for at least 3 weeks. Due to poor approximation and tensile strength, great caution must be used when moving the patient to avoid pulling on the suture line. It's possible to tear open a late-stage surgical repair, which commonly leads to complete flap failure.

Pressure relief is crucial following flap repair. Surgeons usually prescribe air-fluidized beds or low-air-loss beds for 2 to 6 weeks. Be sure the patient is not removed from the bed without the surgeon's permission (for example, sent for an X-ray procedure). Large skin flaps are especially prone to failure because of tension on the distal edges of the flap. If fecal incontinence is likely, the patient may be placed on a low-residue diet and constipating medications. Diverting colostomy may be required prior to flap closure in extreme cases to prevent contamination of the surgical site with stool. Usually bed pans are contraindicated for the first few weeks.

The patient must be compliant with off-loading strategies after a surgical flap for wound closure to prevent breakdown of the surgical repair. This involves not only immediate postoperative pressure redistribution but continued interventions of pressure relief and reduction after complete healing has occurred, especially in patients confined to wheelchairs. Proper chair cushions and weight shifts are essential.[15]

LEG RECONSTRUCTION

Tissue defects of the leg can be reconstructed with muscle flap covered with skin grafts, myocutaneous flaps, or free flaps, depending on the location of the wound and available donor tissue. Attempts are made to salvage the leg unless there is irreversible nerve or vessel damage. Major soft tissue injuries with or without bone involvement provide an environment favorable for infection. Wound care is commonly completed in the operating room, where debridement can be performed in a sterile, controlled atmosphere. Definitive wound coverage often includes rectus abdominis, gluteus, rectus femoris, gastrocnemius, and soleus muscle.

Following surgery, it's imperative to monitor the flap for signs of vascular compromise. These situations are emergent; without immediate intervention, the limb may be lost due to ischemia. Unusual findings must be reported promptly and accurately to the attending surgeon.

> ### PRACTICE POINT
>
> Monitor for the following signs of vascular compromise:
> - pallor and coolness
> - lack of pulses
> - pain with movement
> - slow or absent capillary refill
> - inability to move extremity.

NECROTIZING FASCIITIS

Necrotizing fasciitis, also known as synergistic gangrene and "flesh-eating bacteria" infection, is a rapidly progressive soft tissue infection.

Although beta-hemolytic *Streptococcus pyrogenes* is the most common causative organism, no single organism is responsible for the infection. Frequently, necrotizing fasciitis is caused by two organisms acting in concert, called synergistic gangrene. Gram-positive bacteria (including *Staphylococcus*), gram-negative bacteria, anaerobic bacteria (including gas gangrene caused by *Clostridium perfringens*), marine *Vibrio*, and fungi have been identified. Necrotizing fasciitis caused by beta-hemolytic streptococcal organisms is highly sensitive to antibiotics. However, antibiotics don't penetrate necrotic tissue so delays in treatment can lead to a 75% mortality.[18]

Necrotizing fasciitis appears to develop following a breach in the integrity of a mucous membrane barrier, especially in the abdomen and perineum. The extremities are also commonly involved. A malignancy may also give rise to a portal of entry. In males, leakage into the perineal region can result in a syndrome called Fournier's gangrene, which is characterized by massive swelling and tissue loss of the scrotum and penis with extension into the perineum, the abdominal wall, and legs.

Pain out of proportion to the size and extent of the skin wound is the hallmark sign. Early presentation also includes a reddened, painful, swollen area of cellulitis and fever. More generalized swelling develops and is followed by brawny edema. With progression, dark red induration of the epidermis appears, along with bullae (filled with blue or purple fluid). Later, the skin becomes friable and takes on a bluish, maroon, or black color. By this stage, thrombosis of blood vessels in the dermal papillae is extensive. Extension of infection to the level of the deep fascia causes this tissue to take on the brownish-gray appearance of frank gangrene. Skin is normally a very effective barrier preventing bacteria from invading the body; likewise, immune cells in the skin are also able to trap organisms, preventing rapid spread along fascial planes and through venous channels and lymphatics. Patients in the later stages are toxic and frequently manifest septic shock and multiorgan failure. Progression may be rapid. Skin inflammation is rapidly followed by necrosis of superficial fascia, subcutaneous fat, and in some cases, muscle. Necrotizing fasciitis is commonly seen in conjunction with severe systemic toxicities.

> **PRACTICE POINT**
>
> The hallmark of necrotizing fasciitis is pain out of proportion to physical findings.

Diagnosis and treatment

Aspiration cultures from the wound edge or punch biopsy with frozen section may be helpful if the results are positive, but false-negative results occur in approximately 80% of cases. There is some evidence that aspiration alone may be superior to injection and aspiration using normal saline solution. However, deep biopsy and frozen section histopathology may confirm diagnosis. Frozen sections are especially useful in distinguishing necrotizing fasciitis from other skin infections such as toxic epidermal necrolysis.

> **PRACTICE POINT**
>
> In cases of suspected necrotizing fasciitis, myositis, or gangrene, early and aggressive surgical exploration is necessary to:
>
> - visualize deep structures
> - remove necrotic tissue
> - open compartments to decrease pressure
> - obtain tissue for Gram stain for aerobic and anaerobic organisms.

Repeated débridements are usually necessary until all devitalized tissue is removed. Intravenous broad-spectrum antibiotics are started pending more specific culture results. Appropriate empirical antibiotic treatment for necrotizing fasciitis from group A streptococcal organisms is commonly clindamycin plus penicillin G and cephalosporin (first- or second-generation). Mixed aerobic-anaerobic infections can be treated with ampicillin and sulbactam, cefoxitin, or combinations of either clindamycin, metronidazole, and ampicillin or ampicillin, sulbactam, and gentamicin. Group A streptococcal and clostridial infection of the fascia or muscle carries a mortality rate of 20% to 50% even with penicillin treatment. Although honey dressings were used successfully in patients with Fournier's gangrene in one study, this work needs replication.[19] Hyperbaric oxygen treatment may also be useful as many of these infections have an anaerobic or micro-aerophilic component. Antibiotic treatment should be continued until all signs of systemic toxicity have resolved, all devitalized tissue has been removed, and granulation tissue has developed. Multiorgan system failure is not uncommon.

Following debridement, wounds are left open and packed. The packing can be extensive and may be completed in the operating room with daily debridement. Definitive treatment may include amputation or extensive skin grafting after the infection is under control and the wounds show evidence of granulation. It's essential that the dressings stay moist to prevent desiccation of tissue. It may be helpful to use products with a higher absorptive capacity than gauze to manage fluid from draining wounds.

In one retrospective study, patients who survived an episode of necrotizing fasciitis had an increased risk of premature death due to infection, such as pneumonia, cholecystitis, urosepsis, or sepsis.[20] Women died much earlier than men in the study. In our experience, patients with necrotizing fasciitis have an increased frequency of colon cancer, and colonoscopy prior to dismissal has become part of the routine care provided.

SUMMARY

Understanding the etiology of complex wounds is a critical first step in developing an effective treatment plan. Recognition of the unique characteristics of each of these wound categories will enable the clinician to correctly identify the wound. The goal of care for acute wounds is wound closure with the return of form and function. Use of the reconstructive ladder can assist clinicians in the decision-making process. Surgical management may be part of the care plan for complex acute and chronic wounds. Monitoring for signs of failure is imperative for patients with skin flaps and grafts.

PATIENT SCENARIO

Clinical Data

Andre is a 22-year-old who became a T-12 paraplegic following a motor vehicle crash 2 years ago. Andre had been the driver of the car, and his best friend was killed in the crash. Andre has been struggling with his residual paralysis and accepting responsibility for his injuries and his friend's death. He was treated initially at a trauma center for repair of a fractured spine, followed by rehabilitation at a spinal cord center. He often expressed the hope to "walk again" doing "whatever it takes." He uses a wheelchair with a gel cushion to allow for sliding transfers.

This admission to acute care began with treatment in the emergency department for fever and chills. He was diagnosed with sepsis, the source of which was determined to be his ischial pressure ulcers. At the time of admission, the wounds were found to be dressed with newspaper. Andre said he did not have the money to buy dressings and uses paper towels or newspaper to absorb the drainage. He has no other chronic illnesses. He is protein malnourished and smokes 1 to 1½ packs of cigarettes daily.

Examination of Andre's wounds reveals extensive pressure ulcers throughout the perineum (see Figure 18-1). Both unstageable ischial pressure ulcers and healing pressure ulcers are present. Surgical consultation is recommended.

Case Discussion

Let's consider the following four questions as the basis for our clinical decision making regarding Andre's plan of care.

1. **What surgical treatment is likely to be recommended now?** Because the source of his sepsis is his wounds, these ulcers need to be debrided. Ideally, the debridement should be done in the operating room; however, if he is hypotensive from the sepsis, the wounds could be unroofed at the bedside. Eventually, the wounds will need to be evaluated to determine whether osteomyelitis is present. Infectious disease consultation should be obtained. Once certain anaerobic infection is controlled, NPWT could be used to promote healing.

2. **What type of pressure redistribution system is needed in the bed and in the chair?** An integrated bed system with low air loss and patient movement or an air-fluidized system is needed. While these ulcers could be seen as affecting only one turning surface, the use of a standard foam mattress will likely not be adequate because his risk for new ulcers is also high enough to justify the expenditure for an upgraded surface.

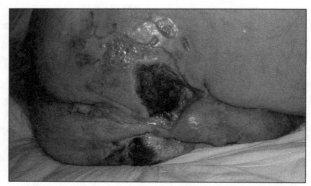

Figure 18-1. Extensive pressure ulcers throughout the perineum in a 22-year-old paraplegic man. (See *color section*, *Patient Scenarios*, page C47, for the color version of this image.)

3. **Is flap closure advisable? Why or why not?** Technically, there are flaps that could be raised to close these ulcers. However, it would likely be a multistage procedure and the flaps can only be used once. Unless Andre becomes more complaint with an off-loading program, the flaps are likely to fail. He has obviously had several ulcers and even a surgical debridement in the past 2 years. He may still be angry over the physical impact on his body and would benefit from mental health evaluation. A quick surgical fix to close these wounds would likely not benefit him in the long run.

4. **What social support is imperative in order for these wounds to stabilize? Heal?** Andre's social support network needs to be explored. If he lives alone, he might benefit from a group home with other persons confined to wheelchairs. The positive role modeling from others with spinal cord injury may be able to engage him to do off-loading and examine his skin for signs of breakdown. Social services should be working with Andre to ensure that he has a medical benefit program that can provide appropriate supplies. He also needs to be evaluated by physical and occupational therapists to assess his wheelchair, wheelchair cushion, methods of transfer, and off-loading and other potential rehabilitation strategies.

SHOW WHAT YOU KNOW

1. Which of the following situations depicts the use of the simplest method for closure of a wound?
   A. A skin graft of a venous stasis ulcer
   B. Secondary healing of a calcium extravasation
   C. Primary closure for a sternal incisional dehiscence
   D. A free fasciocutaneous flap for a stage III pressure ulcer

   ANSWER: B. *Secondary healing is the simplest method for any wound, but in many deep wounds secondary healing may be lengthy and result in excessive scarring. Venous stasis ulcers and sternal dehiscence can sometimes heal secondarily, so skin grafting would be more complex. A stage III ulcer should be able to heal with other methods than free flaps, which are the "top of the line" for surgical options.*

2. Which of the following wounds might require a musculocutaneous flap for closure?
   A. Large burn on the face
   B. Calciphylaxis of the lower legs
   C. Radiation necrosis of the chest wall
   D. A stage II pressure ulcer on the trochanter

   ANSWER: C. *Only the radiation of the chest wall is a wound with muscle involvement.*

3. Which of the following signs might indicate arterial impairment in a flap?
   A. Pain and coolness
   B. Pallor and warmth
   C. Slow capillary refill and pain
   D. Slow capillary refill and pallor

   ANSWER: D. *The loss of arterial inflow will render a flap pulseless (often only by Doppler), so delays in capillary refill are seen first, and then pallor. If the early signs are not recognized, the flap can become cyanotic and eventually lose tissue.*

4. You discharged a patient with ischial ulcers from the hospital after 6 weeks of local wound care. Upon return to the clinic, the wounds have recurred and are necrotic. Which of these causes of recurrence should be investigated first?

(continued)

REFERENCES

1. Levine, J. "Historical Notes on Pressure Ulcers: The Cure of Ambrose Pare," *Decubitus* 5(2):23-24, 26, 1992.
2. Scheppach, W. "Abdominal Compartment Syndrome," *Best Practice and Research in Clinical Gastroenterology* 23(1):25-33, 2009.
3. Paylidis, T.E., et al. "Complete Dehiscence of the Abdominal Wound and Incriminating Factors," *European Journal of Surgery* 167(5):351-55, 2001.
4. Doughty, D. "Preventing and Managing Surgical Wound Dehiscence," *Home Health Nurse* 22:364-67, 2005.
5. Moz, T. "Wound Dehiscence and Evisceration," *Nursing* 34(5):88, 2004.
6. Argenta, L., et al. "Vacuum-assisted Closure: State of the Clinical Art," *Plastic and Reconstructive Surgery* 117(7S):127S-142S, 2006.
7. Bell, P.L. and Gabriel, V. "Evidence Based Review for the Treatment of Post-Burn Pruritus," *Journal of Burn Care and Research* 30:55-61, 2009.
8. Breuing, K.H., et al. "Early Experience Using Low-frequency Ultrasound in Chronic Wounds," *Annals of Plastic Surgery* 55(2):183-87, 2002.
9. Maciver, R.H., et al. "Topical Application of Bacitracin Ointment Is Associated with Decreased Risk of Mediastinitis after Median Sternotomy," *Heart Surgery Forum* 9(5):E750-33, 2006.
10. Fowler, V., et al. "Clinical Predictors of Major Infections after Cardiac Surgery," *Circulation* 112(9 Suppl):I358-65, 2005.
11. Finkelstein, R., et al. "Surgical Site Infection Rates Following Cardiac Surgery: The Impact of a 6-year Infection Control Program," *American Journal of Infection Control* 33(8):450-54, 2005.
12. Ahumada, L.A., et al. "Comorbidity Trends in Patients Requiring Sternotomy and Reconstruction," *Annals of Plastic Surgery* 54(3):264-68, 2005.
13. Seyfer, A. "Chest Wall Reconstruction," in *Plastic Surgery: Indications, Operations and Outcomes.* Edited by Achauer, B. St. Louis: Mosby-Year Book, Inc., 2001.
14. Black, S.B. and Eastman, S. "Repair and Care of Chest Wall Defects," *Plastic Surgical Nursing* 21(1):13-19, 2001.
15. Black, S., Black, J., and Brem, H. "Surgery for Pressure Ulcers," *EPUAP-NPUAP Guidelines for Prevention and Treatment of Pressure Ulcers.* Washington, DC: National Pressure Ulcer Advisory Panel, 2009.
16. National Pressure Ulcer Advisory Panel and European Pressure Ulcer Advisory Panel. "Prevention and Treatment of Pressure Ulcers: Clinical Practice Guideline." Washington, DC: National Pressure Ulcer Advisory Panel, 2009.
17. Krause, J.S., and Broderick, L. "Patterns of Recurrent Pressure Ulcers after Spinal Cord Injury: Identification of Risk and Protective Factors 5 or More Years after Onset." *Archives of Physical Medicine and Rehabilitation* 85:1257-64, 2004.
18. Chapnick, E.K. and Albert, E.I. "Necrotizing Soft Tissue Infections," *Infectious Disease Clinics of North America* 10:838-43, 1996.
19. Efem, S.E. "Recent Advances in the Management of Fournier's Gangrene: Preliminary Observations. *Surgery* 113(2):200-4, 1993.
20. Light, T.D., et al. "Long Term Outcomes of Patients with Necrotizing Fasciitis," *Journal of Burn Care and Research* 31:93-9, 2010.

CHAPTER 19

Tube, Drain, and Fistula Management

Paula Erwin-Toth, MSN, RN, CWOCN, CNS

Linda J. Stricker, MSN/ED, RN, CWOCN

Objectives

After completing this chapter, you'll be able to:

- describe different types of tubes and drains
- state the etiology of fistulae
- discuss management options for drains, tubes, and fistulae.

Tube, drain, and fistula care may seem out of place in a wound care text. However, the realities of clinical practice sometimes dictate that a wound care clinician be consulted in the management of these special patients. In fact, it is not uncommon for people with wounds to have an assortment of concomitant conditions that include a fistula or the use of tubes and drains. Wound care is a science; drain, tube, and fistula management is an art based in science. As with all aspects of patient care, a holistic approach is essential.

TUBES AND DRAINS

The purposes of tubes and drains include the promotion of drainage from a wound or body cavity, decompression, lavage, and medication administration. Placement of tubes and drains will depend on the type, location, and purpose of the tube or drain being used. Determining a management plan starts with an assessment of the type of tube being used and the manufacturer's guidelines for care; the location of the tube, including any associated skin folds that can impede the stability of the device; and a medical record review to determine the internal location and purpose of the tube and how well the device is functioning.[1] Depending on the type, purpose, and location of the tube or drain, the insertion process will be facilitated by computed tomography, fluoroscopic illumination, or endoscopic guidance. (See *Categories of tubes and drains,* page 478.) In the case of open or laparoscopic surgery, the tube or drain generally is placed during the procedure.[1]

Pre-marking the drain site prior to insertion is sometimes helpful. With an enteral feeding tube, for example, pre-marking the drain site minimizes the possibility of the tube residing within a skin fold or crease. Tubes situated on a level plane of skin are easier to stabilize and manage.

A gap often exists in patient and family education regarding drains and tubes. Most people are aware of what to expect as far as an incision is concerned, but the presence of a tube or drain is unanticipated and unwelcomed. Preparing the patient for the potential outcome of tube or drain placement reduces anxiety and gives the patient the opportunity to plan ahead.[1]

Patient Teaching

Tell the patient and family the location and the number of tubes and drains that might be needed after surgery or to treat their medical condition.

Categories of Tubes and Drains

- **Simple tube/drain:** A catheter or a soft, flat, rubber drain. A rectal tube is an example of a simple tube that is inserted into the rectal cavity to relieve flatus, stool, or postoperative drainage. Simple tubes can be used for enema or medication administration.
- **Closed drainage catheter:** A catheter connected to a drainage container. In most cases, the collection container is considered sterile and sealed during the manufacturing process. Chest tubes, Jackson-Pratt drains, Hemovac drains, and indwelling urinary catheters (IUCs) are examples of closed drainage systems that attach to a bedside collection system.
- **Chest tube:** A sterile, closed drainage and suction system used in an emergency or surgical setting to relieve air or fluid from the pleural space. The closed drainage system is sterile and includes a water seal and negative pressure for suction.
- **Simple sump:** A catheter inserted into the abdominal cavity following surgery. It can be connected to a suction device at the distal end of an incision or can be used to instill an irrigant such as saline.
- **Nasogastric tube:** A tube that accomplishes nasogastric decompression when inserted through the mouth or nares into the stomach to remove gastric contents or administer food or medications.
- **Feeding tube:** A tube that is inserted into the stomach or small intestine for enteral feeding.
- **Indwelling urinary catheter:** A type of catheter that is inserted, using a sterile process, into the bladder to drain urine and decompress the bladder. A Lubricath Coude Catheter has a curved tip to ease insertion past the prostate.[1,2]

Types of tubes and drains
FEEDING TUBES

Patients who require enteral feeding are debilitated by disease, traumatic injury, extensive surgery, or malnourishment. Enteral feeding following a surgical procedure in which the patient is unable to take food by mouth is desirable to treat and prevent nutritional deficits and prevent atrophy of mucosal villi in the small intestine.[2] Types of enteral feeding systems include nasogastric, gastrostomy, percutaneous endoscopic gastrostomy (PEG), and jejunostomy. Tubes can be placed using several methods, including surgical, endoscopic, radiological, or manual by way of the nares. (See *Nursing care of feeding tubes*.)

Nasogastric tubes
Nasogastric tubes are inserted manually and are the least stable of the enteral feeding options. The procedure involves selecting the appropriate feeding tube, measuring the patient's anatomy to determine the length of insertion, lubricating the tube, placing the patient in a high Fowler's position, having the patient swallow water (if responsive) during

---

Nursing care of feeding tubes

Successful nursing care of feeding tubes depends on:

- ensuring that the device is stable
- providing appropriate nutritional management
- meeting the patient's hydration needs
- using the proper technique for instillation of medications.

the insertion process, and educating the patient about the procedure. Be sure to maintain tube stability at the nares used for insertion, and check throughout the insertion procedure and before instilling the liquid feeding that the tube does indeed end distally in the stomach.

Gastrostomy tubes

Gastrostomy tubes (G tubes) are surgically inserted directly into the stomach and exit at the anterior abdominal wall. This type of procedure allows for proximal decompression with simultaneous distal enteral feeding. A number of commercially manufactured G tubes are available for use. The typical design includes a disk to stabilize the tube exteriorly against the abdominal wall and a balloon tip at the distal end to ensure internal stability.[2]

Percutaneous endoscopic gastrostomy tubes

Percutaneous endoscopic gastrostomy (PEG) tubes are inserted directly into the abdominal wall using an endoscope. The tube exits proximally at the abdominal wall. The main purpose of PEG tubes is to treat and prevent nutritional deficits associated with chronic illness complications, extensive surgery, and abdominal trauma. Tube stabilization is achieved with internal and external bumpers placed along the abdominal wall.[2]

Jejunostomy tubes

Jejunostomy tubes are surgically or endoscopically inserted directly into the jejunum for the purpose of long-term enteral feeding in patients who are at risk for aspiration or for patients with esophageal, gastric, or duodenal disease processes. Tube stability is achieved with internal and external bumpers.[2]

Biliary tubes

Biliary tubes are used to relieve obstruction and facilitate drainage from the bile ducts of the liver. The catheter is inserted into the liver and bile duct either as part of a surgical procedure or via fluoroscopy using contrast and a guidewire. Catheter holes are positioned above and below the obstruction. Biliary tract drains include cholecystectomy tubes, percutaneous drains of the biliary tract, T tubes, and endoscopically placed nasobiliary tubes. Nursing management of biliary tubes includes maintaining tube stability, containing the effluent (output), caring for the skin around the tube, and monitoring output.[2]

Esophagostomy tubes

During esophagostomy, which involves surgical resection of the diseased part of the esophagus, the proximal end of the esophagus is brought to skin level and forms a stoma. The stoma is generally flush with the skin and located lateral to the trachea, resulting in an uneven surface that is difficult to pouch. Creative management solutions involve skin preparation and the use of moldable skin barriers attached to a pouching system to contain the drainage. A decompression tube can be added to aid patient comfort in cases of intractable nausea and vomiting.[2]

INDWELLING URINARY CATHETERS

Indwelling urinary catheters (IUCs) are used to monitor urinary output, manage urinary retention, decompress the bladder following surgery, and manage wounds complicated by urinary incontinence; in addition, they are used occasionally for long-term management of urinary incontinence.[1,3,4,5] A large variety of IUCs are available for use, including catheters made from latex or silicone and catheters coated with hydrogel, Teflon, or a silver alloy.[3] Common IUC properties include a double lumen, a balloon tip at the proximal end to maintain placement in the bladder, a distal end that will accommodate connection to a closed drainage system, and sufficient length to extend from the bladder and through the urethra to connect to a closed drainage system. The double lumen allows for balloon inflation and deflation as well as urinary drainage.

IUCs are one of the most frequent causes of nosocomial infection in acute care settings. Selecting the appropriate IUC begins with assessment of the patient. Considerations include allergies (such as latex) that will preclude the use of some types of catheters, the length of time the IUC is expected to be in place, and the mobility of the patient. In general, the smallest French size needed should be selected because the elastic urinary mucosa will conform to the catheter. Using larger French size catheters can cause erosion of the uroepithelium and result in leakage of urine and permanent damage to the urethra. The newer silver alloy–coated catheters are intended to reduce bacterial growth. A review of the literature demonstrates effective reduction of catheter-associated urinary tract infection (CAUTI) with short-term IUC use.[1,3]

Nursing management of IUCs incorporates measures to prevent infection and limit the length of time the catheter is used.[1,3,4,5] The longer the catheter is in place, the higher the risk will be for bacteria to infiltrate the bladder. Most IUCs should be considered for short-term use (20 to 30 days). Local care of the urinary meatus with soap and water on a daily basis along with use of a closed drainage system have been shown to reduce bacterial migration as well as provide an opportunity for the nurse to monitor the condition of the perineal area.[1,4,5] Balloon size and inflation have also been discussed in the literature as important aspects of care. The purpose of the balloon is to stabilize the catheter in the bladder. For most adults, this can be achieved with a 5-ml balloon. Larger balloons (up to 30 ml) are manufactured with the intent of providing hemostasis by adding internal pressure following prostatectomy.[1,3,4,5] Additional nursing management strategies center on monitoring the patient for leakage (usually a result of bladder spasms), catheter-associated pain or discharge, and the color, odor, and amount of urine. Assess the patient for symptoms of CAUTI. Anchoring the catheter to the internal area of the patient's leg will provide additional stabilization and comfort and reduce the risk of accidental removal.[1,3,5]

> **▶ PRACTICE POINT**
>
> Presenting symptoms of CAUTI include fever, chills, diaphoresis, hematuria, and pain (flank and suprapubic).

NEPHROSTOMY TUBES

Nephrostomy tubes are used to relieve obstructive uropathy of the lower urinary tract. They are placed into the renal pelvis of the kidney at the flank using fluoroscopy in interventional radiology with the patient under conscious sedation.[2] Nephrostomy tubes provide temporary or permanent drainage for the urinary collection system. They also provide for insertion of stents, divert urine from urethral fistulae, and allow access for kidney stone removal or biopsy.

Nursing plan of care

The nursing plan of care for patients with tubes or drains is developed using an holistic approach, which requires a thorough understanding of the anatomy and physiology of the body systems involved as well as the rationale for the selected tube or drain. Knowledge of these factors combined with assessment of the external factors affecting the patient provides a clear picture of what is needed to manage patient needs. External factors include the physical environment of care, socioeconomic issues, family support, and psychosocial concerns.[1–5] A comprehensive plan of care involves an interdisciplinary team approach that includes daily assessment and care of the skin around the tube or drain as well as thorough patient education.

Interdisciplinary team approach

Achieving a comprehensive plan of care to meet the complex needs of patients with tubes or drains requires a collaborative team. This team can include, but is not limited to, the primary care physician, surgeon, radiologist, gastroenterologist, physical therapist, social worker, case manager, registered dietitian, primary nurse, and wound, ostomy, and continence (WOC) nurse. The care plan needs to include interventions aimed at tube stabilization, containment and measurement of effluent, skin management, nutritional support, patient mobilization, and effective communication practices with the medical team.[1,2]

The registered dietitian plays a vital role on the interdisciplinary team because he or she is educationally prepared to determine the appropriate formula for enteral feeding, hydration needs, and management of diarrhea. Nurses caring for patients receiving enteral tube feedings need to develop policies that include monitoring hydration, assessing for patient tolerance by evaluating gastric aspirates, maintaining the stability of the device, and engaging with the physician and pharmacist for optimal medication management.[2]

EDUCATION

Education and discharge planning are the next step in the plan of care. Each member of the collaborative team will contribute to the education needs of the patient or caregiver; understanding these needs in turn helps the team to determine discharge needs.[2] Education should be based on the principles of adult learning and include an explanation of the purpose of the drain or tube, the need for and how to stabilize the tube, management of the containment device, skin care, any feeding schedules and procedures, and the signs and symptoms of complications. Determine whether the complexity of care is beyond the ability of the patient and, if so, ascertain whether a caregiver is willing and able to provide support.[2] The details of care should be demonstrated, reviewed, and evaluated, and written instructions should be provided. What, if any, support will be needed after discharge? How stable is the patient? Is discharge to the home a realistic option?

SKIN CARE AROUND THE TUBE

The skin around the insertion site should be assessed daily for signs of skin breakdown, infection, or excoriation. Leakage of gastric contents onto the skin is not uncommon; when it occurs, the tube must be examined for leaks and stabilized to prevent movement in and out of the abdomen. If the tube migrates or stretches, leakage of gastric contents from the puncture site can damage the skin. For the first week after tube placement, the insertion site and external retention device should be cleaned with normal saline. Half-strength hydrogen peroxide can be used to remove crusts. After the first week, the stoma site and the area beneath the external retention device should be cleaned daily with a pH-balanced skin cleanser. pH-balanced solutions do not damage the skin, leave little residue, and protect the skin without changing its pH.

G tubes should be checked for their ability to be moved in and out of the abdominal wall; ¼ inch (0.5 cm) of movement is normal. If the tube

cannot be moved even slightly, notify the physician. Often called "buried bumper syndrome," the inability to move the tube may indicate that it has become embedded in the tissues and can erode into the stomach wall. G-tube insertion sites should not be packed tightly with dressings between the tube and skin. Occasionally, hypergranulation tissue will develop at the puncture site. This tissue is not harmful and usually results from irritation from the tube.

Tube blockage is common with crushed medication, inadequate flushing (particularly with nasojejunal tubes, which tend to be longer and of finer bore), or precipitation of protein in the feeding. To avoid a clogged feeding tube, thoroughly flush enteral feeding devices every 4 to 6 hours during continuous feedings and whenever feedings are on hold, before and after administration of feedings and medications, and after checking residuals. Always use a large syringe (30 to 60 ml) for flushing to prevent rupture of the tube. Irrigate the tube with 20 to 30 ml of tepid water. Tubes can generally be unblocked using a variety of solutions, such as water, carbonated soda, pancreatic enzymes, or commercially available products. No fluid has been found to be superior to water for maintaining patency. If the feeding tube has a Y-port connector, flush through the side port. Otherwise, disconnect the feeding infusion device and flush directly into the tube.

> ### ▸ PRACTICE POINT
>
> Medications that can be administered in liquid form are best suited for enteral feeding tubes. Water flushes between medications and feedings will help prevent tube obstruction.

ENTEROCUTANEOUS FISTULAE

An enterocutaneous fistula (ECF) is an abnormal connection between two epithelial surfaces.[6,7] This connection can occur between two internal organs or can lead from an internal organ to a body surface. The physiological origin and exit point of the fistula are the basis for naming and evaluating a fistula. (See *Types of fistulae,* page 482.)

Types of fistulae	
Fistula	**Connection**
Colocutaneous	Colon to skin
Rectovaginal	Rectum to vagina
Entero-entero	Small intestine to small intestine
Enterocutaneous	Small intestine to skin

Although ECFs are not common, certain diseases or conditions will predispose a person to develop an ECF. Inflammatory bowel disease, such as Crohn's disease, can cause spontaneous fistula development and increase the risk of a postoperative fistula.[6–8] These patients require medical support and regular monitoring for complications. Other predisposing factors include traumatic abdominal injury, peritonitis, small bowel obstruction, malnutrition (especially prior to abdominal surgery), the presence of de-vascularized tissue, and radiation enteritis.[6] Many times these conditions can result in a large, deep abdominal wound with or without exposure of the bowel wall.

An ECF is one of the most challenging complications for the nurse to manage and devastating for the patient. Fluid and electrolyte imbalances, erosion of adjacent skin secondary to the corrosive nature of the effluent, malnutrition, dehydration, and the psychosocial well-being of the patient all require ongoing monitoring and evaluation for the best outcomes. The mortality rate for patients with ECF ranges from 12% to 25%, usually the result of sepsis, malnutrition, and dehydration.[7–9] Advances in nutritional support options, antibiotics, containment devices, and managing fluid and electrolyte balance have contributed to improved care and patient recovery from this type of event.[9]

Classification of ECFs

ECFs can be classified in a number of ways based on the type and amount of effluent present, the anatomy involved, and the complexity of the tract.[6] Classifying the fistula provides assessment and documentation parameters as well as clues to interventions aimed at both stabilizing and managing the patient. A simple fistula has a direct tract without an abscess. A type I complex fistula is associated with abscesses and multiple organ involvement.[6] Type II complex fistulae open into the base of an open wound; these are among the most challenging and devastating fistulae to care for.[6]

The amount of effluent is also important. Low-volume fistulae are defined by drainage amounts of less than 500 ml in a 24-hour period, while high-volume fistulae have drainage in excess of 500 ml over 24 hours.[7,9] Effective monitoring and measuring of ECF output are critical in managing fluid balance. Generally, the more proximal the fistula is located, the higher the amount of output will be.[6,7,9]

The color and consistency of the effluent provide clues to the origin of the ECF. Gastric drainage is clear to light yellow-green in color with a watery consistency; the pH will be about 3.0.[6] Biliary drainage is a gold to deep green viscous liquid with a pH of 7.5.[6] Pancreatic drainage is clear and watery with a pH of 8.3.[6] Considering that the normal pH of skin is 4.5 to 5.5, the issue of protection of adjacent skin is a primary goal of care.[6,7]

Goals of management

The goals of management for a patient with an ECF are complex and require the skills and attention of a collaborative team.[9] Early identification of the presence of an impending fistula provides an opportunity to manage complications in a timely fashion.[6,10] While an ECF is not a common event, paying attention to certain signs in the patient at risk provides clues to the need for early care. Following abdominal surgery or in cases of inflammatory bowel disease, signs such as fever, localized edema, induration, progressive local discomfort, changes in fluid and electrolyte balance, and altered mental state should be monitored closely and communicated to the physician or surgeon.[6,10,11] Once a person is predisposed to develop an ECF, some direct causes include a breakdown of the anastomotic site due to sepsis or tension, peritoneal abscess, altered blood supply, steroid therapy, and malnutrition.[12,13]

Once an ECF is suspected, it is important to identify the extent and source of the fistula. This can be accomplished through a fistulogram, computerized tomography, magnetic resonance imaging (MRI), or positron emission tomography (PET) scan.[6,12] Determining the extent of the ECF provides the information needed to develop a plan of care and guides surgical intervention if needed. Immediate stabilization of the patient by managing his or her electrolytes and fluids is a critical step.[6,12,14,15] The drainage from an ECF includes sodium, potassium, magnesium, zinc, proteins, digestive enzymes, and fluid, the loss of which will cause fluid and electrolyte depletion, and malnutrition.[6,7,9,12,15] The corrosive nature of the effluent will erode the surrounding skin and cause pain.[6,7,10,12,13] Supportive efforts are aimed at correcting these problems through intravenous support as well as quantification and containment of effluent.[6] It may be necessary to withhold oral intake (NPO) initially until all factors are identified and the extent of the ECF is determined.[12,13]

MEDICAL MANAGEMENT

The medical management of fistulae has four primary goals: stabilize fluid and electrolyte imbalance, provide nutritional support, manage sepsis, and determine the exact location of the fistula. Supporting these goals provides optimal care for the patient and increases the chance of spontaneous closure of the fistula.[12,15] Although spontaneous closure of ECFs occurs in only about a third of cases, this is still the desired outcome. A number of strategies are recommended to achieve these goals. Involving a registered dietitian is critical. Along with the physician, he or she will monitor electrolytes and fluids for replacement needs as well as determine required nutritional support.[14,15] Initially the patient may be NPO while total parenteral nutrition (TPN) is initiated. Resuming feedings either through the oral or enteral route will prevent mucosal villa

atrophy in the small bowel and promote optimal nutritional absorption.[7,12,14–16] TPN is a viable option if enteral feeding is not possible; however, the risk of hyperglycemia is always present.[16–18] Continued monitoring of serum electrolytes and nutritional markers such as prealbumin and transferrin provides important clues to the effectiveness of the nutritional plan of care.[16] Pharmacologic treatments are also useful medical management strategies. The use of octreotide or somatostatin has been shown to decrease the volume from a high-output fistula in some cases,[6,7,16,17] although the results are not always predictable. Mortality rates increase with sepsis, so the identification and treatment of sepsis in these situations is an important aspect of care.[19]

Spontaneous closure of an ECF is defined as closing with medical management in 6 to 8 weeks.[17,18,20–22] If spontaneous closure does not occur within this time frame, surgical intervention may be indicated.[17,21,22] Situations that preclude spontaneous closure include sepsis, malnutrition, distal obstruction, a matured fistula (that is, the fistula tract has epithelialized), mucosa exposure, and consistently high output of effluent. Recent attention has been placed on the use of biological fibrin glue (a combination of fibrinogen and thrombin) to close the fistula.[15] The procedure initially involves debridement of devitalized tissue and saline irrigation followed by injection of fibrin glue directly into the fistula[15,23,24]; more than one injection may be required. The expected result of this process is stimulation of coagulation within the fistula tract.

When all medical management options fail to result in closure of the fistula, surgical intervention may be needed.[25] Surgery must be planned carefully and be preceded by fluid and electrolyte balance, nutritional support, and sepsis and inflammation control. This will reduce the complications of peritonitis and the development of additional fistulae.[26–28] Timing of surgical intervention is critical. Surgical approaches are aimed at identification of the origin of the fistula and a surgical takedown. For those patients who are not stable enough for surgery, medical management should continue.

NURSING MANAGEMENT

An holistic approach to patient care begins with a thorough patient assessment prior to implementation of interventions.[6,7] Review the medical record for the history of the problem as well as the current situation. What baseline tests are available, and what should be continuously monitored? Assessment and documentation of issues surrounding the ECF include physical assessment of the affected area as well as the patient's psychosocial needs and discharge planning needs.[6,7] Take time at this point to consider options that will best facilitate the needs of the patient as a plan of care is developed. Skin care is of primary concern in these patients. Maintaining skin integrity reduces the need for pain management due to erosion of the skin, reduces infection, and improves the integrity of the management system.[6,7]

WOC nurses can be invaluable in caring for a patient with an ECF because these nurses add knowledge of a variety of pouching systems and skin care products to the plan of care.[6,7] Care is centered on containment and measurement of effluent, odor control, peri-fistula skin care, cost containment, and education of those involved in care.[6,7,29,30] Management options include the use of ostomy pouches and accessories, skin barriers, wound care pouches and accessories, catheter holders, odor controlling agents, and suction. Many times a combination of these measures will be needed for optimal care. ECFs with an output of less than 100 ml per day can be managed with standard dressings, including charcoal-based dressings if odor is an issue.[6,7,29,30]

When the effluent is of high output and if the fistula is located within an abdominal wound, the containment plan becomes complex, and more than one person may be required to help in the application of the management system. Consider the high-output ECF located within a skin crease. The amount of effluent, the location of the ECF, and the skin crease pose serious challenges to maintaining a predictable seal of a pouching system. WOC nurses will employ the use of solid skin barriers, skin barrier paste, and powder as well as pouching system that facilitates accurate quantification of the output.[6,7] Fistulae presenting within an abdominal wound pose a particular challenge from the standpoint that not only is the fistula draining into the wound, but the wound must be managed and containing the effluent requires creativity and fistula management pouches for effective care.[6,7,30] Some authors recommend the use of an isolation technique in which the fistula is isolated using a combination of solid skin barriers, skin barrier paste, pouching, and accessory products followed by the application of negative-pressure wound therapy (NPWT) for wound healing.[31,32] By creating a predictable wear time with pouches, dressings, suction, and NPWT, a budget can be set up based on how many dressing changes are required on a weekly basis and additional care goals can be achieved.[32–35] The complications of immobility are well documented in the literature, and a predictable wear time allows the patient more freedom to participate in therapy or other activities.

NPWT was introduced to wound care nearly 20 years ago; its use as an adjunct in the management of ECFs has evolved more recently. While further study is needed to define the efficacy of NPWT in the management of ECFs, recent literature demonstrates the value of this option in reducing effluent in high-output fistulae as well as in optimizing the care of the patient. It is unclear whether NPWT increases the chances of spontaneous closure, but the improved tissue oxygenation and reduction of effluent are factors that improve outcome.[32–35] Also not clear are the circumstances under which NPWT is most helpful. Some authors use the criteria of exposed bowel to preclude the use of this option, while others suggest the use of petrolatum-impregnated gauze as a contact layer prior to the application of the sponge, and negative pressures of 75 mm Hg.[34] The use of NPWT in the care of ECF has been demonstrated in some cases to reduce effluent and allow the patient improved mobility and may be considered as a possible treatment modality. If NPWT will be used, it is important for the clinician to follow manufacturer guidelines for use. Consistent monitoring of serum electrolytes, nutritional status, effluent, and response to care coupled with physician communication provide information that can help determine the effectiveness of the plan of care.[32,34,35]

PRINCIPLES OF POUCHING

In cases in which NPWT is not an option or has failed, pouching systems are available to support the plan of care by containing effluent and odor and providing for wound care. Evaluation of abdominal topography in the supine, sitting, and standing positions will expose any skin folds, creases, and scars that will undermine the pouch seal.[6,7] The use of skin barrier paste and moldable solid skin barriers will even out the skin contours and promote a level pouching surface. Solid skin barriers trimmed to form a wedge shape assist in evening out contours. The use of radial slits (darts) offers flexibility while simultaneously evening skin contours.[6,7] Each layer of wedges should be ½" larger than the preceding layer to prevent effluent from leaking between the wedges and pouch barrier. Apply the skin barrier as close to the wound margins as possible. If peri-fistula skin was left exposed, add protection to the exposed skin with barrier ointments and powders once the system in place.[6] The use of pouches with windows facilitates this process.

> ### PRACTICE POINT
>
> Even the most skilled nurse will be challenged pouching a wound with an ECF, but an individualized approach, assessment of skin contours, creativity, and persistence will yield a predictable system that meets management goals.

CASE MANAGEMENT

At some point in the care of the patient with an ECF, case management/discharge planning must occur. The high cost of care and implications for psychosocial well-being necessitate involving a case manager before the patient is discharged to home.[7,10] Certain questions should be asked in deciding when discharge

to home is a viable option. Can an effective pouching/containment system be achieved for a predictable time (at least 24 hours)? Is someone available and willing to care for the patient and learn the management system? Can the caregiver demonstrate the procedures of care? Also consider the availability of supplies, the durable medical supplier, and whether insurance will cover the needed products. If the needed products are not covered, what financial arrangements can be made? Is home health care needed and an option?

Patients who develop an ECF are at high risk for complications from sepsis, malnutrition, dehydration, and skin breakdown.[6,7,12,15] The mortality associated with ECF demonstrates the need for early identification and management, which begins with assessing for patients with predisposing factors and early signs of ECF development.[6] The goals of care include stabilizing the nutrition and fluid and electrolyte status, containing effluent, managing sepsis, and employing medical and surgical management where needed.[6,7,12,15] Nursing care centers on continuous monitoring of serum electrolytes, communicating with the registered dietitian and surgeon, patient assessment and planning, and containment and quantification of effluent.[6,7,12,15,16] While wound dressings and pouching systems provide options in the care of these patients, newer treatments such as NPWT are fast becoming a standard option to consider to help reduce volume in high-output ECFs.[35–37] Continued review of current literature is recommended for healthcare providers caring for patients with ECF.

SUMMARY

Understanding the various types of drains and tubes and when they are used is a critical first step in developing an effective treatment plan. Maintaining the patency of drains and tubes as well as assessing and protecting the skin around them are imperative. Fistulae are classified by the tissue involved, whether they are external or internal and simple or complex, and by the amount of effluent draining from them. The name given to the fistula provides information about which two body areas are connected. Because fistula effluent is so odorous and caustic to the skin, skin protection is very important. Consideration must be given to fluid and electrolyte balance and nutritional management. Care of the patient with tubes, drains, or fistulae is challenging and requires the care of an interdisciplinary team.

PATIENT SCENARIO

Coleen Potts and Chizu Sakai-Imoto

Clinical Data

Ms. BH is a 50-year-old woman with a complex medical and surgical history that includes laparoscopic repair of a recurrent ventral hernia. Postoperatively, Ms. BH became hypotensive and was transferred to the intensive care unit, where she developed acute respiratory failure, pneumonia, and sepsis. Her condition continued to deteriorate, and she underwent an emergency laparotomy with a diverting colostomy and removal of mesh. After this surgery, she was transferred to a tertiary care facility. She presented with a colocutaneous fistula (CCF) in her dehisced abdominal incision, mucocutaneous junction separation of her colostomy, a chronic abdominal abscess, and infected mesh. Ms. BH was medically stabilized and given parenteral nutritional support before conservative management of her ostomy and stomatized (epithelialized) CCF with pouching systems.

Case Discussion

One year after her original surgery, Ms. BH was deemed a good candidate for surgical closure of her CCF. She underwent an exploratory laparotomy, extensive lysis of adhesions, takedown of the CCF, takedown of her colostomy with transverse-to-descending anastomosis, removal of the remaining infected mesh, drainage of an intra-abdominal abscess, and creation of a loop ileostomy.

After a lengthy hospital recovery, Ms. BH was successfully discharged home. Her midabdominal wound was managed using NPWT, and she was placed on a gastrointestinal (GI) soft diet. She returned to the hospital a month later with shortness of breath. Workup revealed a pulmonary embolism, for which she was treated with Lovenox (enoxaparin) with a transition to Coumadin (warfarin). She returned home and a month later came back to the hospital with abdominal pain and GI bleeding. Her anticoagulant was stopped and an inferior vena cava filter was placed. Ms. BH was subsequently sent home but returned a week later with decreased ileostomy output and green liquid drainage from her midline wound; a new ECF had developed. The NPWT dressing was discontinued and the wound/fistula was pouched. After numerous modifications to the initial pouching system, a 48- to 72-hour seal was maintained. The patient's husband was knowledgeable about pouching the ECF, and the patient was discharged with home care nursing.

After a week at home, Ms. BH went to her local emergency department complaining of frequent pouch leakage and severe irritation to the peri-fistular skin (Fig. 19-1A). A consistent seal had never been obtained with the initial patch. The patient and her husband tried a variety of techniques, resulting in consistent leakage requiring up to 10 changes in a 24-hour period. This led them to manage the fistula/wound with petrolatum gauze and dressings. Ms. BH returned to our facility where she was ordered NPO and placed on total parenteral nutrition.

The goals of WOC care during this visit were to:

1. contain effluent from the ECF to protect the periwound skin and decrease pain
2. increase the patient's activities of daily living

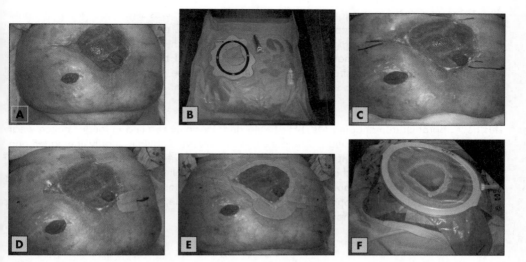

Figure 19-1. (A) The patient's skin condition when she arrived at the hospital. Irritant dermatitis resulted from frequent leakage of effluent. (B) Pouch equipment used. (C) The contour of the abdomen was checked with the patient in a sitting position. Deep creases around the wound were marked. (D) Creases were filled with CMC skin barrier wedges. (E) The "petalling" method was used to build up the wound edges. (F) Finished pouching product. (See *color section*, *Patient Scenarios*, page C48, for color versions of these images.)

3. monitor strict measurement of ECF output to evaluate the patient's fluid/nutritional requirements
4. promote an optimal environment for wound healing
5. improve the patient's quality of life and psychological stability by obtaining and maintaining an intact pouch seal.

ECF repair

WOC nursing recommendations were to continue using a medium fistula/wound pouch system with a solid carboxymethylcellulose (CMC) skin barrier that has tack on both sides. The CMC was cut into wedges, as were the skin barrier pieces that remained after cutting the pouch aperture. CMC paste and a solid CMC flat skin barrier ring were used (Fig. 19-1B). The pouching method was as follows:

1. Multiple creases were filled in with CMC wedges, followed by "petaling" of the skin barrier around the wound bed to even the skin surface (Figs. 19-1C–E).
2. The pouch was applied and the inner margins caulked with CMC skin barrier paste. The caulking was reinforced with strips of solid CMC flat skin barrier ring from the 5- to 7-o'clock positions to reinforce the seal. This was an area identified by the patient as being especially problematic (Fig. 19-1F).
3. The inner seal was then recaulked with CMC paste and powder.
4. Hypoallergenic woven tape was added to reinforce all pouch edges.
5. Both pouch drainage spouts were connected to gravity drainage (Fig. 19-1F).

Loop ileostomy repair

Because the ECF was proximal to her loop ileostomy, the stoma only produced mucus. The amount was enough to undermine the margin of her fistula pouch and macerate the peristomal skin. The ileostomy located in the right lower quadrant was red, moist, and flush to Ms. BH's skin. The mucocutaneous junction was intact, the peristomal skin was slightly denuded, and mild erythema was noted. The peristomal skin was dusted with CMC powder and the ostomy refitted with a flat CMC skin barrier ring and a pediatric ostomy pouch.

Because it was critical that the patient and her husband be educated on the pouching methods before discharge, instructions were given and both the patient and her husband were able to return the demonstration without difficulty.

Conclusion

This new approach in managing Ms. BH's fistula and ileostomy resulted in longer pouch wear time and improved skin condition. The patient was able to ambulate shortly thereafter and placed on strict intake and output monitoring. Her quality of life improved greatly not only as a result of decreased pain and anxiety but also because she felt more in control. This case provides an example of how the application of skin, wound, and pouching principles, along with a creative and individualized approach, can improve the outcome, cost-effectiveness, and quality of life for a patient with a complex ECF.

SHOW WHAT YOU KNOW

1. Which statement about fistula care is TRUE?
   A. NPWT is contraindicated for treating fistulae.
   B. External fistulae empty into an organ.
   C. Low-output fistulae produce less than 200 ml of effluent per day
   D. Fistulae that open into granulating wounds have the best chance of healing.

   ANSWER: C. *Effluent from a low-output fistula is less than 200 ml/day, whereas high-output fistulae produce more than 500 ml/day. B is incorrect because external fistulae empty to the environment; internal fistulae empty into an organ. A is incorrect because NPWT can now be used to treat patients with fistulae. D is incorrect.*

2. Optimal functioning of enteral feeding tubes depends on which primary nursing considerations?
   A. Hydration, location of tube, diagnosis
   B. Skin care, hydration, location of tube
   C. Tube stabilization, hydration, nutrition
   D. Nutrition, location of tube, continuum of care

   ANSWER: C. *If the tube is stabilized, the skin is less likely to break down; if adequate hydration is maintained, there will be fewer problems with the tube; nutritional support is the primary goal.*

3. Which of the following conditions predisposes a patient to formation of an enterocutaneous fistula?
   A. Normal nitrogen balance
   B. Albumin level of 4.0 g/dl
   C. Blood glucose of 80 mg/dl
   D. Crohn's disease

   ANSWER: D. *Crohn's disease is an inflammatory bowel disease that affects all layers of the bowel wall, predisposing the patient to fistula formation. A, B, and C are all within normal range.*

(continued)

4. A patient with an enterocutaneous fistula is averaging an output of 9,600 ml over a 24-hour period. The direct care staff is concerned about pouch overflow and leakage. What would you advise?

A. Discontinue the pouch and switch to gauze dressings

B. Connect the pouch to bedside gravity drainage

C. Add more skin barrier paste and tape to caulk the leaks

D. Restrict enteral and intravenous fluids

ANSWER: B. *Using a bedside gravity drainage system will prevent overfilling the pouch and reduce leakage. Answers A and C expose the skin to corrosive fistula drainage. Answer D runs the risk of dehydrating the patient and reducing caloric intake.*

REFERENCES

1. Smith M.J. "Current Concepts in Catheter Management," in *Urinary and Fecal Incontinence: Current Management Concepts*, 3rd ed. Edited by Doughty D. St. Louis, Mo.: Mosby/Elsevier; 2006.

2. Carmel, J.E., Scardillo, J. "Tube Management," in Colwell, J., Goldberg, M., and Carmel, J. (eds), *Fecal and Urinary, Diversions: Management Principles*, 2nd ed., pp. 351-380. St. Louis: Mosby/Elsevier, 2004.

3. Parker, D., Callan, L., Harwood, J., Thompson, D.L., Wilde, M., Gray, M. "Nursing Interventions to Reduce the Risk of Catheter-Associated Urinary Tract Infection. Part I. Catheter Selection," *Journal of Wound, Ostomy and Continence Nursing* 36(1):23-34, 2009.

4. Wilson, M., Wilde, M., Webb, M.L., Thompson, D., Parker, D., Harwood, J., Callan, L., Gray, M. "Nursing Interventions to Reduce the Risk of Catheter-Associated Urinary Tract Infection. Part II Staff Education, Monitoring, and Care Techniques," *Journal of Wound, Ostomy and Continence Nursing* 36(2):137-54, 2009.

5. Newman, K. "The Indwelling Urinary Catheter: Principles for Best Practice," *Journal of Wound, Ostomy and Continence Nursing* 34(6):655-61, 2007.

6. Erwin-Toth, P., Hocevar, B., Landis-Erdman, J. Fistula Management. In *Fecal and Urinary Diversions: Management Principles*, ed 2. Edited by Colwell, J., Goldberg, M., and Carmel, J. St. Louis, Mo.: Mosby/Elsevier; 2004.

7. McNaughton, V. "Summary of Best Practice Recommendations for Management of Enterocutaneous Fistulae from the Canadian Association for Enterostomal Therapy ECF Best Practice Recommendations Panel," *Journal of Wound, Ostomy and Continence Nursing* 37(2):173-84, 2010.

8. Sahu, S.K., Raghuvanshi, S., Bahl, D.V., Sachan, P.K. "Spontaneous Colocutaneous Fistula," *Internet Journal of Surgery* 15(2), 2008.

9. Wainstein, D.E., Fernandez, E., Gonzalez, D., Chara, O., Berkowski, D. "Treatment of High-output Enterocutaneous Fistula with a Vacuum-compaction Device: A Ten Year Experience," *World Journal of Surgery* 32:430-35, 2008.

10. Phillips, M., Walton, M. "Caring for Patients with Enterocutaneous Fistulae," *British Journal of Nursing* 2(9):496-500, 1993.

11. Skovard, R., Keiding, H. "A Cost-effective Analysis of Fistula Treatment in the Abdominal Region Using a New Integrated Fistula and Wound Management System," *Journal of Wound, Ostomy and Continence Nursing* 35(6):592-95, 2008.

12. Schecter, W.P., Hirshberg, A., Chang, D.S., Harris, H.W., Napolitano, L.M., Wexner, S.D., Dudrick, S.J. "Enteric Fistulas: Principles of Management," *Journal of the American College of Surgeons* 209(4):484-91, 2009.

13. Kool, B. "The Wound that Nearly Got Away: A Case Presentation," *Pediatric Nursing* 26(1):55-65, 2000.

14. Slater, R. "Nutritional Management of Enterocutaneous Fistula," *British Journal of Nursing* 18(4):225-30, 2009.

15. Draus, J.M., Huss, S.A., Harty, N.J., Cheadle, W.G., Larson, G.M. "Enterocutaneous Fistula: Are Treatments Improving?" *Surgery* 140(4):570-78, 2006.

16. Austin, T. "Nutritional Management of Enterocutaneous Fistulas," *Support Line* 28(6):10-13, 2006.

17. Schein, M. "What's New in Postoperative Enterocutaneous Fistulas?" *World Journal of Surgery* 32:336-38, 2008.

18. Martinez, A., Ferron, F., Gal, M.L., Torrent, J.J., Capdet, J., Querleu, D. "Management of Ileocutaneous Fistulae Using TPN after Surgery for Abdominal Malignancy," *Journal of Wound Care* 18(7):282-88, 2009.

19. Mawdsley, J.E., Hollington, P., Bassett, P., Windsor, A.J., Forbes, A., Gabes, M. "An Analysis

of Predictive Factors for Healing and Mortality in Patients with Enterocutaneous Fistulas," *Alimentary Pharmacology and Therapeutics* 28:1111-21, 2008.

20. Teixeira, P., Inaba, K., Dubose, J., Salim, A., Brown, C., Rhee, P., Browder, T., Demetriades, D. "Enterocutaneous Fistula Complicating Trauma Laparotomy: A Major Resource Burden," *American Journal of Surgery* 75:30-32, 2009.

21. Gupta, M., Sonar, P., Kakodkar, R., Kumaran, V., Mohanka, R., Soin, A., Nundy, S. "Small Bowel Enterocutaneous Fistulae: The Merits of Early Surgery," *Indian Journal of Surgery* 70:303-07, 2008.

22. Kushimoto, S., Miyauchi, M., Yokota, H., Kawaii, M. "Damage Control Surgery and Open Abdominal Management: Recent Advances and Our Approach," *Journal of Nippon Medical School* 76(6):280-90, 2009.

23. Blaker, J.J., Pratten, J., Ready, D., Knowless, J.C., Forbes, A., Day, R.M. "Assessment of Antimicrobial Microspheres as a Prospective Novel Treatment Targeted Towards the Repair of Perianal Fistula," *Alimentary Pharmacology and Therapeutics* 28: 614-22, 2008.

24. Garcia-Olmo, D., Herreros, D., Pascual, M., Pascual, I., De-La-Quintana, P., Trebol, J., Garcia-Arranz, M. "Treatment of Enterocutaneous Fistula in Crohn's Disease with Adipose-Derived Stem Cells: A Comparison of Protocols with and without Cell Expansion," *International Journal of Colorectal Disease* 24:27-30, 2009.

25. Fischer, P.E., Fabian, T.C., Magnotti, L.J., Schroeppel, T.J., Bee, T.K., Maish, G.O., Savage S.A., Laing, A.E., Barker, A.B., Croce, M.A. "A Ten-Year Review of Enterocutaneous Fistulas after Laparotomy for Trauma," *Journal of Trauma* 67(5): 924-28, 2009.

26. Wind, J., Koperen, P.J., Slors, F.M., Bemelman, W.A. "Single-Stage Closure of Enterocutaneous Fistula and Stomas in the Presence of Large Abdominal Wall Defects Using the Components Separation Technique," *American Journal of Surgery* 197:24-29, 2009.

27. Connolly, P.T., Teubner, C.A., Lees, N.P., Anderson, I.D., Scott, N.A., Carlson, G.L. "Outcome of Reconstructive Surgery for Intestinal Fistula in the Open Abdomen," *Annals of Surgery* 247(3):440-44, 2008.

28. Andreani, S.M., Dang, H.H., Grondona, P., Khan, A.Z., Edwards, D.P. "Rectovaginal Fistula in Crohn's Disease," *Diseases of the Colon & Rectum* 50:2215-22, 2007.

29. Hawthorn, M. "Caring for a Patient with a Fungating Malignant Lesion in a Hospice Setting: Reflecting on Practice," *International Journal of Palliative Nursing* 16(2):70-76, 2010.

30. Woodward, L.M. "Management of an Enterocutaneous Fistula in a Patient with a Gastrointestinal Stromal Tumor." *Journal of Wound, Ostomy and Continence Nursing* 37(3):314-17, 2010.

31. Datta, V., Engledow, A., Chan, S., Forbes, A., Cohen, C.R., Windsor, A. "The Management of Enterocutaneous Fistula in a Regional Unit in the United Kingdom: A Prospective Study," *Diseases of the Colon & Rectum* 53(2):192-99, 2010.

32. Brindle, C.T., Blankenship, J. "Management of Complex Abdominal Wounds with Small Bowel Fistulae," *Journal of Wound, Ostomy and Continence Nursing* 36(4):396-403, 2009.

33. Hess, C.T. "Managing an External Fistula, Part 2," *Nursing* 32(9):22-24, 2002.

34. Heller, L., Levin, S., Butler, C. "Management of Abdominal Wound Dehiscence Using Vacuum Assisted Closure in Patients with Compromised Healing," *American Journal of Surgery* 191:165-72, 2006.

35. Bovill, E., Banwell, P., Teot, L., Eriksson, E., Song, C., Mahoney, J., Gustafsson, R., Horch, R., Deva, A., Whitworth, I. "Topical Negative Pressure Wound Therapy: A Review of its Role and Guidelines for its Use in the Management of Acute Wounds," *International Wound Journal* 5(4):511-29, 2008.

36. Murphree, R.W. "Allogenic Acellular Dermal Matrix in the Management of an Enterocutaneous Fistula," *Journal of Wound, Ostomy and Continence Nursing* 36(6):674-78, 2009.

37. Gunn, L.A., Follmar, K.E., Wong, M.S., Lettieri, S.C., Levin, L.S., Erdmann, D. "Management of Enterocutaneous Fistulas Using Negative-Pressure Dressings," *Annals of Plastic Surgery* 57(6):621-25, 2006.

CHAPTER 20

Atypical Wounds

David Weinstein, MD
Tami de Araujo, MD
Robert S. Kirsner, MD, PhD

Objectives

After completing this chapter, you'll be able to:

- recognize the importance of identifying atypical wounds
- explain the need for wound biopsies in determining the etiology of an atypical wound
- describe the various clinical manifestations of atypical wounds.

TYPES OF ATYPICAL WOUNDS

Prolonged pressure (pressure ulcers), venous insufficiency (venous leg ulcers), complications of longstanding diabetes mellitus (diabetic foot ulcers), and poor vascular supply (arterial ulcers) are the most common causes of chronic wounds. Wounds resulting from uncommon etiologies, called *atypical wounds,* are less frequently encountered and less well understood. Their prevalence has not been studied extensively, but it is estimated that at least 10% of the more than 500,000 leg ulcers in the United States may be due to unusual causes.[1,2] A variety of etiologies may cause atypical wounds,[3] such as infections, external or traumatic causes, metabolic disorders, genetic diseases, neoplasms, or inflammatory processes.

It is critical to recognize when a wound is caused by an etiology other than prolonged pressure, neuropathy, or abnormal vascular supply so that a correct diagnosis can be made and the appropriate therapy provided. A wound should be evaluated for an atypical etiology if:

- it is present in a location different from that of a common chronic wound
- its appearance varies from that of a common chronic wound
- it does not respond to conventional therapy.

For example, the thigh is an atypical location for a pressure, venous, arterial, or diabetic ulcer and should raise the suspicion of an atypical cause. A wound on the medial aspect of the leg but extending deep to the tendon would be considered atypical despite being in a common location because the depth of this wound is atypical for venous ulcers. Finally, any wound that is not healing after 3 to 6 months of appropriate treatment should raise the consideration of an atypical cause, even if the distribution and clinical appearance are classic for a common chronic wound.

Once a wound is deemed atypical, a tissue sample is critical for histologic evaluation with special stains, tissue culture (for infectious causes), and immunofluorescence testing (for some inflammatory or immune-based causes).

Potential etiologies of atypical wounds

Although not all-inclusive, this list presents some of the most commonly encountered etiologies for an atypical wound.

Inflammatory causes
- Vasculitis
- Pyoderma gangrenosum

Infections
- Atypical mycobacteria
- Deep fungal infections

Vasculopathies
- Cryoglobulinemia
- Cryofibrinogenemia
- Antiphospholipid anti- body syndrome

Metabolic and genetic causes
- Calciphylaxis
- Sickle cell anemia

Malignancies
- Squamous cell carcinoma
- Basal cell carcinoma
- Lymphoma
- Kaposi's sarcoma

External causes
- Burns
- Bites
- Stings
- Radiation

Evidence-Based Practice

Tissue samples are mandatory for atypical wounds because many of the unusual causes of wounds can resemble each other, making visual diagnosis alone difficult and risky.

ETIOLOGIES OF ATYPICAL WOUNDS

Some of the most commonly encountered etiologies for an atypical wound include inflammatory causes, infections, vasculopathies, metabolic and genetic factors, malignancies, and external causes. (See *Potential etiologies of atypical wounds*.) However, a thorough medical history, including epidemiological exposure, family history, personal habits, and concomitant systemic diseases, along with a thorough physical examination, histologic evaluation, and laboratory testing, will provide critical information necessary for a correct diagnosis of an atypical wound.

Inflammatory causes

Among the most interesting—and probably more common—causes of atypical wounds are the inflammatory ulcers. Although a variety of inflammatory and immunologic diseases affect the skin, two relatively common causes of inflammatory ulcers are vasculitis and pyoderma gangrenosum.

VASCULITIS

Vasculitis is defined as inflammation and necrosis of the blood vessels, which can ultimately result in end organ damage.[4] Often idiopathic, vasculitis is a reaction pattern that may be triggered by certain reactants, among which are underlying infections, malignancy, medications, and connective tissue diseases. (See *Potential etiologies of vasculitis*.) Clinically, vasculitis varies depending on the size of the underlying vessel affected. For example, lesions may include a reticulated erythema due to disease of the superficial cutaneous plexus, or they may present as widespread purpura, necrosis, and ulceration due to disease in larger, deeper vessels. (See *color section, Vasculitis*, page C28.) Patients also may have similar involvement of different end organs such as the kidney, lung, central nervous system, and gastrointestinal tract.[5]

Circulating immune (antibody-antigen) complexes, which deposit in blood vessel walls, are the cause of many types of vasculitis.[6] Tissue biopsies will confirm the presence of vasculitis if performed early, and biopsies of

Potential etiologies of vasculitis

Although not all-inclusive, the most common causes of vasculitis are listed below.

Infections
- *Streptococcus* spp.
- *Mycobacterium tuberculosis*
- *Staphylococcus* spp.
- *Mycobacterium leprae*
- Hepatitis viruses A, B, and C
- Herpes virus
- Influenza virus
- *Candida* spp.
- *Plasmodium* spp.
- Schistosomiasis

Medications
- Penicillin
- Sulfonamides
- Tamoxifen
- Streptomycin
- Oral contraceptives
- Thiazides

Chemicals
- Insecticides
- Petroleum products

Foods
- Milk
- Gluten

Connective tissue and other inflammatory diseases
- Systemic lupus erythematosus
- Dermatomyositis
- Sjögren's syndrome
- Rheumatoid arthritis
- Behçet's syndrome
- Cryoglobulinemia
- Scleroderma
- Primary biliary cirrhosis
- Human immunodeficiency virus infection

Malignancies
- Lymphomas
- Leukemias
- Multiple myeloma

---

perilesional skin may detect the type of immunoglobulin involved in the process. Biopsies performed later in the course of lesion development may fail to reveal immunoreactants or inflammatory cells, and their by-products will degrade immunoglobulins. Tissue culture may be helpful if the vasculitis is due to an infectious process. A histologically confirmed diagnosis mandates evaluation of other organ systems and an attempt to determine the etiologic factor.

If identified—and if possible—the causative agent should be addressed. Additionally, treatment of the vasculitis is based on the extent of the disease. (See *Diagnostic tests for vasculitis,* page 494.) Mild disease that is limited to the skin can be treated with only supportive care, such as leg elevation and dressings. Treatments with limited adverse effects, such as colchicine, dapsone, antihistamines, or nonsteroidal anti-inflammatory agents, also may be used. If skin disease is extensive or systemic involvement is present, more aggressive treatment such as systemic steroids, anti-inflammatory agents, or immunosuppressants may be needed.[7] (See *Vasculitis treatment options,* page 494.)

PYODERMA GANGRENOSUM

The term *pyoderma gangrenosum* actually refers to a disorder that is neither infectious nor gangrenous. Rather, it is an inflammatory process of unknown etiology that leads to painful skin ulcers. Pyoderma gangrenosum is characterized by the appearance of one or more chronic ulcerations with violaceous undermined borders.[8] (See *color section, Pyoderma gangrenosum,* page C28.) It mainly affects adults and its usual course is that of recurring, destructive ulcers, which begin as pustules and resolve with cribriform scars. Several clinical variants of pyoderma gangrenosum have been described, including ulcerative, pustular, bullous, vegetative, and peristomal types.

▶ PRACTICE POINT

Because a diagnostic test to confirm pyoderma gangrenosum does not exist and a number of other conditions may resemble it clinically, a correct diagnosis relies on the clinical presentation and exclusion of other causes.

Diagnostic tests for vasculitis

Use the following tests to determine the etiology of vasculitis.

- Anti-neutrophilic cytoplasmic antibody
- Rheumatoid factor
- Anti-nuclear antibody
- Hepatitis A, B, C profile
- Complete blood count
- Anti-streptolysin O titer
- Cryoglobulin level
- Serum protein electrophoresis
- Chest radiograph
- Purified protein derivative test
- Throat culture
- Tissue culture.

To determine the extent of disease, use these tests:

- Urinalysis
- Stool guaiac
- Chest radiograph
- Renal function tests
- Liver function tests
- Complete blood count.

Vasculitis treatment options

Extent of disease	Treatment options
Mild	• Leg elevation • Compression dressings • Antihistamines • Nonsteroidal anti-inflammatory drugs • Anti-inflammatory antibiotics • Topical steroids • Support stockings • Dapsone • Colchicine • Potassium iodide
Extensive or systemic	• Dapsone • Systemic steroids • Stanozolol • Cyclophosphamide • Methotrexate • Azathioprine • Cyclosporine • Plasmapheresis • Mycophenolate mofetil • Tacrolimus • Other anti-inflammatory or immunosuppressant drugs

It is important for the clinician to search for underlying diseases when a diagnosis of pyoderma gangrenosum is rendered because it is associated with other conditions in more than 50% of patients.[9] (See *Systemic diseases associated with pyoderma gangrenosum.*) Among these are inflammatory bowel disease, arthritis (seropositive and seronegative), monoclonal gammopathies, and other hematologic disorders and malignancies. Pyoderma gangrenosum lesions can occur around the stoma in persons with inflammatory bowel disease.[10] (See *color section, Pyoderma gangrenosum,* page C28.)

The mechanism by which pyoderma gangrenosum lesions develops is unknown; however, it is believed that pathergy (the development of lesions in areas of trauma) plays a role. In susceptible people, even minimal trauma to the skin can result in the production of pyoderma gangrenosum lesions, such as pustules or ulcers.

Curative treatment does not exist. The course of pyoderma gangrenosum waxes and wanes; however, corticosteroids usually are helpful.[11] For limited or mild disease, topical or intralesional steroids may be used. For more severe or widespread disease, systemic steroids can be used, although their adverse effects limit long-term use. A variety of systemic therapies can be used, including antibiotics with anti-inflammatory properties or systemic steroids. In addition, immunosuppressant or anti-inflammatory agents may also be of value; for example, cyclosporine also

Systemic diseases associated with pyoderma gangrenosum

No diagnostic test exists to confirm the presence of pyoderma gangrenosum. In addition, pyoderma gangrenosum is typically associated with other conditions.[8] Reported associations are listed below.

Inflammatory bowel disease
- Ulcerative colitis
- Regional enteritis
- Crohn's disease

Arthritis
- Seronegative arthritis
- Rheumatoid arthritis
- Osteoarthritis
- Psoriatic arthritis

Hematologic abnormalities
- Myeloid leukemia
- Hairy cell leukemia
- Myelofibrosis
- Myeloid metaplasia
- Immunoglobulin A monoclonal gammopathy
- Polycythemia rubra, polycythemia vera
- Paroxysmal nocturnal hemoglobinuria
- Myeloma
- Lymphoma

Immunologic abnormalities
- Systemic lupus erythematosus
- Complement deficiency
- Hypogammaglobulinemia
- Hyperimmunoglobulin E syndrome
- Acquired immunodeficiency syndrome

Pyoderma gangrenosum treatment options

Type of treatment	Treatment options
Topical	• Topical steroids • Topical tacrolimus • Nicotine patch • Intralesional steroids
Systemic	• Steroids • Antibiotics (dapsone and minocycline) • Cyclosporine • Clofazamine • Azathioprine • Methotrexate • Chlorambucil • Cyclophosphamide • Thalidomide • Tacrolimus • Mycophenalate • Mofetil • Intravenous immunoglobulin • Plasmapheresis • Infliximab

appears quite effective in treating this disorder. (See *Pyoderma gangrenosum treatment options*.) Infliximab (Remicade), a monoclonal antibody to tumor necrosis factor-α, has been reported to be useful.[12] Infliximab is FDA-approved to treat Crohn's disease and rheumatoid arthritis. A randomized study evaluating the efficacy of different treatment modalities for pyoderma gangrenosum has not been done.

Infectious causes

Infectious causes of atypical wounds may be due to a variety of different organisms, some of which are not commonly encountered in the United States. For example, atypical mycobacterial infections (other than leprosy and tuberculosis) and fungal infections (other than dermatophytes and *Candida*) occasionally are detected upon diagnostic testing. Infection caused by *Vibrio vulnificus* may be responsible for lower leg ulcers in geographic areas where there is warm salt water.

ATYPICAL MYCOBACTERIAL INFECTION

Atypical mycobacteria are ubiquitous in the environment and were not generally viewed as human pathogens until the 1950s, when several cases of disease caused by these organisms were reported.[13] Cutaneous infection usually results from exogenous inoculation, and predisposing factors include a history of preceding trauma, immunosuppression, or chronic disease. While *Mycobacteria marinum* is the most common agent of skin infection by atypical mycobacteria,[14] many others have been reported in recent decades. (See *Mycobacterium species that cause skin ulcers*.) The cutaneous lesions vary depending on the causative agent and may present as granulomas, small superficial ulcers, sinus tracts, or large ulcerated lesions localized in exposed areas. (See *color section*, *Hansen's disease*, page C29.)

Histologically, mycobacterial infections present as granulomas and abscesses that are difficult to distinguish from those of leprosy and cutaneous tuberculosis. Diagnosis invariably will depend on tissue culture or more recent techniques, such as polymerase chain reaction and gene rearrangement studies.

The appropriate therapy will depend on the causative agent because susceptibility to antibiotics varies. In some cases, simple excision of the cutaneous lesions or a combination of excision and chemotherapy often is most beneficial to the patient.

BURULI ULCER

Buruli ulcer is a health problem in the tropical areas of many developing countries. Since 1980, Buruli ulcer has emerged as an important cause of human suffering. It was first encountered in 1897 when Sir Albert Cook described large ulcers in patients in Uganda. In the late 1940s,

Mycobacterium species that cause skin ulcers

Mycobacterium species	Clinical manifestations	Diagnosis	Treatment
M. marinum	• Swimming pool granuloma	Tissue culture	• Antituberculous drugs
M. ulcerans	• Subcutaneous nodule • Deep ulcers	Tissue culture	• Surgical excision
M. scrofulaceum	• Cervical lymphadenitis • Fistulae	Tissue culture	• Surgical excision
M. avium-intracellulare	• Small ulcers with erythematous borders	Tissue culture	• Surgical excision • Chemotherapy
M. kansasii	• Crusted ulcerations	Tissue culture	• Antituberculous drugs • Minocycline
M. chelonae	• Painful nodules and abscesses • Surgical wound infection	Tissue culture	• Erythromycin • Tobramycin • Amikacin • Doxycycline
M. fortuitum	• Painful nodules and abscesses • Surgical wound infection	Tissue culture	• Amikacin • Doxycycline • Ciprofloxacin • Sulfamethoxazole

MacCallum identified an organism similar to *Mycobacterium ulcerans* in an ulcer in a 15-year-old in Bairnsdale, Australia. Large ulcers were subsequently observed in patients living along the Nile River in Buruli County, Uganda in the 1960s, hence the name of the disease. Buruli ulcer is caused by *M. ulcerans*, from the family of bacteria that causes tuberculosis and leprosy.

The World Health Organization (WHO) has defined Buruli ulcer as an infectious disease of the skin and subcutaneous tissue characterized by painless nodules, papules, plaque, or edema evolving into a painless ulcer with undermined edges and edema. Progression of the disease is associated with extensive sloughing and massive ulceration, particularly over joints, that may lead to contractures. Significant areas of the torso, face, or an entire limb may be involved. Amputation is often required when a limb is involved.[15]

Extensive cutaneous ulcers occur as the disease progresses from the early, more treatable, nodular form to the ulcerative form, which can result in the loss of skin and soft tissue. Although Buruli ulcer is rarely fatal, the associated disabilities and disfigurement are extensive and have a profound impact on quality of life in affected patients.[15,16] (See *color section*, *Buruli ulcer*, page C29.)

The majority of those suffering from Buruli ulcer are younger than age 15. Early diagnosis is key to treating this disease. A recent prospective trial showed that antibiotic therapy for early, limited lesions can result in healing in more than 90% of patients in less than a year.[17] In more extensive cases, wide excision and grafting are often recommended, although limited excision followed by small islet grafts may be successful. Aminoglycosides also are helpful in preventing the extensive ulcers, contractures, edema, and other late sequelae of this devastating disease.[15,16]

Healing often is slow and is associated with significant functional incapacity due to contractures and amputation. Treatment is complicated by the resistance of the organism to most medical regimens due to the ability of the organism to suppress the immune system of the host. Disease progression is related directly to a decrease in the level of interferon-γ, a Th1 cytokine, as well as a concomitant increase in the Th2 cytokine interleukin-10.[15] Buruli ulcer has been clearly identified as an immunodeficiency disease. Reversing the deficiency of interferon-γ and/or decreasing the interleukin-10 level has been identified as a novel therapeutic target for interventional development.

The disease, its treatment, and the resulting disabilities are a significant burden to patients, their families, and their society. In some countries such as Ghana, patients and families are reluctant to seek treatment due to lack of money or misunderstanding that treatment can lead to amputation.[16] Educational sessions for clinicians to recognize Buruli ulcer early and to change patient, family, and societal resistance to seeking early treatment have met with success, and the number of late cases of this disease in Ghana has declined over the past decade.[15,16]

DEEP FUNGAL INFECTIONS

Deep fungal infections of the skin can be divided into subcutaneous and systemic mycoses. The subcutaneous mycoses result from traumatic implantation of the etiologic agent into the subcutaneous tissue, development of localized disease, and eventual lymphatic spread. In rare instances, hematogenous dissemination can occur, especially in immunocompromised hosts. As may occur with sporotrichosis or chromomycosis, ulcers from deep fungal infections are found worldwide and can present in a wide variety of clinical settings.[18]

Systemic mycoses are the result of systemic penetration of pathogenic fungi, with the lungs being the most common port of entry. These infections are restricted to the geographic areas where the fungi occur, especially tropical regions such as Central and South America. After an initial pulmonary infection, the fungi can spread hematogenously or via lymphatic vessels to other organs, including the skin. A decrease in immunity will lead to expression of the fungal infection, as is commonly observed in patients infected with human immunodeficiency virus (HIV).

PRACTICE POINT

A thorough patient history assists the clinician in considering a diagnosis of systemic mycosis because of the limited area in which the causative fungi occur.

SPOROTRICHOSIS

Sporotrichosis is a subacute or chronic fungal infection caused by the fungus *Sporothrix schenckii*. Occurring as a consequence of traumatic implantation of the fungus into the skin, it is often associated with lymphangitis. Less commonly, inhalation of the conidia can lead to pulmonary infection and subsequent spread to the bones, eyes, central nervous system, and viscera. Systemic disease is seen in individuals with impaired immunity, such as alcoholic and HIV-infected patients.[19]

S. schenckii, a saprophyte in the environment, has been isolated in a variety of plants and other fauna as well as in animals (bites or scratches from animals, such as armadillos and cats). Individuals whose professional or leisure activities expose them to the environment are at greater risk of acquiring the infection. Sporotrichosis is treated with systemic medications, including saturated solution of potassium iodide, itraconazole, fluconazole, terbinafine, and amphotericin B. Topically applied heat also may be used because the organism grows at low temperatures.

Evidence-Based Practice

Because it is difficult to distinguish the presence of sporotrichosis directly from host tissue, culture on Sabouraud dextrose agar medium should be performed.[19] .

CHROMOBLASTOMYCOSIS

Chromoblastomycosis is a subcutaneous mycosis caused by several pigmented fungi, including *Fonsecaea pedrosoi*, *Fonsecaea compacta*, *Phialophora verrucosa*, *Cladosporium carrionii*, and *Rhinocladiella aquaspersa*. These fungi are acquired through inoculation of the causative agents in the skin, after which a mycotic infection develops at the site of entry. These microorganisms can be found in soil throughout the world; however, the disease is most common in tropical and subtropical climates, with the majority of cases seen in South America.[20]

Primarily affecting men ages 30 to 50, the principal lesion is a slow-growing papule that eventuates into a verrucous nodule. Exposed areas are involved, with extremities—especially the lower limbs—being affected in 95% of the cases.[20] The surface of the lesion may be covered by scales or may be ulcerated with serosanguineous crusts. Black dots can be often observed; these dots are rich in fungi and represent the site of transepidermal elimination of necrotic tissue.

Diagnostic examinations should include scrapings from the lesion with potassium hydroxide 20%; tissue samples should be obtained from biopsies for tissue culture and histology.

The disease tends to be chronic and difficult to treat, and may lead to lymphedema and elephantiasis. Ulcerated and cicatricial lesions have been reported to develop into carcinoma. Small lesions can be cured by surgical excision; however, chronic lesions are often resistant to treatment.

Systemic antifungal agents, such as ketoconazole, itraconazole, terbinafine, and amphotericin B, have been used, both alone and in combination, with variable results. Pulse therapy with either itraconazole or terbinafine and itraconazole combination therapy is currently recommended.[21] The new-generation triazole antifungals show promise, as demonstrated by the positive results with posaconazole, although they may be prohibitively expensive.[22] Cryosurgery has also been used alone and in combination with antifungal chemotherapy. In addition, local heat therapy of 42°C to 45°C can also be an effective therapeutic modality.

PARACOCCIDIOIDOMYCOSIS

Paracoccidioidomycosis (South American blastomycosis) is a chronic, infectious disease caused by the fungus *Paracoccidioides brasiliensis*, a saprophyte of soil and decaying vegetation found in tropical and subtropical climates. Infection occurs via a respiratory route with occasional dissemination to other organs, including the skin. Patients present with painful ulcerative lesions of the mouth, the face or, less frequently, the extremities. Involvement of regional lymphatics is characteristic.[23]

Diagnosis can be established by isolation and identification of the etiologic agent with direct mycologic examination, histopathologic or cytopathologic examination, or culture. Treatment includes trimethoprim–sulfamethoxazole, azole derivatives such as itraconazole and ketoconazole, and amphotericin B for severe cases.

MYCETOMA

Mycetoma is a chronic infection of the skin and subcutaneous tissue characterized by local edema, sinus tract formation, and the presence of grains—hard concretions representing colonies of the etiologic agent. It occurs worldwide, but most commonly in tropical and subtropical regions. Mycetomas can be divided into eumycetomas, caused by fungi, and actinomycetomas, caused by actinomycetes. The most common agent in Central and South America is the bacteria *Nocardia brasiliensis*, which is found in soil.[24] This agent is rarely found in the United States but when it does occur, the fungus *Pseudallescheria boydii* is the most commonly isolated agent.

Male rural workers ages 20 to 40 are most frequently affected. After trauma, a slow-growing, painless nodule develops, which may discharge purulent material and grains. Neighboring lesions may interconnect with each other, giving rise to the sinus tracts that are characteristic of the disease.

Diagnosis can be established based on clinical findings; additional examinations may include visualization of grains or filaments in discharge or biopsy and tissue culture. On ultrasonographic evaluation, the mycetoma grains, capsules, and the resulting inflammatory granulomas have characteristic appearances.[25] Treatment is difficult. Surgical excision, commonly in combination with chemotherapy, may be effective. Sulfonamides, tetracycline, aminoglycosides, rifampin, ciprofloxacin, amoxicillin–clavulanate, and oral azoles may be used depending on sensitivities of the etiologic agent. Recent preliminary evidence suggests that linezolid, imipenem, and the newer triazoles voriconazole and posaconazole also may be efficacious.[26]

VIBRIO VULNIFICUS INFECTION

V. vulnificus, a bacterium, is found widely in raw shellfish in Atlantic Coast waters .[27] It produces extracellular proteolytic and elastolytic enzymes and collagenases that favor tissue invasiveness. Wound infection with *V. vulnificus* occurs when contaminated seawater enters the body through a break in the epidermal barrier, commonly during fishing or water sport activities. Pustular lesions, lymphangitis, lymphadenitis, and cellulitis may ensue; in some cases, rapid progression to myositis and skin necrosis follows. Treatment of *V. vulnificus* wound infections consists of antibiotics, such as the combination of doxycycline and ceftazidime, and wound care.[28]

Primary septicemia from *V. vulnificus* occurs 24 to 48 hours after the ingestion of raw oysters, especially in patients with hepatic cirrhosis, diabetes, renal failure, or immunosuppression. Clinically, fever and hypotension may be present, along with the development of bullous cellulitis and necrotic skin ulcers.

NECROTIZING FASCIITIS

Necrotizing fasciitis (NF) is an uncommon but life-threatening soft tissue infection characterized by rapidly spreading inflammation and necrosis of the skin, subcutaneous fat, and fascia.[29] (See *color section, Necrotizing fasciitis*, page C30.) Mortality rates have exceeded 70% in the past,[30] although recent data have shown a dramatic decrease, with mortality rates below 10%.[31] Rapid, early intervention, including surgical debridement and antimicrobial therapy, is imperative to reduce morbidity and mortality.

The incidence of necrotizing fasciitis has been reported to be 0.40 cases per 100,000 population.[31] Although it is rare, certain conditions can predispose patients to developing the disease, including immunocompromised states such as diabetes mellitus (the most common), acquired immunodeficiency syndrome (AIDS), and malignancy as well as obesity, peripheral vascular disease,[32] and trauma, such as burns, lacerations, or minor trauma. (See *Conditions leading to necrotizing fasciitis,* page 500.)

Necrotizing fasciitis is categorized as type 1, type 2, or type 3 depending on which

Conditions leading to necrotizing fasciitis

The conditions listed below place patients at risk for necrotizing fasciitis.[29,33,34]

- Age 50 and older
- Alcoholism
- Anogenital infection: anorectal, perianal, scrotal, ischiorectal, periurethral abscess
- Atherosclerosis: coronary artery disease, peripheral vascular disease
- Chronic obstructive pulmonary disease
- Cirrhosis or chronic liver disease
- Compromised skin integrity: psoriasis, herpes zoster, chronic leg ulcers
- Diabetes mellitus
- Hypertension
- Immunosuppression: HIV, corticosteroid therapy
- Intravenous drug use
- Malignancy
- Malnutrition
- Obesity
- Renal failure
- Smoking
- Surgery
- Trauma: needle puncture, insect bites, fish-fin injury, burns, lacerations, surgical wounds

organisms are cultured. Type 1 necrotizing fasciitis is caused by a polymicrobial infection from aerobic and anaerobic bacteria such as *Clostridium* and *Bacteroides* species. Type 2 necrotizing fasciitis consists of group A *Streptococcus* (*S. pyogenes*) with or without a coexisting staphylococcal infection. Type 3 necrotizing fasciitis is caused by a *Vibrio* infection from a puncture wound due to fish or marine insects.

Necrotizing fasciitis can affect any area of the body, but it most commonly occurs on the extremities. Involvement of the genitalia is referred to as Fournier's gangrene and usually results from a polymicrobial infection. There is a higher mortality rate when the head, neck, chest, and abdomen are involved because those areas tend to be refractory and, as such, are more difficult to treat.

Early on, patients generally present with a clinical picture similar to cellulitis. As with less aggressive cases of cellulitis, redness and edema can be seen at the site, with a spreading, diffuse inflammatory reaction that blends into the surrounding tissue. The overlying skin is shiny and tense without any clear lines of demarcation. However, patient complaints of severe pain are usually out of proportion to the clinical lesion. This characteristic clue of necrotizing fasciitis may be the only hint of a deeper, more aggressive infection. It is critical to be alert for this sign because the earlier the diagnosis is made, the earlier treatment can be instituted and the better the chance of survival will be.

Over time, frank cutaneous gangrene may extend beyond the skin and into the subcutaneous fat and fascial planes below. Separation of the necrotic tissue along the fascial planes with suppuration may occur. Myonecrosis develops in the underlying muscle. Lymphadenitis, lymphangitis, crepitation, and venous thrombosis are seen less often.

Metastatic abscesses have been reported in the liver, lung, spleen, brain, and pericardium, but these are rare. In addition to cutaneous manifestations of necrotizing fasciitis, there are systemic findings as well as those associated with progression of disease. Patients usually will appear toxic with high fever, chills, and constitutional symptoms. In fulminant cases, multiorgan system failure occurs.

Vasculopathies

A heterogeneous group of disorders is classified under this category. Vasculopathy is characterized by occlusion of small vessels within the skin due to thrombi or emboli, which leads to tissue hypoxia and the clinical manifestations of purpura, livedo reticularis, and painful ulcers. Cryofibrinogenemia, monoclonal cryoglobulinemia, and antiphospholipid antibody syndrome are among the causes of vasculopathies that commonly present as atypical skin ulcerations of the lower extremities.

CRYOFIBRINOGENEMIA

Cryofibrinogenemia occurs as a primary (idiopathic) disorder or in association with underlying diseases, such as infectious processes, malignancy, or collagen, vascular, or thromboembolic disease. The clinical presentation is painful cutaneous ulcerations located on the leg and foot; these lesions are usually unresponsive to treatment. (See *color section, Cryofibrinogenemia,* page C30.) Other cutaneous findings include livedo reticularis (a netlike erythema), purpura, ecchymoses, and gangrene. The pathogenesis of the lesions is related to the in vivo occlusion of small blood vessels initiated in the distal extremities by the abnormal precipitate. This hypothesis is corroborated by the pathology findings of cryofibrinogen, consisting of thrombi within superficial dermal vessels due in part to protein deposition. Cryofibrinogen is a circulating complex of fibrin, fibrinogen, and fibronectin along with albumin, cold-insoluble globulin, and factor VIII. The complex is soluble at 98.6°F (37°C) but forms a cryoprecipitate at 39.2°F (4°C).[35] Additionally, this complex can be made to clot with thrombin. The mechanism by which cryofibrinogen is produced is not well understood.

Treatment is symptomatic or, in secondary disease, directed to the underlying cause.[36] Agents that lyse fibrin thrombi are helpful.

Stanozolol, streptokinase, and streptodornase have been used with success.

CRYOGLOBULINEMIA

Cryoglobulinemia occurs when deposits of cryoglobulins lead to the formulation of thrombi in medium and small vessel walls.[37] Three types of cryoglobulinemia have been identified; type I or monoclonal cryoglobulinemia may be seen in patients with malignant diseases, such as myeloma, or benign lymphoproliferative conditions, such as Waldenström's macroglobulinemia. This classically leads to thrombotic phenomena but can clinically resemble vasculitis. Type II or mixed cryoglobulinemia combines polyclonal and a monoclonal immunoglobulin; this type of cryoglobulinemia is seen less often in association with malignancies and more frequently with infectious or inflammatory diseases. Type III is comprised of only polyclonal immunoglobulin and is most commonly associated with hepatitis C infection. Both type II and III cryoglobulinemia cause vasculitis, which can lead to skin ulcers.[38] Other skin manifestations include acral cyanosis, Raynaud's phenomenon, livedo reticularis, altered pigmentation of involved skin, and palpable purpura, which may progress to blistering and frank ulceration. Some patients may have systemic manifestations, such as arthritis, peripheral neuropathy, and glomerulonephritis. Diagnosis is based on skin biopsies, which show either vasculopathy or vasculitis, and subsequent detection of cryoprecipitate and analysis of cryoglobulins by immunoelectrophoresis.

> **▶ PRACTICE POINT**
>
> Evaluate the patient with vasculitis for type II or III cryoglobulinemia; these conditions can cause vasculopathy.

Treatment should be directed at the underlying cause when cryoglobulinemia is associated with hepatitis C. Either pegylated interferon-α or ribavarin is used to treat hepatitis C and may result in resolution of the associated cryoglobulinemia. Corticosteroids alone or in combination with immunosuppressive drugs (cyclophosphamide or mycophenolate mofetil) have been used to induce remission in patients with cryoglobulinemia. Plasmapheresis and rituximab can be used as well to treat severe cases of cryoglobulinemic vasculitis.[39]

ANTIPHOSPHOLIPID ANTIBODY SYNDROME

Antiphospholipid antibody syndrome (APS) is characterized by elevated titers of different antiphospholipid antibodies in association with venous or arterial thrombosis, recurrent fetal loss, and often thrombocytopenia. Antiphospholipid antibodies include lupus anticoagulant, anticardiolipid antibodies, and anti-β2-glycoprotein-1 antibodies. All or any of the antibodies are part of the syndrome.[40,41] APS may present as primary disease or may be secondary to an underlying autoimmune disease such as systemic lupus erythematosus (seen in about 50% of cases). Elevated antiphospholipid antibody titers also have been associated with malignancy and infectious states. The exact pathogenic mechanism of APS remains unknown.

The clinical hallmark of this disease is the presence of livedo reticularis. Arterial and venous thrombosis may elicit a variety of skin lesions, including ulcerations (most commonly), superficial thrombophlebitis, and cutaneous infarcts. Any organ system can be affected. Placental vessel thrombosis and ischemia can result in miscarriage precipitated by placental insufficiency. A proposed mechanism responsible for this event is a disruption of annexin A5 (a cell-surface protein with anticoagulant properties) binding of phospholipids on the trophoblast cells by antiphospholipid antibodies, thus promoting a procoagulant state that leads to thrombosis at the maternal-fetal interface followed by damage to the placenta and eventual fetal loss.[42] Treatment includes the use of aspirin, warfarin, and prednisone, but response is not uniform.

Metabolic disorders

Metabolic diseases are uncommon causes of chronic wounds. One condition, called calciphylaxis, is commonly seen in a subset of patients undergoing long-term hemodialysis who develop secondary hyperparathyroidism.[43]

This leads to deposition of calcium within soft tissue and the vasculature and, eventually, tissue death.

CALCIPHYLAXIS

Calciphylaxis is a rare, often fatal condition that is characterized clinically by progressive cutaneous necrosis, which frequently occurs in patients with end-stage renal disease. Many eliciting factors have been suggested, but the most common linking phenomenon is the development of secondary hyperparathyroidism.[44] Secondary hyperparathyroidism causes elevated calcium-phosphate product and the development of vascular, cutaneous, and subcutaneous calcification that, in turn, leads to tissue death. Calciphylaxis typically develops after beginning dialysis and is seen in approximately 1% of patients with chronic renal failure[45] and in 4.1% of patients receiving hemodialysis.[46] The prognosis for patients who develop calciphylaxis is grim, with an estimated 1-year survival rate of approximately 46%.[47,48] In addition to skin involvement, the pathophysiologic process may also occur within internal organs; this, along with sepsis from infected skin wounds, is a major cause of morbidity and mortality in patients with this condition.

The cutaneous manifestations begin as red or violaceous mottled plaques in a livedo reticularis-like pattern. This signifies a vascular pattern, and these early ischemic lesions often progress to gangrenous, ill-defined, black plaques. With time, the plaques ulcerate and become tender; indurated ulcers can lead to auto-amputation. The ulcers of calciphylaxis are usually bilateral and symmetric and may extend deep into muscle. Vesicles frequently appear at the periphery of the ulcers. (See *color section*, *Calciphylaxis*, page C31.)

The term *calciphylaxis* is considered a misnomer that originated from experiments in rats that resulted in interstitial calcification.[49] "Calciphylaxis" originally was coined by Selye in 1962 [49] after he produced ectopic calcifications in experimental animals using variety of sensitizing agents, including parathyroid hormone, vitamin D, and a diet high in calcium and phosphorus. Calciphylaxis should be distinguished from calcinosis cutis, which may be associated with significant morbidity but typically not mortality. Calciphylaxis has been given a number of other names, including uremic gangrene syndrome, metastatic calcinosis, azotemic calcific arteriopathy, and calcific uremic arteriopathy. Some authors prefer the term *calcific uremic arteriopathy*[50] because it reflects the histologic findings of calcium deposits in the walls of the small- and medium-sized vessels of lesions. The important distinction is that calcific uremic arteriopathy involves small vessel calcifications with intimal hypertrophy and small vessel thrombosis. (See *color section, Calcific uremic arteriopathy*, page C32.)

The pathogenesis of calciphylaxis is still poorly understood. Recent studies have shown increases in the expression of bone-specific proteins, including collagen I, bone morphogenic protein 2 and 3, matrix Gla protein, osteopontin, osteonectin, and ostecalcin, in calcified arteries. These proteins, together with elevated calcium and inorganic phosphate levels, may induce calcification or osteoblastic differentiation in pluripotent vascular smooth muscle cells.[43,44,50,51]

Diagnosis can usually be made based on clinical findings. Although vascular processes may present similarly, laboratory evaluation for the presence of an elevated calcium, phosphate, or calcium $\times$ phosphate product confirms calciphylaxis. An elevated intact parathyroid hormone level along with radiographic evidence and consistent histology also help confirm a diagnosis. Calcification of the intima and media of small- and medium-sized vessels in the dermis and subcutaneous tissue are characteristic of calciphylaxis. Radiographic findings include pipe stem calcifications resulting from the calcium deposits outlining the vessels in these patients.

As secondary infections may have tragic sequelae, treatment of infected ulcers is critical. Swab and tissue cultures from the wound may aid in guiding antibiotic therapy.

The treatments used for patients with calciphylaxis can be divided into either medical or surgical therapies[43,44,50,51] and are often used in tandem. (See *Calciphylaxis treatment options*.)

Calciphylaxis treatment options

Medical treatment options
- Phosphate binders
- Decreased calcium in dialysate
- Antibiotics
- Low phosphate diet
- Cinacalcet
- Bisphosphonates
- Sodium thiosulfate
- Avoidance of challenging agents
- Avoidance of systemic steroids
- Hyperbaric oxygen
- Anticoagulation
- Cyclosporine
- Stanozolo

Surgical treatment options
- Parathyroidectomy
- Wound care and debridement
- Amputation
- Renal transplantation
- Skin grafting using either autologous or tissue engineered skin

Malignancies

Malignancies may present either as wounds or developing from wounds. Nonmelanoma skin cancer, lymphomas, and sarcomas may ulcerate as they outgrow their blood supply. (See *color section, Malignancies,* page C33.) Alternatively, chronic wounds may develop into a malignancy, most commonly squamous cell carcinoma. This phenomenon is termed *Marjolin's ulcer* after the author who first described cells from an edge of a chronic wound that had undergone malignant change—an occurrence that can be seen in up to 2% of chronic wounds.[52] (See *color section, Marjolin ulcer,* page C33.) A similar phenomenon may also occur in scars, burn wounds, sinus tracts, chronic osteomyelitis, and even vaccination sites.

The precise mechanism of malignant degeneration in chronic wounds is not known, although several theories have been proposed.[53,54] In addition to squamous cell carcinoma, basal cell carcinomas and other neoplasms, such as Kaposi's sarcoma and lymphoma, have also been found in chronic wounds.

Early identification of malignancy, typically via biopsy of suspected lesions, is critical. Treatment of biopsy-confirmed neoplasia includes excision with margins (usually at least 2 cm), possibly adjuvant therapy with radiation, topical 5-fluorouracil, methotrexate, L-phenylalanine mustard, and even lymph node dissection; amputation of the affected limb may be necessary in some cases.[53] Mohs surgery to ensure complete removal of the primary lesion has been used successfully to treat malignancy arising from chronic osteomyelitis.[55]

External causes

External causes of atypical wounds include spider bites, chemical injury, chronic radiation exposure, trauma, and factitial ulcers.[56] A thorough patient history is the most valuable tool in determining the etiologic agent in ulcers caused by external factors.

SPIDER BITES

At least 50 spider species in the United States have been implicated in causing significant medical conditions; however, the *Loxosceles* (brown recluse or violin spider) and the *Latrodectus* (black widow) species are the most well known to cause skin necrosis and ulcers in the Americas.

Loxoscelism

The bite of *Loxosceles reclusa* is usually painless and often goes unnoticed; however, some patients will experience progression to more significant wounds. In these patients, enlargement of the bite site occurs within 2 to 6 hours, with associated pain and general symptoms, such as fever, malaise, headache, and arthralgia. As the disease progresses, a pustule, blister, or large plaque forms at the bite site. These wounds may present as a deep purple plaque surrounded by a clear halo (vasoconstriction) and surrounding erythema—the so-called red, white, and blue sign (See *color section, Loxoscelism,* page C34.) Viscerocutaneous loxoscelism, a systemic illness that can include diarrhea, nausea, vomiting, petechia, urticaria, and disseminated intravascular coagulation, can occur in 0.7% to 27% of patients depending on the geographic region.[57]

With bites occurring in areas of greater fat content, such as the abdomen, buttocks, and thighs, necrosis develops more frequently. When the eschar is shed, an ulcer may result. Healing of the ulcer is generally very slow and may take up to 6 months.

The differential diagnosis includes foreign body reaction, infections, trauma, vasculitis, pyoderma gangrenosum, and methicillin-resistant *Staphylococcus aureus* infection. Treatment consists of cooling the bite site, elevation (if possible), and analgesics. The use of systemic steroids may prevent enlargement of the necrotic areas. Dapsone also has been recommended at a dose of 100 mg per day in adults.

Latrodectism

The black widow spider, or *Latrodectus mactans,* is easily recognized by a bright red hourglass marking on the abdomen. The painless bite is followed by severe pain, swelling, and tenderness at the site where the bite occurred. Systemic symptoms may follow, including headaches and abdominal pain, but they subside in 1 to 3 days. Treatment includes local ice, calcium gluconate, and the administration of specific antivenin. Black widow bites are rarely fatal; death may occur in children, those with comorbidities, or elderly people.

CHEMICAL BURNS

A variety of chemical products are capable of producing skin wounds.[58] Cutaneous injury caused by caustic chemicals progresses continually after the initial exposure and, if not properly cared for, may produce painful ulcers that are difficult to heal. The lesions caused by alkalis are usually more severe than those caused by acids; however, the severity of the burn is determined by the mode of action and concentration of the chemical as well as the duration of contact before treatment is initiated.[58] Prolonged irrigation with water for 30 minutes or longer is the most important initial treatment, followed by standard burn care.

Certain chemicals possess unique properties that require special additional therapy, such as hydrofluoric acid (application of 25% magnesium sulfate), chromic acid (excision of the affected area), and phenol (application of polyethylene glycol mixed with alcohol 2:1).[56]

RADIATION DERMATITIS

After exposure to ionizing radiation exceeding 10 Gy, local skin reactions characterized by mild erythema, edema, and pruritus may occur. This acute radiation dermatitis usually begins 2 to 7 days after exposure, peaks within 2 weeks, and gradually subsides. With exposure to higher doses, intense erythema with vesiculation, erosion, and superficial ulceration may ensue. Postinflammatory pigmentary abnormalities, telangiectasia, and atrophy are common.[59]

Excision of the affected area and hyperbaric oxygen have been suggested as possible treatment options.

FACTITIAL DERMATITIS

The term *factitial dermatitis* denotes a self-imposed injury. The clinical appearance of these ulcers is usually particular, with sharp or linear edges in an area of easy access such as the extremities, abdomen, and anterior chest. (See *color section, Factitial dermatitis*, page C34.)

The care includes evaluation and treatment of underlying psychological diseases and limitation of accessibility to the wound, such as placing a dressing or cast over the wound.

Drug-induced causes
COUMADIN NECROSIS

Coumadin (warfarin)-induced skin necrosis is a rare complication of anticoagulant treatment. It is estimated that 1 in every 1,000 to 10,000 patients treated with anticoagulants experiences this complication. Coumadin skin necrosis occurs almost exclusively between the 3rd and 10th day after beginning anticoagulation therapy in association with the administration of a large initial dose of the drug. Although the precise nature of the disease is still unknown, advances in knowledge about protein C, protein S, and antithrombin III anticoagulant pathways have led to a better understanding of the mechanisms involved in pathogenesis.[60]

Postpartum women have a unique risk due to reduced levels of free protein S during the antepartum and immediate postpartum periods.[61] Manifestations range from ecchymoses and purpura to hemorrhagic necrosis; maculopapular, vesicular urticarial eruptions; and purple toes in all affected patients.

Wounds are painful and usually evolve into full-thickness skin necrosis within a few days. Differentiating between warfarin/coumadin-induced skin necrosis and necrotizing fasciitis, gangrene, and other causes of skin necrosis may be difficult.[60]

Local wound care can be conservative but may include debridement and grafting, depending on the extensiveness of the wound. Previously uncomplicated courses of warfarin therapy do not obviate the possibility of skin necrosis with future warfarin administration. Initiation of low-dose warfarin with heparin can reduce the likelihood of this disorder.

EXTRAVASATION

Solutions of calcium, potassium, bicarbonate, hypertonic dextrose, cardiac drugs, chemotherapeutic drugs, cytotoxic drugs, and antibiotics can lead to extravasation injury. Tissue loss can evolve into extensive wounds. Local wound care with debridement and eventual skin grafting is usually required for extensive skin and tissue loss. (See *color section, Extravasation*, page C35.)

Patient Teaching

Patients don't always give a complete history or believe that certain information is relevant to a clinician pertaining to their wound. Because certain diseases or treatments, travel to certain locations, or even contact with certain insects and animals can be associated with some atypical wounds, telling a clinician about these factors can be important in determining the correct etiology of the wound. Instruct patients to always tell the clinician if they:

- have inflammatory bowel disease, as this is often an underlying etiology in pyoderma grangrenosum
- lived in a developing country, as there could be a risk for Buruli ulcers
- visited or lived in a tropical region of Central or South America, as deep fungal infections, systemic mycoses, or exposure to soil (such as being on a farm in a subtropical location, especially in South America) could lead to chromoblastomycosis or paracoccidioidomycosis
- have eaten raw oysters or been fishing or participated in water activities in Atlantic Coast waters, as this can lead to *V. vulnificus* infection
- have a history of chronic renal failure and/or been on hemodialysis, as calcific uremic ateriopathy ulcers (calciphylaxis) can occur
- have an impaired immune system, such as from HIV or alcoholism, as sporotrichosis may be present
- are taking certain medications, such as warfarin (Coumadin), as this can cause necrosis.

Wounds with less tissue loss can be managed conservatively with the same outcome.[62] Because many extravasation injuries occur on the hands, scar management and return of function remain a problem. Proper administration through the correct needle size (small), vein size (large), and dilution of the medication is best. Infusion should be performed as slowly as possible to allow adequate dilution into the blood. Any complaints of pain during infusion warrant immediate cessation of the solution, assessment of the intravenous site, and adherence to treatment protocols for extravasation as deemed necessary. Calcium gluconate is less likely to extravasate and should be used instead of calcium chloride for the management of low serum levels, especially those levels that are not life-threatening. Because many of these cases may elicit external review and sometimes legal review, documentation is crucial to determine what care was given prior to and after the medication was given. Nurses need to be especially vigilant when administering medications prone to extravasation.

SUMMARY

Treating the underlying cause, when possible, is the initial step in caring for patients with atypical wounds. Anti-infective agents may be used for infectious ulcers, malignancies may require surgical removal, and anti-inflammatory agents may be used for inflammatory ulcers. In addition, the use of a moist healing environment, compression dressings (in the absence of arterial insufficiency) for leg lesions, off-loading areas at risk for prolonged pressure, and maximizing patients' nutritional status are essential.

Despite these measures, healing is often slow in patients with atypical wounds. Prolonged healing leads to increased morbidity and decreased quality of life as well as an increase in direct and indirect costs of care. Adjunctive therapies are often used, aimed at both increasing the number of patients who will heal (effectiveness of therapy) and the speed at which they heal (cost-effectiveness of therapy).

Clinical Data

Ms. VS is a 43-year-old patient who comes to your clinic for the first time for treatment of a painful leg ulcer. She has had the ulcer for approximately 3 months. She states that it started as a small pustule on the lateral aspect of her lower left leg that ulcerated and slowly became larger. Two months ago she went to a wound clinic close to her house. The doctor told her the wound appeared infected and needed to be debrided; she would also need antibiotics. Within the week after debridement, the wound almost doubled in size. Upon further questioning you find out that Ms. VS has a history of ulcerative colitis. On physical exam, the ulcer is approximately 6 cm in diameter with irregular, violaceous, undermined borders. The base of the ulcer is purulent with ample exudate present.

Case Discussion

Several aspects of the history and physical exam should clue you in to the correct diagnosis of pyoderma gangrenosum. Pyoderma gangrenosum classically starts as a pustule that ulcerates and enlarges, although not all ulcers start this way. The appearance of the wound is also classic, with violaceous, undermined borders with a purulent base.

The patient's past medical history is very important in this case. Nearly 50% of patients with pyoderma gangrenosum have an underlying disease, the most common of which is inflammatory bowel disease. Other associated diseases include hematologic malignancies and inflammatory arthritis.

Ms. VS clearly demonstrates pathergy, the development of ulcers in an area of trauma. In this case it was evident by the severe worsening of the ulcer following debridement. Other patients may report the development of ulcers following seemingly trivial trauma, such as hitting one's leg against a coffee table.

Treatment consisted of cleansing the wound with normal saline and dressing the wound with an absorbent dressing. High-dose systemic steroids were started and the ulcer gradually resolved over the next 3 weeks, at which point the steroids were tapered.

1. Which of the following is the most important reason to recognize a wound as atypical?
   A. The wound may be contagious.
   B. Treatment varies based on etiology.
   C. Standard wound healing therapies don't apply.
   D. To bill correctly.

   ANSWER: B. *It's critical to recognize when a wound is caused by an etiology other than prolonged pressure, neuropathy, or abnormal vascular supply so that appropriate measures may be undertaken to make a correct diagnosis and provide appropriate therapy. Although an infectious agent that's contagious may be a cause of an atypical ulcer, this isn't common. Although oftentimes specific therapies for atypical wounds exist, these are usually coupled with principles of good wound care, such as compression, off-loading, moist wound healing, and others. Billing for medical therapies is based on Evaluation and Management Codes as opposed to CPT codes.*

2. Which of the following may be performed on tissue biopsies of wounds?
   A. Histology
   B. Culture
   C. Immunofluorescence
   D. All of the above

(continued)

SHOW WHAT YOU KNOW *(continued)*

ANSWER: D. *As a variety of etiologies cause atypical wounds, a variety of techniques are used to confirm these etiologies. Histology is critical for diagnosing inflammatory, malignant, and infectious causes. Biopsies for tissue culture aid in diagnosing infectious causes, and biopsies for immunofluorescence will aid in diagnosing some inflammatory and autoimmune diseases.*

3. Which of the following should not typically be debrided?
    A. Diabetic foot ulcer
    B. Ulcers due to infectious causes
    C. Pyoderma gangrenosum ulcers
    D. Ulcers due to vasculitis

ANSWER: C. *In susceptible people, even minimal trauma to the skin can result in the production of pyoderma gangrenosum lesions, such as pustules and ulcers. This phenomenon is called pathergy. Therefore, debridement of an ulcer secondary to pyoderma gangrenosum may lead to severe worsening of the ulcer.*

4. Sporotrichosis is a fungal infection caused by:
    A. *S. schenckii*
    B. *M. ulcerans*
    C. *F. pedrosoi*
    D. *M. marinum*

ANSWER: A. *S. schenckii causes sporotrichosis. M. ulcerans and M. marinum are species of mycobacteria. F. pedrosoi is a pigment fungi related to chromoblastomycosis.*

5. Cryofibrinogenemia is classified as a:
    A. *mycobacterium.*
    B. pyoderma gangrenosum.
    C. vasculopathy.
    D. metabolic disease.

ANSWER: C. *Cryofibrinogenemia is a painful cutaneous ulceration classified as a vasculopathy. Mycobacterium is a bacterium. Pyoderma gangrenosum is an inflammatory ulcer, and metabolic disease is an uncommon cause of chronic wounds.*

6. Which type of wound is a rare, often fatal condition characterized by progressive cutaneous necrosis that occurs in patients with end-stage renal disease?
    A. Calciphylaxis
    B. Vasculopathy
    C. Radiation dermatitis
    D. Chemical burn

ANSWER: A. *Calciphylaxis is the correct answer. Vasculopathy, radiation dermatitis, and chemical burns are all other types of atypical wounds.*

7. Factitial dermatitis is a:
    A. rare condition.
    B. self-imposed injury.
    C. red rash.
    D. dry, scaly scab.

ANSWER: B. *Factitial dermatitis is a self-imposed injury usually found in easily accessible areas such as the extremities, abdomen, and anterior chest. The other options are incorrect.*

REFERENCES

1. Coon, W.W., Willis, P.W., 3rd, and Keller, J.B. "Venous Thromboembolism and Other Venous Disease in the Tecumseh Community Health Study," *Circulation* 48(4):839-46, 1973.
2. Srinivasaiah, N., Dugdall, H., Barrett, S., et al. "A Point Prevalence Survey of Wounds in North-East England," *J Wound Care* 16(10):413-6, 18-9, 2007.
3. Patel, G.K., Grey, J.E., and Harding, K.G. "Uncommon Causes of Ulceration," *BMJ* 332(7541):594-6, 2006.
4. Carlson, J.A. "The Histological Assessment of Cutaneous Vasculitis," *Histopathology* 56(1):3-23, 2010.
5. Chen, K.R., and Carlson, J.A. "Clinical Approach to Cutaneous Vasculitis," *Am J Clin Dermatol* 9(2):71-92, 2008.
6. Carlson, J.A., Ng, B.T., and Chen, K.R. "Cutaneous Vasculitis Update: Diagnostic Criteria, Classification, Epidemiology, Etiology, Pathogenesis, Evaluation and Prognosis," *Am J Dermatopathol* 27(6):504-28, 2005.
7. Lapraik, C., Watts, R., and Scott, D.G. "Modern Management of Primary Systemic Vasculitis," *Clin Med* 7(1):43-7, 2007.
8. Callen, J.P., and Jackson, J.M. "Pyoderma Gangrenosum: an Update," *Rheum Dis Clin North Am* 33(4):787-802, vi, 2007.
9. Bennett, M.L., Jackson, J.M., Jorizzo, J.L., et al. "Pyoderma Gangrenosum. A Comparison of Typical and Atypical Forms with an Emphasis on Time to Remission. Case Review of 86 Patients from 2 Institutions," *Medicine (Baltimore)* 79(1):37-46, 2000.
10. Sheldon, D.G., Sawchuk, L.L., Kozarek, R.A., et al. "Twenty Cases of Peristomal Pyoderma Gangrenosum: Diagnostic Implications and Management," *Arch Surg* 135(5):564-8; discussion 68-9, 2000.
11. Ruocco, E., Sangiuliano, S., Gravina, A.G., et al. "Pyoderma Gangrenosum: an Updated Review," *J Eur Acad Dermatol Venereol* 23(9):1008-17, 2009.
12. Geren, S., Kerdel, F., Falabella, A., et al. "Infliximab: A Treatment Option for Ulcerative Pyoderma Gangrenosum," *Wounds* 15(2):49-53, 2003.
13. Groves, R. "Unusual Cutaneous Mycobacterial Diseases," *Clin Dermatol* 13(3):257-63, 1995.
14. Dodiuk-Gad, R., Dyachenko, P., Ziv, M., et al. "Nontuberculous Mycobacterial Infections of the Skin: A Retrospective Study of 25 Cases," *J Am Acad Dermatol* 57(3):413-20, 2007.
15. Kwyer, T.A., and Ampadu, E. "Buruli Ulcers: an Emerging Health Problem in Ghana," *Adv Skin Wound Care* 19(9):479-86, 2006.
16. Ampadu, E., Kwyer, T.A., and Otcher, Y. "Buruli Ulcer: Picture of an Emerging Health Challenge and the Response in Ghana," *JWCET* 26(4):30-36, 2006.
17. Nienhuis, W.A., Stienstra, Y., Thompson, W.A., et al. "Antimicrobial Treatment for Early, Limited Mycobacterium Ulcerans Infection: a Randomised Controlled Trial," *Lancet* 375(9715):664-72, 2010.
18. Lupi, O., Tyring, S.K., and McGinnis, M.R. "Tropical Dermatology: Fungal Tropical Diseases," *J Am Acad Dermatol* 53(6):931-51, quiz 52-4, 2005.
19. Ramos-e-Silva, M., Vasconcelos, C., Carneiro, S., et al. "Sporotrichosis," *Clin Dermatol* 25(2):181-7, 2007.
20. Lopez Martinez, R., and Mendez Tovar, L.J. "Chromoblastomycosis," *Clin Dermatol* 25(2):188-94, 2007.
21. Ameen, M. "Managing Chromoblastomycosis," *Trop Doct* 40(2):65-7, 2010.
22. Negroni, R., Tobon, A., Bustamante, B., et al. "Posaconazole Treatment of Refractory Eumycetoma and Chromoblastomycosis," *Rev Inst Med Trop Sao Paulo* 47(6):339-46, 2005.
23. Ramos, E.S.M., and Saraiva Ldo, E. "Paracoccidioidomycosis," *Dermatol Clin* 26(2):257-69, vii, 2008.
24. Lichon, V., and Khachemoune, A. "Mycetoma: a Review," *Am J Clin Dermatol* 7(5):315-21, 2006.
25. Fahal, A.H., Sheik, H.E., Homeida, M.M., et al. "Ultrasonographic Imaging of Mycetoma," *Br J Surg* 84(8):1120-2, 1997.
26. Ameen, M., and Arenas, R. "Developments in the Management of Mycetomas," *Clin Exp Dermatol* 34(1):1-7, 2009.
27. de Araujo, M.R., Aquino, C., Scaramal, E., et al. "Vibrio Vulnificus Infection in Sao Paulo, Brazil: Case Report and Literature Review," *Braz J Infect Dis* 11(2):302-5, 2007.
28. Bross, M.H., Soch, K., Morales, R., et al. "Vibrio Vulnificus Infection: Diagnosis and Treatment," *Am Fam Physician* 76(4):539-44, 2007.
29. Salcido, R.S. "Necrotizing Fasciitis: Reviewing the Causes and Treatment Strategies," *Adv Skin Wound Care* 20(5):288-93; quiz 94-5, 2007.
30. McHenry, C.R., Piotrowski, J.J., Petrinic, D., et al. "Determinants of Mortality for Necrotizing Soft-tissue Infections," *Ann Surg* 221(5):558-63; discussion 63-5, 1995.
31. Ogilvie, C.M., and Miclau, T. "Necrotizing Soft Tissue Infections of the Extremities and Back," *Clin Orthop Relat Res* 447:179-86, 2006.
32. Bellapianta, J.M., Ljungquist, K., Tobin, E., et al. "Necrotizing Fasciitis," *J Am Acad Orthop Surg* 17(3):174-82, 2009.
33. Unalp, H.R., Kamer, E., Derici, H., et al. "Fournier's Gangrene: Evaluation of 68 Patients

and Analysis of Prognostic Variables," *J Postgrad Med* 54(2):102-5, 2008.

34. Angoules, A.G., Kontakis, G., Drakoulakis, E., et al. "Necrotising Fasciitis of Upper and Lower Limb: a Systematic Review," *Injury* 38(Suppl 5): S19-26, 2007.

35. Saadoun, D., Elalamy, I., Ghillani-Dalbin, P., et al. "Cryofibrinogenemia: New Insights Into Clinical and Pathogenic Features," *Am J Med* 122(12): 1128-35, 2009.

36. Falanga, V., Kirsner, R.S., Eaglstein, W.H., et al. "Stanozolol in Treatment of Leg Ulcers Due to Cryofibrinogenaemia," *Lancet* 338(8763):347-8, 1991.

37. Tedeschi, A., Barate, C., Minola, E., et al. "Cryoglobulinemia," *Blood Rev* 21(4):183-200, 2007.

38. Ferri, C. "Mixed Cryoglobulinemia," *Orphanet J Rare Dis* 3 25, 2008.

39. Iannuzzella, F., Vaglio, A., and Garini, G. "Management of Hepatitis C Virus-Related Mixed Cryoglobulinemia," *Am J Med* 123(5):400-8, 2010.

40. Eby, C. "Antiphospholipid Syndrome Review," *Clin Lab Med* 29(2):305-19, 2009.

41. Lim, W. "Antiphospholipid Antibody Syndrome," *Hematology Am Soc Hematol Educ Program* 233-9, 2009.

42. Rand, J.H., Wu, X.X., Quinn, A.S., et al. "The Annexin A5-Mediated Pathogenic Mechanism in the Antiphospholipid Syndrome: Role in Pregnancy Losses and Thrombosis," *Lupus* 19(4):460-9, 2010.

43. Dauden, E., and Onate, M.J. "Calciphylaxis," *Dermatol Clin* 26(4):557-68, ix, 2008.

44. Guldbakke, K.K., and Khachemoune, A. "Calciphylaxis," *Int J Dermatol* 46(3):231-8, 2007.

45. Budisavljevic, M.N., Cheek, D., and Ploth, D.W. "Calciphylaxis in Chronic Renal Failure," *J Am Soc Nephrol* 7(7):978-82, 1996.

46. Angelis, M., Wong, L.L., Myers, S.A., et al. "Calciphylaxis in Patients on Hemodialysis: a Prevalence Study," *Surgery* 122(6):1083-9; discussion 89-90, 1997.

47. Weenig, R.H., Sewell, L.D., Davis, M.D., et al. "Calciphylaxis: Natural History, Risk Factor Analysis, and Outcome," *J Am Acad Dermatol* 56(4):569-79, 2007.

48. Fine, A., and Zacharias, J. "Calciphylaxis is Usually Non-Ulcerating: Risk Factors, Outcome and Therapy," *Kidney Int* 61(6):2210-7, 2002.

49. Selye, H., Gabbiani, G., and Strebel, R. "Sensitization to Calciphylaxis by Endogenous Parathyroid Hormone," *Endocrinology* 71 554-8, 1962.

50. Rogers, N.M., and Coates, P.T. "Calcific Uraemic Arteriolopathy: an Update," *Curr Opin Nephrol Hypertens* 17(6):629-34, 2008.

51. Weenig, R.H. "Pathogenesis of Calciphylaxis: Hans Selye to Nuclear Factor Kappa-B," *J Am Acad Dermatol* 58(3):458-71, 2008.

52. Yang, D., Morrison, B.D., Vandongen, Y.K., et al. "Malignancy in Chronic Leg Ulcers," *Med J Aust* 164(12):718-20, 1996.

53. Copcu, E. "Marjolin's Ulcer: a Preventable Complication of Burns?" *Plast Reconstr Surg* 124(1):156e-64e, 2009.

54. Enoch, S., Miller, D.R., Price, P.E., et al. "Early Diagnosis is Vital in the Management of Squamous Cell Carcinomas Associated with Chronic Non Healing Ulcers: a Case Series and Review of the Literature," *Int Wound J* 1(3):165-75, 2004.

55. Chang, A., Spencer, J.M., and Kirsner, R.S. "Squamous Cell Carcinoma Arising from a Nonhealing Wound and Osteomyelitis Treated with Mohs Micrographic Surgery: a Case Study," *Ostomy Wound Manage* 44(4):26-30, 1998.

56. Newcomer, V.D., and Young, E.M., Jr. "Unique Wounds and Wound Emergencies," *Dermatol Clin* 11(4):715-27, 1993.

57. Hogan, C.J., Barbaro, K.C., and Winkel, K. "Loxoscelism: Old Obstacles, New Directions," *Ann Emerg Med* 44(6):608-24, 2004.

58. Bates, N. "Acid and Alkali Injury," *Emerg Nurse* 7(8):21-6, 1999.

59. Hymes, S.R., Strom, E.A., and Fife, C. "Radiation Dermatitis: Clinical Presentation, Pathophysiology, and Treatment 2006," *J Am Acad Dermatol* 54(1):28-46, 2006.

60. Nazarian, R.M., Van Cott, E.M., Zembowicz, A., et al. "Warfarin-Induced Skin Necrosis," *J Am Acad Dermatol* 61(2):325-32, 2009.

61. Cheng, A., Scheinfeld, N.S., McDowell, B., et al. "Warfarin Skin Necrosis in a Postpartum Woman with Protein S Deficiency," *Obstet Gynecol* 90(4 Pt 2):671-2, 1997.

62. Doellman, D., Hadaway, L., Bowe-Geddes, L.A., et al. "Infiltration and Extravasation: Update on Prevention and Management," *J Infus Nurs* 32(4):203-11, 2009.

CHAPTER 21

Wounds in Special Populations

Objectives

After completing this chapter, you'll be able to:

- identify the unique risk factors for pressure ulcer development in the critically ill patient
- describe risk assessment tools and methods appropriate for use with the critically ill patient
- list special considerations for pressure ulcer treatment in the critically ill patient
- describe successful strategies for reducing the incidence of pressure ulcers in the patient who has a spinal cord injury (SCI)
- identify risk factors of pressure ulcers in the patient with an SCI
- discuss the major health complications of an SCI
- describe the impact of highly active antiretroviral therapy (HAART) on the prevalence of skin disorders in the patient with human immunodeficiency virus (HIV) or acquired immunodeficiency syndrome (AIDS)
- describe six common infectious skin disorders and two common noninfectious skin disorders in the patient with HIV or AIDS that results in altered skin integrity
- discuss two of the neoplastic skin disorders seen in the patient with HIV or AIDS
- discuss bariatric and obesity healthcare facility concerns
- identify skin problems commonly found in the bariatric patient
- discuss unique risk factors and pressure ulcer prevention strategies for the bariatric patient.

With the vast variety of special patient populations, proper consideration and care are paramount in the treatment of skin conditions, particularly pressure ulcers. In the intensive care setting, some pressure ulcers may be unavoidable. Vigilant monitoring is necessary to find and treat these ulcers as soon as they develop. Remember, pressure ulcers may be a source of sepsis in an already compromised patient. Assess the patient and determine his or her wishes as well as those of the family, and adapt your goals accordingly. Aggressive treatment may be necessary to minimize tissue damage and relieve pain. Some patients may be too physiologically unstable for interventions such as turning. In such cases the priority is saving the patient, sometimes at the expense of the skin.

The patient with a spinal cord injury faces a lifelong risk for the development of pressure ulcers. Although mostly preventable, pressure ulcers are a deterrent to achieving rehabilitation goals, may contribute to a loss of independence, and interfere with the pursuit of educational, vocational, and leisure activities after a spinal cord injury. It's now possible to identify patients with a spinal cord injury who are at highest risk for pressure ulcers so that effective prevention strategies can be incorporated into their lifestyles.

In patients with human immunodeficiency virus (HIV) and acquired immune deficiency syndrome (AIDS), skin disorders are common. Accurate identification of skin lesions is critical so appropriate treatment can be implemented. Consultation with an HIV or AIDS clinician is helpful in the comprehensive care of these patients.

Finally, proactive planning, preparation, proper equipment, interdisciplinary teamwork, and sensitivity are important hallmarks in providing appropriate care to bariatric patients.

This chapter addresses four special populations: intensive care patients, spinal cord injury patients, patients with HIV/AIDS, and bariatric patients.

INTENSIVE CARE POPULATION

Janet E. Cuddigan, PhD, RN, CWCN

PRESSURE ULCER INCIDENCE AND PREVALENCE

Pressure ulcer incidence may be higher in patients in the intensive care unit (ICU) than in patients in other units. In a series of international multisite pressure ulcer surveys, facility-acquired pressure ulcer (FAPU) rates were highest in adult intensive care units.[1] In 2009, critical care FAPU rates ranged from 8.8% in general cardiac care units to 10.3% in surgical ICUs. These rates contrast sharply with the FAPU rates in medical, surgical, and medical-surgical units, where FAPU rates ranged from 3.9 to 4.3%. Pressure ulcers acquired in critical care units tend to be more severe, with 3.3% of these patients developing stage III, stage IV, unstageable, or suspected deep tissue injury (sDTI) ulcers.[1]

Similar disparities are seen between FAPU rates for children in pediatric ICUs (PICUs; 5.1%) and children on medical-surgical units (1.6%).[1] Pediatric patients, especially babies and toddlers, tend to develop pressure ulcers on the occiput more often than adult patients due to the higher proportion of body weight in the head.[2,3] In addition, high-frequency oscillation ventilation is used more frequently in pediatric than in adult patients, often creating friction and shear injuries to the head.[4]

RISK FACTORS

All too often, the critically ill patient survives a life-threatening illness with the aid of advanced technology, yet faces weeks or months of additional treatment for a painful, disfiguring, and potentially preventable complication—a pressure ulcer. The ICU population encompasses a broad range of physiologically unstable patients.

The key component of a pressure ulcer prevention program for an ICU patient is an initial risk assessment to identify the specific level and type of risk the patient faces. Frequent follow-up assessments are also essential for prevention. If pressure ulcers develop, you should supplement aggressive treatment with continued preventive measures, including frequent reassessment.

Risk assessment tools

Debate in the research literature and clinical arena is ongoing with regard to the most valid and reliable method of evaluating pressure ulcer risk status in the critically ill patient. Options include standard risk assessment tools (for example, the Braden,[5] Norton,[6] and Waterlow[7] Scales), risk assessment tools designed specifically for the critically ill patient (for example, the Jackson-Cubbin Scale for adults[8–10] and the Braden Q Scale for children[11]), individual risk factors unique to the critically ill patient (for example, conditions creating poor local and systemic oxygenation, poor local and systemic perfusion), and professional judgment. The answer to this debate is "all of the above."

Standardized risk assessment tools such as the Braden Scale still provide good general screening for risk status in the critically ill patient. They also help focus our preventive interventions on the type and level of modifiable risk (for example, mobility, nutrition, moisture). In a prospective study of 186 neurological ICU patients, the Braden Scale was a better predictor of pressure ulcers than any factor other than low body mass index on admission.[12] With a cut-off score of 16, all patients developing stage II or greater pressure ulcers were considered at risk; however, the false-positive rate was 81.9%. The high false-positive rate may have been due to over-prediction by the Braden Scale or to the fact that the staff may have succeeded in preventing pressure ulcers in some patients whose scores indicated risk. In the same study, a cut-off score of 13 more accurately predicted pressure ulcers, with a sensitivity of 91.4% but a false-negative rate of 1.8%. Other authors have recommended different Braden Scale cut-off scores.[13] Clinical practice is moving away from using the total Braden Scale score as a basis for intervention and moving instead toward risk-based prevention programs that focus on moderating or eliminating the specific type of risk identified by subscale scores. Subscale scores also provide information about the degree of risk, so we can modify the intensity of interventions accordingly.

How do risk assessment tools specifically designed for the critically ill patient measure up? Several investigators have developed risk assessment scales specific to the ICU population.[8,16,20,23–27] These tools show varying levels of accuracy, yet none has undergone the degree of validation testing of the Braden Scale. The most thoroughly tested of the "designer tools" is the Jackson-Cubbin Pressure Ulcer Risk Calculator. The Jackson-Cubbin Scale compares favorably with the Braden Scale in predicting pressure ulcer development in critically ill adults[9,10,28,29]; however, it is a more complex tool containing 10 items.

Several studies correlate higher Acute Physiological Assessment and Chronic Health Evaluation (APACHE) II or III scores among ICU patients with pressure ulcer development.[14,17,22,23,30] The APACHE Scale is based on physiological factors, age, and chronic health conditions. It's predictive of patient mortality, so it isn't surprising that a scale that predicts the death of a patient would also predict the tissue death associated with pressure ulcers.

Are there individual risk factors for pressure ulcers that are unique to the critical care population and highly predictive of pressure ulcer development? In a comprehensive literature review, deLaat and colleagues[31] identified more than 50 risk factors from epidemiological

Pressure ulcer risk factors in intensive care patients

Epidemiological studies of critically ill patients show that the following individual risk factors are strongly associated with the development of pressure ulcers:

- being "too unstable to turn"[14] or "turned less often"[15]
- days in bed and days without nutrition[16]
- longer length of stay[17–19]
- low albumin levels[19]
- infection[17]
- use of vasoconstrictive agents[14,20–22]
- High APACHE II scores.[14,17,22]

Many of these risk factors can be included under the more general categories of the Braden Scale. For example, "too unstable to turn" could fit into the Braden subscale of mobility. None of these individual risk factors carry enough "statistical weight" to be included in a risk assessment scale; however, keep them in mind as you're assessing the unique risks of critically ill patients.

studies and concluded that "no discriminatory risk factor for pressure ulcer development could be identified in the critically ill population.[31] (See *Pressure ulcer risk factors in intensive care patients*.) A subsequent review in 2009 found similar results.[32]

Several authors have looked for the "one or two additional risk factors" that would make the Braden Scale more predictive of pressure ulcer development in the critically ill patient, yet none has developed a tool that has clinical utility and predictive validity. The most validated is Quigley and Curley's study of PICU patients. They adapted the descriptions in the Braden Scale for the pediatric population and added a tissue perfusion and oxygenation subscale. Their findings demonstrate high predictive validity for PICU patients; however, the tissue perfusion and oxygenation subscale has not been tested in adult populations.[2]

Risk assessment depends on a finely integrated combination of risk assessment tools, such as the Braden Scale, to screen for type and level of risk as well as knowledge of population-specific risk factors from the research literature and clinical judgment. To develop a successful preventive plan, each risk factor or abnormal Braden subscore should be addressed comprehensively in light of the patient's physiological condition. Risk should be assessed daily in the ICU setting and reassessed with major changes in the patient's condition.

RISK-BASED PREVENTION

Although allocating resources according to the overall level of risk estimated by a total Braden Scale score is useful, a risk-based prevention program should be based on each patient's unique level and type of risk. Target your interventions to address low subscale scores. For example, if mobility and activity subscores are low (1 or 2) and moisture subscores are high (4), focus your interventions on mobility and activity issues. The following discussion focuses on the unique needs of the critically ill patient within the common categories of risk, including mobility, activity, and nutrition, among others.

Mobility

The critically ill patient's level of mobility must be taken into consideration when assessing pressure ulcer risk. Although the standard of care recommends repositioning high-risk patients every 2 hours, a study of 74 ICU patients indicated that only 2.7% of the patients had a change in body position every 2 hours.[33] If the patient's condition prevents position changes, provide a bed that allows additional pressure redistribution. If the patient can't be turned completely due to hemodynamic instability, small shifts in position may be effective as an adjunct to more complete position changes.[34] Too frequently, the memory of a patient desaturating or becoming hypotensive during turning prevents us from resuming a turning schedule. Reassess the patient to determine when you *can* resume turning. Starting with slower, more gradual turns may allow the patient time to compensate for hemodynamic instability related to turning. Measures to restore hemodynamic stability and oxygenation will of course support a quicker return to mobility. Decreased mobility may also result from paralytics, sedation, coma, or spinal instability. Early mobilization programs have been shown to reduce the length of stay in critical care units and may also help reduce the incidence of pressure ulcers.[35]

> ### ▶ PRACTICE POINT
>
> Use caution when turning a patient. Is he or she lying on any tubes or medical devices? Are endotracheal tubes putting pressure on the lips or mouth? Check these points before you turn the patient.[36]

Patients in respiratory distress may be placed in the prone position to improve the partial pressure of arterial oxygen–to–fraction of inspired oxygen ratio. However, prone positioning creates a whole new set of pressure points, including the chin, jaw, breasts, anterior ribs, pelvic bones, genitalia (for males), anterior knees, and toes. Ensure that pressure is off-loaded in these areas. Using pressure-redistributing mattresses and "bridging" to off-load pressure points may be helpful. Several special prone positioning devices are commercially available. Be aware that significant facial edema may develop in a patient while in the prone position. Without proper oral care, the skin around the mouth and cheeks may become macerated from saliva. Assess the patient for tubes, devices, or positioning strategies that may increase pressure in this position. Patients in respiratory distress may also be placed on rotation beds to improve pulmonary status. Make sure that the patient is secure in the bed and that friction and shear injuries don't occur with rotation. Monitor the patient through at least one complete turning cycle to assess for friction and shear problems as well as crimping of tubes (especially endotracheal) during rotation.[32,36]

Bed selection

Selecting the optimal bed can be vital in the care of a critically ill patient. It may be cost-effective to have pressure-redistributing mattresses on all beds in an ICU if patient acuity and pressure ulcer incidence tend to be high.[37-39] The cost-benefit ratio may vary according to overall patient acuity in your unit. The decision to order a bed with such features as alternating pressure, low air loss, or fluidized air should be triggered by low scores on the Braden mobility-activity subscales or in the presence of certain conditions, such as pharmacologic paralysis, sedation, poor local and systemic perfusion (e.g., history of peripheral vascular disease, vasopressor use, prolonged capillary refill time, or prolonged hypotension), poor local and systemic oxygenation, and early signs of multiorgan system failure. Patient needs including moisture and temperature control should also be considered. An analysis of randomized controlled trials published prior to 2004 suggested that high-specification foam mattresses may be more effective than regular mattresses for moderate- to high-risk patients and low-air-loss beds may reduce ulcers in ICU patients.[40,41] Literature reviews completed since then have not identified a type of support surface that is clearly superior for this population.[32]

Beds with lateral rotation features may be used to improve oxygenation for patients with severe respiratory failure; however, they also increase the risk of shear injury. Make sure that the patient is aligned properly in the center of the bed with supporting bolster pads. Observe the patient through at least one complete rotation to ensure that he or she is not sliding in the bed with each rotation, creating shear injury. Continue to turn the patient regularly and assess carefully for shear injury, particularly over the buttocks. Reassess risk and benefits of using the bed periodically.[32]

> **PRACTICE POINT**
>
> Don't counteract the pressure-redistributing effects of a specialized bed by using extra layers of sheets and underpads. Also, don't use padding because it increases pressure. However, you should:
>
> - use incontinence pads recommended by the bed manufacturer for patients who need moisture management
> - make sure that any powered specialty bed is turned on and adjusted for maximum pressure redistribution for each individual patient.
>
> Remember, specialty beds don't replace turning and positioning, nor do they adequately relieve heel pressure.

Positioning

Patient positioning is another important consideration for the critically ill patient. Although the sacrum and the coccyx are the most frequent sites of pressure ulcers in these patients, heels are a close second and the incidence of heel ulcers is increasing. Therefore, vigilant protection of the heels in the critically ill patient is essential.[42] Your patient assessment should include findings that alert you to vascular insufficiency (pulses [palpated or Doppler], capillary refill time, color, warmth, shiny hairless skin, ankle-brachial pressure index, toe pressure, pulse wave-form analysis, and vascular studies). Patients in shock experience constricted vessels in their extremities, accentuating the problem. Devices such as Rooke boots may keep the heels warm (supporting perfusion) and protected, but they don't relieve pressure. Likewise, cloth heel protectors may decrease the risk of skin injury from friction, but they do not relieve pressure. A number of commercial heel protectors are designed to relieve heel pressure by "suspending" the heel. Cadue and colleagues[43] conducted a randomized controlled trial of a heel-suspending foam device in high-risk medical intensive care patients. The number of pressure ulcers was significantly lower in the experimental group and the time to pressure ulcer development was significantly longer. Correct placement is essential to prevent additional rubbing or pressure. Remove heel protectors regularly to inspect the skin. Placing a pillow or bath blanket under the calves to elevate the heels is an effective technique in patients who aren't agitated. Avoid placing pressure under the Achilles tendon, and slightly flex the knee.[32] Remember, heels are the one area where you can truly relieve pressure.

Proper positioning can also help the patient with a critical respiratory condition. There is convincing research evidence that a 45-degree backrest elevation reduces the incidence of ventilator-associated pneumonia. Head-of-bed elevation is also recommended for patients at high risk for aspiration, even if they are not mechanically ventilated.[44] Positioning a patient with respiratory difficulty in an elevated head of bed position is a tried-and-true method of facilitating breathing, yet all of these essential interventions may increase sacral injury from shear as the patient slides down in bed. Placing pillows under the patient's arms may help support him or her in the upright position and may also improve respiratory excursion.

Activity

The patient's level of activity needs to be taken into consideration as well. Getting a critically ill patient into a chair—even a stretch or geri-chair—can be challenging due to the potential problems with postural hypotension, oxygenation, coordination of multiple tubes and invasive lines, and dependence on ventilators. Some bed manufacturers make beds that adjust to a sitting position, which may be an effective alternative for improving early activity. Regardless of these devices, the patient should progress to sitting in a chair.

PRACTICE POINT

If you can get the patient into a chair, don't forget a seat cushion. A foam cushion 3″ to 4″ (7.5 to 10 cm) thick is usually adequate. In a study involving interface pressure measurement, sheepskin and gel cushions were found to have little pressure-reducing effect.[45]

In a study in healthy volunteers, the seating position with the lowest interface pressure was the sitting back (seat tilted) posture with lower legs on a rest. If the seat can't be tilted back, an upright seating posture with feet on the ground is preferable.[46] Check for slouching, and reposition the patient as needed. Periodically adjust the patient's position (for example, with lift-offs or mechanical adjustments of the head-of-bed elevation), and don't leave him or her in the chair for more than 1 hour at a time. When the patient has returned to bed, check his or her skin carefully for areas of redness. If possible, do not place the patient on any reddened area. Reddened skin is a sign that the tissue has not recovered from its last episode of pressure loading.[32]

Sensory perception

Reduced sensory perception can significantly increase a patient's risk of pressure ulcers. Patients scoring low on the sensory perception subscale include those with spinal cord injuries, head trauma, pharmacological paralysis, heavy sedation, and coma. In a Braden Scale validation study, Carlson et al.[30] found the sensory perception subscale to be the most predictive of pressure ulcer risk in 136 critically ill patients. Patients with a low sensory score may not feel pressure-induced discomfort and may not be able to change position. As long as the patient lacks this ability, the nursing staff must assume the responsibility for anticipating pressure-induced discomfort and ensuring routine repositioning and pressure redistribution. Special attention should be paid to checking under the various medical devices (such as splints, tubes, and oxygen masks) for proper fit and signs of pressure-induced injury.[36]

Moisture

Moisture can put the critically ill patient at risk for pressure ulcers. There are numerous reasons why excess moisture might be produced in the critically ill patient, the most obvious being fecal and urinary incontinence. Typical measures for preventing excess moisture include correcting incontinence (when possible), using pads or briefs that wick moisture away from the skin, using moisture barrier creams, changing and cleansing the patient frequently, and assessing the skin for maceration and yeast infections.

Don't underestimate other sources of moisture damage that may macerate skin and increase the risk for pressure ulcers. For example, wound drainage may be excessive and require absorptive dressings, such as foams and alginates. Critically ill patients may exhibit massive, generalized edema. Small injuries such as skin tears may lead to leakage of large amounts of exudates and serum proteins, particularly in patients with low serum albumin levels. Use absorptive dressings and pads to wick moisture away from the skin. Skin protectants may be appropriate for some patients.

Nutrition

Poor nutrition is another risk factor for pressure ulcer development in the critically ill patient.[16] Initiate oral or enteral feeding as soon as possible. If these methods of feeding aren't feasible, weigh the risks and benefits of total parenteral nutrition. Recommend a dietary consult within 48 hours of admission if the patient's Braden nutrition subscale score is 3 or less. Even if nutritional supplementation is provided, be aware that it may be inadequate to meet the increased metabolic needs of a critically ill patient despite your best efforts.

Friction and shear

The factors of friction and shear must also be considered as pressure ulcer risk factors in the critically ill patient. Friction injury may occur with agitation or with insufficient help with turning. Shear injury in the sacrum is a major problem when the patient slides down in the bed or chair; however, some degree of shear exists whenever there is pressure.[47] Make sure you have enough help when turning and positioning. Use lift sheets and slide boards. When the patient is sitting in a chair or in bed, place pillows under the patient's arms to support his or her weight and lessen the chance of shear injury.

SKIN ASSESSMENT

Total skin assessment should be performed on every shift, with precise documentation of all breaks in skin integrity. The National Pressure Ulcer Advisory Panel (NPUAP)/European Pressure Ulcer Advisory Panel (EPUAP) 2009 guideline[32] recommends that pressure ulcers be assessed and measured weekly. Pressure ulcers may deteriorate more rapidly in the medically unstable, critically ill patient; therefore, assessment should be done more frequently in this population.

> **PRACTICE POINT**
>
> Pressure ulcers can be a source of sepsis in a critically ill, immunocompromised patient.

Damage related to medical devices

Be aware of unusual sites of pressure injury, such as under medical devices (casts, splints, external pelvic fixators, pins, traction devices, or heel lifters). Areas of the body affected by placement of bi-level positive airway pressure (Bi-PAP) masks, indwelling catheters, and endotracheal tubes—common sources of pressure injury in the intensive care environment—can also be easily overlooked as potential sites for pressure ulcer development.[36] Check anterior surfaces of the patient who has been placed in a prone position.

Pressure injuries can occur internally from tracheostomy and endotracheal tubes; use the minimal occlusive volume to prevent tracheal damage. Assess the intubated patient's oral cavity and lips with a flashlight by shifting his or her position slightly without disrupting the tube's level. Tape or commercial tube tamers may be used. Likewise, inspect the site of tracheostomy stoma; excessive exudate around the stoma can cause skin breakdown. Under tracheostomy tubes with a lot of mucus and drainage, consider more absorptive dressings, such as foam or alginates, rather than a low-absorptive split-gauze dressing. Whenever you can, avoid using rigid equipment on the critically ill patient; for example, switch to a soft cervical collar when possible.

> **PRACTICE POINT**
>
> Always provide thorough oral care for the intubated patient to prevent pressure-related wounds.

Suspected deep tissue injury

The exact nature of sDTI is still being investigated.[48] (See chapter 13, Pressure ulcers, for more information. See also *color section, Suspected deep tissue injury,* page C19.) Be careful when assessing early sDTIs, which can be mistaken for stage I pressure ulcers. For example, a patient who develops a deep purple area on the buttocks following a sustained period of hypotension and immobility might not have a stage I pressure ulcer, even if the skin is intact. Such a wound is consistent with deep-tissue damage, which will become apparent as dead superficial tissue sloughs off. The area should be off-loaded to prevent further damage and should be reassessed frequently. Early off-loading may allow reperfusion and recovery of ischemic or injured tissues in some cases of sDTI. In other cases, the tissue is already dead and you can expect to see signs of deterioration as the skin sloughs off and deeper damage is revealed.

SUMMARY

Pressure ulcers may be more common in the critically ill patient. Prevention is certainly more challenging. However, with a special eye for the unique needs of the critically ill patient, pressure ulcer incidence can be reduced in this high-risk population.

SHOW WHAT YOU KNOW—INTENSIVE CARE POPULATIONS

1. Risk assessment for pressure ulcer development in the critically ill patient should include:
   A. a validated screening tool.
   B. assessment of unique risk factors common in the ICU.
   C. professional judgment.
   D. all of the above.

   ANSWER: D. *Critically ill patients are at extremely high risk for pressure ulcers. A combination of approaches should be used in appraising risk.*

2. A risk-based prevention program for pressure ulcers in the ICU should be based on each subscale of a risk assessment tool.
   A. True
   B. False

   ANSWER: A. *Each critically ill patient has a unique level and type of risk. Each subscale should be addressed separately with appropriate interventions.*

REFERENCES: INTENSIVE CARE POPULATION

1. VanGilder, C., Amlung, S., Harrison, P., and Meyer, S. "Results of the 2008 - 2009 International Pressure Ulcer Prevalence Survey and a 3-Year, Acute-care, Unit-specific Analysis," *Ostomy Wound Management* 55(11):39-45, 2009.
2. Curley, M.A., et al. "Predicting Pressure Ulcer Risk in Pediatric Patients: The Braden Q Scale," *Nursing Research* 51(1): 22-33, January-February 2003.
3. Willock, J., et al. "Pressure Sores in Children—the Acute Hospital Perspective," *Journal of Tissue Viability* 10(2):59-62, April 2000.
4. Schmidt, J.E., et al. "Skin Breakdown in Children and High Frequency Oscillatory Ventilation," *Archives of Physical Medicine and Rehabilitation* 79:1565-69, 1998.
5. Braden, B.J., and Bergstrom, N.A. "Clinical Utility of the Braden Scale for Predicting Pressure Sore Risk," *Decubitus* 2(3):44-51, July-August1989.
6. Norton, D., et al. *An Investigation of Geriatric Nursing Problems in Hospital.* London: National Corporation for the Care of Old People, 1992.
7. Waterlow, J. "Pressure Sores: A risk Assessment Card," *Nursing Times* 81(48):49-55, 1985.
8. Jackson, C. "The Revised Jackson/Cubbin Pressure Area Risk Calculator," *Intensive Critical Care Nursing* 15(3):169-75, June 1999.

9. Kim, E., Lee, S., Lee, E., and Eom, M. "Comparison of the Predictive Validity Among Pressure Ulcer Risk Assessment Scales for Surgical ICU Patients," *Australian Journal of Advanced Nursing* 26(4):87, 2009.

10. Kosmidis, D., and Koutsouki, S. "Pressure Ulcer Risk Assessment Scales in ICU Patients: Validity Comparison of Jackson/Cubbin (Revised) and Braden Scales [Greek]," *Nosileftiki* 47(1), 86-95, 2008.

11. Quigley, S.M, and Curley, M.A.Q. "Skin Integrity in the Pediatric Population: Preventing and Managing Pressure Ulcers," *Journal for Specialists in Pediatric Nursing* 1(1):7-18, 1996.

12. Fife, C., et al. "Incidence of Pressure Ulcers in a Neurologic Critical Care Unit," *Critical Care Medicine* 29(2):283-90, February 2001.

13. Lewicki, L.J., et al. "Sensitivity and Specificity of the Braden Scale in the Cardiac Surgical Population," *Journal of Wound Ostomy Continence Nursing* 27(1):36-41, January 2000.

14. Theaker, C., et al. "Risk Factors for Pressure Sores in the Critically Ill," *Anesthesia* 55(3):221-24, March 2000.

15. Kaitani, T., Tokunagak, K., et al. "Risk Factors Related to Development of Pressure Ulcers in the Critical Care Setting," *Journal of Clinical Nursing* 19(3-4):414-21, 2010.

16. Eachempati, S.R., et al. "Factors Influencing the Development of Decubitus Ulcers in Critically Ill Surgical Patients," *Critical Care Medicine* 29(9):1678-82, September 2001.

17. Yepes, D., Molina, F., Leon, W., and Perez, E. "Incidence and Risk Factors Associated with the Presence of Pressure Ulcers in Critically Ill Patients," *Medicina Intensiva* 33(6):276, 2009.

18. Terekeci, H., Kucukardali, T., et al. "Risk Assessment Study of Pressure Ulcers in Intensive Care Unit Patients," *European Journal of Internal Medicine* 20(4):394-97, 2009.

19. Sayar, S., Turgut, S., Dogan, H., et al. "Incidence of Pressure Ulcers in Intensive Care Unit Patients at Risk According to the Waterlow Scale and Factors Influenceing development of Pressure Ulcers," *Journal of Clinical Nursing* 18(5):65-774, 2009.

20. Batson, S., et al. "The Development of a Pressure Area Scoring System for Critically Ill Patients: A Pilot Study," *Intensive Critical Care Nursing* 9(3):146-51, September 1993.

21. Boyle, M., Green, M. "Pressure Sores in Intensive Care: Defining Their Incidence and Associated Factors and Assessing the Utility of Two Pressure Sore Risk Assessment Tools," *Australian Critical Care* 14(1):24-30, 2001.

22. Nijs, N., Toppets, A., Defloor, T., Bernaerts, K., and Milisen, K. "Incidence and Risk Factors

for Pressure Ulcers in the Intensive Care Unit." *Journal of Clinical Nursing* 18(9):1258-66, 2009.

23. Inman, K.J., et al. "Clinical Utility and Cost-effectiveness of an Air Suspension Bed in the Prevention of Pressure Ulcers," *Journal of the American Medical Association* 269(9):1139-43, March 3, 1993.

24. Jiricka, M.K., et al. "Pressure Ulcer Risk Factors in a Critical Care Unit Population," *American Journal of Critical Care* 4(5):361-67, September 1995.

25. Lowery, M.T. "A Pressure Sore Risk Calculator for Critical Care Patients: 'The Sunderland Experience'," *Intensive Critical Care Nursing* 11(6):344-53, December 1995.

26. Weststrate, J.T., et al. "The Clinical Relevance of the Waterlow Pressure Sore Risk Scale in the Critical Care Unit," *Critical Care Medicine* 24(8):815-20, August 1998.

27. Compton, F., et al., "Pressure Ulcer Predictors in ICU Patients: Nursing Skin Assessment Versus Objective Parameters," *Journal of Wound Care* 17(10):417, 2008.

28. Eun-Kyung, K., Sun-Mi, L., Eunpyo, L., and Mi-Ran, E. "Comparison of the Predictive Validity Among Pressure Ulcer Risk Assessment Scales for Surgical ICU Patients," *Australian Journal of Advanced Nursing* 26(4):87-94, 2009.

29. Seongsook, J., et al. "Validity of Pressure Ulcer Risk Assessment Scales; Cubbin and Jackson, Braden and Douglas Scale," *International Journal of Nursing Studies* 41(2):199-204, February 2004.

30. Carlson, E.V., et al. "Predicting the Risk of Pressure Ulcers in Critically Ill Patients," *American Journal of Critical Care* 8(4):262-69, July 1999.

31. deLaat, E.H.E.W., et al. "Epidemiology, Risk and Prevention of Pressure Ulcers in Critically Ill Patients: A Literature Review," *Journal of Wound Care* 15(6):269-75, June 2006.

32. National Pressure Ulcer Advisory Panel and European Pressure Ulcer Advisory Panel. *Prevention and Treatment of Pressure Ulcers: Clinical Practice Guideline*. Washington, DC: National Pressure Ulcer Advisory Panel, 2009.

33. Krishnagopalan, S., Johnson, E.W., Low, L.L., and Kaufman, L.J. "Body Positioning of Intensive Care Patients: Clinical Practice versus Standards," *Critical Care Medicine* 30(11): 2588-92, 2002.

34. Oertwich, P.A., et al. "The Effects of Small Shifts in Body Weight on Blood Flow and Interface Pressure," *Research in Nursing & Health* 18(6): 481-88, December 1995.

35. Kress, J. P. "Clinical Trials of Early Mobilization of Critically Ill Patients," *Critical Care Medicine* 37(10 Suppl), S442-47, 2009.

36. Black, J.M., Cuddigan, J.E. Walko, M.A., Didier, L. A., Lander, M.J., Kelpe, M.R. "Medical Device

Related Pressure Ulcers in Hospitalized Patients," *International Wound Journal* 7(5):358-65, 2010.

37. Hibbert, C.L., et al. "Cost Considerations for the Use of Low-air-loss Bed Therapy in Adult Critical Care," *Intensive Critical Care Nursing* 15(3):154-62, June 1999.

38. Inman, K.J., et al. "Pressure Ulcer Prevention: A Randomized Controlled Trial of Two Risk-directed Strategies for Patient Surface Assignment," *Advances in Wound Care* 12(2):72-80, March 1999.

39. Jastremski, C.A. "Pressure Relief Bedding to Prevent Pressure Ulcer Development in Critical Care," *Journal of Critical Care* 17(2):122-25, June 2002.

40. Cullum, N., et al. "Beds, Mattresses and Cushions for Pressure Sore Prevention and Treatment," (Cochrane Review). In: *The Cochrane Library,* Issue 1. Chichester, UK: John Wiley & Sons, Ltd., 2004.

41. Reddy, M., et al. "Preventing Pressure Ulcers: A Systematic Review," *Journal of the American Medical Association* 296(8):974-84, August 23-30, 2006.

42. Burdette-Taylor, S.R., and Kass, J. "Heel Ulcers in Critical Care Units: A Major Pressure Problem," *Critical Care Nursing Quarterly* 25(2):41-53, August 2002.

43. Cadue, J.-F., Karolewicz, S, Tardy, C., Barrault, C., Robert, R., and Pourrat, O. "Prevention of Heel Pressure Sores with a Foam Body-support Device. A Randomized Controlled Trial in a Medical Intensive Care Init [in French]." *Presse Mẽdicale* (Paris, France: 1983) 37(1 Pt 1):30-6, 2008.

44. Grap, M.J., and Munro, C.L. "Quality Improvement in Backrest Elevation: Improving Outcomes in Critical Care," *AACN Clinical Issues* 16(2): 133-39, 2005.

45. Defloor, T., and Grypdonck, M.H. "Do Pressure Relief Cushions Really Relieve Pressure?" *Western Journal of Nursing Research* 22(3):335-50, April 2000.

46. Defloor, T., and Grypdonck, M.H. "Sitting Posture and Prevention of Pressure Ulcers," *Applied Nursing Research* 12(3):136-42, August 1999.

47. Baharestani, M.M., Black, J., Carville, K., Clark, M., Cuddigan, J., Dealey, C., et al. *International Guidelines. Pressure Ulcer Prevention: Pressure, Shear, Friction and Microclimate in Context. A Consensus Document.* London: Wounds International, 2010.

48. Black, J.M., and the National Pressure Ulcer Advisory Panel. "Moving Toward Consensus on Deep Tissue Injury and Pressure Ulcer Staging," *Advances in Skin & Wound Care* 18(8):415-16, 418, 420-21, October 2005.

SPINAL CORD INJURY POPULATION

Susan L. Garber, MA, OTR, FAOTA, FACRM

SPINAL CORD INJURY INCIDENCE AND PREVALENCE

Approximately 262,000 persons are living with spinal cord injury (SCI) in the United States today, of whom 17% (42,000) are veterans[1]; 12,000 new SCI cases are reported every year.[2] The National Spinal Cord Injury Statistical Center provides statistics on five major categories of etiology:

- motor vehicle crashes (41.3%)
- falls (27.3%)
- acts of violence (15%)
- recreational sporting activities (7.9%)
- causes that don't fit into any of these categories (8.5%).[2]

SCI occurs most frequently in males ages 16 to 30 (55%).[2] The average age at injury today is 42 years, up from 29 years at the end of the 1970s. More than 80% of the patients in the National Spinal Cord Injury Statistical Center database are male.[2] Among those injured since 1990, 66% are white, 27% are black, 8% are Hispanic, 2% are Asian, 0.4% are American Indian, 0.5% are of unknown ethnicity, and 2.5% are unclassified.[2] Almost half of the SCI population had completed high school at the time of injury. Given the young age at onset of injury, more than half were single. Although most were employed at the time of injury, more than 14% are unemployed following SCI.[2]

People with an SCI are at risk for a number of complications. For instance, pulmonary complications are the most common cause of death during both the acute and chronic phases after SCI.[3] Other potential complications arising soon after injury—some of which may become lifelong problems—include pressure ulcers, urinary tract infections (UTIs), osteoporosis, fractures, and heterotopic ossification.

Pressure ulcers are among the most common long-term secondary medical complications observed at annual follow-up visits.[4] As such, they are a serious, costly, and potentially life-threatening complication of SCI. Clinical observations and research studies have confirmed staggering costs and human suffering, including a profoundly negative impact on the patient's general physical health, socialization, financial status, and body image, compounded by a loss of independence and control.[5]

Reliable and current data on the incidence and prevalence of pressure ulcers in the patient with an SCI have been difficult to obtain, primarily because limitations in the data collection methods used limit or prevent standardization of the statistics. These limitations include the use of different classification systems to stage pressure ulcers, the inability to compare varied populations (for example, acute or chronic SCI) presenting with or developing pressure ulcers, and the use of different methods of obtaining data, such as direct observation or retrospective chart review.[6]

SCOPE OF THE PROBLEM

The database of the Spinal Cord Injury Model Systems is one of the most reliable resources from which to obtain data that reflect the scope of the problem. The National Institute on Disability and Rehabilitation Research[7] sponsors the Model Systems Program, a federal extramural grant program of selected research and demonstration sites. Model System sites provide exemplary, state-of-the-art care from the time of injury through acute medical care, comprehensive rehabilitation, and long-term follow-up and health maintenance services. An individual is included in the database only if he or she was admitted to a system facility within 24 hours of trauma. The Model System database has included statistics on pressure ulcers in patients with SCI since 1981.[8]

According to the 1998 National Spinal Cord Injury Statistical Center Annual Report, 34% of patients admitted to a Model System facility within 24 hours of an SCI developed at least one pressure ulcer during acute care or rehabilitation,[9] with pressure ulcer prevalence increasing over time following injury. On follow-up, 15% had a pressure ulcer at their first annual examination, 20% at year 5, 23% at year 10, 24% at year 15, and 29% at year 20. These numbers are based on 4,065 patients, 2,971 of whom developed pressure ulcers. In 2005, Chen and colleagues[10] reported that 27% (910) of 3,361 patients from nine Spinal Cord Injury Model System facilities had one or more episodes of pressure ulcers of stage II or greater between 1986 and 2002. Other investigators have reported prevalence rates ranging from 17% to 33% in populations of SCI patients residing in the community.[8,11,12] The occurrence of pressure ulcers is among the most common long-term secondary medical complications identified during annual follow-up visits[13] in individuals with paraplegia (T1-S5, neurological level),[2] who are more likely to be rehospitalized for pressure ulcers.[14] Risk factors include complete injury (classified as A, B, or C by the

American Spinal Injury Association (ASIA) impairment scale

A—Complete: No motor or sensory function is preserved in the sacral segments S4-5.

B—Incomplete: Sensory but not motor function is preserved below the neurological level and includes the sacral segments S4-5.

C—Incomplete: Motor function is preserved below the neurological level, and more than half of key muscles below the neurological level have a muscle grade less than 3.

D—Incomplete: Motor function is preserved below the neurological level, and at least half of key muscles below the neurological level have a muscle grade of 3.

E—Normal: Motor and sensory functions are normal.

American Spinal Injury Association to denote complete vs. incomplete injury), tetraplegia, older age, comorbidities, and violent injury.[13] (See *American Spinal Injury Association [ASIA] Impairment Scale,* page 521.)

RECURRENCE RATE

High rates of pressure ulcer recurrence also have been reported, ranging from 21% to 79% regardless of treatment.[15,16] Epidemiological studies have found that 36% to 50% of all patients with SCI who develop pressure ulcers will develop a recurrence within the first year after initial healing.[11,12,16–18] Niazi and colleagues[16] reported a recurrence rate of 35% regardless of the type of treatment (medical or surgical) provided. Holmes et al.[19] found that 55% of their sample, most of whom had a history of severe previous ulcers, experienced a recurrence within 2 years after surgical repair. In a 20-year study in Canada (1976 to 1996), Schryvers and colleagues[15] studied 168 spinal cord injury patients admitted 415 times for treatment of 598 severe recurring pressure ulcers. Of these ulcer recurrences, 31% (185) occurred at the same site as the previous ulcer and 21% (125 ulcers) occurred at a different site. Goodman et al.[20] observed a recurrence or new ulcer development rate of 79% within a 1- to 6-year follow-up time frame.

Pressure ulcer history seems to be a more viable measure of pressure ulcer outcome than measures taken at any single point in time over a brief period. Other studies reveal the protective mechanisms against pressure ulcer recurrence. For example, Krause and Broderick[21] reported that 13% of their sample of 633 subjects had recurring pressure ulcers (one or more per year) over a 5-year period. Their findings suggested that lifestyle, exercise, and diet were protective mechanisms against pressure ulcer recurrence.

Pressure ulcer recurrence in the patient with an SCI has been associated with gender (male), age (older), ethnicity (black), unemployment, residence in a nursing home, and previous pressure ulcer surgery.[16,22,23] Most of the literature describing recurrence following surgery focuses on surgical techniques.[24–27] Investigators have reported recurrence rates of 11% to 29% in patients with postoperative complications and 6% to 61% in patients without postoperative complications.[23,28–30] Relander and Palmer[29] recommended that social factors be studied to determine the causes of pressure ulcer recurrence after surgical repair and suggested that patients who don't display the appropriate knowledge regarding pressure ulcer prevention should be counseled before consideration for surgery. Disa and colleagues[23] reported that high recurrence rates among patients with traumatic paraplegia were associated with substance abuse and the absence of an adequate social support system. They suggested developing more effective educational programs for both patients and caregivers.[23] In other studies, Mandrekas and Mastorakos,[30] Baek et al.,[31] and Rubayi et al.,[32] reported that inadequate patient education with regard to pressure ulcer prevention contributed to the recurrence rates.

Recurrence also is a significant problem for veterans with SCI. Guihan et al.[33] reported that the most significant predictors of pressure ulcer recurrence in veterans are race (being black), more comorbidities indicating a higher burden of illness, Salzburg PrU Risk Assessment Scale score (which measures 15 items associated with SCI, cardiovascular and pulmonary disease, albumin and hematocrit, and impaired cognition), and longer sitting time at discharge from the hospital following the treatment of a pressure ulcer.[33]

FINANCIAL CONCERNS

The financial burden of pressure ulcers is undoubtedly immense, although estimates of the cost of preventing and treating pressure ulcers in the patient with an SCI are not readily available. In 1994, Miller and DeLozier[34] reported that the total cost of treating stage II, III, and IV pressure ulcers in hospitals, nursing homes, and home care was approximately $1.335 billion per year. One could extrapolate from these data the financial implications of pressure ulcers for patients with SCI. However, the financial burden does not begin to reflect the personal and social costs experienced by patients and their families. These include loss of independence and self-esteem;

time away from work, school, or family; and, ultimately, diminished quality of life.

Throughout their lifetime, persons with SCI are at risk for the development of pressure ulcers.[6] Most of the reported costs deal with investigations of various treatment interventions, especially dressings.[35] In 2003, Garber and Rintala[36] reported that 39% (215 of 553) of the veterans on the SCI roster at the Michael E. DeBakey VA Medical Center in Houston were found to have visited the clinic or received home care for the treatment of pressure ulcers during the 3-year study period (1997-1999). Of these, 102 veterans' charts met the inclusion criteria for the study (complete data sets). A total of 625 visits were made to treat 400 pressure ulcers at a cost of $250 per outpatient visit (approximate costs from 1998; costs are higher now). Stage IV was the most prevalent pressure ulcer seen, and pelvic ulcers accounted for almost two-thirds of the worst ulcers reported. Most of the ulcers did not heal during the study period. The average number of clinic or home visits for pressure ulcer treatment was more than six per person. More than half of the study sample was admitted to the hospital for pressure ulcer treatment at least once during the study period. The average number of hospital admissions was two; almost 30% of veterans were admitted three times or more. Fifty-seven patients were hospitalized for pressure ulcer treatment, with an average number of hospitalization days for pressure ulcer treatment being 150 at $1,000 per day, not counting the cost of surgical intervention (which, at the time, could exceed $70,000).

Xakellis and Frantz[37] assessed pressure ulcer management from initial occurrence in long-term care through their natural history, including hospitalization for complications. Including hospital costs, the mean cost, reported in 1996, of treating each ulcer was $2,731 and the per-patient cost was $4,647. In this small study (30 patients), 80% of the total cost of pressure ulcer treatment was generated by the 4% of patients who required hospitalization. The mean length of stay for treatment was 116 days.[37] Javitz and colleagues[38] identified the following "cost drivers" in treating pressure ulcers: wound-care nursing time, time to turn or reposition patients, dressings,

pressure-reducing support surfaces for wheelchair and bed, antibiotics, room and doctor visits, surgical debridement, hospital admissions for medical and/or surgical treatment, and treatment of comorbid conditions.

RISK FACTORS

More than 200 risk factors for the development of pressure ulcers have been reported in the literature. Most of the risk factors were derived from studying elderly nursing home residents. However, many of the risk factors for these patients differ from those experienced by patients with SCI. Immobility increases the risk of pressure ulcer development in both populations. Unlike nursing home residents, however, patients with SCI are encouraged to oversee or direct their own daily care and are expected to take primary responsibility for pressure ulcer prevention. As a result of the limitations imposed by the variables among studies, the literature is often contradictory regarding the effects of a particular risk factor or set of factors potentially responsible for the development of pressure ulcers. Different populations (for example, acute or chronic SCI patients), inadequate sample sizes, different ways of standardizing the dependent measures, and poor or uncontrolled study designs all add confusion to the interpretation of study results.[39,40]

According to Chen et al.,[10] the risk of pressure ulcers seems to be steady in the first 10 years but increases 15 years post-injury. Males, the elderly, blacks, singles, individuals who have less than a high school education, the unemployed, persons with complete SCI, and those with a history of pressure ulcers, rehospitalization, nursing home stay, and other medical comorbidities are at greater risk of developing pressure ulcers.[10] Although the number of days hospitalized and frequency of rehospitalizations decreased, the number of pressure ulcers increased over time.[10] Charlifue and colleagues[41] found that although the number of pressure ulcers increased as time passed, the best predictor of pressure ulcers over time was a previous history of pressure ulcers.

Despite these limitations, a number of pressure ulcer risk factors specific to the patient with SCI have been identified and described in the literature. Byrne and Salzberg[39] summarized the major pressure ulcer risk factors for the patient with an SCI as follows:

- severity of the SCI (immobility, completeness of the injury, urinary incontinence, and severe spasticity)
- preexisting conditions (advanced age, smoking, lung and cardiac disease, diabetes and renal disease, and impaired cognition)
- residence in a nursing home
- malnutrition and anemia.

Characteristics associated with better pressure ulcer outcomes include maintaining normal weight, returning to work and family roles, and not smoking or having a history of tobacco use, suicidal behavior, incarceration, or alcohol or drug abuse.[42] The Consortium for Spinal Cord Medicine Clinical Practice Guideline ("Pressure Ulcer Prevention and Treatment Following Spinal Cord Injury")[6] categorized pressure ulcer risk factors in patients with SCI as follows:

- demographic factors (age, gender, ethnicity, marital status, and education)
- physical or medical and SCI-related factors (level and completeness of the injury; activity and mobility; bladder, bowel, and moisture control; and comorbidities, such as diabetes and spasticity)
- psychological and social factors (psychological distress, financial problems, cognition, substance abuse, adherence to recommended prevention behaviors/strategies, and health beliefs and practices).[6]

As far back as 1979, Anderson and Andberg[43] identified psychological factors associated with the development of pressure ulcers, including the patient's unwillingness to take responsibility for his or her skin care, low self-esteem, and dissatisfaction with life activities. Gordon and colleagues[44] also found poor social adjustment in the patient with an SCI and a pressure ulcer.

> **PRACTICE POINT**
>
> Innovative educational programs are needed to provide persons with SCI with information and the motivation necessary to regain control over their lives.

RISK-BASED PREVENTION

A person with an SCI is at risk for the development of pressure ulcers from the moment of injury. Prolonged immobilization during the hours and days immediately after injury significantly increases the risk. Pressure reduction strategies to protect vulnerable areas of the body should be implemented soon after emergency medical intervention and spinal stabilization.

> **PRACTICE POINT**
>
> Pressure ulcer development is a lifelong concern for the individual with an SCI.

Preventing pressure ulcers is a major component of both informal and formal educational sessions during rehabilitation of the SCI patient. A regimen of preventive strategies usually is developed for each patient and includes information and instructions that are given to patients and their families.[45] (See *Patient Teaching: Preventing pressure ulcers in SCI patients at home*.)

Printed materials or visual media (videotapes, CDs, DVDs) are used frequently to augment educational sessions, and some of these materials may be sent home with patients when they are discharged. Because most patient education programs are hospital-based, little is known about what information the patient retains, which behaviors or activities are practiced routinely, and the compatibility of the patient's lifestyle with prevention strategies. In the 1970s and 1980s, a number of SCI centers established comprehensive pressure ulcer prevention education programs.[46–48] Both inpatient and outpatient programs advocated multidisciplinary, coordinated, structured, and wide-ranging approaches to prevention. Some of these programs still serve as models for practice today.[49]

Several educational needs have been described recently. These include (rank-ordered by the authors of the study[50]):

- awareness of the lifelong risk for developing pressure ulcers (including the ability to assess personal risk factors and how risk changes over time)

Patient Teaching
Preventing Pressure Ulcers in SCI Patients at Home

Persons with SCI are at risk for developing pressure ulcers, especially after they leave your care. Teach patients and their families the following strategies to help them prevent pressure ulcers after they have returned home.

- Perform daily visual and tactile skin inspection.
- Maintain good personal hygiene.
- Turn and reposition often, and perform frequent weight shifts.
- Use appropriate and well-maintained support surfaces for the bed and wheelchair.
- Maintain adequate nutrition.
- Maintain a healthy lifestyle (avoid alcohol, tobacco, and illegal drugs).

- ability to take charge of personal skin care regimen and to partner with healthcare providers
- ability to perform prevention strategies consistently that are compatible with level of function and activity, and update practices as risk changes
- ability to coordinate social supports

Effective prevention education and early detection of pressure ulcers are critical.[50]

SKIN ASSESSMENT

The SCI patient with a pressure ulcer should undergo two assessment phases. The first phase is a comprehensive evaluation and examination, including:

- complete social and medical history
- physical examination
- laboratory tests
- assessment of psychological health, behavior, and cognitive status
- information on social and financial resources and the availability and utilization of personal care assistance
- assessment of positioning, posture, and related equipment
- assessment of lifestyle, including use of tobacco, past and present, and alcohol and drug use/abuse.[6]

The second phase of assessment consists of a detailed description of the pressure ulcer itself and the surrounding tissues, including the following factors:

- anatomical location and general appearance
- size (length, width, depth, and wound area)
- stage or severity
- exudate
- odor
- necrosis
- undermining
- sinus tracts
- infection
- granulation and epithelialization
- wound margins and surrounding tissue.[6]

Photographs can be useful in these assessments and in monitoring.

 PRACTICE POINT

Patients with darkly pigmented skin are particularly vulnerable to undetected pressure ulcers. Although areas of damaged skin appear darker than the surrounding skin, tactile information must be used in addition to visual data when assessing persons with darker skin. The skin may be taut and shiny, indurated, and warm to the touch. Color changes may range from purple to blue. Remember, pressure-damaged dark skin doesn't blanch when compressed.[51]

TREATMENT

Prevention and treatment are inextricably linked across the continuum of care for the person with a pressure ulcer.[52] During rehabilitation following an SCI, the patient is exposed to a great deal of information about the major physiological changes that have occurred as well as how to prevent or manage potential secondary complications, such as pressure ulcers and UTIs. Unfortunately, much of this information isn't absorbed during this early post-traumatic phase, resulting in episodes of potentially life-threatening conditions once the patient returns to his or her home and community. Coupled with non-retention of information is today's significant decrease in length of stay, which makes structured education sessions during hospitalization very limited at best or totally absent.

Nonsurgical treatment

The treatment of pressure ulcers is a complex process, based on a number of patient-related and pressure ulcer–related factors. Nonsurgical treatment for pressure ulcers consists of a number of sequential steps that become the treatment plan for that patient with his or her specific ulcer. The elements of a comprehensive treatment plan include cleaning, debriding, applying dressings, and assessing the need for (and appropriateness of) new technologies aimed at wound healing. Education, in the form of printed materials or discussions with healthcare professionals, is intended to prevent recurrence in the patient with a SCI. Enhanced, individualized pressure ulcer prevention and management education is effective in improving pressure ulcer knowledge during hospitalization for surgical repair of a pressure ulcer.[53,54] Furthermore, initial individualized preventive intervention combined with structured follow-up within a person's individual everyday life setting may reduce the risk of pressure ulcers in persons with SCI.[55]

Surgical treatment

Stage III and IV pressure ulcers are frequently treated surgically in patients with SCI. The goals of surgical closure include:

- preventing protein loss through the wound
- reducing the risk of progressive osteomyelitis and sepsis

- preventing renal failure
- reducing costly and lengthy hospitalization
- improving hygiene and appearance
- expediting time to healing.[6,56,57]

The surgical process includes:

- excision of the ulcer and surrounding scar, underlying bursa, soft-tissue calcification, and underlying necrotic or infected bone
- filling dead space with fascia or muscle flaps
- improving vascularity and distribution of pressure over bony prominences
- resurfacing the area with a large flap so that the suture line is away from areas of direct pressure
- providing a flap that leaves options for future surgeries.[56,57]

Preoperatively, the rehabilitation and surgical teams coordinate their efforts to control local wound infection, improve and maintain nutrition, regulate the bowels, control spasms and contractures, and address comorbid conditions. Previous pressure ulcer surgery, smoking, UTI, and heterotopic ossification could affect surgical outcomes.[6]

New surgical techniques to repair pressure ulcers have been developed and are being used to improve surgical outcomes. Although these techniques are being evaluated,[58–62] reports of long-term follow-up of the status of the skin and recurrence have been limited. One study by Lee[58] used a new wound closure technique and followed patients for 102 days, after which 18 of 21 (86%) wounds in 13 patients remained closed. Sorensen and colleagues[63] suggested that thorough preoperative debridement, patient compliance, control of comorbidities, professional postoperative support, and sufficient pressure relief are essential if surgical success is to be achieved.

Evidence-Based Practice

Post-surgical care includes keeping the surgical site pressure-free, using specialty beds to maximize pressure reduction, mobilizing the patient progressively, and providing patient and family education.[6]

Support surfaces

Support surfaces are devices or systems intended to reduce the interface pressure between a patient and his or her bed or wheelchair.[52] Support surfaces don't heal pressure ulcers; rather, they are prescribed by a clinician and incorporated into a comprehensive pressure ulcer prevention and management program. Pressure redistribution products, such as static or dynamic mattresses, mattress overlays, or specialty beds, may be used at various times to reduce the patient's risk of developing pressure ulcers. Materials such as foams and gels, used alone or in combination, and elements such as air and water, also used alone or in combination, are being used across inpatient and home environments. Wheelchair cushions and seating systems of various materials and designs are intended to reduce pressure and maximize balance and stability when a patient is in a wheelchair. (For further discussion on support surfaces, see chapter 11, Pressure redistribution: Seating, positioning, and support surfaces.)

Adverse effects of pressure on tissue are a major source of morbidity and mortality in persons with SCI.[6] Issues surrounding wheelchair sitting and associated seating devices have been studied extensively and therapeutic strategies developed to minimize pressure on the skin, especially in anatomical areas overlying bony prominences.[64–66] These efforts have led to major improvements in the technology of seating support and pressure-reducing devices such as wheelchair cushions and in mattresses for the supine patient.

Another area remains as yet uninvestigated, namely the adverse effects of pressure exerted while sitting on a commode chair during bowel care procedures necessary for persons with SCI. Chronic constipation, difficulty in evacuation, incontinence, and damage to mucosa are all complications associated with neurogenic bowel in persons with SCI. One attempt to deal with the adverse effects of pressure during bowel management programs is the padded commode seat. This has led to some success in safety and in reducing the risk of pressure ulcers during the bowel management procedures.[67–71] Rates of rehospitalization following SCI remain high and result from complications in the genitourinary system, respiratory complications, and pressure ulcers.[14] Unfortunately, very little data exist on the specific nature of pressure ulcer development in association with bowel care sitting time or process. Research is needed on an equally relevant therapeutic approach that would focus on duration of sitting time during each evacuation attempt.

New interventions

A number of adjunctive therapies have been reported in the literature with varying degrees of success in treating pressure ulcers in the patient with a SCI, including:

- electrical stimulation
- ultraviolet and laser therapy
- normothermia
- hyperbaric oxygen and ultrasound
- negative-pressure wound therapy
- nonantibiotic drugs
- topical agents
- skin equivalents
- growth factors.

Among these, only electrical stimulation has enough reported scientific evidence supporting it to justify its use as a treatment for pressure ulcers in the patient with a SCI.[72,73]

SUMMARY

Although SCI research has increased tremendously in recent years, designing and conducting randomized, controlled trials that are capable of producing compelling observational evidence on which to base management of pressure ulcers have been disappointing. Despite advances in pressure ulcer treatment, little scientific evidence points the way to preventing pressure ulcers in the SCI population. Randomized, controlled trials in real-world settings are the gold standard for assessing the effectiveness of prevention and treatment strategies. However, in complex, rapidly changing healthcare settings, blinding is infeasible and it may be impractical to control for every variable that influences a study's outcome. Furthermore, any assumptions that usual care is static are probably mistaken. Innovative approaches to maintain the integrity of the study design must be used, including flexibility in inclusion and exclusion criteria to support accrual, obtaining a better understanding of the important aspects of usual care that may need to be standardized, continuous improvement within the intervention arm, and anticipation and minimization of risks from organizational changes.[33] Research efforts should focus on prospective studies to prevent recurrence that include long-term follow-up programs promoting self-management.

PATIENT SCENARIO: SPINAL CORD INJURY POPULATION

Clinical Data

Mr. K is a 36-year-old black man who sustained a complete SCI at the T8 level from a motor vehicle crash 4 years ago that resulted in paraplegia. He lives independently, is unmarried and unemployed, and has a history of hypertension. During his rehabilitation hospitalization, Mr. K was told about pressure ulcers and things he could do to prevent them. However, within 1 year after discharge, he developed a stage III right ischial pressure ulcer for which he was hospitalized for surgical repair. The surgery resulted in a healed ulcer, and Mr. K. was discharged. Although pressure ulcer prevention was reviewed during this hospitalization, he returned home and resumed previous habits, including sitting in front of the television for long hours, driving around with friends, not eating well, and smoking. Less than a year after the first surgery, Mr. K developed a stage IV pressure ulcer with osteomyelitis on his left ischium. He was readmitted to the hospital for the surgical repair of this ulcer. Compounding Mr. K's pressure ulcer history are the following: he does not have a support system to help and encourage him to be more proactive in preventing pressure ulcers; he seems depressed and unable to take control of his physical health; he would like to return to work as a computer programmer but has not put much effort into looking for a job; he often does not take his prescribed medication for hypertension; and he smokes and sometimes uses alcohol and illegal drugs.

Case Discussion

The first priority is to treat the infection (osteomyelitis) and surgically repair the ulcer. During this hospitalization, a case manager was assigned to coordinate discharge and follow-up plans. The case manager requested that an occupational therapist knowledgeable about SCIs and pressure ulcers work with Mr. K to develop strategies to prevent future pressure ulcers, take control of the things he can control, identify appropriate support systems within the community and the healthcare system, and improve his quality of life. The occupational therapist worked with Mr. K to develop a pressure ulcer prevention plan that was acceptable and appropriate to Mr. K's lifestyle. Relevant actions and behaviors were included in a written plan so Mr. K could refer to it daily. These included weight shifts and turns, skin checks (with special attention to the changes in his darkly pigmented skin), nutrition, hygiene, limiting sitting in one place for long periods of time, limiting smoking and drinking, and not using drugs. Additionally, the occupational therapist performed a complete assessment of Mr. K's wheelchair and support surfaces used in the bed and wheelchair. His wheelchair and wheelchair cushion were in very poor condition. A new wheelchair was ordered and a pressure evaluation performed to identify the most effective wheelchair cushion for him.

Mr. K was instructed on the routine care of his new equipment (wheelchair and cushion), especially with regard to changes in his skin that might reflect the deterioration of the support surfaces. He was reevaluated for management of his hypertension, and a new medication regimen was designed. A home visit by the occupational therapist identified ways to minimally adapt Mr. K.'s home environment to maximize his independence and safety. He was referred to a psychologist for counseling that seemed to result in better insight into his behaviors and lifestyle. Finally, Mr. K. was given a list of resources he could contact with problems, including the case manager, equipment vendor, physician, and clinics. He also was given information on how to seek employment.

SHOW WHAT YOU KNOW—SPINAL CORD INJURY POPULATION

1. All of the following are major risk factors for pressure ulcer development in the SCI population except:
   A. preexisting conditions.
   B. severity of the SCI.
   C. gender.
   D. nutrition.

   ANSWER: C. *Although more males have SCI, gender isn't a major risk factor for pressure ulcer development. Preexisting conditions, severity of the SCI, and nutrition are all major risk factors for pressure ulcer development.*

2. The most commonly occurring complication of an SCI is:
   A. fracture.
   B. urinary tract infection.
   C. pressure ulcer development.
   D. osteoporosis.

   ANSWER: B. *Urinary tract infection is the most commonly occurring complication of an SCI. Pressure ulcer development is second. Fractures and osteoporosis are also other complications that may occur.*

REFERENCES: SPINAL CORD INJURY POPULATION

1. Weaver, F.M. "Spinal Cord Injury QUERI Center Strategic Plan," Hines, IL: Edward Hines Jr. VA Hospital, December 2009; Available at http://www.queri.research.va.gov/about/strategic_plans/sci-strategic-plan.pdf. Accessed January 19, 2011.

2. National Spinal Cord Injury Statistical Center. "Spinal Cord Injury: Facts and Figures at a Glance." Birmingham, AL: Author, February 2010. Available at https://www.nscisc.uab.edu/public_content/pdf/Facts%20and%20Figures%20at%20a%20Glance%202010.pdf. Accessed January 19, 2011.

3. Ragnarsson, K.T., et al. "Management of Pulmonary, Cardiovascular, and Metabolic Conditions after Spinal Cord Injury," in Stover, S.L., et al. (eds.), *Spinal Cord Injury: Clinical Outcomes from the Model Systems.* Gaithersburg, MD: Aspen Publishers, Inc., 1995.

4. McKinley, W.O., et al. "Long-term Medical Complications after Traumatic Spinal Cord Injury: A Regional Model Systems Analysis," *Archives of Physical Medicine Rehabilitation* 80(11):1402-10, November 1999.

5. Langemo, D.K., et al. "The Lived Experience of Having a Pressure Ulcer: A Qualitative Analysis," *Advances in Skin & Wound Care* 13(5):225-35, September-October 2000.

6. Garber S.L., et al. *Pressure Ulcer Prevention and Treatment Following Spinal Cord Injury: A Clinical Practice Guideline for Health-care Professionals, Consortium for Spinal Cord Medicine Clinical Practice Guidelines.* Washington, DC: Paralyzed Veterans of America, 2000.

7. The National Institute on Disability and Rehabilitation Research. Available at www2.ed.gov/legislation/FedRegister/announcements/2006-1/022706b.pdf. Accessed June 22, 2010.

8. Young, J.S., and Burns, P.E. "Pressure Sores and the Spinal Cord Injured: Part II," *Spinal Cord Injury Digest* 3:11-26, 48, 1981.

9. Yarkony, G.M., and Heinemann, A.W. "Pressure Ulcers," in Stover, S.L., et al. (eds.), *Spinal Cord Injury: Clinical Outcomes from the Model Systems.* Gaithersburg, MD: Aspen Publishers, 1995.

10. Chen, Y., DeVivo, M.J., Jackson, A.B. "Pressure Ulcer Prevalence in People with Spinal Cord Injury: Age-period-duration Effects." *Archives of Physical Medicine and Rehabilitation* 86:1208-13, 2005.

11. Fuhrer, M.J., et al. "Pressure Ulcers in Community-resident Persons with Spinal Cord Injury: Prevalence and Risk Factors," *Archives of Physical Medicine and Rehabilitation* 74(11):1172-77, November 1993.

12. Carlson, C.E., et al. "Incidence and Correlates of Pressure Ulcer Development after Spinal Cord

Injury," *Journal of Rehabilitation Nursing Research* 1(1):34-40, 1992.

13. McKinley, W.O., Jackson, A.B., Cardenas, D.D., DeVivo, M.J. "Long-term Medical Complications after Traumatic Spinal Cord Injury: A Regional Model Systems Analysis," *Archives of Physical Medicine and Rehabilitation* 80:1402-10, 1999.

14. Cardenas, D.D., Hoffman, J.M., Kirshblum, S., McKinley, W. "Etiology and Incidence of Rehospitalization after Traumatic Spinal Cord Injury: A Multicenter Analysis," *Archives of Physical Medicine and Rehabilitation* 85:1757-63, 2004.

15. Schryvers, O.I., et al. "Surgical Treatment of Pressure Ulcers: A 20-year Experience," *Archives of Physical Medicine and Rehabilitation* 81(12): 1556-1562, December 2000.

16. Niazi, Z.B., et al. "Recurrence of Initial Pressure Ulcer in Persons with Spinal Cord Injuries," *Advances in Wound Care* 10(3):38-42, May-June 1997.

17. Goldstein, B. "Neurogenic Skin and Pressure Ulcers," in Hammond, M.C. (ed.), *Medical Care of Persons with Spinal Cord Injury*. Washington, DC: DVA Employee Education System and Government Printing Office, 1998.

18. Salzberg, C.A., et al. "Predicting and Preventing Pressure Ulcers in Adults with Paralysis," *Advances in Wound Care* 11(5):237-46, September 1998.

19. Holmes, S.A., et al. "Prevention of Recurrent Pressure Ulcers after Myocutaneous Flap," *Journal of Spinal Cord Medicine* 25:S23, 2002.

20. Goodman, C.M., et al. "Evaluation of Results and Treatment Variables for Pressure Ulcers in 48 Veteran Spinal Cord-injured Patients," *Annals of Plastic Surgery* 43(6):572-74, June 1999.

21. Krause, J.S., Broderick, L. "Patterns of Recurrent Pressure Ulcers after Spinal Cord Injury: Identification of Risk and Protective Factors 5 or More Years after Onset," *Archives of Physical Medicine and Rehabilitation* 85:1257-64, 2004.

22. Yasenchak, P.A., et al. "Variables Related to Severe Pressure Sore Recurrence," [Abstract]. Orlando, FL: Annual Meeting of the American Spinal Injury Association (ASIA), 1990.

23. Disa, J.J., et al. "Efficacy of Operative Cure in Pressure Sore Patients," *Plastic and Reconstructive Surgery* 89(2):272-78, February 1992.

24. Scheflan, M. "Surgical Methods for Managing Ischial Pressure Wounds," *Annals of Plastic Surgery* 3(3):238-47, March 1982.

25. Romm, S., et al. "Pressure Sores: State of the Art," *Texas Medicine* 78(4):52-60, 62, April 1982.

26. Pers, M. "Plastic Surgery for Pressure Sores," *Paraplegia* 25(3):275-78, June 1987.

27. Buntine, J.A., and Johnstone, B.R. "The Contributions of Plastic Surgery to Care of the Spinal Cord Injured Patient," *Paraplegia* 26(2): 87-93, April 1988.

28. Hentz, V.R. "Management of Pressure Sores in a Specialty Center—A Reappraisal," *Plastic and Reconstructive Surgery* 64(4):683-91, October 1979.

29. Relander, M., and Palmer, B. "Recurrence of Surgically Treated Pressure Sores," *Scandinavian Journal of Plastic Reconstructive Surgery* 2(1): 89-92, 1988.

30. Mandrekas, A.D., and Mastorakos, D.P. "Management of Decubitus Ulcers by Musculocutaneous Flaps: A Five-year Experience," *Annals of Plastic Surgery* 28(2):167-74, February 1992.

31. Baek, S., et al. "The Gluteus Maximus Myocutaneous Flap in the Management of Pressure Sores," *Annals of Plastic Surgery* 5(6): 471-76, December 1980.

32. Rubayi, S., et al. "Proximal Femoral Resection and Myocutaneous Flap for Treatment of Pressure Ulcers in Spinal Cord Injury Patients," *Annals of Plastic Surgery* 27(2):132-37, August 1991.

33. Guihan, M., Garber, S.L., Bombardier, C.H., Durazo-Arizu, R., Goldstein, B., Holmes, S.A. "Lessons Learned While Conducting Research on Prevention of Pressure Ulcers in Veterans with Spinal Cord Injury," *Archives of Physical Medicine and Rehabilitation* 88:858-61, 2007.

34. Miller, H., and DeLozier, J. "Cost Implications," in Bergstrom, N., and Cuddigan, J. (eds.), *Treating Pressure Ulcers: Guideline Technical Report*, Vol II, No. 15, Rockville, MD: US Department of Health and Human Services, Public Health Service, Agency for Health Care Policy and Research. Publication 96-N015, 1994.

35. Kerstein, M.D. "Unexpected Economics of Ulcer Care Protocols," *Southern Medical Journal* 97:135-6, 2004.

36. Garber, S.L., Rintala, D.H. "Pressure Ulcers in Veterans with Spinal Cord Injury: A Retrospective Study," *Journal of Rehabilitation Research and Development* 40:433-442, 2003.

37. Xakellis, G.C., Frantz, R. "The Cost of Healing Pressure Ulcers across Multiple Health Care Settings," *Advances in Wound Care* 9:18-22, 1996.

38. Javitz, H.S., Ward, M.M., Martens, L. "Major Costs Associated with Pressure Sores," *Journal of Wound Care* 7:286-90, 1998.

39. Byrne, D.W., and Salzberg, C.A. "Major Risk Factors for Pressure Ulcers in the Spinal Cord Disabled: A Literature Review," *Spinal Cord* 34(5):255-63, May 1996.

40. Rintala, D.H. "Quality-of-life Considerations," *Advances in Wound Care* 8(4):71-83, July-August 1995.

41. Charlifue, S., Lammertise, D.P., Adkins, R.H. "Aging with Spinal Cord Injury: Changes in Selected Health Indices and Life Satisfaction," *Archives of Physical Medicine and Rehabilitation* 85:1848-53, 2004.

42. Krause, J.S., Vines, C.L., Farley, T.L., Sniezek, J., Coker, J. "An Exploratory Study of Pressure Ulcers after Spinal Cord Injury: Relationship to Protective Behaviors and Risk Factors," *Archives of Physical Medicine and Rehabilitation* 82:107-13, 2001.

43. Anderson, T.P., and Andberg, M.M. "Psychosocial Factors Associated with Pressure Sores," *Archives of Physical Medicine and Rehabilitation* 60(8): 341-46, August 1979.

44. Gordon, W.A., et al. "The Relationship between Pressure Sores and Psychosocial Adjustment in Persons with Spinal Cord Injury," *Rehabilitation Psychology* 27:185-91, 1982.

45. Garber, S.L., et al. "A Structured Educational Model to Improve Pressure Ulcer Prevention Knowledge in Veterans with Spinal Cord Dysfunction," *Journal of Rehabilitation Research and Development* 39(5):575-88, September-October 2002.

46. Andberg, M.M., et al. "Improving Skin Care through Patient and Family Training," *Topics in Clinical Nursing* 5(2):45-54, July 1983.

47. Krouskop, T.A., et al. "The Effectiveness of Preventive Management in Reducing the Occurrence of Pressure Sores," *Journal of Rehabilitation Research and Development* 20(1):7483, July 1983.

48. King, R.B., et al., eds. "The Skin," in *Rehabilitation Guide*. Chicago, IL: The Rehabilitation Institute of Chicago, 1977.

49. Bergstrom, N., et al. *Pressure Ulcers in Adults: Prediction and Prevention*, Guideline Report No. 3. Rockville, MD: US Department of Health and Human Services, Public Health Service, Agency for Health Care Policy and Research. AHCPR Publication No. 93-0013, May 1992.

50. Schubart, J.R., Hilgart, M., Lyder, C. "Pressure Ulcer Prevention and Management in Spinal Cord-injured Adults: An Analysis of Educational Needs," *Advances in Skin & Wound Care* 21:322-9, 2008.

51. Bennett, M.A. "Report of the Task Force on the Implications for Darkly Pigmented Intact Skin in the Prediction and Prevention of Pressure Ulcers," *Advances in Wound Care* 8(6):34-35, November-December 1995.

52. Bergstrom, N., et al. *Treatment of Pressure Ulcers,* Guideline Report No. 15. Rockville, MD: US Department of Health and Human Services, Public Health Service, Agency for Health Care Policy and Research. AHCPR Publication No. 96-N014, December 1994.

53. Garber, S.L., Rintala, D.H., Holmes, S.A., Rodriguez, G.P., Friedman, J. "A Structured Educational Model to Improve Pressure Ulcer Prevention Knowldege in Veterans with Spinal Cord Dysfunction," *Journal of Rehabilitation Research and Development* 39:575-88, 2002.

54. Rintala, D.H., Garber, S.L., Friedman, J.D., Holmes, S.A. "Preventing Recurrent Pressure Ulcers in Veterans with Spinal Cord Injury: Impact of a Structured Education and Follow-up Intervention," *Archives of Physical Medicine and Rehabilitation* 89:1429-41, 2008.

55. Dunn, C.A., Carlson, M., Jackson, J.M., Clark, F.A. "Response Factors Surrounding Progression of Pressure Ulcers in Community-residing Adults with Spinal Cord Injury," *American Journal of Occupational Therapy* 63:301-9, 2009.

56. Netscher, D., et al. "Surgical Repair of Pressure Ulcers," *Plastic Surgery Nursing* 16:225-33, 239, Winter 1996.

57. Clamon, J., and Netscher, D.T. "General Principles of Flap Reconstruction: Goals for Aesthetic and Functional Outcome," *Plastic Surgery Nursing* 14:9-14, Spring 1994.

58. Lee, E.T. "A New Wound Closure Achieving and Maintaining Device Using Serial Tightening of Loop Suture and Its Clinical Applications in 15 Consecutive Patients for Up to 102 Days," *Annals of Plastic Surgery* 53(5):436-41, 2004.

59. Akyurek, M., et al. "A New Flap Design: Neural-island Flap," *Plastic and Reconstructive Surgery* 114(6):1467-77, 2004.

60. Ichioka, S., et al. "Triple Coverage of Ischial Ulcers with Adipofascial Turnover and Fasciocutaneous Flaps," *Plastic and Reconstructive Surgery* 14(4): 901-5, 2004.

61. Ichioka, S., et al. "Regenerative Surgery for Sacral Pressure Ulcers Using Collagen Matrix Substitute Dermis (Artificial Dermis)," *Annals of Plastic Surgery* 54(4):383-89, 2003.

62. Lin, M.T., et al. "Tensor Fasciae Latae Combined with Tangentially Split Vastus Lateralis Musculocutaneous Flap for the Reconstruction of Pressure Sores," *Annals of Plastic Surgery* 53(4): 343-47, October 2004.

63. Sorensen, J.L., et al. "Surgical Treatment of Pressure Ulcers," *American Journal of Surgery* 188(suppl 1A):42-51, 2004.

64. Garber, S.L. "Wheelchair Cushions: A Historical Review," *American Journal of Occupational Therapy* 39:453-59, 1985.

65. Garber, S.L. "Wheelchair Cushions for Spinal Cord-injured Individuals," *American Journal of Occupational Therapy* 39:722-5, 1985.

66. Garber, S.L., Dyerly, L.R. "Wheelchair Cushions for Persons with Spinal Cord Injury: An Update," *American Journal of Occupational Therapy* 45:550-4, 1991.

67. Malassigne, P., Nelson, A., et al. "Toward the Design of a New Bowel Care Chair for the Spinal Cord Injured: A Pilot Study," *SCI Nursing* 10: 84-90, 1993.

68. Malassigne, P., Nelson, A.L., et al. "Design of the Advanced Commode-shower Chair for Spinal Cord-injured Individuals," *Journal of Rehabilitation Research and Development* 37: 373-82, 2000.

69. Nelson, A., Malassigne, P., et al. "Promoting Safe Use of Equipment for Neurogenic Bowel Management," *SCI Nursing* 17:119-24, 2000.

70. Nelson, A.L., Malassigne, P., Murray, J. "Comparison of Seat Pressures on Three Bowel Care/Shower Chairs in Spinal Cord Injury," *SCI Nursing* 11:105-7, 1994.

71. Nelson, A., Malassigne, P., et al. "Descriptive Study of Bowel Care Practices and Equipment in Spinal Cord Injury," *SCI Nursing* 10:65-7, 1993.

72. Baker, L., et al. "Effect of Electrical Stimulation Waveform on Healing of Ulcers in Human Beings with Spinal Cord Injury," *Wound Repair and Regeneration* 4(1):21-28, January-February 1996.

73. Wood, J.M., et al. "A Multicenter Study on the Use of Pulsed Low-intensity Direct Current for Healing Chronic Stage II and III Decubitus Ulcers," *Archives of Dermatology* 129(8):999-1009, August 1993.

HIV/AIDS POPULATION

Carl A. Kirton, DNP, RN, ANP-BC, ACRN

SKIN ALTERATION IN HIV AND AIDS PATIENTS

More than 90% of HIV-infected patients will develop at least one type of dermatologic disorder during the course of their HIV infection.[1] In fact, in the early 1980s it was the identification of an unusual skin lesion in young homosexual men that prompted the search for the virus that causes AIDS. A broad range of infectious and noninfectious skin lesions may develop during both the asymptomatic and symptomatic course of the disease. Alteration in the skin is often the first manifestation of an impaired immune system and may be a sign or symptom of a serious opportunistic infection. Skin alterations can also indicate advancing HIV disease.

Several points regarding HIV, skin disease, and its treatments are noteworthy. Lesions that are common in the non–HIV-infected adult population may present atypically in HIV-infected persons. In addition, skin disorders often aren't responsive to the usual treatments, may be present for longer than expected, and may develop into chronic, disfiguring disorders. Skin lesions may also be the precursor of a life-threatening illness.

> **PRACTICE POINT**
>
> Prompt and accurate investigation of skin lesions in the HIV-infected patient is essential and often warrants collaboration with an HIV specialist.

The effective combination of several antiretroviral drugs to suppress viral replication with consequent repletion of the CD4+ lymphocyte count is often known as highly active antiretroviral therapy (HAART). HAART-based regimens and drugs that prevent or treat opportunistic infections have contributed to a significant decline in HIV-associated morbidity and mortality. Previously common skin disorders also decreased in incidence with the common use of HAART, including Kaposi's sarcoma, eosinophilic folliculitis, molluscum contagiosum, bacillary angiomatosis, and condylomata acuminata. One study estimated that

TABLE 21-1	Adverse Cutaneous Reactions in HIV Disease
Drug class	**Dermatologic manifestations**
Nucleoside reverse-transcriptase inhibitors (NRTI), especially zidovudine, abacavir	Mucocutaneous pigmentation, drug hypersensitivity DRESS (Drug Rash, Eosinophilia, and Systemic Symptoms)
	Hypertrichosis, leukocytoclastic vasculitis
	Life-threatening skin diseases: Stevens-Johnson syndrome (SJS) and toxic epidermal necrolysis (TEN)
Non-nucleoside reverse-transcriptase inhibitors (NRTI), especially nevirapine	Skin rash, most often an exanthematous eruption
	Other less frequently reported reactions that may manifest in the skin, including SJS and potentially life-threatening conditions such as TEN and DRESS
Protease inhibitors	Maculopapular eruption, urticaria, acute generalized exanthematous pustulosis, asteatotic dermatitis, acute porphyria, DRESS, SJS, and single or multiple pyogenic granulomas
Fusion inhibitors	Injection-site reactions: erythema, cysts, and nodules at injection sites
Entry inhibitors	No significant reactions reported
Integrase inhibitors	Pruritus, rash

HAART has reduced the total number of HIV patients with skin problems by 40%.[2] Although HAART and regimens to treat opportunistic infections have improved the quality of life for patients by controlling HIV replication, the increased use of pharmaceutical agents has led to an increased incidence of adverse reactions to these drugs. The risk for adverse cutaneous reactions to certain drugs is greatly increased in patients with HIV compared with that of the general population (as much as 100 times) and occurs in tandem with the level of immunosuppression.[3] Drugs often associated with adverse effects include sulfonamides, co-trimoxazole, and tuberculostatics as well as many of the antiretrovirals. (See Table 21-1.)

CUTANEOUS DRUG ERUPTIONS

Cutaneous drug-induced eruptions, not due to antiretroviral therapy, can occur with some drugs used to prevent opportunistic infections. Bactrim (trimethoprim-sulfamethoxazole), the most effective drug in the prevention and treatment of *Pneumocystis jiroveci* pneumonia, is known to cause cutaneous eruption in patients with HIV infection. The rate of cutaneous eruption associated with trimethoprim-sulfamethoxazole in HIV patients is 20% to 80% compared with 1% to 3% in persons without HIV infection, possibly due to altered drug metabolism, decreased glutathione levels, or both.[4]

In its severe form, Stevens-Johnson syndrome (SJS) and toxic epidermal necrolysis (TEN) may also develop. SJS is characterized by fever as well as widespread blisters of the skin and mucous membranes of the eye, mouth, or genitalia. TEN is a more serious manifestation of SJS that involves widespread areas of the skin with confluent bullae that can lead to loss of skin in massive sheets.

IMMUNE RECONSTITUTION INFLAMMATORY SYNDROME (IRIS)

The introduction of HAART has in recent years resulted in the emergence of the immune reconstitution inflammatory syndrome (IRIS). This syndrome is characterized by a paradoxical clinical deterioration in or an exacerbation of certain conditions, some of which may potentially manifest in the skin and may occur in 15% to 25% of all patients on HAART.[5] IRIS is thought to be the result of an overzealous immunologic response to infectious or self-antigens as the immune system is restored with HAART. IRIS results in frank disease but often results in moderate to severe cutaneous eruptions, including follicular inflammatory eruptions, mycobacterial skin infections, and viral infections such as human herpes virus infection (e.g., herpes zoster). IRIS may even exacerbate an underlying autoimmune disease such as lupus erythematosus.

INFECTIOUS SKIN DISORDERS

The immunocompromised status of patients with HIV or AIDS puts them at greater risk for infectious bacterial or viral skin disorders, such as herpes virus, cytomegalovirus (CMV), human papillomavirus, molluscum contagiosum, *Staphylococcus* and *Streptococcus* infection, and bacillary angiomatosis.

Herpes virus

Breakouts of grouped blister-like lesions typically caused by the common herpes virus are easily recognized and common in patients with HIV at all stages of the disease. Herpes zoster may occur either early or late in the course of HIV-induced immunosuppression and may be the first clinical clue to suggest undiagnosed HIV infection. Herpes infection may occur on the oral and genital mucosa as well as in the perianal region. Lesions typically manifest as painful, grouped vesicles on an erythematous base that rupture and become crusted. History and clinical presentation are often all that's necessary to establish the disorder; therefore, confirmatory tests, such as the Tzanck smear preparation, biopsy, or viral culture are rarely necessary. In patients with advanced HIV, a herpetic infection may develop into chronic ulcers and fissures with a substantial degree of edema.

The incidence of herpes zoster is more than 14 times higher in HIV-infected adults than in age-matched controls.[6] Herpes zoster can occur in HIV-infected adults at any CD4+ count, but the frequency of disease is highest in those with

Patient Teaching
Herpes virus teaching tips

- Scrupulous hand washing helps prevent the spread of infection.
- Use individual washcloths and linens.
- Mild analgesics may be necessary for pain associated with herpes infection.
- Topical soaks (such as Domeboro solution) can be used to help dry wet lesions.
- Impetiginization of skin lesions may be treated with warm compresses.

CD4+ counts less than 200 cells/µl. Unlike other skin disorders, the incidence of herpes zoster infection is *not* reduced by HARRT.

Uncomplicated zoster outbreaks should be treated for 7 to 10 days with acyclovir (Zovirax), famciclovir (Famvir), or valacyclovir (Valtrex). Painful atrophic scars, persistent ulcerations, and acyclovir-resistant chronic verrucous lesions may also develop. (See *Patient Teaching: Herpes virus teaching tips*.)

PRACTICE POINT

Healing of herpetic lesions is usually complete in less than 2 weeks. If they haven't healed within 3 to 4 weeks, the patient may have a drug-resistant virus. Acyclovir-resistant cases of varicella-zoster virus or herpes simplex virus infection require treatment with IV foscarnet (Foscavir).

PRACTICE POINT

A patient with herpes zoster involving V1, the ophthalmic division of the trigeminal nerve, should be referred to an ophthalmologist immediately due to the risk of corneal ulceration. Signs or symptoms of this condition, such as painful vesicular lesions on the tip of the nose or lid margins, should be considered an ocular emergency.

Cytomegalovirus

CMV is a double-stranded DNA virus in the herpes virus family that can cause disseminated or localized end-organ disease among patients with advanced immunosuppression. The incidence of new cases of CMV end-organ disease has declined by 75% to 80% with the advent of HAART and now is estimated to be fewer than 6 cases per 100 person-years.[6] When the skin is involved, CMV may cause a number of different clinical manifestations, including ulcers, verrucous lesions, and palpable purpuric papules. Effective treatments for a CMV infection include oral valganciclovir (Valcyte) or IV ganciclovir (Cytovene), foscarnet (Foscavir), or cidofovir (Vistide).

PRACTICE POINT

Ulcers are commonly secondarily colonized with CMV, and many patients have combined herpes simplex and CMV infections.

Human papillomavirus

The most common skin complaint of HIV-positive patients is warts caused by the human papillomavirus (HPV). It has been shown that immune deficiency is associated with increased frequency of HPV infections, suggesting that the emergence of HPV is modulated by the patient's immune status.

Verruca vulgaris warts (common warts) appear as dull-colored papules that can erupt anywhere on the skin; verruca plana warts are flat-topped, skin colored papules on the face and dorsal hands. Condyloma acuminata warts (genital warts) are characterized by soft, skin-colored cauliflower papules on the genital areas. Their appearance, size, and number vary with the site. Warts can range in size from less than 1 mm to 2 cm "cauliflower lesions." Verruca plantaris warts are hyperkeratotic papules and plaques that appear on the soles of the feet. Certain types of HPV have oncogenic potential and are associated with cervical cancer in women, bowenoid papulosis of the penis, anal cancers, and invasive carcinoma. HPV-16 alone accounts for approximately 50% of cervical cancers in the general population and HPV-18 for another 10% to 15%, whereas the other oncogenic HPV types each individually account for less than 5% of tumors.[6] Unlike other HIV-associated infections, treatment with HAART has not affected the incidence of HPV infection.

Treatment, although effective, rarely eradicates HPV entirely. Destructive measures—such as the application of topical chemicals (for example, salicylic or trichloroacetic acid), cryotherapy with liquid nitrogen, and ablative surgery—are standard measures used for common verrucae (warts). Condyloma acuminata can be treated by using podophyllin resin 10% to 50% in tincture of benzoin, 3% cidofovir ointment, intralesional interferon-a, liquid nitrogen cryotherapy, electrodesiccation and curettage, or carbon dioxide laser.

Patient Teaching

Imiquimod 5% (Aldara Cream) is often prescribed to prevent recurrence of HPV infection. Instruct the patient to apply the medication to his or her warts at night three times per week for up to 16 weeks.

Patients who use Aldara Cream may experience application-site reactions such as itching and/or burning. Skin reactions may be of such intensity that patients *may require rest periods from treatment*. Teach the patient to use the cream exactly as prescribed; using too much Aldara Cream, or using it too often or for too long, can increase chances of having a severe skin reaction.

Patient Teaching

Recent literature and anecdotal evidence suggests that the application of duct tape is successful at removing common warts; however, this strategy has not been tested formally in HIV-infected patients.[7]

Patient Teaching
Post-procedure care after HPV surgical excision

Post-procedure patient teaching should include the following.

- Medication usually isn't needed after removal of lesions. Topical anesthetic ointments may be used to minimize discomfort. Sitz baths may aid resolution when large areas are treated; silver sulfadiazine (Silvadene) ointment or antibiotic ointment may not only be soothing but may also reduce the possibility of superficial infection. No dressing is required, but some patients may request a sanitary napkin for treated genital lesions. Ice packs are helpful.
- Cryonecrosed lesions will progress from erythema to edema and then will turn black. The lesions will disappear within a few days, and healing should be complete in 7 to 8 days. For chemically cauterized lesions, the healing process is usually less than 1 week.
- Treated areas should be washed and dried gently each day of the healing process. Post-cryotherapy management is similar to that for a superficial partial-thickness burn.
- Counsel the patient to report excessive discomfort or any signs of infection.[8]

Plantar verrucae are generally treated with topical 40% salicylic acid plaster applied daily, with paring of hyperkeratotic areas, although intralesional bleomycin and liquid nitrogen therapy have also been used. Verruca plana warts are commonly treated with topical tretinoin alone or in combination with 5-fluorouracil. Light electrodessication or liquid nitrogen application may be used as an adjunct therapy. Verrucous carcinoma requires excisional surgery. (See *Patient Teaching: Post-procedure care after HPV surgical excision.*)

Molluscum contagiosum

Molluscum contagiosum is a benign, usually asymptomatic viral skin infection caused by the poxvirus; it is spread by direct contact and causes no systemic manifestations. The diagnosis can usually be made from the characteristic appearance of dome-shaped, umbilicated, translucent papules that may develop on any cutaneous site, especially the genital areas and the face. In the patient with AIDS, lesions may become widespread, disfiguring, and resistant to treatment. The lesions appear verrucous, pruritic, or eczematous. Once they become confluent, they can be difficult to treat. Although the exact incidence of molluscum contagiosum in patient with AIDS is unknown, it is estimated to be 5% to 18%.[9] Treatment is generally by destructive measures, including cryotherapy or curettage. (See *Patient Teaching: Molluscum contagiosum.*)

Staphylococcus or *Streptococcus*

In general, most bacterial infections are caused by *Staphylococcus* and *Streptococcus* organisms and are commonly encountered in immunocompetent patients. Primary bacterial lesions manifest as vesicles, papules, and pustules and are often pruritic. It's the pruritic feature that often leads the patient to scratching, subsequently resulting in a break in the epithelial surface followed by excoriation of the lesion. Some lesions (such as impetigo) may contain purulent fluid. Diffusely red, warm, tender areas in the skin suggest soft-tissue cellulitis or a deep-seated infected wound.

In recent years there has been an increase in the number of HIV patients with community-acquired methicillin resistance *Staphylococcus aureus* (CA-MRSA) infection. More importantly, MRSA-associated bacteremia is also on the rise: from 5.3 cases per 1,000 person-years in 2000 and 2001 to 11.9 cases per 1,000 person-years in 2003 and 2004.[10] It is now established that HIV disease is a major risk for CA-MRSA,[11] possibly related to immunodeficiency. Lower CD4+ cell counts are an independent risk factor for MRSA colonization, and lifestyle factors such as high-risk sexual behaviors and injection drug use may also play a role. Nasal colonization could be another factor. In a prospective Veterans Affairs study of more than 200 HIV-infected patients who were followed for at least 2 years, 49% had at least one nasal culture positive for *S. aureus*.[12]

Treatment with dicloxacillin, cephalexin, or ciprofloxacin is indicated in bacterial infections. Clindamycin or linezolid remains a commonly used treatment option for CA-MRSA. Wounds caused by bacterial infections should be assessed regularly and treated accordingly; incision and draininge may be indicated. (See *Patient Teaching: Preventing staphylococcal*

Patient Teaching
Molluscum contagiosum

- Molluscum contagiosum can be transmitted through direct contact.
- The lesions are prone to autoinoculation, and in male patients, shaving the beard area has been reported to cause particularly severe infections, with lesions encompassing the entire face.
- Cryonecrosed lesions will progress from erythema to edema, and then will turn black. The lesions will disappear within a few days, and healing should be complete in 7 to 8 days.
- For chemically cauterized lesions, the healing process is usually less than 1 week.

Patient Teaching
Preventing staphylococcal or CA-MRSA skin infections

Practice good hygiene:

- Keep hands clean by washing thoroughly with soap and water or using an alcohol-based hand sanitizer.
- Keep cuts and scrapes clean and covered with a bandage until healed.
- Avoid contact with other people's wounds or bandages.
- Avoid sharing personal items, such as towels, washcloths, razors, clothing, or uniforms, that may have come into contact with an infected wound or bandage. Wash soiled sheets, towels, and clothes with water and laundry detergent. Use a dryer to dry clothes completely.

or CA-MRSA skin infections.) (Also see chapter 7, Wound bioburden and infection.)

Bacillary angiomatosis

Bacillary angiomatosis is a bacterial infection caused by organisms of the genus *Bartonella* (formerly *Rochalimaea*), specifically *Bartonella quintana* and *Bartonella henselae*. These cutaneous vascular lesions are characteristically small, reddish to purple papules that are tender to the touch. Lesions may ulcerate and then become covered by a crust. Complicated bacillary angiomatosis infections occur when the lesion is located deep in the subcutis, extending to involve soft tissue and bone. Infection with bacillary angiomatosis leads to systemic involvement. Biopsy followed by special staining is often necessary to definitively identify the organism. Treatment with erythromycin or doxycycline provides a prompt response. (See *Patient Teaching: Bacillary angiomatosis*.)

PRACTICE POINT

With the advent of HAART, bacillary angiomatosis infections seem to have almost disappeared. However, these infections may mimic Kaposi's sarcoma, which should therefore remain the differential diagnosis until the actual causative agent is identified.

NONINFECTIOUS SKIN DISORDERS

The immunocompromised status of patients with HIV and AIDS also puts them at greater risk for noninfectious skin disorders.[14]

Pruritic Rash

A rash that is predominantly papular may be due to pruritic papular eruption (PPE),

Patient Teaching
Bacillary angiomatosis

The most common reservoirs for the bacilli that cause bacillary angiomatosis are domestic cats and cat fleas. Clients with AIDS should avoid rough play with cats and situations in which scratches from cats are likely to occur. Cats shouldn't be allowed to lick open wounds or cuts. All cats should be treated for fleas, or other flea control measures should be followed.[13]

eosinophilic folliculitis, nodular prurigo, drug reaction, syphilis, granuloma annulare, and atopic-like dermatitis.

PPE is often reported as the most common rash seen in HIV infection. The typical primary lesion is a firm, discrete, erythematous, urticarial papule. Anywhere from 18% to 46% of patients with HIV have this condition at some time.[1] Severe pruritus and subsequent scarred excoriations subject patients to HIV-related stigma. Topical or intralesional glucocorticoids are the treatment of choice. Other topical treatments, such as topical vitamin D_3 and topical capsaicin, have also been reported to be effective. Often treatments provide minimal relief and can be disappointing.

NEOPLASTIC DISORDERS

Patients with HIV and AIDS are at risk for a variety of neoplastic disorders.

Lymphoma

Although lymphomas generally start in the lymph nodes or collections of lymphatic tissue in organs, such as the stomach or intestines, the skin may also be affected. Non-Hodgkin's lymphoma usually manifests as pink to purplish papules or nodules. Deeply seated soft-tissue involvement may expand superficially, forming dome-shaped nodules that often ulcerate. Cutaneous Hodgkin's disease appears similar to non-Hodgkin's lymphoma. The diagnosis is made by the identification of atypical cells having a Reed-Sternberg–like morphology. Treatments include methotrexate, prednisone, bleomycin, adriamycin, cyclophosphamide, and vincristine.

Kaposi's sarcoma

Kaposi's sarcoma is a vascular neoplastic disorder. Prior to the use of HAART, Kaposi's sarcoma was the most common skin disorder seen in men who have sex with men (MSM) with AIDS. The pathogenesis of Kaposi's sarcoma has now been identified as human herpes virus type 8. This virus is transmitted sexually, which explains in part the epidemiology of Kaposi's sarcoma predominantly in MSM.

Clinically, Kaposi's sarcoma skin lesions may be pink, red, brown, or purple macules, patches, plaques, nodules, or tumors and can appear almost anywhere on the body, including the mucous membranes. (See *color section*, *Kaposi's sarcoma*, page C36.) The appearance of many cutaneous lesions typically predicts visceral organ involvement. When pressure-bearing areas such as the base of the spine are involved, lesions often ulcerate. Marked edema may develop when tumors involve the lymphatics, leading to diffuse swollen areas of skin and subsequent breaks in the skin.

Diagnosis of Kaposi's sarcoma is usually based on the finding of purplish skin lesions. Biopsy is rarely necessary but may be performed to rule out bacillary angiomatosis. HAART is considered the first-line treatment for Kaposi's sarcoma lesions, and when CD4+ cells improve lesions tend to regress. Other treatments include liquid nitrogen cryotherapy for small cutaneous lesions; radiation treatment and electron-beam therapy are used in selected cases. Radiotherapy is effective for painful lesions of the palms and soles. Intralesional injections of vinblastine sulfate at biweekly intervals are also effective, especially if the patient has only a few small lesions; however, the injections are painful. With more advanced disease, systemic therapy with interferon and liposomally encapsulated doxorubicin and daunorubicin are effective agents.

Squamous cell carcinoma of the anal mucosa

A growing body of evidence suggests a high prevalence of anal HPV infection and dysplasia in HIV-infected individuals. Some studies in HIV-infected individuals have shown that anal HPV infection is present in 93% of MSM and 76% of women, and anal dysplasia (any grade) is present in 56% of MSM and 26% of women.[15–17] Receptive anal intercourse may increase the likelihood of anal HPV infection but is not a prerequisite for anal HPV or dysplasia.[17] Patients with lower CD4+ cell counts appear to be at higher risk of developing anal dysplasia. Tumors in the anal area typically present as a mass associated with bleeding and pain. Anal neoplasia must be ruled out in anyone with HIV infection who presents with anorectal complaints. Investigation of any abnormal discharge, bleeding, bowel irregularity, pruritus, dysuria, or pelvic pain should include screening for anal neoplasia. HAART and immune reconstitution do not offer protection against anal dysplasia.[18] A person with HIV infection who develops anal neoplasia should receive the standard therapy for the specific stage of disease.

SUMMARY

Skin disorders are common in patients with HIV and AIDS. Accurate identification of skin lesions is critical so appropriate treatment can be implemented. Consultation with an HIV or AIDS clinician is helpful in the comprehensive care of these patients.

PATIENT SCENARIO: HIV/AIDS POPULATION

Clinical Data

PK is a 23-year-old black man who was diagnosed with HIV 5 years ago. He is seeing his nurse practitioner (NP) today for his 3-month HIV visit, which includes an assessment of his viral load and CD4+ cell count. At his last visit, PK's viral load was below the limits of detection (<48 copies) and his CD4+ cell count was 653 cell/mm^3. He is 100% adherent with his HIV medications and tells the NP that he is feeling well overall. Since this is also his annual exam, the NP performs a complete physical examination as well as an anal Pap smear. There are no visble lesions around the anus, and PK has no anorectal complaints. Several days later the NP receives the results of PK's anal Pap, which reveals low-grade squamous intraepithelial lesions (LSIL).

Case Discussion

Anal cancer, like cervical cancer, is a member of a broader group of anogenital cancers known to be associated with sexually transmitted viral HPV infection. HPV is extremely prevalent, particularly in young, sexually active populations. Sexual practices involving receptive anal intercourse lead to a significantly elevated risk for anal dysplasia and cancer, particularly in those with HIV/AIDS. Unlike cervical cancer, there are no universally accepted guidelines or standards of care for anal dysplasia. Expert opinion suggests that annual testing be performed, particularly in high-risk groups. An anal Pap screening involves the blind insertion of a swab into the anal canal and fixing the retrieved cells either on a slide or in fluid for cytological examination.

With the finding of dysplasia, PK will need to be referred for an anoscopic examination and biopsy, the procedure for which is as follows. After an initial application of acetic acid, Lugol's iodine solution is applied. Then an anoscope, a high-resolution microscope, is used to inspect visually the entire anal canal, particularly the transformation zone, an area of increased risk for dysplastic changes. High-grade lesions do not take up the iodine solution because of the lack of glycogen in the dysplastic cells; they appear yellow to tan, whereas normal or low-grade lesions appear dark brown or black. Any abnormalities such as aceto-whitening (a temporary change to a white color when acetic acid is applied topically), papillation (raised bumps) and ulceration, or irregular surface changes noted in the inspection are biopsied. The classification system for anal cytology similarly includes normal or atypical squamous cells of undetermined significance (ASCUS). Atypical findinds are further classified as low-grade (LSIL) or high-grade (HLSL) dysplasia. PK's lesions were LSIL. For PK's small, localized lesions, treatment included application of trichloroacetic acid but could have included various ablative therapies with lasers, infrared coagulation, or cryosurgery. Surgical excision is generally reserved for deeper or more diffusely spread lesions.

1. Highly active antiretroviral therapy (HAART) has impacted skin disorders in patients with human immunodeficiency virus (HIV) in which one of the following ways:
   A. Adverse effects of HAART have led to an increase in the number of skin disorders seen in the patient infected with human immunodeficiency virus.
   B. There has been a decrease in the incidence of skin disorders seen in the patient with HIV.
   C. There has been an increase in the number of noninfectious skin disorders in the patient with HIV.
   D. Viral infections are the only skin disorders affected by HAART.

   ANSWER: B. *HAART-based regimens have contributed to a significant decrease in HIV-associated morbidity and mortality, including many of the cutaneous manifestations of HIV infection. The other options are incorrect.*

2. Community-acquired methicillin-resistant *Staphylococcus aureus* (CA-MRSA) infection can best be prevented by teaching patients to:
   A. Take antiretroviral drugs every day.
   B. Wipe surfaces with alcohol-based sanitizers.
   C. Share only visibly clean items.
   D. Keep the hands clean.

   ANSWER: D. *Frequent hand washing or using an alcohol-based hand sanitizer is the best method of preventing transmission of community-acquired methicillin-rersistant* Staphylococcus aureus *(CA-MRSA).*

3. What is the causative agent for dysplastic changes in the anal canal?
   A. HIV
   B. Hepatitis B virus (HBV)
   C. Human papillomavirus (HPV)
   D. CA-MRSA

   ANSWER: C. *HPV is the causative agent for anal dysplasia and anal carcinoma.*

REFERENCES: HIV/AIDS POPULATION

1. Zancaro, P., McGirt, L., Mamelak, A., Nguyen, R., Martins, C. "Cutaneous Manifestations of HIV in the Era of Highly Active Antiretroviral Therapy: An Institutional Urban Clinic Experience," *Journal of American Academy of Dermatology* 54:581-88, 2006.
2. Calista, D., Morri, M., Stagno, A., Boschini, A. "Changing Morbidity of Cutaneous Diseases in Patients with HIV after the Introduction of Highly Active Antiretroviral Therapy Including a Protease Inhibitor," *American Journal of Clinical Dermatology* 3:59-62, 2002.
3. Grayson, W. "The HIV-positive Skin Biopsy," *Journal of Clinical Pathology* 61:802-17, 2008.
4. Farrell, J., Naisbitt, D.J., Drummond, N.S., Depta, J.P., Vilar, F.J., Pirmohamed, M., Park, B.K. "Characterization of Sulfamethoxazole and Sulfamethoxazole Metabolite-specific T-cell Responses in Animals and Humans," *Journal of Pharmacology and Experimental Therapeutics* 306:229-37, 2003.
5. Hurias, E., Preda, V., Maurer, T. & Whitfle, M. "Cutaneous Manifestations of Immune Reconstituition Inflammatory Syndrome," *Current Opinion in HIV and AIDS* 3:453-60, 2008.
6. Centers for Disease Control and Prevention. "Guidelines for Prevention and Treatment of Opportunistic Infections in HIV-Infected Adults and Adolescents," *Morbidity and Mortality Weekly Report* 58(No. RR-44), 2009.
7. Focht, D.R. III, Spicer, C., Fairchok, M.P. "The Efficacy of Duct Tape vs Cryotherapy in the Treatment of Verruca Vulgaris (the Common Wart)," *Archives of Pediatric and Adolescent Medicine* 156:971-74, 2002.

8. Apgar, S.A., and Pfenninger, J.L. "Treatment of Vulvar, Perianal, Vaginal, Penile and Urethral Condyloma Acuminata," in Pfenninger, J.L. and Fowler, G.C. (eds)., *Procedures for Primary Care Physicians,* 2nd ed. St. Louis: Mosby-Year Book, Inc, 2003.

9. Strauss, R.M., Doyle, E.L., Mohsen, A.H., and Green, S.T. "Successful Treatment of Molluscum Contagiosum with Topical Imiquimod in a Severely Immunocompromised HIV-positive Patient," *International Journal of STD & AIDS* 12:264-66, 2001.

10. Burkey, M.D., Wilson, L.E., Moore, R.D., Lucas, G.M., Francis, J., Gebo, K.A. "The Incidence of and Risk Factors for MRSA Bacteraemia in an HIV-infected Cohort in the HAART Era," *HIV Medicine* 9:858-62, 2008.

11. Miller, M., Cespedes, C., Vavagiakis, P., Klein, R.S., Lowy, F.D. "*Staphylococcus aureus* Colonization in a Community Sample of HIV-infected and HIV-uninfected Drug Users," *European Journal of Clinical Microbiology & Infectious Diseases* 22: 463-69, 2003.

12. Nguyen, M.H., Kauffman, C.A., Goodman, R.P., Squier, C., Arbeit, R.D., Singh, N., Wagener, M.M., Yu, V.L. "Nasal Carriage of and Infection with *Staphylococcus aureus* in HIV-infected Patients," *Annals of Internal Medicine* 2:130-221, 1999.

13. Zwolski, K., and Talotta, D. "Bacterial Infections," in Kirton, C. (ed.), *Handbook of HIV/AIDS Nursing.* St. Louis: Mosby-Year Book, Inc., 2001.

14. Goldstein, B., Berman, B., Sukenik, E., Frankel, S.J. "Correlation of Skin Disorders with CD4 Lymphocyte Counts in Patients with HIV/AIDS," *Journal of the American Academy of Dermatology* 36:262-64, 1997.

15. Chin-Hong, P.V., and Palefsky, J.M. "Natural History and Clinical Management of Anal Human Papillomavirus Disease in Men and Women Infected with Human Immunodeficiency Virus," *Clinical Infectious Disease* 35:1127-34, 2002.

16. Palefsky, J.M., Holly, E.A., Ralston, M.L., Jay, N. "Prevalence and Risk Factors for Human Papillomavirus Infection of the Anal Canal in Human Immunodeficiency Virus (HIV)-positive and HIV-negative Homosexual Men," *Journal of Infectious Disease* 177:361-67, 1998.

17. Piketty, C., Darragh, T.M., Da Costa, M., Bruneval, P., Heard, I., Kazatchkine, M.D. Palefsky, J.M. "High Prevalence of Anal Human Papillomavirus Infection and Anal Cancer Precursors Among HIV-infected Persons in the Absence of Anal Intercourse," *Annals of Internal Medicine* 138:453-59, 2003.

18. Berry, J. M., Palefsky, J.M., & Welton, M.L. "Anal Cancer and Its Precursors in HIV-positive Patients: Perspectives and Management," *Surgical Oncology Clinics of North America* 13:355-73, 2004.

BARIATRIC POPULATION

Janet E. Cuddigan, PhD, RN, CWCN, and Sharon Baranoski, MSN, RN, CWCN, APN-CCNS, DAPWCA, FAAN

AN IMPORTANT HEALTHCARE CONCERN

The population of bariatric patients is increasing, and with it the need for solutions that fit these patients' needs. The term "bariatrics" comes from the Greek word *barros*, meaning large or heavy. It is used to describe the area of medicine/healthcare concerning people who are overweight or obese.[1] The National Center for Health Statistics reports that 34% of American adults—approximately 60 million people—are obese.[2] Morbid obesity is defined as weighing a minimum of 100 lb more than ideal body weight or having a body mass index (BMI) of 40 or higher.[3] Healthcare costs for morbidly obese patients are nearly double those of normal-weight patients due to the additional costs of obesity-linked chronic health conditions, such as diabetes, hypertension, and cardiovascular disease.[4]

Healthcare facilities specializing in bariatric surgeries have been aware of the need for appropriate equipment and special skin care protocols for this population for years.[5,6] Facilities without bariatric specialty services are challenged to meet the needs of an ever-increasing bariatric population. Failure to address the needs of this patient population may lead to an increased risk of pressure ulcers and skin integrity challenges. Clinicians encountering bariatric patients need to be aware of these challenges and the special needs of caring for the bariatric patient.[7]

CLASSIFYING THE BARIATRIC PATIENT

What makes a person bariatric? This category can be based on the amount of body weight compared with height as well as where the person's weight is located on his or her body. The National Heart, Lung, and Blood Institute (NHLBI) provides the following classifications for obesity based on BMI, which is calculated as body weight in kilograms/body height in meters squared[8,9]:

- Overweight: BMI 25 to 29.9
- Class I obesity: BMI 30.0 to 34.9
- Class II obesity: BMI 35.0 to 39.9
- Class III (extreme) obesity: BMI over 40

The NHLBI is updating its data and expects to have new classifications available in late 2011.

The distribution of body weight should also be assessed. Health risks (and skin care needs) vary between those with "apple-shaped" versus "pear-shaped" physiques. (See *Identifying body shapes*.) The waist-to-hip circumference ratio is often used to describe these differences. The patient with an apple-shaped physique has a greater waist-to-hip ratio and is at greater risk for cardiovascular disease. The pear-shaped individual has a lower ratio but may need special chairs and commodes to accommodate a larger hip size.[6] Bariatric patients run a high-risk of developing pressure ulcers due to their body weight.

MEETING PATIENT NEEDS

With ever-increasing obesity rates in the United States, all healthcare facilities need to have bariatric skin care protocols in place

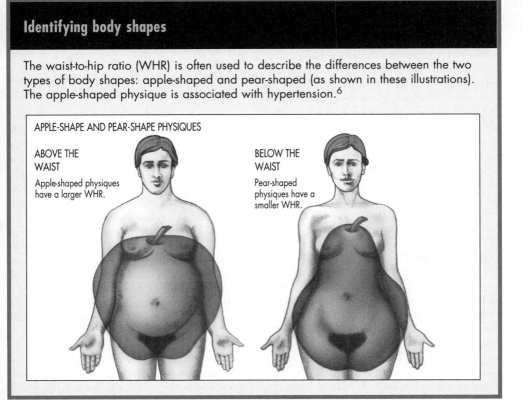

Identifying body shapes

The waist-to-hip ratio (WHR) is often used to describe the differences between the two types of body shapes: apple-shaped and pear-shaped (as shown in these illustrations). The apple-shaped physique is associated with hypertension.[6]

APPLE-SHAPE AND PEAR-SHAPE PHYSIQUES

ABOVE THE WAIST

Apple-shaped physiques have a larger WHR.

BELOW THE WAIST

Pear-shaped physiques have a smaller WHR.

and "ready access" to beds, chairs, commodes, walkers, and other equipment appropriate for bariatric patients. Advanced preparation with regard to protocols and equipment is essential to meet the needs of these patients. Bariatric patients frequently have significant healthcare problems, such as hypertension, type 2 diabetes, coronary artery disease, stroke, gallbladder disease, osteoarthritis, sleep apnea, respiratory problems, an increased risk for certain cancers, and numerous skin manifestations.[10] Despite these risks, bariatric patients may delay medical treatment out of fear or embarrassment. Ask yourself these questions as you develop your institutional readiness:

• Is your facility prepared to handle the special needs of these patients as they enter the emergency department?
• Is your staff prepared to provide safe, respectful patient care while avoiding injuries in both patients and staff members?

Many complex considerations are involved in treating bariatric patients, including multiple comorbidities; the potential for non-healing surgical wounds due to dehiscence or infection; a higher risk of venous disease, pressure ulcer development, and diabetic foot wounds; and nutritional concerns.[11] In a prospective study of 31 patients following Roux-en-Y anastomosis bypass surgery that measured knowledge of incision care as well as discharge concerns, Pieper et al. found increased patient fear with lower levels of knowledge.[12] The discharge and educational needs of post-surgical bariatric patients have been summarized by Pieper et al.[13] The focus of our discussion is skin assessment and care of the bariatric patient, with the goal of maintaining skin integrity.

SKIN ASSESSMENT

A complete skin assessment is the first step in any skin care protocol. A cursory assessment of the skin is not sufficient. Bariatric patients may have changes in skin physiology due to a greater skin-to-weight ratio, reduced vascularity, and perfusion in adipose tissue that can result in poor wound healing.[1] Skin inspection should be completed on admission with the patient wearing a hospital gown and lying flat, if condition tolerates, in bed. All skin folds should be separated gently and examined for erythematous, moist denuded areas or pressure ulcers. These areas can be extremely painful, so care and assistance (two or more persons) are needed to complete a thorough exam. Common skin fold areas include behind the neck, under the arms and breasts, under the abdomen or pannus, the flank area, the perineal and rectal area, the upper and lower thighs, and the calf and ankle areas.[11] (See *color section*, *Skin folds*, page C36.)

The abdominal fat and skin fold apron is called a pannus (see *color section*, *Pannus*, page C36). A bariatric patient with a BMI of 60 (5'4" weighing 350 lb) can have a pannus weighing 55 lb or more.[11] The pannus is the only skin fold on the body that has its own grading system to describe size and extent.[11] A scale of 1 to 5 is cited in the literature[11]:

• Grade 1: pannus covers the pubic hairline but not the entire mons pubis
• Grade 2: pannus extends to cover the entire mons pubis
• Grade 3: pannus extends to cover the upper thigh
• Grade 4: pannus extends to mid-thigh
• Grade 5: pannus extends to the knee and below

The weight created by skin folds and skin-to-skin contact can create forces that enable pressure ulcers to develop in areas that are *not* normally considered to be at high risk, such as the hips, buttocks, trunk, or torso.[1] Ongoing skin assessment and appropriate interventions are critical in maintaining and healing any skin manifestations or ulcers. The NPUAP/EPUAP Pressure Ulcer Prevention and Treatment Guideline[14] for Bariatric (Obese) Individuals provides assessment and positioning recommendations. (See *Assessment and positioning recommendations for bariatric patients*.)

When examining the skin you may find certain benign conditions that more commonly occur in obese individuals. These include:

• Acanthosis nigricans: hyperpigmented (often brown) irregular plaques in skin folds (especially the axilla and back of the neck).

Assessment and positioning recommendations for bariatric patients

- Get adequate assistance to fully inspect all skin folds.
- Pressure ulcers may develop in unique locations, such as underneath folds of skin and in locations where tubes and other devices have been compressed between skin folds.
- Pressure ulcers develop over bony prominences but may also result from tissue pressure across the buttocks and other areas of high adipose-tissue concentration.
- Avoid pressure on skin from tubes and other medical devices
- Use pillows or other positioning devices to off-load pannus or other large skin folds and prevent skin-on-skin pressure.

National Pressure Ulcer Advisory Panel and European Pressure Ulcer Advisory Panel. *Prevention and Treatment of Pressure Ulcers: Clinical Practice Guideline.* Washington, DC: National Pressure Ulcer Advisory Panel, 2009.

(See *color section*, *Acanthosis nigricans*, page C37.) The plaques often feel like velvet when touched but may eventually become rougher in texture. Although acanthosis nigricans is usually a benign condition, changes that may indicate malignancy (for example, bleeding or inflammation) should be referred to the primary care provider for follow-up. This condition is associated with obesity as well as other systemic diseases, such as hyperinsulinemia and cancer. A 12% ammonium lactate cream applied twice daily may improve the condition.[15]

- Skin tags: common in obese patients and usually benign. They may be surgically removed for cosmetic reasons.[15]
- Androgen effects: adipose tissue synthesizes testosterone. Obese female patients may show male-pattern baldness, excessive hair growth in other areas, and acne.[15]
- Stretch marks (striae distensae): from stretching of connective tissue, collagen rupture, and dermal scarring.[15]
- Plantar hyperkeratosis—excessive weight on the feet leads to thickening of the weight-bearing surfaces on the soles. (See *colo section*, *Plantar hyperkeratosis*, page C37.) Treatment includes weight loss and orthotic shoe inserts to protect bony prominences from breakdown.[15]

More serious skin problems are often found during the initial assessment of obese patients, such as cellulitis, skin infections, lymphedema, hemosiderosis, and other skin changes associated with venous insufficiency of the lower extremities; venous ulcers; infection, seroma, poor healing, or dehiscence of surgical wounds; intertrigo; and pressure ulcers.[15,16] Many of these conditions are covered in other chapters of this book. Here we give special consideration to prevention and treatment of intertrigo and pressure ulcers as they relate to bariatric patients.

INTERTRIGO

Intertrigo is inflammation of the skin folds.[17] The inflammatory changes often present as mirror images where one skin surface touches another. Intertrigo and intertriginous dermatitis are actually fairly broad terms that cover a variety of skin disorders found between the folds of the skin. Although this condition can be found in any patient, obese patients are at higher risk because multiple large skin folds create conditions ideal for inflammation and infection. These conditions include moisture (as perspiration is trapped under skin folds, creating maceration); pressure of large skin folds on underlying skin, creating areas of pressure-induced injury; friction (as one skin surface moves across another); shear, with movement resulting in fissures at the base of the skin fold; physical challenges in maintaining hygiene; and the warm, dark, moist conditions that favor growth of yeast and fungal infections. Secondary bacterial skin infections may also develop, and progression to cellulitis is certainly a risk if the condition is not treated. (See *color section*, *Intertrigo*, page C38.)

Intertrigo can develop in any skin fold but is most common under the breasts, abdominal skin folds (pannus), and axillae as well as in the submaxillary area and groin or perineum. Obese patients may report a history of skin irritation under skin folds. Confounding factors, such as bed rest, immobility, fever, and the use of such medications as antibiotics and steroids, often increase the risk of recurrence once the patient is hospitalized.

Preventing intertrigo

Prevention of intertrigo is a key component of any bariatric skin care protocol. Preventive interventions focus on keeping the skin clean, dry, and well supported and minimizing the effects of moisture, pressure, friction, and shear. Use a gentle soap or no-rinse skin cleanser for bathing.[15] Pat skin dry with a soft cloth. Moisture accumulation between skin folds is an ongoing problem between bathing. Soft absorbent pads, such as soft linen or non-occlusive high-air-flow incontinence pads, can be placed between skin folds to off-load pressure, absorb moisture, and lessen friction and shear with movement. Some facilities have had success with a product called InterDry, which is designed to be placed in the skin folds of bariatric patients (Fig. 21-1). A properly fitted non-synthetic brassiere may also help achieve these goals in large-breasted women. Any material placed between skin folds should be changed frequently.

When repositioning bariatric patients in bed, make sure that the pannus is well supported with a pillow and separate the legs by placing a pillow between the knees to make sure there is adequate airflow to skin fold areas. Low-air-loss beds may help dry moist areas; however, a less expensive alternative is

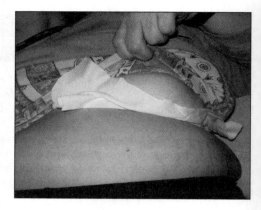

Figure 21-1. InterDry, a product used to prevent intertrigo in bariatric patients.

placing air tubing under the sheets to enhance air circulation.

Some authors recommend the use of cornstarch, talc, moisture barriers, and prophylactic antifungal powders and creams.[15–18] Powders often cake, creating more skin damage when removed. Moisture barriers are most effective when placed on skin that is subjected to external sources of moisture, such as urine, feces, and wound drainage. Products containing dimethicone may reduce friction. There is no evidence to support the use of prophylactic antifungal agents. At the first signs of *Candida intertrigo*, topical antifungals should be started. (See *color section,* page C38, bottom photo.)

Treating intertrigo

A wide variety of products have been used to treat intertigo[18]; however, the most effective treatments are based on an analysis of the underlying etiology. *Candida* should be treated with topical antifungal products; systemic antifungal agents such as fluconazole may be necessary in severe cases. Likewise, bacterial infections of the skin may be treated with topical antibiotics or, if not improving or if progressing to cellulitis, systemic antibiotics. Topical and systemic steroids may be useful in cases of atopic or contact dermatitis.[17]

Unfortunately, intertrigo may continue to plague obese patients even after weight loss. Panniculectomy and other forms of recontouring surgery may be necessary to remove excessive skin folds after weight loss has been achieved.[19]

PRESSURE ULCERS

Prevention

Pressure ulcer prevention is discussed in chapter 13, Pressure ulcers. This discussion focuses on the unique risk factors and needs of the bariatric patient in preventing pressure ulcers.

Unique risk factors

Several factors increase pressure ulcer risk in the bariatric patient. Because adipose tissue is not well vascularized, it is more susceptible to the ischemic effects of pressure. Pressure mapping studies indicate that pressure is distributed somewhat differently in obese patients. In patients of normal weight, high-pressure areas in the supine position are predominantly over bony prominences (for example, the head, sacrum, and heels). In the obese patient, a large amount of weight-induced force is distributed over the entire supine surface. Pressures may be high over bony prominences, but high-pressure areas are also seen in traditionally soft-tissue areas such as the buttocks. Even though the surface area is larger in an obese patient, there is still often greater tissue weight than normal on traditionally soft-tissue areas. (See *Pressure distribution*.)

RISK ASSESSMENT

Standard risk assessment tools such as the Braden Scale are still important as general screening measures for pressure ulcer risk status. However, you should delve more deeply into each subscale when caring for an obese

---

Pressure distribution

High-pressure areas are more focused over bony prominences in patients with a lower body mass index (BMI). A more diffuse pattern of high pressure distribution is evident in the patient with a higher BMI. High-pressure areas occur over soft-tissue areas as well as bony prominences.

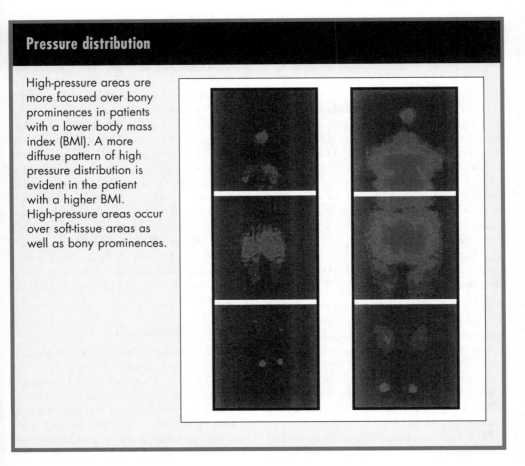

patient. Consider the following questions when planning care for your bariatric patients:

- For patients on bed rest, what positioning strategies will improve respiration without increasing shear risk?
- Can pillows be placed under the arms to prevent sliding and shear? Would a trapeze over the bed help with patient mobility?
- Is the bed wide enough for the patient to turn?
- Even though the patient may appear overweight, is his or her nutritional status really adequate?
- If moisture from incontinence is an issue, could it be improved by providing a bariatric bedside commode or walker to ambulate to the bathroom?
- Because stress incontinence is frequently a problem in obese patients due to greater weight on the pelvic floor, are you also creating functional incontinence because you have not provided the appropriate toileting equipment?

BARIATRIC EQUIPMENT

In order to meet the individualized needs of your bariatric patients, a full range of bariatric support equipment must be used in addition to, of course, the correct size bed. These include bariatric chairs, commodes, toilets, walkers, wheelchairs, and canes. Proper equipment should be made available well in advance of the patient's arrival. Both rental and purchase arrangements are available from a wide variety of manufacturers.

When selecting a bariatric bed, some basic criteria should be considered. Ask yourself these questions:

- Is the bed wide enough? Fit the individual to the bed from the time of admission.[14]
- Can the patient turn in the bed? Confirm that the bariatric patient's girth does not touch the side rails of the bed when the patient is turned from side to side.[14]
- What is the weight capacity for the bed? This is important for the safety and dignity of the patient.
- Even if the usual weight capacity of the bed is appropriate for your patient's weight, does

your patient "bottom out" or leave indentations in the bed over areas of higher weight distribution? (Remember the discussion about apple-shaped versus pear-shaped physiques.)

- Is a trapeze (or other supportive structure) available so that the patient can assist with turning?
- Does the bed have a turn-assist mode?
- Does the bed have features to assist with moisture control if indicated? Consider using features that provide air flow over the surface of the skin to facilitate fluid evaporation if the skin is excessively moist.[14]
- Is the bed designed for easy patient egress to help facilitate remobilization?
- Are wheelchairs and chairs in the room wide enough to accommodate the individual's girth?[14]

STAFF CONCERNS

Equipment characteristics and safety features are of equal concern for the staff. Can staff transport the patient in the bed? Can the bed fit through the doors in the hospital? Can the bed be steered easily? Are bariatric-size lifts and air transfer mattresses available? Has the staff been properly trained to use bariatric equipment to ensure both staff and patient safety? Eliminating the fear of being injured while providing care requires education of the staff with regard to proper lifting and handling techniques as well as available equipment. It should be a part of an organization's educational program to fully prepare all patient care staff on safe handling of the bariatric patient. This will prevent injuries and provide a high level of care that diminishes tissue damage and reduces the inherent risks associated with bariatric patients.[1]

REPOSITIONING AND CARE

Repositioning the bariatric patient is both an art and a science. Routine turning should be accomplished by a team of trained caregivers in a manner that preserves the patient's dignity. When possible, enlist the patient's help in turning. Patients and their families often have very useful suggestions for achieving and maintaining mobility despite challenges. The frequency of repositioning should be based on the individual's ability to tolerate turning and repositioning. Bariatric patients who cannot reposition themselves should be assessed frequently and repositioned as often as needed.

When repositioning bariatric patients in bed, several strategies are particularly important. Be sure to off-load bony prominences the patient has been lying on. Rather than repositioning pillows under the patient's shoulders and hips, you should turn the patient off bony prominences. Several people or the use of turn-assist devices may be required to accomplish repositioning without creating friction or shear injuries. Without adequate assistance, you are more likely to drag rather than lift the patient. Grabbing and pulling on a patient may also cause skin tears. Small shifts in body weight may be effective based on the research of Oertwich and colleagues.[20] However, small shifts are intended as an adjunct, not a replacement, to regular repositioning in high-risk patients.

OFF-LOADING HEELS

Heels should be floated off the surface of the bed by placing pillows under the calf or with the use of positioning devices. Examine the unique anatomy of your patient's lower extremities. Patients with large calves may be naturally suspending their heels off the surface of the bed. Feel under the heel and leg to note any high-pressure areas that can be relieved with properly placed pillows that redistribute weight. When using heel-positioning devices, make sure they are properly sized for your patient and can be applied without creating high-pressure areas under straps or other areas of the device.

PANNUS CARE

The pannus, or "abdominal apron," and other areas of adipose tissue are suspended by gravity when the patient is standing. While on bed rest, these tissues create pressure on the underlying skin. Place pillows or soft folded bath blankets under the pannus and other skin folds to keep the area dry and off-load pressure. If the patient has any tubes or other medical devices, make sure they are not under the weight of the pannus or other skin folds. An object as simple

as a pillow between the legs can help prevent damage from a Foley catheter.

ULCER LOCATIONS AND CHARACTERISTICS

Pressure ulcers that do develop in obese patients often have slightly different characteristics. They develop not only over bony prominences but also over other areas of high tissue pressure, such as the buttocks. (See *Pressure distribution.*) Bilateral hip ulcers are commonly seen in patients placed in chairs that are too narrow for their hip size.[6] Bariatric patients seem to be at higher risk for pressure damage related to medical devices (such as tubes, oxygen tubing, endotracheal tubes, oximetry probes, and tight narrow tracheostomy ties). Many of these pressure ulcers can be prevented with proper selection of bariatric-sized equipment, proper application of equipment, and frequent inspection of the skin under the equipment for high-pressure areas or tissue damage.

Deep tissue injury

There is some clinical speculation that suspected deep tissue injury (sDTI) may also be more common in obese patients. Deep pressure may predispose the patient to deep injury. When assessing the skin of bariatric patients, check carefully for subtle signs of sDTI, such as slight discoloration of the skin, and changes in skin temperature and texture. If deep tissue injury is suspected, off-load the affected area in an attempt to reduce pressure and salvage any tissue that is injured but not ischemic.

SUMMARY

Strategies based on expert opinion, patient and family experiences, and the limited published scientific evidence of the bariatric patient population have been presented. The use of an interdisciplinary team is key to understanding more fully the interdepartmental impact of caring for overweight patients in all healthcare settings. Little research has been conducted on appropriate skin care and pressure ulcer prevention in this population. Research has been cited when available, yet much remains to be done. Research to evaluate the outcomes of care and implementation of bariatric protocols are needed. The National Association of Bariatric Nurses was formed several years ago. This group is diligently working on establishing bariatric guidelines for this special population.[21]

SHOW WHAT YOU KNOW—BARIATRIC POPULATION

1. Mirror-image inflammation in the skin folds of the obese patient is called:
   A. a skin tag.
   B. stretch marks.
   C. intertrigo.
   D. hyperkeratosis.

   ANSWER: C. *Intertrigo is an inflammation in the skin folds and often presents as a mirror image from the skin in one area touching the other. A, B, and D are skin manifestation seen in bariatric patients.*

2. Acanthosis nigricans is always a benign condition for which there is no treatment.
   A. True
   B. False

   ANSWER: B. *Acanthosis nigricans is usually benign but occasionally undergoes malignant changes. Ammonium lactate cream may improve the condition.*

3. Proper positioning for the bariatric patient confined to bed includes:
   A. using small shifts in body weight to replace turning.
   B. keeping the head of the bed flat at all times to prevent shear.
   C. avoiding pillows between the legs.
   D. supporting the pannus and other large skin folds.

   ANSWER: D. *The pannus and other skin folds should be supported. "Off-load" turns are necessary; small shifts may be an adjunct but do not replace turning. The head of the bed may need to be elevated for proper respiration; supporting the arms with pillows will lessen the chance of sliding and sacral shear. Pillows should be placed between the legs to provide air and pressure redistribution and avoid compression and pressure damage to a Foley catheter.*

REFERENCES: BARIATRIC POPULATION

1. Rush, A. "Bariatric Pressure Ulcer Prevention," *Bariatric Nursing & Surgical Patient Care* 3(2): 125-8, 2008.
2. Centers for Disease Control and Prevention. *Overweight and Obesity.* Atlanta, GA: Author, 2008.
3. Flegal, K.M., Carroll, M.D., Ogden, C.I., Johnson, C.L. "Prevalence and Trends in Obesity Among US Adults," *Journal of the American Medical Association* 288(14):1723-27, 2002.
4. Arterbum, D.E., Maciejewski, M.L., Tsevat, J. "Impact of Morbid Obesity on Medical Expendiurers in Adults," *International Journal of Obesity (Lond)* 29(31):334-39, 2005.
5. Gallagher, S.M. "Restructuring the Therapeutic Environment to Promote Care and Safety for Obese Patients," *Journal of Wound, Ostomy & Continence Nursing* 26:292-97, 1999.
6. Gallagher, S. "Taking the Weight Off with Bariatric Surgery," *Nursing 2004* 34(3): 58-64, 2004.
7. Gallagher, S. "The Challenges of Obesity and Skin Integrity," *Nursing Clinics of North America* 40(2):325-35, 2005.
8. Centers for Disease Control and Prevention. *Overweight and Obesity: Defining Overweight and Obesity.* Atlanta, GA: Author, 2006.
9. National Heart Lung and Blood Institute. *Clinical Guidelines on the Identification, Evaluation, and Treatment of Overweight and Obesity in Adults.* Washington, DC: Author, 1998, p 262.

10. Centers for Medicare and Medicaid Services. *Decision Memo for Bariatric Surgery for the Treatment of Morbid Obesity* (CAG-00250R). Washington, DC: Author, 2006.

11. Kennedy-Evans, K.L., Henn, T., Levine, N. "Skin and Wound Care for the Bariatric Patient," in Krasner, D.L., Rodeheaver, G.T., Sibbald, R.G. (eds.), *Chronic Wound Care: A Clinical Source Book for Healthcare Professionals*, 4th ed. Malvern, PA: HMP Communications, 2007, pp 695-99.

12. Pieper, B., et al. "Bariatric Surgery: Patient Incision Care and Discharge Concerns," *Ostomy Wound Management* 52(6):48-61, 2006.

13. Pieper, B., et al. "Discharge Information Needs of Patients after Surgery," *Journal of Wound, Ostomy & Continence Nursing* 33(3):281-90, 2006.

14. National Pressure Ulcer Advisory Panel and European Pressure Ulcer Advisory Panel. *Prevention and Treatment of Pressure Ulcers: Clinical Practice Guideline*. Washington, DC: National Pressure Ulcer Advisory Panel, 2009.

15. Hahler, B. "An Overview of Dermatological Conditions Commonly Associated with the Obese Patient," *Ostomy Wound Management* 52(6): 34, 2006.

16. Wilson, J.A., and Clark, J.J. "Obesity: Impediment to Postsurgical Wound Healing," *Advances in Skin & Wound Care,* 17(8):426-35, 2004.

17. Janniger, C.K., et al. "Intertrigo and Common Secondary Skin Infections," *American Family Physician,* 72(5):833-38, 2005.

18. Mistiaen, P., et al. "Preventing and Treating Intertrigo in the Large Skin Folds of Adults: A Literature Overview," *Dermatology Nursing* 16(1):43, 2004.

19. Gallagher, S. and Gates, J.L. "Obesity, Panniculitis, Panniculectomy, and Wound Care: Understanding the Challenges," *Journal of Wound, Ostomy and Continence Nursing* 30(6):334-41, 2003.

20. Oertwich, P.A., Kindschuh, A.M., and Bergstrom, N. "The Effects of Small Shifts in Body Weight on Blood Flow and Interface Pressure," *Research in Nursing & Health* 18(6):481-88, 1995.

21. Rose, M.A., and Drake, D.J. "Best Practice for Skin Care of the Morbid Obese," *Bariatric Nursing and Surgical Patient Care*, 3(2)129-130, 2008.

CHAPTER 22

Pressure Ulcers in Neonatal and Pediatric Populations

Mona Mylene Baharestani, PhD, ANP, CWON, CWS

Objectives

After completing this chapter, you will be able to:

- identify pediatric pressure ulcer risk assessment tools
- describe factors that place neonates and children at risk for pressure ulcers
- discuss disparities between adult patients and neonatal and pediatric patients that may lead to potential problems in providing skin and wound care.

Very few research articles related to the neonatal or pediatric wound care populations have been published. Therefore, clinical guidelines and literature to support best practices in preventing and treating pressure ulcers in small children are sparse.

Epidermal stripping, extravasation injuries, incontinence-associated perineal dermatitis, and pressure ulcers are some of the most common injuries seen in this very young population. This chapter focuses mainly on pressure ulcers in the neonatal and pediatric populations.

INTEGUMENTARY DEVELOPMENT

The premature neonate, at 24 weeks' gestation, has minimal stratum corneum and rete ridges are very thin and small. Premature neonates are born with red, wrinkled, translucent skin that is almost gelatinous in appearance. Subcutaneous tissue has not yet developed, so the dermal tissue (dermis) is lying over the muscle. Skin stripping from the removal of tape or adhesive products can result in a full-thickness injury.

As subcutaneous fat deposit begins to form (weeks 26 to 29), skin wrinkling starts to decrease. Maturity of the integumentary system is complete at approximately 33 weeks' gestation. As the infant continues to develop (40 weeks' gestation), the stratum corneum begins to increase in thickness. The skin remains extremely fragile and easily insulted.

PRESSURE ULCER PREVALENCE AND INCIDENCE

Pressure ulcer prevalence rates as high as 27% and 20% have been reported in pediatric intensive care units (PICUs) and neonatal intensive care units (NICU), respectively, with the majority of these ulcers occurring within 2 days of admission.[1-5] Among hospitalized children in non-critical areas, variable prevalence rates of 0.47% to 27.7% have been cited.[6-8] These rates increase dramatically in children with myelomeningocele (37% to 97%)[9,10] and spinal cord injuries (22% to 55%).[11]

Pressure ulcer incidence rates among hospitalized non-critical children range from 0.29% to 6%,[6,12] while PICU incidence rates range from 3.4% to 27%[1-5] (see *Table 22-1*). Reports of pressure ulcer incidence in the NICU range from 19% to 23%.[3,13]

TABLE 22-1	Pressure Ulcer Incidence in the Pediatric Intensive Care Unit (PICU)	
Investigator	**Year**	**Incidence**
Neidig et al.[15]	1989	16.9% (pre-guideline) 4.8% (post-guideline)
Zollo et al.[64]	1996	26%
Willock et al.[65]	2000	15.6%
Curley et al.[5]	2003	27%
McLane et al.[1]	2004	3.4%
Bahrestani et al.[3]	2004 2005	20% (pre-guideline) 5.8% (post-guideline)

FINANCIAL IMPACT

In a 4-year longitudinal study at the Children's Hospital Medical Center of Akron, the skin status of patients with spina bifida and spinal cord injuries was tracked.[14] Of the 4,533 hospital days studied, 994 (22%) were attributed to pressure ulceration at a cost of over $1.3 million.[14]

ANATOMICAL DISTRIBUTION

The occiput is the most common anatomical site for pressure ulcer formation in patients from birth to age 3, as the head comprises a disproportionately higher percentage of the total body weight at this age.[13,15] When lying supine, the occiput is the primary pressure point with the greatest interface pressure.[16,17] In older children, similar to adults, the sacrum and heels are the most common sites for pressure ulceration. Among children with myelomeningocele, pressure ulcers are most frequently seen over the gibbus, ischial sectionregion, and perineum.[10] (See *color section, Occiput pressure ulcer,* page C39.)

> ### ▶ PRACTICE POINT
>
> The occiput is the most common site for pressure ulcers in children from birth to age 3.

COMPLICATIONS

Pressure ulcer formation in neonatal and pediatric populations can result in increased morbidity, mortality, infection, sepsis, osteomyelitis, pain, scarring alopecia, altered body image, grief, anxiety, depression, social isolation, and parental and family stress.[14,18–21]

RISK FACTORS

Pressure ulcer development has traditionally been viewed as uncommon among neonatal and pediatric populations given the presumed relative ease of repositioning and frequency of movement.[22,23] However, as survival rates among critically and chronically ill premature neonates and children increase through technological advances, so too does the risk for pressure ulcer formation.[24] Premature neonates with edematous, dry skin, attenuated rete ridges, little to no subcutaneous tissue, and immature organ systems are especially susceptible to the deleterious effects of pressure and shear forces.[25–28] Their anatomically immature skin is further challenged by multiple negative physiological responses to repositioning. In fact, repositioning of premature neonates can result in agitation, apnea, bradycardia, emesis, airway obstruction, tachycardia, and slower oxygenation recovery time than any other form of handling.[29–31] Consequently, prolonged periods of immobilization may be maintained, especially among those on extracorporeal membrane oxygenation (ECMO) and high-frequency oscillatory ventilation (HFOV).[29–31]

Medical equipment or devices

Pressure exerted on the soft tissue from monitoring and respiratory equipment also greatly increases the risk for ulcer formation in this highly vulnerable population. In fact, Willock and colleagues found that 50% of neonatal and pediatric pressure ulcers were directly associated with equipment pressing on the skin.[32] (See *Common devices that cause pressure ulcers in neonates and children*.) The high risk for ala, caudal septal, columnar, and nasal bridge pressure ulceration, which can occur secondary to nasal prong and mask continuous positive air pressure (CPAP), is of concern in all NICUs.[33–35] Preventive measures, such as hourly prong or mask repositioning with skin assessments and the use of protective hydrocolloid or silicone dressings, often prevent the occurrence of these devastating ulcers.[34,35]

Interestingly, in a retrospective cohort study of 64 NICU patients by Schmidt and colleagues, univariate analyses revealed that while more patients on HFOV developed pressure ulcers than those on conventional ventilation (53% vs. 12.5%), multivariate and life-table analyses found that PICU length of stay (LOS) was statistically more significant than ventilator type in predicting pressure ulcer risk.[36] Among prone children with acute respiratory distress syndrome (ARDS), increased risk of pressure ulcer development on the chin, chest, shoulders, knees, iliac crests, sternum, pretibial crests, ears, and corners of the mouth has been reported.[2]

In a case-controlled study of 118 PICU patients by McCord and colleagues, edema, PICU length of stay longer than 96 hours, increased positive end-expiratory pressure (PEEP), weight loss, and not turning the patient or using a specialty bed in turn mode were all identified as risk factors for pressure ulcer development.[37] Neidig et al. found that in pediatric open heart surgery patients, turning was not initiated postoperatively until hemodynamic and respiratory stability were achieved, as turning was not viewed as a priority or risk factor for pressure ulcers.[15] Furthermore, positioning of the head was often limited by internal and external

---

Common devices that cause pressure ulcers in neonates and children

- Arm boards
- Endotracheal tubes
- Head dressings and hats
- Improperly worn or improperly fitted orthotics
- Nasal continuous positive airway pressure (CPAP) and bilevel positive airway pressure (BiPAP) masks
- Nasal cannulae
- Gastrostomy tube bolsters
- Cables, intravenous tubing
- Cervical collars
- Blood pressure cuffs
- Sequential compression devices (SCD)
- Nasogastric or orogastric tubes
- Outgrown wheelchair or cushion
- Plaster casts, splints, braces
- Tracheal plates or ties
- Transcutaneous oxygen tension (TcPO$_2$) probes

jugular catheters, head and neck edema, and air leakage around endotracheal tubes with movement.[15]

Paralysis

Paralysis has been shown to be a risk factor for pressure ulcers in children in several studies.[9,10,38] In an attempt to obtain a more comprehensive understanding of pressure ulcer development among children and adolescents with spinal cord injuries (SCIs), a retrospective study was undertaken at the Chicago Shriners Hospital for Children.[9] Seventy-eight patients who sustained an SCI at age 12 or younger were enrolled. Of these 78 children, 43 (55%) developed at least one pressure ulcer, for a group total of 155 ulcers.[9] The risk factors identified were complete injuries, presence of scoliosis, and paraplegia. Those with paraplegia were more likely to have ulcers than those with tetraplegia, especially if the child was younger than age 12.[9]

Other risk factors

In a longitudinal study spanning more than two decades at the Seattle Children's Orthopedic Hospital and University of Washington's Neurodevelopmental/Birth Defects Clinic, Okamoto et al. analyzed morbidity and risk factors associated with skin breakdown in patients with myelomeningocele.[10] Among the 227 patients who developed pressure ulcers, high paraplegia, high sensory impairment, mental retardation, large head size, kyphosis or kyphoscoliosis, chronic fecal or urinary soiling, and an abnormal upper extremity neurologic examination were all implicated.[10] Okamoto and colleagues also noted that rates of pressure ulcer formation increased with age, until the children were 10 or 11, at which time occurrence leveled off at 20% to 25%.[10]

In a retrospective, exploratory study by Samaniego of 69 pediatric outpatients with a primary diagnosis of myelodysplasia, paralysis, insensate areas, high activity, and immobility were all identified as pressure ulcer risk factors.[38]

Lack of caregiver knowledge regarding risk factors and effective pressure ulcer prevention measures are also critical factors impacting patient risk.[12] In fact, the beliefs held by many clinicians that pressure ulcers are "inevitable," "irrelevant," or "simply not a problem in the neonatal and pediatric populations" are in themselves risk factors.[22,23,39–41]

RISK ASSESSMENT TOOLS

Currently there are 10 published neonatal/ pediatric pressure ulcer risk assessment scales[13,17,40–49] (see *Table 22-2*). (See also *Glamorgan scale*, page 558, and *Table 22-3, Neonatal and pediatric skin condition scales*, pages 556 and 557)[44–46,50–54] However, the only pediatric pressure ulcer risk assessment scales for which there are published sensitivity and specificity data are the Braden Q,[40] Neonatal Skin Risk Assessment Scale (NSRAS),[13] and Glamorgan.[44]

Both the Braden Q[40] and NSRAS[13] were modeled after the adult Braden Scale for predicting pressure ulcer risk. In developing the Braden Q Scale, Quigley and Curley adapted the six subscale descriptions for the pediatric population and added a tissue perfusion and oxygenation subscale.[5,40] In a multisite prospective study of 322 PICU patients, which excluded children with intracardiac shunting or unrepaired congenital heart disease, the Braden Q Scale was found to be 88% sensitive and 58% specific at a cut-off score of 16.[5] The Braden Q is recommended for those age 21 days through 8 years of age. For children older than age 8, Quigley and Curley suggest that the Braden Scale be utilized.[5]

NSARS measures six subscales pertinent to neonates.[13] The subscales are based on validity testing among 32 NICU patients and demonstrated a sensitivity of 83% and a specificity of 81%.[13]

The Glamorgan Scale risk factors were identified through literature review, clinical experts, and a multi-center study. When used in the assessment of pressure ulcer risk in 336 patients (1 day to 18 years of age), the Glamorgan Scale was found to be 98.4% sensitive and 67.4% specific at a cut-off score of 15.[44–46] The higher the Glamorgan total score, the greater the pressure ulcer risk: ≥10 = at risk, ≥15 = high risk, and ≥20 = very high risk.[44–46]

TABLE 22-2	Neonatal and Pediatric Pressure Ulcer Risk Assessment Tools	
Author	**Tool**	**Based on**
Barnes[49]	Barnes	Literature review
Bedi[42]	Bedi	Adult Waterlow
Cockett[47]	Cockett	Literature review
Garvin[43]	Garvin	Not specified
Huffiness and Lodgson[13]	NSRAS	Adult Braden
Olding and Patterson[17]	Pattold Pressure Scoring System	Literature review Key components for maintaining skin
Pickersgill[41]	Derbyshire	Medley and Adult Waterlow
Quigley and Curley[40]	Braden Q	Adult Braden Expert panel
Waterlow[48]	Pediatric Waterlow	Pediatric pressure ulcer risk factor identification and incidence study (Waterlow)
Willock et al.[44–46]	Glamorgan	Literature review Expert panel Pediatric pressure ulcer risk factors study (Willock)

TABLE 22-3	Neonatal and Pediatric Skin Condition Scales		
Author	**Tool**	**Based on**	**N**
Lund and Osborne[51]	Neonatal Skin Condition Scale	AWHONN & NANN Neonatal Skin Care Guidelines[54]	1,006
McGurk et al.[52]	Northampton Neonatal Skin Assessment Tool	Northampton General Hospital Skin Integrity Pressure Ulcer Standards	None
Perez-Woods and Malloy[53]	Loyola University Neonatal Skin Assessment Scale (LUNSAS)	Literature review Panel of experts	None
Suddaby et al.[50]	Starkid Skin Scale	Braden Q	347

N	Setting	Age	Sensitivity	Specificity
None	Pediatric acute care	Not specified	Not performed	Not performed
None	PICU progressive care unit	Neonate > 12 years	Not performed	None
None	PICU	Not specified	Not performed	None
None	PICU	Not specified	Not performed	None
32	NICU	26 to 40 weeks' gestation	83%	81%
None	PICU	Not specified	None	None
None	Not stated	Not specified	No	None
322	PICU	21 days to 8 years	88% (modified version 92%)	58% (modified version 59%)
302	Pediatric acute care	Neonate to 12 years	None	None
336	Pediatric acute care	Birth to 18 years	98.4%	67.5%

Setting	Age	Sensitivity	Specificity	Inter-rater Reliability
NICU, special care unit, well baby nursery	Birth to 28 days of age	None specified	None specified	65.9% to 89%
Not stated	Not stated	None specified	None specified	None specified
NICU	Neonates	None specified	None specified	90%
Pediatric acute care	PICU med-surg oncology adolescents	17.5%	99%	85%

Glamorgan Scale

The Glamorgan Scale[44-46] is comprised of 11 statistically significant pediatric risk factors that include:

- child cannot be moved without great difficulty or deterioration in condition
- child unable to change position without assistance; cannot control body movement; general anesthesia
- some mobility, but reduced for age
- equipment, objects, or hard surface pressing or rubbing on skin
- significant anemia (hemoglobin <9 g/dl)
- persistent pyrexia (temperature >100° F [38° C] for more than 4 hours)
- poor peripheral perfusion (cold extremities; capillary refill >2 seconds; cool, mottled skin)
- inadequate nutrition (unable to take; not absorbing oral or enteral feeds and not supplemented with hyperalimentation)
- low serum albumin (<3.5 g/dl)
- weight <10th percentile
- incontinence (inappropriate for age).

PRACTICE POINT

Use a pressure ulcer risk assessment scale designed for pediatric patients.

PRESSURE REDISTRIBUTION PRODUCTS

Although children are typically placed on support surfaces designed for adults, the clinical efficacy and safety of this practice raises serious concerns.[43,55,56] Low-air-loss beds designed for adults do not have the numerical option to accommodate for the height and weight of an infant or small child.[1] Children and infants often sink in and between cushions.[1] When adult specialty beds are placed in the turn mode, the occiput of small children pivots on the same pressure point, potentially increasing shear and friction and not redistributing pressure.[37] If a low-air-loss bed or alternating overlay is clinically indicated, only those that are age appropriate, clinically efficacious, and safe should be used in accordance with manufacturer's recommendations. A product currently available in this category is the Nimbus® Pediatric System (Huntleigh Healthcare, LLC, Eatontown, NJ), which is an alternating overlay for patients weighing between 13 and 55 lb.

According to the findings of Solis and colleagues, pressure redistribution devices effective for children are statistically different than those used for adults.[16] In their study of 13 healthy children ages 10 weeks to 13.5 years, the highest interface pressure readings were noted under the occiput (average, 59 mm Hg).[16] In older, larger children ages 10 to 14, the highest pressures were in the sacral area.[16] Convoluted foam (2″ to 4″ thick) was effective in decreasing these interface pressures.[16] Similarly, in a 2002 pilot study of 54 children at Texas Children's Hospital by McLane and colleagues, the highest interface readings were on the occiput from infancy to age 6 and on the occiput, coccyx, and heels from ages 6 to 18.[57] For children younger than age 2, use of the Delta foam overlay (Span America, Greenville, SC) resulted in the lowest interface occiput pressures.[57] For children over age 2, use of the Delta foam overlay with a Gel-E Donut pillow (Children's Medical Venture, Norwell, MA) significantly lowered occipital pressure and provided generalized pressure redistribution.[57]

Selection of appropriate support surfaces and positioning devices is adjunctive to manual offloading of pressure, as is medically feasible. In an examination of children undergoing cardiovascular surgery, Neidig and colleagues reported a 3.4-fold decrease in occipital pressure ulcer incidence after placement of 1.5″ foam cushions under all patients' heads in the operating room, followed by postoperative head repositioning in the PICU at least every 2 hours.[15]

Given that upwards of 50% of pressure ulcers are related to pressure from equipment and devices,[32] it's important to perform frequent skin assessments, rotate blood pressure cuffs and transcutaneous oxygen tension (tcPO2) probes, and provide sufficient padding under tracheostomy plates, nasal prongs, CPAP and BiPAP masks, arm boards, plaster casts, and traction boots. Proper fitting of orthotics, wheelchairs, and wheelchair cushions as children grow must also be ensured. Beds and cribs should be inspected to ensure that no tubing, cables, leads, hard toys, or syringe caps are inadvertently left under the patient's skin.[32] Tapes securing nasogastric and orogastric tubes, head dressings, and hats should be gently removed and the skin assessed for pressure injuries.

NUTRITIONAL CONSIDERATIONS

Malnutrition affects 15% to 20% of patients admitted to the PICU.[58] The systemic and immunological ramifications of malnutrition on this compromised population further limits their tissue tolerance to pressure, friction, and shear, especially as third spacing occurs. It's essential that the protein, caloric, and hydration needs of neonates and children be addressed as part of a comprehensive pressure ulcer prevention and treatment plan.

TOPICAL MANAGEMENT

When selecting a topical agent for use in the neonatal and pediatric populations, it is critical to consider the patient's age and degree of integumentary maturity, skin condition, product adherence, potential for skin sensitization, impact of product absorption, and need for avoidance of products containing dyes, fragrances, and preservatives.[22–24,59] Knowledge of product safety and manufacturer's recommendations in the neonatal and pediatric populations is essential.[22–24,60]

Normal saline and sterile water are commonly used for wound cleaning in neonatal and pediatric populations. Amorphous and sheet, preservative-free hydrogels and hydrofibers are utilized for pressure ulcer treatment, while thin hydrocolloids, foams, thin films, and silicone-based dressings may be used in both prevention and treatment. If the ulcer is necrotic and wound closure is the goal of treatment, then an appropriate method of debridement (surgical or autolytic) should be performed. (See chapter 8, Wound debridement.) Although anecdotal case reports exist of topical enzymes having been used in the neonatal and pediatric populations, manufacturer recommendations for topical enzymes are only for those over age 18; safety data for children do not exist.[60]

In the treatment of extensive, full-thickness pressure ulcers, negative-pressure wound therapy may be utilized to achieve wound closure or as a bridge to surgical closure.[61,62] In the presence of osteomyelitis, the need for appropriate systemic antibiotics must be addressed.

PATIENT EDUCATION

Education regarding pressure ulcer risk factors and effective prevention and treatment measures is essential for school nurses, teachers, teacher's aides, professional and lay caregivers, as well as children and their families at high risk. Integral to pediatric education is the recognition of each child's uniqueness, the developmental characteristics of each age group, and the psychological and psychosocial factors they face.[5,32]

Parents of high-risk infants should be taught to perform skin assessments during bathing, diaper changes, and catheterization. They should be warned of the risk of ulcer formation over the knees, ankles, and feet when crawling begins.[9] Toddlers and preschool-age children can be taught how to perform skin checks on their doll or teddy bear and then on themselves.[9] School-age children with upper-extremity abilities should be taught "lift-offs" with the use of mirrors to check the buttocks as well as how to ensure that their wheelchair cushion is functioning properly.[9] Written educational materials, alarm clocks or watches as reminders for lift-offs, and rewards for assuming self-care are beneficial.[9] As parents begin to relinquish control, they should maintain a safety-net role in their child's care.[9] Education of teenagers is best provided on a one-on-one basis with respect for their privacy.[9] Educational materials that are concise and focused on their tasks are best received.[9] Watches with automatic alarms to serve as a reminder for lift-offs are of benefit during this developmental stage as well.[9] Graphic images of pressure ulcers and discussion of the possible need for hospitalizations and surgery and time away from friends and social events will assist in emphasizing the importance of prevention.[9]

> **▶ PRACTICE POINT**
>
> The pressure ulcer prevention teaching plan should be specific to the child's age, developmental level, and individual characteristics.

SUMMARY

Based on available pressure ulcer prevalence and incidence data, neonates and children are at risk for developing pressure ulcers.[22–24,63] Neonates and children face unique problems from the development of pressure ulcers. Support surfaces and topical products manufactured for adults may not be suitable for use in neonates and children because their clinical efficacy and safety in these age groups are unknown.

Neonates and children require skin care specific to their needs. The development of much needed clinical practice guidelines and educational programs focused on pressure ulcers in neonates and children must address the immature integument of the premature neonate, including the potential for absorptive toxicity and disparities in weight distribution, and the physiological and psychological uniqueness of these populations while acknowledging the basic tenets found in adult models.[22–24,60]

1. What percentage of pressure ulcers in children are caused by medical equipment or devices?
   A. None
   B. 25%
   C. 50%
   D. 75%

   ANSWER: C. *Studies support that about 50% of pressure ulcers in children occur under medical devices.*

2. Which one of the following is a pressure ulcer risk assessment scale that can be used for a 5-year-old child?
A. Braden Scale
B. Waterlow Scale
C. Starkid Skin Scale
D. Glamorgan Scale

ANSWER: D. *The Glamorgan Scale is correct. The Braden Scale is not designed for adults but can be used for children older than age 8. The Braden Scale is not the same as the Braden Q Scale, which can be used for young pediatric patients. The Waterlow Scale is for adults; however, the Waterlow Pediatric Scale could be used for a 5-year-old child. The Starkid Skin Scale is used to assess skin condition and not pressure ulcer risk. Remember:* Skin assessment is not the same as pressure ulcer risk assessment.

REFERENCES

1. McLane, K.M., et al. "The 2003 National Pediatric Pressure Ulcer and Skin Breakdown Prevalence Survey," *Journal of Wound, Ostomy & Continence Nursing* 31(4):168-78, 2004.
2. Curley, M.A.Q., et al. "Predicting Pressure Ulcer Risk in Pediatric Patients: The Braden Q Scale," *Nursing Research* 52(1):22-31, 2003.
3. Baharestani, M., et al. "A Neonatal & Pediatric Evidence-linked Pressure Ulcer & Skin Care Performance Improvement Initiative," Poster abstract presented at the Symposium on Advanced Wound Care and Medical Research Forum on Wound Repair, April 21-24, 2005, San Diego, CA, 2005.
4. Curley, M.A. "Prone Positioning of Patients with Acute Respiratory Distress Syndrome: A Systematic Review," *American Journal of Critical Care* 8(6):397-405, November 1999.
5. Curley, M.A., et al. "Pressure Ulcers in Pediatric Intensive Care: Incidence & Associated Factors," *Pediatric Critical Care Medicine* 4(3):284-90, 2003.
6. Baldwin, K. "Incidence and Prevalence of Pressure Ulcers in Children," *Advances in Skin & Wound Care* 15:121-24, 2002.
7. Shluer, A.B., et al. "The Prevalence of Pressure Ulcers in Four Paediatric Institutions," *Journal of Clinical Nursing* 18:3244-52, 2009.
8. Groeneveld, A., et al. "The Prevalence of Pressure Ulcers in a Tertiary Care Pediatric and Adult Hospital," *Journal of Wound, Ostomy & Continence Nursing* 31(3):108-20, 2004.
9. Hickey, K., et al. "Pressure Ulcers in Pediatric Spinal Cord Injury," *Topics in Spinal Cord Injury Rehabilitation* 6(suppl):85-90, 2000.
10. Okamoto, G.N., et al. "Skin Breakdown in Patients with Myelomeningocele," *Archives of Physical Medicine & Rehabilitation* 64:20-23, 1983.
11. Thompson, H., et al. "The Recurrent Neutrotrophic Buttock Ulcer in the Myelomeningocele Paraplegic: A Sensate Flap Solution," *Plastic & Reconstructive Surgery* 108(5):1192-96, 2001.
12. Waterlow, J. "Pressure Sore Risk Assessment in Children," *Paediatric Nursing* 9(6):21-24, 1997.
13. Huffiness, B., Lodgson, M.C. "The Neonatal Skin Risk Assessment Scale for Predicting Skin Breakdown in Neonates," *Issues in Comprehensive Pediatric Nursing* 20:103-14, 1997.
14. Pallija, G., et al. "Skin Care of the Pediatric Patient," *Journal of Pediatric Nursing,* 14(2):80-87, 1999.
15. Neidig, J.R.E., Kleiber, C., Oppliger, R.A. "Risk Factors Associated with Pressure Ulcers in the Pediatric Patient Following Open-heart Surgery," *Progress in Cardiovascular Nursing* 4(3):99-106, 1989.
16. Solis, I., et al. "Supine Interface Pressure in Children," *Archives of Physical Medicinea and Rehabilitation* 69:524-26, 1988.
17. Olding, L., Patterson, J. "Growing Concern," *Nursing Times* 94(38):74-79, 1998.
18. Brook, I. "Microbiological Studies of Decubitus Ulcers in Children," *Journal of Pediatric Surgery* 26(2):207-9, 1991.
19. Gershan, L.A. "Scarring Alopecia in Neonates as a Consequence of Hypoxaemia-hypoperfusion," *Archives of Disease in Childhood* 68:591-93, 1993.
20. Kumar, K.A., Kumar, E. "A Pressure Sore in an Infant," *Journal of Wound Care* 2(3):145-46, 1993.
21. Kozierowski, L. "Treatment of Sacral Pressure Ulcers in an Adolescent with Hodgkin's Disease," *Journal of Wound, Ostomy & Continence Nursing* 23(5):244-47, 1996.
22. Baharestani, M.M., and Pope, E. "Chronic Wound Care in Neonates and Children," in Krasner, D., et al. (eds.), *Chronic Wound Care: A Clinical Source Book for Healthcare Professionals,* 4th ed. Malvern, PA: HMP Communications, 2007.
23. Baharestani, M.M. "Neonatal and Pediatric Issues in Wound Care," in McCulloch, J., and Kloth, L.

(eds.), *Wound Healing: Evidence Based Management*, 4th ed. Philadelphia: FA Davis Company. 2010.

24. Baharestani, M.M. "Neonatal and Pediatric Wound Care: Filling Voids in Knowledge and Practice," *Ostomy Wound Management* 53(6):8-9, 2007.

25. Eichenfield, L.F., Hardaway, C.A. "Neonatal Dermatology," *Current Opinion in Pediatrics* 11(5):471-78, 1999.

26. Campbell, J.M., Banta-Wright, S.A. "Neonatal Skin Disorders: A Review of Selected Dermatological Abnormalities," *Journal of Perinatal and Neonatal Nursing* 14(1):63-83, 2000.

27. Siegfried, E.C. "Neonatal Skin and Skin Care," *Pediatric Dermatology* 16(3):437-46, 1998.

28. Malloy, M.B., Perez-Woods, R.C. "Neonatal Skin Care: Prevention of Skin Breakdown," *Pediatric Nursing* 17(1):41-48, 1991.

29. Jetlefsen, L. "Postcranial Moulding," *Neonatal Network* 5(7):44, 1987.

30. Norris, S., Campbell, L.A., Brenkert, S. "Nursing Procedures and Alterations in Transcutaneous Oxygen Tension in Premature Infants," *Nursing Research* 31(6):330-35, 1982.

31. Long, J.G., et al. "Excessive Handling as a Cause of Hypoxemia," *Pediatrics* 65(2):203-7, 1980.

32. Willock, J., Harris, C., Harrison, J., Poole, C. "Identifying the Characteristics of Children with Pressure Ulcers," *Nursing Times* 101(11):40-43, November 2005.

33. Friedman, J. "Plastic Surgical Problems in the Neonatal Intensive Care Unit," *Clinics in Plastic Surgery* 25(4):599-617, 1998.

34. Smith, Z.K. "Adapting a Soft Silicone Dressing to Enhance Infant Outcomes," *Ostomy Wound Management* 52(4):30-32, 2006.

35. Jatana, K.R., et al. "Effects of Nasal Continuous Poitive Airway Pressure and Cannula Use in the Neonatal Intensive Care Unit Setting," *Archives of Otolaryngology—Head & Neck Surgery* 136(3):287-91, 2010.

36. Schmidt, J.E., et al. "Skin Breakdown in Children and High Frequency Oscillatory Ventilation," *Archives of Physical Medicine & Rehabilitation* 79: 1565-69, 1998.

37. McCord, S., McElvain, V., Sachdeva, R, Schwartz, P., Jefferson, L.S. "Risk Factors Associated with Pressure Ulcers in the Pediatric Intensive Care Unit," *Journal of Wound, Ostomy & Continence Nursing* 31(4):179-83, July-August 2004.

38. Samaniego, I.A. "A Sore Spot in Pediatrics: Risk Factors for Pressure Ulcers," *Pediatric Nursing* 29(4): 278-82, 2003.

39. Storm, K., Lund, J.T. "Skin Care of Preterm Infants: Strategies to Minimize Potential Damage," *Journal of Neonatal Nursing* 5(2):13-15, 1999.

40. Quigley, S.M., Curley, M.A.Q. "Skin Integrity in the Pediatric Population: Preventing and Managing Pressure Ulcers," *Journal for Specialists in Pediatric Nursing* 1(1):7-18, 1996.

41. Pickersgill, J. "Taking the Pressure Off," *Paediatric Nursing* 9(8):25-27, 1997.

42. Bedi, A. "A Tool to Fill the Gap-developing a Wound Risk Assessment Chart for Children," *Professional Nurse* 9(2):112-20, 1993.

43. Garvin, G. "Wound and Skin Care for the PICU," *Critical Care Nursing Quarterly* 20(1):62-71, 1997.

44. Willock, J., Baharestani, M.M., Anthony, D. "The Development of the Glamorgan Paediatric Pressure Ulcer Risk Assessment Scale," *Journal of Wound Care* 18(1):17-21, 2009.

45. Willock, J., Baharestani, M.M., Anthony, D. "A Risk Assessment Scale for Pressure Ulcers in Children," *Nursing Times* 103(14):32-33, 2007.

46. Willock, J., Baharestani, M.M., Anthony, D. "The Development of the Glamorgan Paediatric Pressure Ulcer Risk Assessment Scale," *Journal of Children's & Young People's Nursing* 1(5):211-18, 2007.

47. Cockett, A. "Paediatric Pressure Sore Risk Assessment," *Tissue Viability Society* 8(1):30, 1998.

48. Waterlow, J. "Pressure Sores in Children: Risk Assessment," *Paediatric Nursing* 10(4):22-23, 1998.

49. Barnes, S. "The Use of a Pressure Ulcer Risk Assessment Tool for Children," *Nursing Times Supplement* 100(14):56-8, 2004.

50. Suddaby, E.C., et al. "Skin Breakdown in Acute Care Pediatrics," *Pediatric Nursing* 31(2):132-48, 2005.

51. Lund, C.H., Osborne, J.W. "Validity and Reliability of the Neonatal Skin Condition Score," *Journal of Obstetric, Gynecologic, & Neonatal Nursing* 33(3): 320-27, 2003.

52. McGurk, V., et al. "Skin Integrity Assessment in Neonates and Children," *Paediatric Nursing* 16(3):15-18, 2004.

53. Perez-Woods, R., Malloy, M.B. "Positioning and Skin Care of the Low-birth Weight Neonate," *NAACOGS: Clinical Issues in Perinatal & Womens Health Nursing* 3(1):97-113, 1992.

54. Association of Women's Health, Obstetric and Neonatal Nurses (AWHONN). *Neonatal Skin Care. Evidence-Based Clinical Practice Guideline.* Washington, DC: Author, January 2001, p 54.

55. Willock, J. *A Study to Identify Characteristics Associated with Pressure Injury in Children.* School of Care Sciences, University of Glamorgan, Pontypridd, UK: The General Nursing Council for England and Wales Trust, 2003.

56. Law, J. "Transair® Paediatric Mattress Replacement System Evaluation," *British Journal of Nursing* 11(5):343-46, 2002.

57. McLane, K.M., Krouskop, T.A., McCord, S., Fraley, J.K. "Comparison of Interface Pressures in the Pediatric Population among Various Support Surfaces," *Journal of Wound, Ostomy & Continence Nursing* 29(5):242-51, 2002.

58. Norris, M.K., and Steinhorn, D.M. "Nutritional Management During Critical Illness in Infants and Children," *AACN Clinical Issues in Critical Care Nursing* 5(4):485-92, 1994.

59. Hoath, S., and Narandren, V. "Adhesives and Emollients in the Preterm," *Seminars in Neonatology* 5:289-96, 2000.

60. Baharestani, M.M. "An Overview of Neonatal and Pediatric Wound Care Knowledge and Considerations," *Ostomy Wound Management* 53(6):16-27, 2007.

61. Baharestani, M.M., et al. "V.A.C. Therapy in the Management of Paediatric Wounds: Clinical Guidance and Review" *International Wound Journal* 6 (Suppl. 1):1-26, 2009.

62. Baharestani, M.M. "Use of Negative PressureWound Therapy in the Treatment of Neonatal and Pediatric Wounds: a Retrospective Examination of Clinical Outcomes," *Ostomy Wound Management* 53(6):16-25, 2007.

63. Baharestani, M., Ratliff, C. "Pressure Ulcers in Neonates and Children: An NPUAP White Paper" *Advances in Skin & Wound Care* 20(6): 208-220, 2006.

64. Zollo, M.B., et al. "Altered Skin Integrity in Children Admitted to a Pediatric Intensive Care Unit," *Journal of Nursing Care Quality* 11(2):62-7, 1996.

65. Willock, J., Hughes, J., et al. "Pressure Sores in Children: The Acute Hospital Perspective," *Tissue Viability Society* 10(2):59-62, 2000.

CHAPTER 23
Palliative Wound Care

Diane K. Langemo, PhD, RN, FAAN

Objectives

After completing this chapter, you'll be able to:
- define palliative wound care
- discuss palliative wound treatment
- delineate treatment for a fungating wound
- explain treatment for a radiation wound.

DEFINING PALLIATIVE WOUND CARE

Palliative care is focused on holistically supporting the individual for comfort rather than cure, or healing of a wound, while improving the quality of living and dying for those who are at or near the end of life. In 1990, the World Health Organization (WHO) defined palliative care as care that affirms life and views death and dying as part of a normal process that neither speeds nor delays death, provides relief from pain and other symptoms, and offers support to the patient and family.[1] This definition is still relevant today. The 2002 National Consensus Project for Quality Palliative Care went a step further and added that palliative care is an organized and highly structured system that focuses care on promoting the greatest comfort for and dignity of the patient (www.nationalconsensusproject.org)[2] and is best delivered by a multidisciplinary team.[3] (See chapter 1, Quality of life and ethical issues.) In response to these national efforts, many (not most) hospitals in the United States have palliative care units or teams. However, in spite of these national-level studies and the growth in palliative care programs, public policies that focus on palliation need to be expanded.

Although the usual goal and plan of care is directed toward healing a wound, for individuals at the end of life (with a nonhealing wound), palliative wound care may be desired and the most appropriate goal. While often overlooked as the largest organ of the body, the skin can fail along with the other organs.[4] It is illogical to expect the skin to heal concomitant with the failure of other vital organ systems.[4,5] Most individuals, if not all, at the end of their lives are at risk for developing soft tissue ulceration.[6–13] Most professionals agree that pressure ulcers occurring at the end of life are often unavoidable, largely attributable to the individual's frail, compromised condition.[4,6,10,14–17] In fact, the literature is replete with reports that it is likely impossible to eradicate pressure ulcers in end-of-life patients with their many comorbid conditions and risk factors.[7,10,17–25] However, with education and teaching, which should include a thorough question and answer session between the patient and family and the physician and other healthcare professionals, the goal of care should then be established. The decision to move a patient from a curative to a palliative treatment plan requires that the clinician has determined that the wound is ultimately nonhealing (rather than undertreated) and that palliation is consistent with the patient's goals.[26,27]

EXTENT OF THE PROBLEM

Today, approximately 300 million individuals, or 3% of the world's population, are in need of end-of-life care every year.[28] Estimates are that by the year 2030, 20% of the U.S. population will be age 65 or older[10] and over 157 million Americans will suffer from chronic illnesses.[29,30] Given this demographic shift, a significant increase must be expected in the number of frail, elderly patients for whom cure may not be the goal. Overall, little information is available on wounds at the end of life.[31] Currently, however, wounds affect more than one-third of the nearly 1 million hospice patients in the United States, as well as many more patients at the end of life who are not under hospice care.[31]

Relatively few studies on pressure ulcer prevalence and incidence in end-of-life patients appear in the literature and, of those that do, most report on subjects with a cancer diagnosis. Little evidence on the prevalence and incidence of end-of-life wounds is available.[32] Reported prevalence rates vary between 13%[33] and 47%,[10,15,34] and incidence rates vary from 8%[3] to 17%.[10,15,16,34–36] In a home hospice study, Reifsnyder and Hoplamazian[36] found a 15% to 27% prevalence of pressure ulcers in a population with a 72-year mean age in whom the primary diagnosis was cancer. The primary comorbidity was cognitive-related disorders, with dementia being the primary risk factor.

Tippett[5] conducted a cross-sectional study of 383 hospice patients; 35% had skin wounds, of which 50% were pressure ulcers. The same author did a case-series analysis of 192 consecutive patients referred for wound consultation. The mean age was 82 years, 67% were female, and the subjects had multiple comorbidities, with dementia being the primary disorder. The researcher found that 40% of the wounds were pressure ulcers, with the primary location being the sacrum, followed by the heel, foot, and leg.[5] In both populations, pressure ulcers were almost exclusively stage III and IV, with concomitant necrosis and gangrene.[5] Tippett concluded that "wounds at the end of life are a problem of tragic proportion for the nearly 1 million hospice patients and millions of other frail, elderly persons living with chronic disease."[5]

RISK FACTORS FOR SKIN BREAKDOWN AND PRESSURE ULCER DEVELOPMENT

Several risk factors place individuals at the end of life at risk for the development of skin ulcers as well as impaired healing of skin ulcerations. Advancing age is a well-known risk factor. As one ages, skin becomes drier and more fragile and prone to injury; healing is slowed; the protective function of the epidermis is compromised; and the production of collagen decreases.[7,37–40]

Impaired mobility and repositioning

Any individual at the end of life experiences prolonged periods of inactivity or immobility, which contribute to the occurrence of tissue ischemia from prolonged pressure.[21,41–50] The risk of tissue breakdown increases when the individual is older, has more comorbid conditions, or has pain that decreases movement. Particularly vulnerable to pressure from inactivity are the heels, sacrum, and elbows. Suspending the heels over a pillow while supporting the entire length of the leg or using heel protectors is helpful in decreasing heel pressure.[44,51] A general guideline is to ensure that the individual with impaired mobility is repositioned every 2 to 3 hours. Repositioning is challenging for a patient who is hemodynamically unstable, has a great deal of pain, is nauseous or vomiting, or is unable to lie on one side or on the back.[16,44] Individual choices must be made after explaining the rationale for these interventions. (See chapter 11, Pressure redistribution: seating, positioning, and support surfaces.)

Friction and shear

Along with immobility, friction and shear are risk factors for pressure ulcer development. Shear stress is the "force per unit area exerted parallel to the plane of interest," and shear strain is the "distortion or deformation of tissue as a result of shear stress."[52] Friction is the "resistance to motion in a parallel direction relative to the common boundary of two surfaces."[52] When combined with pressure, these forces can accelerate tissue damage. To protect the buttocks and sacral areas, use a lift sheet or an overhead trapeze.[42,45,53–56] Protect the sacral area or other bony prominences with a transparent film or hydrocolloid to minimize friction.[44] While maintaining the head of the bed at the lowest elevation possible (ideally 30 degrees or less) is recommended to minimize friction and shear to the sacrum and buttocks,[44,51] this may not be consistent with the patient's condition or goals. For example, many individuals at the end of life have impaired ventilation and require the head of the bed to be raised. A pressure-redistributing mattress overlay or a specialty bed may also be helpful.[44,51] (See chapter 11, Pressure redistribution: Seating, positioning, and support surfaces.)

Nutrition and hydration

As the body systems are shutting down at the end of life, food and fluid requirements generally decrease as well. Individuals at the end of life have a diminished hunger and thirst mechanism, leading to dehydration, decreased oral intake, and impaired metabolism.[56] Lessening of oral intake can occur weeks to months before death.[57] Poor hydration impairs skin turgor, leaving tissue vulnerable to new breakdown. A decrease in protein intake leads to protein wasting and malnutrition. Albumin, a component of protein, provides colloid oncotic pressure to hold liquid in the vascular system. When oncotic pressure is decreased, fluid leaves the vascular system and enters interstitial spaces, causing tissue edema, lowered blood pressure, and impaired blood flow. Nutrition and hydration status can be further impaired if a draining wound causes the loss of large amounts of fluids and proteins in the exudate. At the end of life, the swallow reflex is decreased as well, impairing food and fluid intake and leaving the individual vulnerable to aspiration. Helping the family and loved ones to understand this end-of-life process can relieve their anxiety and stress. (See chapter 10, Nutrition and wound care.)

That protein-calorie malnutrition is associated with pressure ulcer development in individuals at the end of life has been demonstrated in several studies.[7,41–44,58–60] In fact, in a large retrospective cohort study of more than 2,400 adult nursing home residents, Horn and colleagues documented that an unintentional weight loss at any body mass index increased the chance of developing a pressure ulcer by 147%.[41] Cytokines, stress response proteins, are produced following tissue injury and contribute to the occurrence of malaise, anorexia, and consequent malnutrition, muscle wasting, and decreased albumin synthesis.[61] (See chapter 10, Nutrition and wound care).

Moisture

Moisture is another risk factor that can arise from perspiration, wound exudate, urine, and/or feces.[62] Incontinence is of particular importance with palliative care patients because of the risk for skin injury and breakdown. When incontinence is present, the primary goals are to prevent and manage skin breakdown, enhance comfort, and control odor. Feces are a chemical irritant to the skin, and their removal adds the element of a mechanical irritant, so gentleness is important. Skin protectants/barriers are also helpful.[44]

PALLIATIVE WOUND TREATMENT

The goals of palliative wound care differ little from those of curative wound care, aside from the goal of healing. Palliative care is the primary focus when it becomes apparent that the wound has failed to progress or when the patient's clinical condition deteriorates to a point at which aggressive measures are no longer appropriate. This can be particularly true in "nursing home residents with flexion contractures, cognitive impairment, and limited quality of life."[35] When it becomes apparent that wound healing would not render the patient's quality of life significantly better, wound stabilization and palliation become the focus of care. Palliative wound care focuses on controlling pain, choosing appropriate dressings, managing infection, and protecting the periwound area.

Skin care needs of the palliative care patient

The goal of palliative care is to optimize quality of life by controlling physical symptoms and monitoring the patient's psychosocial needs. Patients at the end of life are particularly at risk for skin breakdown. They experience a failure of the homeostatic mechanisms, including the skin's ability to counter insults such as pressure, friction, and shear. This includes decreased cutaneous perfusion and local tissue hypoxia, which ultimately reduce oxygen and vital nutrient utilization and removal.[63] The immune system also becomes imparied with skin breakdown. Thus, not all skin breakdown and pressure ulcers are avoidable.[44,63] When breakdown occurs, impaired oxygenation slows healing due to decreased hemoglobin levels, impaired gas exchange, and decreased blood pressure.[64]

Preventing and treating skin breakdown go a long way toward meeting palliative care goals. Skin breakdown can be prevented and treated through risk appraisal and assessment, meticulous skin care, positioning, reducing friction and shear, using support surfaces, providing nutrition and hydration, and managing moisture. Skin emollients applied according to manufacturer's directions are helpful in maintaining adequate skin moisture and preventing dryness.[44] When incontinence is present, it is important to minimize its harmful effects with skin barrier products.

PRACTICE POINT

End-of-life wound care focuses on:

- pain management
- odor control
- management of exudates
- bleeding control
- self-image
- dignity
- quality of life.

Patient and wound assessment

It is essential to perform a complete head-to-toe assessment of the end-of-life patient, including physical and psychosocial health and overall quality of life. A thorough assessment will assist the healthcare professional in realistically evaluating the need for preventive interventions as well as efficacy and cost-effectivenenss of achieving closure, should there be tissue breakdown. The assessment should establish both the risk for and the presence or absence of skin breakdown, including the presence of a pressure ulcer and the risk for developing additional ulcers. The following areas should be included in the patient assessment:[44]

- comorbid health problems
- medications the patient is taking
- risk factors present in the patient
- nutritional status
- diagnostic test results
- psychosocial implications
- environmental resources
- patient/family goals.

The Pressure Sore Risk Assessment Scale for Palliative Care[10] was developed for use in individuals at or near the end of life. Its seven subscales include sensation, mobility, moisture, activity in bed or chair, nutrition and weight change, skin condition, and friction and shear. Scores can range from 7 to 28, with a score of 12 or lower indicating low risk; 13 to 17, medium risk; 18 to 21, high risk; and 22 or over, very high risk. Risk assessment can be done weekly or with significant changes in condition. (See *Hunters Hill Marie Curie Centre Pressure Ulcer Risk Assessment,* pages 568 and 569.) Risk reassessments are important given the likelihood of the patient's deteriorating condition. As the end of life approaches, assessments may be performed less frequently in order to enhance comfort.[44]

Wounds or ulcers in end-of-life patients are often chronic in nature, as healing is significantly impaired due to physical condition and existing comorbidities. A chronic pressure ulcer has a well-defined border with surrounding nonblanchable erythema. When induration is present, it can extend outward from the wound edges. Many chronic wounds have rolled-under edges that impede wound healing and closure. Wound edges roll under when the wound bed is dry. In response, the wound attempts to preserve what little moisture is present and epithelialization is slowed, leaving the wound bed un-epithelializied. Most wounds have drainage, and chronic wound drainage contains destructive enzymes as well as fibroblasts that are less effective at producing collagen to heal the wound.[65] (See chapter 5, Acute and chronic wound healing.)

Patient's Name _____   Patient ID No. _____

SENSORY PERCEPTION Ability to respond meaningfully to discomfort related to pressure	**1 No impairment** Communicates discomfort clearly	**2 Slightly Limited** Responds to verbal commands but cannot always communicate discomfort or has sensory impairment in 1 or 2 extremities
MOISTURE Degree of skin exposure to moisture/fecal matter	**1 Rarely Moist** Skin rarely moist	**2 Occasionally moist** Skin occasionally moist, extra linen required once per day approximately
MOBILITY Ability to mobilize when out of bed	**1 Walks frequently** Walks around bed at least once every 2 hours and outside room at least twice a day	**2 Walks Occasionally** Walks occasionally during day for short distances but may require assistance
ACTIVITY Ability to change body and limb position when in bed or chair	**1 No limitation** Able to change position frequently and unaided	**2 Slightly Limited** Makes slight but frequent changes in body or extremity position
SKIN CONDITION Observed condition of skin in areas exposed to pressure	**1 Skin condition good** Skin appearance good, no evidence of edema, discoloration, etc.	**2 Fragile skin** Skin thin, fragile, dry, flaky, or edematous (e.g., due to age, steroids, edema, inflammation, or lymphedema)
NUTRITION/WEIGHT Food intake or weight change pattern	**1 Satisfactory** Food intake very good OR no significant weight change in last 6 months	**2 Marginally adequate** Weight appears normal Food intake slightly restricted
FRICTION/SHEAR Presence of friction/shear	**1 No apparent friction/ shear** Can lift body or limb completely without sliding when moving in bed or chair	**2 Occasional friction/ shear** Occasionally slides down bed or chair or drags body or limbs—due to position and poor muscle strength or fatigue

Low: 12 and under; Medium: 13 to 17; High: 18 to 21; Very High: 22 and over

Date of Admission _____ Date of First Assessment _____

		Date	Date	Date	Date
3 Very Limited Responds only to painful stimuli (i.e., moans or is restless or has sensory impairment over half of body surface) (e.g., spinal cord compression)	**4 Severely impaired** Unresponsive due to impaired consciousness or analgesia/sedation or has sensory impairment over most of body surface				
3 Very Moist Skin often but not always moist Linen changed at least once per shift	**4 Constantly Moist** Skin constantly moist with perspiration, urine, or lymphorrhea or in contact with fecal matter				
3 Chairfast Ability to walk severely limited Must be assisted into chair or wheelchair Spends more than 16 hours in chair or bed	**4 Completely Immobile** Spends all day in bed or chair—in excess of 20 hours (e.g., due to unconsciousness, pain, dyspnea, fatigue)				
3 Very Limited Only able to make occasional slight changes in body or limb position—usually requires assistance	**4 Immobile** Unable to change body or limb position due to pain, sedation dyspnea, edema, conscious level, etc.				
3 Skin marks easily Skin easily marked by support surface	**4 Skin integrity broken** Skin surface altered (e.g., due to incontinence dermatitis, pressure damage, wound, or skin condition)				
3 Probably inadequate Significantly underweight or overweight OR poor food intake	**4 Nutritional status very poor/severe cachexia** Nutritional status unsatisfactory due to cachexia, obesity, or minimal intake				
3 Frequent sliding Frequently slides down in bed or chair. Patient unable to lift limb or body without dragging (e.g, due to weakness)	**4 Almost constant friction/shear** Continually slides down bed or chair OR severe lymphedema, spasticity or agitation results in almost constant friction				
	TOTAL SCORE				
	SUPPORT SURFACE				

Maintenance of skin integrity

Careful attention to skin care in the end-of-life patient is exceedingly important, as a feeling of cleanliness can enhance an overall sense of comfort and well-being and can address any odor problems that might be present. A low pH skin cleanser is useful along with a moisture barrier to minimize the effects of excess moisture. Excess moisture can cause skin maceration, which interferes with the ability of the skin to withstand friction, shear, and pressure, thus making it vulnerable to injury.[51] Therefore, gently cleanse the skin, paying attention to the sacrum, elbows, and heels, which are prone to friction and pressure injury.[53, 54] Avoid massage over a reddened area as it can further damage tissue with already impaired perfusion.[51] Unless contraindicated, a gentle overall body massage is often appreciated in an individual at the end of life. Emollients and skin protectants are helpful in protecting the skin.[44]

Support surfaces

Support surfaces are "specialized devices for pressure redistribution designed for management of tissue loads, micro-climate, and/or other therapeutic functions (i.e., any mattress, integrated bed system, mattress replacement, overlay, or seat cushion, or seat cushion overlay)."[52] Some support surfaces provide the additional capability of turning or rotation assistance. It is important to match the support surface to the needs of the individual such that the surface redistributes weight over a larger area, thereby minimizing tissue pressures, particularly over bony prominences.[52] These surfaces are helpful for both the bed and the chair. Refer to the NPUAP/EPUAP guidelines[44] for more specific recommendations regarding pressure redistribution in palliative care patients.

PRACTICE POINT

Individualize the patient's turning and positioning schedule based on his or her pain tolerance and comfort level.

Nutrition and hydration

Meeting the nutrition and hydration needs of the palliative care individual can be very challenging and will likely change over the course of the dying process.

Evidence-Based Practice
Pressure redistribution in palliative care patients

1.0. Strive to reposition an individual receiving palliative care at least every 4 hours on a pressure-redistributing mattress such as viscoelastic foam, or every 2 hours on a regular mattress. (Strength of Evidence = B)

Brown, G. "Long-term Outcomes of Full-thickness Pressure Ulcers: Healing and Mortality," *Ostomy Wound Management* 49:42-50, 2003.

Evidence-Based Practice
Nutrition and hydration in palliative care patients

1.0. Allow the individual to ingest fluids and foods of choice. (Strength of Evidence = C)

1.1. Offer several small meals per day. (Strength of Evidence = C)

Brown, G. "Long-term Outcomes of Full-thickness Pressure Ulcers: Healing and Mortality," *Ostomy Wound Management* 49:42-50, 2003.

Pain management

Both prevention and treatment of skin breakdown can be uncomfortable for individuals at the end of life. The majority of patients with a pressure ulcer experience moderate to severe pain,[66-69] especially during dressing changes and wound bed treatments, and the pain can be acute or chronic.[70,71] In fact, 21 of 23 patients (91%) in one study reported a pressure ulcer as painful.[72] Likewise, in a systematic review of 15 studies addressing the impact of pressure ulcer pain, the authors concluded that "pain was the most significant consequence of having a pressure ulcer and affected every aspect of patients' lives."[73] In fact, pain from a pressure ulcer can

be the most distressing symptom an individual might report.[74] It is important to keep in mind that "pain is anything the patient says it is."[75]

Wound pain can be caused by the tumor pressing on nerves and blood vessels or by exposure of dermis.[76] Pain in wounds often arises from painful procedures, including cleansing and dressing removal, particularly if the dressing is dry and adherent.[77] Given that an individual at or near the end of life has a wound that likely will not heal, the wound and wound pain are chronic in nature. Chronic pain is pain that is persistent and can occur even when the wound is not being manipulated.[78] Concomitant acute pain can occur with dressing changes, treatments, and additional trauma to the area.

A mild to moderate opioid, such as 1 mg morphine or diamorphine mixed with 1 mg of a hydrogel,[79,80] or nonopioid medication can be used to relieve wound pain, as can a topical agent that contains a local anesthetic (for example, one with lidocaine, such as EMLA cream, Lidoderm, or Regenecare)[80,81,82] or a foam dressing containing ibuprofen (not available everywhere).[83,84] One hospital solely dedicated to caring for palliative patients has developed a unique mixture of Balmex and lidocaine 2.75%, which may be applied topically to painful and odorous wounds. They have reported success with this strategy.[85] Wound treatment pain can also be minimized by using minimal mechanical force for cleansing (4 to 15 psi irrigation force); using warmed products, such as normal saline or gauze pads;[86] and avoiding antiseptic and cytotoxic agents.[44,52]

PRACTICE POINT

Premedicating the patient with pain medication 20 to 30 minutes before changing the dressing is an important part of palliative wound care management.

Wound dressings

When possible, select a dressing that can remain in place for several days; however, this isn't always possible when a large amount of exudate is present. A dressing that protects

Evidence-Based Practice

Treating open pressure ulcers in palliative care patients

1.0. Diamorphine HDG is an effective treatment for open pressure ulcers [wounds] in the palliative care setting. (Strength of evidence = B)

Brown, G. "Long-term Outcomes of Full-thickness Pressure Ulcers: Healing and Mortality," *Ostomy Wound Management* 49:42-50, 2003.

periwound skin is also desirable, as is one that protects the wound from incontinence. As a rule, nonadherent and/or silicone dressings are best. Maintain a moist wound care environment to prevent exposure of delicate nerve endings,[87] as dry, desiccated wound beds and dressings are nearly always painful.[88] (See wound treatment options, chapter 9.)

Wound infection, odor, and exudate

Tissue deprived of oxygen and nutrients becomes devitalized and nonviable,[89] and bacteria thrive on this moist, devitalized tissue.[90] As the bacteria colonize, necrotic material appears in the wound and creates an odor, which varies depending on the bacteria present. Nonviable tissue eventually serves as a culture medium to support bacterial growth and inhibit leukocyte phagocytosis of bacteria.[89] Anaerobic bacteria are usually present in necrotic material, thrive in the absence of oxygen, and can become buried deeper within the wound. Anaerobic bacteria[88] also have a stronger, more offensive odor that can be particularly distressing to the patient. The wound appearance becomes black and leathery with exposure to air or yellow-gray when exposed to moisture, which occurs over varying lengths of time depending on the underlying disorder.[88]

It is the odor, drainage, and pain arising from the infection that are often the most distressing to the individual and therefore should be treated. Wound odor can be embarrassing to the individual and lead to isolation and poor quality of life.[2,19,91] Treatment is aimed at removing the cause of the odor and the odor itself. Because saturated dressings can hold odor, more frequent changing may help control the odor as well as the pain from the weight of the dressing. Frequent irrigation also helps remove exudate and odor. Nonviable tissue can be debrided, and autolytic debridement is often the least painful for the individual. Sharp debridement is more or less a last resort, and caution must be exercised to prevent excessive bleeding and/or pain.[91,92]

Nonsurgical (autolytic or enzymatic) debridement is recommended due to the tendency for bleeding and "seeding" of malignant cells in fungating and radiation wounds.[88] Topical metronidazole has also been used successfully to control odor.[2,62] Activated charcoal dressings are effective in controlling odor quickly,[19,91,93,94] as are occlusive dressings and frequent dressing changes.[19] Cadexomer iodine is an effective antiseptic,[95] as is povidone-iodine.[96] Silver dressings are effective for treating infections and thus in controlling odor. Dakin's solution (0.25% sodium hypochlorite) is another effective odor controller; it is saturated into gauze and placed in the wound for a limited time and may cause some discomfort.[96] Placement of larvae is another effective method of eliminating infection and controlling odor from wounds with extensive necrotic tissue.[97] Room deodorizers are also helpful. Sugar paste and honey are once again being used for their antibacterial and debriding properties.[98,99] The high sugar content produces a hyperosmotic wound environment to inhibit bacterial growth and assist in debridement.[98,99]

Periwound skin protection is crucial because exudate, which is liquid and sometimes caustic, can exacerbate skin damage[100] by causing maceration, breakdown, and itching.[44] Dressings that appropriately control exudate without unnecessarily increasing wetness or dryness are recommended, such as an alginate, hydrofiber, foam, or a nonadherent dressing, often with a secondary absorbent pad.[88,101,102] Be sure to change dressings when they become saturated, as heavy or overly saturated dressings can cause wound bed pain and irritate periwound skin. Alternatively, if exudate is minimal, a

Evidence-Based Practice
Wound dressing and odor control options for palliative care patients

1.0. Manage the pressure ulcer [wound] and periwound area on a regular basis as consistent with the individual's wishes. (Strength of Evidence = C)

1.1. Use antimicrobial agents as appropriate to control known infection and suspected critical colonization.[2,85,105,106] (Strength of Evidence = C)

1.2. Consider the use of properly diluted antiseptic solutions for limited periods of time to control odor. (Strength of Evidence = C)

1.3. Consider the use of topical metronidazole to effectively control pressure ulcer [wound] odor associated with anaerobic bacteria and protozoal infections.[2,85,106–110] (Strength of Evidence = C)

1.4. Consider the use of dressings impregnated with antimicrobial agents (for example, silver, cadexomer iodine, medical-grade honey) to help control bacterial burden and odor.[99] (Strength of Evidence = C)

1.5. Consider the use of charcoal or activated charcoal dressings to help control odor.[19,106,111,112] (Strength of Evidence = C)

1.6. Consider the use of external odor absorbers for the room (for example, activated charcoal, kitty litter, vinegar, vanilla, coffee beans, burning candle, potpourri).[2,107,113] (Strength of Evidence = C)

1.7. Cleanse the wound with each dressing change using potable water (i.e., water suitable for drinking),[114] normal saline, or a noncytotoxic cleanser to minimize trauma to the wound and help control the odor.[51,115] (Strength of Evidence = C)

1.8. Debride the ulcer [wound] of devitalized tissue to control infection and odor.[51,116,117] (Strength of Evidence = C)

1.9. Avoid sharp debridement with fragile tissue that bleeds easily.[51,100,113] (Strength of Evidence = C)

Brown, G. "Long-term Outcomes of Full-thickness Pressure Ulcers: Healing and Mortality," *Ostomy Wound Management* 49:42-50, 2003.

---

low-absorbency dressing, such as a hydrocolloid or semi-permeable film, is recommended.[103] A barrier film around the periwound area is helpful in controlling damage from moisture. See chapter 9, Wound treatment options, for further information on dressings.

PRACTICE POINT

Odor control is vital for enhancing quality of life for wound patients receiving palliative care.

The inflammatory fluid that seeps from the extracellular spaces is what is known as exudate. All bacteria produce exudate, the color and odor of which vary according to the causative organism.[88] For example, green exudate generally indicates gram-negative, aerobic bacteria, which respond well to silver found in many dressings now on the market.[88] The more persistent the inflammation or infection is, the more exudate that will be produced. Exudate frequently contains proteins; when combined with inadequate oral intake of protein commonly seen in the end-of-life individual, the degree of hypoproteinemia can increase. Managing exudates can be a major challenge.[104]

FUNGATING WOUNDS

Fungating wounds occur when the skin and its supporting blood and lymph vessels are infiltrated by a local tumor or by metastatic spread from a primary tumor, resulting in oxygen starvation to the tissue and eventual necrosis.[118–121] It's reported that approximately 5% to 10% of patients with metastatic cancer will develop a fungating wound.[122] The incidence in elderly individuals over age 70 is higher.[102,114] Although these wounds often develop during the last months of life, they can be present for years.[19] The most common site for development of a fungating wound is the breast, but they can also be found on the head and neck as well as in an area of melanoma. The anatomical location and the delicacy of the surrounding tissue make it challenging to address these wounds.

The term fungating refers to a malignant process of both ulcerating and proliferative growth through direct invasion.[116,117] An ulcerating wound will produce a crater-like wound, whereas a lesion with a predominantly proliferative growth pattern often develops into a nodular "fungus"- or "cauliflower"- appearing lesion.[123,124] Mixed-appearing lesions can also develop.[124,125] Skin tumors tend to become ulcerated because the skin is a bacterially contaminated surface.[126] Common symptoms of fungating wounds include exudate, pain, odor, pruritus, and bleeding as well as psychosocial issues.[120,121]

► PRACTICE POINT

Families, support persons, and caregivers may need emotional support when viewing patients with fungating wounds.

Fungating wounds rarely heal[127]; thus management is centered on symptom control, promotion of comfort, and maintenance or improvement of quality of life.[122,128] Assessment and management by healthcare providers, especially the nurse and physician, are most challenging.[129] Therefore, excellent interdisciplinary care and ongoing patient-caregiver communication are essential.

Care of fungating wounds

Nonsurgical (autolytic or enzymatic) debridement is recommended due to the tendency for bleeding and "seeding" of malignant cells.[88,101,120] Fungating lesions are friable and predisposed to bleeding. Hemorrhage due to erosion of blood vessels is the most common emergency seen in fungating wounds and can also be related to the decreased platelet function within the tumor.[116,119] Blood vessels can become eroded from the tumor cells themselves or secondary to necrosis or sloughing of tissues after radiotherapy.[130] To minimize bleeding, use a nonadherent or soft silicone dressing, maintain a moist wound bed, and clean by gentle irrigation rather than swabbing.[102] Dry dressings can cause bleeding when they adhere to the wound bed and should be avoided.[88,120] Alginate dressings have a high seaweed content and exchange sodium ions for calcium ions in the wound bed, thus encouraging the clotting cascade. Alginates must be used with caution in fragile tumors, however, because these dressings can also cause bleeding.[79] Hemostatic surgical sponges can also be used and left in place for a time.[19]

RADIATION WOUNDS

Radiation therapy targets a high-energy X-ray beam to an area of treatment. The target area is usually a tumor, the area surrounding a tumor, or an area where a tumor has been surgically removed. While each treatment is designed to target tissue at a particular depth, the tissues overlying the site can be affected as well.[131,132]

Radiation-related skin changes or ulcerations can occur in soft tissues during the course of therapy, immediately after therapy, or a long time following therapy.[131,132] Skin problems can also be noted in individuals who underwent treatments years ago before technological improvements in radiation machines were implemented. The skin reactions seen are generally specific to the area that was irradiated, and the inflammation can occur almost immediately.[132,133] Acute erythematous wounds result from the dilated blood vessels in the irradiated area. The ulceration may be large and may present initially as a draining sinus.[134]

The more common skin reactions associated with radiation therapy include flaking or peeling, redness, changes in pigmentation, loss of hair, decreased or absent perspiration,

TABLE 23-1	Oncology Nursing Society Classification for Skin Reactions
0	None
1	Faint erythema or dry desquamation
2	Moderate to brisk erythema or patchy moist desquamation, mostly confined to skin folds and creases; or moderate edema
3	Confluent moist desquamation ≥1.5 cm in diameter and not confined to skin folds; pitting edema
4	Skin necrosis or ulceration of full-thickness dermis; may include bleeding not induced by minor trauma or abrasion

Adapted from Oncology Nursing Society. *Radiation Therapy Patient Care Record: A Tool for Documenting Nursing Care.* Pittsburgh, PA: Author, 2002, with permission of the publisher.

superficial blood vessel changes, edema, ulceration, and scarring.[126,132,135] (See *Common radiation wound skin reactions.*)

Changes at the cellular level can be reflected by poor healing at the site. Healing is impeded related to atrophy of the epidermis and epidermal accessory structures, microvascular occlusions, exuberant connective tissue, decreased fibroblast reproduction, and significant amounts of cellular damage.[126,134]

Common radiation wound skin reactions

- Flaking or peeling (dry desquamation)
- Erythema
- Alteration in pigmentation
- Hair loss
- Loss of perspiration or sebaceous excretion
- Changes in superficial blood vessels
- Edema
- Ulceration (moist desquamation)
- Scarring

From: Smith, S. *Skin Care Following Radiation Therapy: The Clinician's Notebook.* Carrington Laboratories, Inc. Newsletter;1(3):1-3. Available at: http://www.woundcare.org/newsvol2 n2./ar3.htm. Accessed July 13, 2010.

Most radiation-related lesions are superficial. In 1994, the Oncology Nursing Society created a classification system for radiation ulcers. This system was refined in 2002. The five-level classification system ranges from "0" or no skin problem within a radiation field to "4" or skin necrosis or ulceration of full-thickness dermis[136] (see *Table 23-1.*)

Treatment of a radiation-induced skin lesion is essentially like treatment for other types of wounds. Any tissue within a radiation field must be considered at high risk for potential breakdown and should be kept clean, appropriately moistened, and protected from potential injury. Skin can also be protected by avoiding restrictive clothing, adhesives, harsh chemicals, heat or sunlight, and trauma. Should a minor skin reaction such as erythema or dry desquamation occur, the same guidelines apply, along with use of a topical hydrogel or a steroid cream.[126] Moist desquamation is also treated in the same manner as described above, with the addition of a nonadherent or foam dressing to manage the wound environment. It's important to cover the wound to prevent evaporation of fluid, control pain, and reduce risk of infection.[132,133]

Severe ulceration or necrosis needs to be treated as an open wound, using moist wound healing principles.[132,126] However, it's important to first rule out a new malignancy in the area.[133] Skin grafting or growth factor application may be required.[115] As a consequence of the vascular changes and resultant hypoxia, irradiated tissues have a decreased ability to fight infection. Avoiding or controlling infection is important, and antibiotics are best delivered topically.[134] The vascular changes and hypoxia also are responsible for pain being present in these ulcerations.[134] These wounds are typically difficult to manage and slow to heal. In all instances, systemic support is necessary to enhance the patient's healing potential in order to minimize further trauma to the wound site.[132]

SUMMARY

While cure is not always realistic, it's possible to provide compassionate and symptom-relieving treatment for palliative care patients who have wounds. This includes balancing the management of local wound symptoms, such as pain, odor, exudate, and bleeding, while preserving patient dignity and self-esteem and maximizing quality of life. Few randomized clinical trials or other research studies exist in the area of palliative wound care. However, there is a consensus document from the International Palliative Wound Care Initiative that looks at managing these wounds across the life continuum.[137] Continued study is needed to more clearly understand when a palliative care goal is appropriate. A comprehensive palliative wound care program needs to be developed in clinical agencies that work with these patients. The interdisciplinary team would include the physician, nurses, wound care specialists, dietitian, chaplain services, social services, and pain and hospice consultants.[54] Palliative care units are increasing in number, particularly for patients who are chronically, but not terminally, ill.[138] Wounds treated appropriately, even when the goal is not healing, can markedly improve in 50% of the cases, even on a hospice unit.[4]

PATIENT SCENARIO

Clinical Data

Mr. M is an 86-year-old widow who has end-stage cancer with bone metastasis. Because he is quite coherent, refuses to be hospitalized, and insists on staying in his home, his family is caring for him with the assistance of hospice. While Mr. M is consuming liquids fairly well, his food intake is very minimal; he eats very little, even with encouragement. With his small frame, his current weight is 109 lb, down from his usual weight of about 165 lb. He remains continent and uses a bedside commode with assistance. Upon assessment, the hospice nurse identifies a stage III pressure ulcer over the left greater trochanter measuring 2.5 × 2.3 × 0.3 cm, and there is a moderate amount of tan/green exudate with a slightly foul odor emanating from it. He also has a stage IV pressure ulcer measuring 0.25 × 0.25 cm on the left ear.

The family has tried both a sheepskin and an air overlay on his bed, but Mr. M insisted they be removed because he didn't like them. Mr. M informs the hospice nurse that he is "ready to go, and doesn't wish for any fancy or heroic treatments. Just let me be."

Case Discussion

Based on the initial assessment, the hospice nurse identified a number of problems that needed to be addressed. The assessment included ascertaining both Mr. M's goals of care and those of his family. Mr. M expressed his desire to just be kept comfortable. His wish was to remain in his own bed with a "pillow top" mattress rather than in a "hospital" bed, and he was adamant that he did not wish to have any other pressure-redistributing devices on his bed. While a plan of care would include regular repositioning, Mr. M verbalized that "it hurt less to lie on my left side on the ulcer than in any other position." The nurse educated him on the risk for further breakdown of the ulcer and ear as well as other areas of his skin. With encouragement from his family, Mr. M agreed to lie on his back and right side for 30 minutes each and on his left side for 2 hours at a time, on a rotating basis. Bilateral heel protectors were used, and his legs were elevated with pillows placed lengthwise in the bed.

Mr. M's ulcer was cleansed at each dressing change with an antiseptic solution to assist with odor management and covered with a composite dressing. A foam dressing was used on the ear to cushion and protect it. A pie tin with charcoal was placed under his bed to absorb room odor. A skin protectant was used, particularly over bony prominences, to help prevent further breakdown and protect his fragile skin.

Mr. M's dietary likes and dislikes were also assessed. After being educated on the need for protein for strength and energy to get up to the bedside commode, he agreed to consume three high-protein liquid drinks per day, along with popsicles, ice cream, and occasionally oatmeal and a piece of cold meat rolled with a slice of cheese, as tolerated.

After pain assessment as well as 30 minutes prior to dressing changes, Mr. M was medicated using a non-opioid medication. Mr. M was encouraged to request a "time-out" during dressing changes if needed.

While the pressure ulcer over the left greater trochanter did not heal, it only increased in size to $3.5 \times 3.5 \times 0.3$ cm prior to his death. This outcome was within the goal of the patient and family. The ulcer on the left ear did not heal either, nor did it increase in size. Taking care to position Mr. M's head when he was on his left side proved helpful in preventing deterioration. Mr. M remained coherent up until his death. Two days prior to his death, Mr. M expressed his appreciation for allowing him to do things "his way."

SHOW WHAT YOU KNOW

1. Which of the following defines palliative care?
   A. An organized and highly structured system to deliver care focused on promoting the greatest comfort and dignity of the patient
   B. Care that affirms life yet strives to deliver highly organized care to an individual who is focused on regaining a former health state
   C. A care delivery system focused on wound healing and elimination of symptoms
   D. Care that is delivered at home by loved ones without the involvement of healthcare providers

   ANSWER: A. *Palliative care is focused on holistically supporting an individual for comfort rather than care or healing of a wound, while improving both quality of both living and dying. Palliative care affirms life and views death as part of a normal process and is implemented to neither delay nor speed death. Palliative care provides relief from pain and other symptoms yet is not focused on the complete elimination of these symptoms. Answers B, C, and D do not define palliative care.*

2. Which of the following situations would constitute palliative wound care?
   A. Wet-to-dry dressing changes every 4 hours around the clock
   B. Calcium alginate dressings used on a necrotic-appearing wound with minimal exudate
   C. Silver-impregnated dressings used on a wound with little evidence of inflammation and essentially no evidence of infection
   D. A hydrogel dressing placed on a wound every 3 days and as needed

   ANSWER: D. *A hydrogel dressing that is placed on a wound every 3 days and as needed is recommended in a palliative care patient with a wound, as the hydrogel provides for a moist wound environment, which is soothing and comforting to the patient. It assists in protecting the periwound skin from maceration and is nonadherent, which is desirable. A silver-impregnated or calcium alginate dressing is not necessary unless there is heavy exudate or signs of infection or moderate to severe inflammation. Wet-to-dry dressings that are changed every 4 hours could likely contribute to periwound maceration and cause pain.*

(continued)

SHOW WHAT YOU KNOW *(continued)*

3. Which of the following orders should the clinician question in caring for a fungating wound?
   A. Using nonadherent dressings
   B. Using cold saline when irrigating the wound
   C. Using a mixture of morphine with amorphous hydrogel
   D. Using music and other relaxation techniques when providing care

   ANSWER: B. *Warm rather than cold saline is recommended when irrigating wounds in palliative care patients. Answers A, C, and D are appropriate management strategies.*

4. A patient with a grade 3 (Oncology Nursing Society classification system) skin reaction would require which the following interventions:
   A. None, skin is normal
   B. Frequent application of skin moisturizer
   C. Use of a protective skin barrier
   D. Enzymatic debridement ointment three times per day

   ANSWER: C. *The skin is moist and desquamated, so it needs protection from injury caused by the edema and wetness. Answer A is incorrect because the skin is compromised and needs care. Answer B is incorrect as the skin is too moist already. Answer D is incorrect because debridement is not indicated. In addition, debridement agents do not need to be applied as frequently as three times per day.*

REFERENCES

1. World Health Organization. *Cancer Pain Relief,* 2nd ed. Geneva: Author, 1996.
2. National Institutes of Health. *Improving End-of-Life Care. State-of-the-Science Conference Statement.* Bethesda, MD: Author, December 6-8, 2004.
3. Alvarez, O., et al. "Chronic Wounds: Palliative Management for the Frail Population," *Wounds* 2002:14(8 Suppl):1-27.
4. Langemo, D.K., and Brown, G. "Skin Fails Too: Acute, Chronic, and End-Stage Skin Failure," *Advances in Skin & Wound Care* 19(4):206-11, 2006.
5. Tippett, A.W. "Wounds at the End of Life," *Wounds* 17(4):91-98, 2005a.
6. Naylor, W. "Malignant Wounds: Aetiology and Principles of Management," *Nursing Standard* 16:45-56, 2002.
7. Henoch, I., Gustafsson, M. "Pressure Ulcers in Palliative Care: Development of a Hospice Pressure Ulcer Risk Assessment Scale," *International Journal of Palliative Nursing* 9:474-84, 2003.
8. Bale, S. "The Contribution of the Wound Care Nurse in Developing a Diabetic Foot Clinic." *British Journal of Clinical Governance* 7:22-6, 2002.
9. van Rijswijk, L., Lyder, C.M. "Pressure Ulcer Prevention and Care: Implementing the Revised Guidance to Surveyors for Long-Term Care Facilities," *Ostomy/Wound Management* 4(Suppl):7-19, 2005.
10. Chaplin, J. "Pressure Sore Risk Assessment in Palliative Care," *Journal of Tissue Viability* 10(1):27-31, 2000.
11. Colburn, L. "Pressure Ulcer Prevention for the Hospice Patient. Strategies for Care to Increase Comfort," *American Journal of Hospice Care* 4:22-6, 1987.
12. Froiland, K.G. "Wound Care of the Advanced Cancer Patient," *Hematology and Oncology Clinics of North America* 16:629-39, 2002.
13. Langemo, D.K., Anderson, J., Hanson, D., Hunter, S., Thompson, P. "Understanding Palliative Wound Care," *Nursing* 37:65-6, 2009.
14. Baharestani, M.M. "The Lived Experience of Wives Caring for Their Frail, Home Bound, Elderly Husbands with Pressure Ulcers," *Advances in Skin & Wound Care* 7:40-52, 1994.
15. Bale, S., et al. "Pressure Sore Prevalence in a Hospice," *Journal of Wound Care* 4(10):465-66, 1995.
16. Hatcliffe, S., and Dawe, R. "Monitoring Pressure Sores in a Palliative Care Setting," *International Journal of Palliative Nursing* 2(4):182-86, 1995.
17. Langemo, D.K., Black, J. "Pressure Ulcers in Individuals Receiving Palliative Care: A National Pressure Ulcer Advisory Panel White Paper," *Advances in Skin & Wound Care* 23(2):59-72, 2010.

18. National Pressure Ulcer Advisory Panel. "Avoidable versus Unavoidable Pressure Ulcers." (in press)

19. Naylor, W. World Wide Wounds: Part 1: Symptom Control in the Management of Fungating Wounds. Available at: http://www.worldwidewounds.com/2002/march/Naylor/Symptom-Control-Fungating-Wounds.html. Accessed May 15, 2010.

20. Bennett, R.G., et al. "Medical Malpractice List Related to Pressure Ulcers in the United States," *Journal of the American Geriatric Society* 48:73-81, 2000.

21. DeConno, F., Ventafridda, V., Saita, L. "Skin Problems in Advanced and Terminal Cancer Patient," *Journal of Pain Symptom Management* 6:247-56, 1991.

22. Gilchrist, B., Corner, J. "Pressure Sores: Prevention and Management – A Nursing Perspective," *Palliative Medicine* 3:257-61, 1989.

23. Moss, R.J., LaPuma, J. "The Ethics of Pressure Sore Prevention and Treatment in the Elderly: A Practical Approach," *Journal of the American Geriatric Society* 39:905-8, 1991.

24. Walding, M., Andrews, C. "Preventing and Managing Pressure Sores in Palliative Care," *Professional Nurse* 11:33-8, 1995.

25. Waller, A., Caroline, N.L. "Pressure Sores," In: *Handbook of Palliative Care in Cancer*. Boston, MA: Butterworth Heinemann; 2001, 91-98.

26. Weissman, D.E. *End-of-Life Cares Eases Pain and Prepares Patient for Death*. Health Link, Medical College of Wisconsin 2003. Available at: http://healthlink.mcw.edu/article/100171698.html. Accessed June 22, 2010.

27. Langemo, D.K. "When the Goal is Palliative Care," *Advances in Skin & Wound Care* 19(3):148, 150-54, 2006.

28. Singer, P.A., Bowman, K. "Quality End-of-Life Care: A Global Perspective." *BMS Palliative Care* 1:4, 2002.

29. Rice, K.N., et al. "Factors Influencing Models of End-of-Life Care in Nursing Homes: Results of a Survey of Nursing Home Administrators," *Journal of Palliative Medicine* 7(5):668-75, 2004.

30. Covinsky, K.E, et al. "The Last 2 Years of Life: Functional Trajectories of Frail Older People," *Journal of the American Geriatric Society* 51(4):492-98, 2003.

31. Tippett, A.W. "Wounds at the End of Life," *Journal of Palliative Medicine* 8(1):243, 2005.

32. Schim, S.M., and Cullen, B. "Wound Care at End of Life," *Nursing Clinics of North America* 40(2):281-94, 2005.

33. Hanson, D., et al. "The Prevalence and Incidence of Pressure Ulcers in the Hospice Setting: Analysis of Two Methodologies," *American Journal of Hospice Palliative Care* 8(5):18-22, 1991.

34. Galvin, J. "An Audit of Pressure Ulcer Incidence in a Palliative Care Setting," *International Journal of Palliative Nursing* 8(5):214-21, 2002.

35. Olson, K., et al. "Preventing Pressure Sores in Oncology Patients," *Clinical Nursing Research* 7(2):207-24, 1998.

36. Reifsnyder, J., and Hoplamazian, L. "Incidence and Prevalence of Pressure Ulcers in Hospice," *Journal of Palliative Medicine* 8(1):244, 2005.

37. Vanderwee, K., Clark, M., Dealey, C., Defloor, T., et al. "Development of Clinical Practice Guideline on Pressure Ulcers." *EWMA Journal* 7:44-6, 2007.

38. Ersser, S., et al. "Best Practice in Emollient Therapy: A Statement for Health Care Professionals," *Dermatology Nursing* 6:S2-19, 2007.

39. Davies, A. "Management of Dry Skin Conditions in Older People," *Nursing Standard* 13:250-7, 2008.

40. Lawton, S. "Effective Use of Emollients in Infants and Young People," *Nursing Standard* 19:44-50, 2004.

41. Horn, S.D., et al. "The National Pressure Ulcer Long-term Care Study: Pressure Ulcer Development in Long-Term Care Residents," *Journal of the American Geriatric Society* 52(3):359-67, 2004.

42. Brown, G. "Long-term Outcomes of Full-thickness Pressure Ulcers: Healing and Mortality," *Ostomy Wound Management* 49:42-50, 2003.

43. Reifsnyder, J., Magee, H. "Development of Pressure Ulcers in Patients Receiving Home Hospice Care," *Wounds* 17:74-9, 2005.

44. National Pressure Ulcer Advisory Panel & European Pressure Ulcer Advisory Panel. *Prevention and Treatment of Pressure Ulcers: Clinical Practice Guideline*. Washington, DC: National Pressure Ulcer Advisory Panel; 2009.

45. Bergquist, S., Frantz, R.A. "Pressure Ulcers in Community-based Older Adults Receiving Home Care: Prevalence, Incidence, and Associated Risk Factors," *Advances in Skin & Wound Care* 12:339-51, 1999.

46. Brink, P., Smith, T.F., Linkewich, B. "Factors Associated with Pressure Ulcers in Palliative Home Care," *Journal of Palliative Medicine* 9:1369-75, 2006.

47. Ferrell, B.A., Josephson, K., Norvid, P. "Pressure Ulcers Among Patients Admitted to Home Care," *Journal of the American Geriatric Society* 48:1042-47, 2000.

48. Pang, S.M., Wong, T.K. "Predicting Pressure Sore Risk with the Norton, Braden, and Waterlow Scales in a Hong Kong Rehabilitation Hospital," *Nursing Research* 47:147-53, 1998.

49. Perneger, T.V., Gaspoz, J.M., Rae, A.C., et al. "Contribution of Individual Items to the Performance of the Norton Pressure Ulcer Prediction Scale," *Journal of the American Geriatric Society* 46:1282-86, 1998.

50. Salzburg, C.A., Byrne, D., Cayten, C.G., et al. "Predicting and Preventing Pressure Ulcers in Adults with Paralysis," *Advances in Skin & Wound Care* 11:237-46, 1998.

51. Wound, Ostomy, Continence Nurses Society. *Guideline for Prevention and Management of Pressure Ulcers.* Glenview, IL: Author, 2003.

52. National Pressure Ulcer Advisory Panel. *Support Surface Standards Initiative: Terms and Definitions Related to Support Surfaces.* Available at: http://www.npuap.org/s3i.htm. Accessed June 28, 2010.

53. Chaplin, J., and McGill, M. "Pressure Sore Prevention," *Palliative Care Today* 8(3):38-39, 1999.

54. Dealey, C. *The Care of Wounds.* Oxford, UK: Blackwell, 1999.

55. Peerless, J., et al. "Skin Complications in the Intensive Care Unit," *Clinics in Chest Medicine* 20(2):453-67, 1999.

56. Emanuel, L., Ferris, F.D., von Gunten, C.F., Von Roenn, J.H. "End-of-Life Care in the Setting of Cancer: Withdrawing Nutrition and Hydration," *EPEC-O: Education in Palliative and End-of-Life Care for Oncology* (Module 11: Withdrawing Nutrition, Hydration). Chicago, IL: The EPEC Project, 2005.

57. End-of-Life Nursing Education Consortium (ELNEC). *Training Program: Faculty Guide.* Washington, D.C.: American Association of College of Nursing and City of Hope National Medical Center, 2002.

58. Bergstrom, N., and Braden, B. "A Prospective Study of Pressure Sore Risk Among Institutionalized Elderly," *Journal of the American Geriatric Society* 40(8):747-58, 1992.

59. Berlowitz, D.R., and Wilking, S.V. "Risk Factors for Pressure Sores: A Comparison of Cross-Sectional and Cohort-Derived Data," *Journal of the American Geriatric Society* 37:1043-59, 1989.

60. Pinchovsky-Devin, G., and Kaminski, M.V. "Correlation of Pressure Sores and Nutritional Status," *Journal of the American Geriatric Society* 34:435-40, 1986.

61. Posthaurer, M.E., Thomas, D.R. "Nutrition and Wound Care," in Baranoski, S., and Ayello, E.A., eds. *Wound Care Essentials: Practice Principles.* 2nd ed. Philadelphia: Lippincott Williams & Wilkins; 2008, 197.

62. Grey, J., Enoch, S., Harding, K.G. "Wound Assessment," *British Medical Journal* 332:285-8, 2006.

63. Sibbald, R.G., Krasner, D.L., Lutz, J. "SCALE©: Skin Cchanges at Life's End: Final Consensus Statement: October 1, 2009," *Advances in Skin & Wound Care* 23:225-38, 2010.

64. Sussman, C. "Wound Healing Biology and Chronic Wound Healing," in Sussman, C., and Bates-Jensen, B., eds. *Wound Care: A Collaborative Practice Manual for Physical Therapists and Nurses.* Gaithersburg, MD: Aspen Publishers, 1998.

65. Maklebust, J., and Sieggreen, M. *Pressure Ulcers: Guidelines for Prevention and Management,* 3rd ed. Philadelphia: Lippincott Williams, & Wilkins, 2001.

66. Langemo, D.K., Melland, H., Hanson, D., Hunter, S., Burd, C. "The Lived Experience of Having a Pressure Ulcer: A Qualitative Study," *Advances in Skin & Wound Care* 13:225-235, 2000.

67. Fox, C. "Living with a Pressure Ulcer: A Descriptive Study of Patients' Experiences," *British Journal of Community Nursing* 7:10,12,14,16,20,22, 2002.

68. Rastinehad, D. "Pressure Ulcer Pain," *Journal of Wound Ostomy & Continence Nursing* 33:252-56, 2006.

69. Bale, S., et al. "The Experience of Living with a Pressure Ulcer," *Nursing Times* 103:42-3, 2007.

70. Dallam, L., et al. "Pain Management and Wounds," in Baranoski, S. and Ayello, E.A., eds. *Wound Care Essentials: Practice Principles,* 2nd ed. Philadelphia: Lippincott Williams & Wilkins, 2008, 229-251.

71. Pasero, C.L. "Procedural Pain Management," *American Journal of Nursing* 98(7):18-20, 1998.

72. Spilsbury, K., Nelson, A., Cullum, N., et al. "Pressure Ulcers and Their Treatment and Effects on Quality of Life: Hospital Inpatient Perspective," *Journal of Advanced Nursing* 57:494-504, 2007.

73. Gorecki, C., et al. "Impact of Pressure Ulcers on the Quality of Life in Older Patients: A Systematic Review," *Journal of the American Geriatric Society* 57:1175-83, 2009.

74. Price, P. "An Holistic Approach to Wound Pain in Patients with Chronic Wounds," *Wounds* 17:55-7, 2005.

75. McCaffrey, M., and Pasero, C. *Pain: Clinical manual,* 2nd ed. St. Louis: Mosby, 1999.

76. Manning, M.P. "Metastasis to Skin," *Seminars in Oncology Nursing* 14(3):240-43, 1998.

77. Jones, M., et al. "Dressing Wounds," *Nursing Standard* 12(39):47-52; quiz 55-56, 1998.

78. Krasner, D. "The Chronic Wound Pain Experience: A Conceptual Model," *Ostomy/Wound Management* 41(3):20-29, 1995.

79. Grocott, P. "Controlling Bleeding in Fragile Fungating Tumors," *Journal of Wound Care* 7(7):342, 1998.

80. Twillman, R.K., et al. "Treatment of Painful Skin Ulcers with Topical Opioids," *Journal of Pain Symptom Management* 17(4):39-42, 1997.

81. Smith, N.K., et al. "Non-Drug Measures for Painful Procedures," *American Journal of Nursing* 97(8):18-20, 1997.

82. Briggs, M., and Nelson, E.A. "Topical Agents or Dressings for Pain in Venous Leg Ulcers," Oxford: The Cochrane Library, 2001.

83. Jorgensen, B., Friis, G.I., Gottrup, F. "Pain and Quality of Life for Patients with Venous Leg Ulcers: Proof of Concept of Efficacy of Biatain-Ibu, a New Pain Reducing Wound Dressing," *Wound Repair & Regeneration* 14:233-39, 2006.

84. Sibbald, R.G., et al. "A Pilot (Real-life) Randomized Clinical Evaluation of a Pain-relieving Foam Dressing: Ibuprofen-foam versus Local Best Practice," *International Wound Journal* 4:16-23, 2007.

85. Kalinski, C., et al. "Effectiveness of Topical Formulation Containing Metronidazole for Wound Odor and Exudates Control." *Wounds* 17:74-9, 2005.

86. Hollingworth, H. "Wound Care—Less Pain, More Gain," *Nursing Times* 93(46):89-91, 1997.

87. Hallett, A. Fungating Wounds, *Wound Care Society Education Leaflet*. Huntingdon, U.K.: Wound Care Society, 1993.

88. Hampton, S. "Managing Symptoms of Fungating Wounds," *Journal of Cancer Nursing* 20(1):21-28, 2006.

89. Slavin, J. "Wound Healing: Pathophysiology." *Surgery* 17(4):I-IV, 1999.

90. Rodeheaver, G. "Wound Cleaning, Wound Irrigation, Wound Disinfection," in Krasner, D.L., Rodeheaver, G.T., Sibbald, R.G., et al., eds. *Chronic Wound Care: A Clinical Sourcebook for Healthcare Professionals*, 4th ed. Wayne, PA: HMP Communications; 2008.

91. McDonald, A., Lesage, P. "Palliative Management of Pressure Ulcers and Malignant Wounds in Patients with Advanced Illness." *Journal of Palliative Medicine* 9:285-95, 2006.

92. Eisenberger, A., Zeleznik, J. "Pressure Ulcer Prevention and Treatment in Hospices: A Qualitative Analysis." *Journal of Palliative Care* 19:9-14, 2003.

93. Grocott, P. "Palliative Management of Fungating Malignant Wounds." *Journal of Community Nursing* [online] 14(3):2000. Available at: http://www.jcn.co.uk.backiss.asp?YearNum=2000&MonthNum=03&ArticleID=221. Accessed July 14, 2010.

94. Williams, C. "Role of CarboFlex in the Nursing Management of Wound Odour." *British Journal of Nursing* 10:123-35, 2001.

95. Falanga, V. "Iodine-containing Pharmaceuticals: A Reappraisal." *Proceedings of the 6th European Conference on Advances in Wound Management.* London, UK: Macmillian Mags Ltd.; 1997.

96. Ferris, F., vonGuten, C. Malignant wounds. 2nd ed. 2005. *Fast Facts and Concepts* #46. End-of-Life Physician Education Resource Center. Available at: http://www.eperc.mcw.edu. Accessed September 9, 2009.

97. Thomas, S., et al. "Odour Absorbing Dressings." *Journal of Wound Care* 7:246-50, 1998.

98. Cooper, R., Molan, P. "The Use of Honey as an Antiseptic in Managing *Pseudomonas* Infection," *Journal of Wound Care* 8(4):161-64, 1999.

99. Molan, P.C. "Re-introducing Honey in the Management of Wound and Ulcers – Theory and Practice," *Ostomy Wound Management* 48:28-40, 2002.

100. Cameron, J., Powell, S. "Contact Kept to a Minimum," *Nursing Times Wound Care Supplement* 92:39:85-6, 1996.

101. Grocott, P. "The Management of Fungating Malignant Wounds," *Journal of Wound Care* 5:232-34, 1999.

102. Pudner, R. "The Management of Patients with Fungating or Malignant Wounds," *Journal of Community Nursing* 12(9):1998. Available at: http: // www. jcn. co. uk / backiss. asp ? Y earNum = 1998&MonthNum=09&ArticleID=82. Accessed July 13, 2010.

103. Baranoski, S. "Wound and Skin Care, Choosing a Wound Dressing, Part 2," *Nursing 2008* 38(2): 14-15, 2008.

104. White, R., Cutting, K.G. "Modern Exudates Management: A Review of Wound Treatments," *World Wide Wounds* 2006. Available at: http:// www.worldwidewounds.com/2006/September/ White/Modern-Exudate-Management.html. Accessed December 21, 2010.

105. Paul, J.C., Pieper, B.A. "Topical Metronidazole for the Treatment of Wound Odor: A Review of the Literature," *Ostomy Wound Management* 54(3):18-27, 2008.

106. McDonald, A., Lesage, P. "Palliative Management of Pressure Ulcers and Malignant Wounds in Patients with Advanced Illness," *Journal of Palliative Medicine* 9:285-95, 2006.

107. Barton, P., Parslow, N., Savage, P. "Malignant Wound Management: A Patient-centered Approach," in Krasner, D.L., et al. *Chronic Wound Care: A Clinical Sourcebook for Healthcare Professionals.* 4th ed. Wayne, PA: HMP Communications, 2008.

108. Bale, S., Tebbie, N., Price, P. "A Topical Metronidazole Gel Used to Treat Malodorous Wound," *British Journal of Nursing* 13:S4-11, 2004.

109. Cutting, K. *Wound and Infection Education Leaflet.* Huntingdon, UK: Wound Care Society, 1998.

110. Pierleoni, E.E. "Topical Metronidazole Therapy for Infected Decubitus Ulcers," *Journal of the American Geriatric Society* 32:775, 1984.

111. Goldberg, M., Tomaselli, N.L. "Management of Pressure Ulcers and Fungating Wounds," in Berger, A.M., Portenoy, R.K., Weissman, D.E., eds. *Principles and Practice of Palliative Care and Supportive Oncology,* 2nd ed. Philadelphia: Lippincott Williams & Wilkins, 2002, 321-322.

112. Williams, C. "Clinisorb Activated Charcoal Dressing for Odour Control," *British Journal of Nursing* 8(15):1016-1019, 1999.

113. Ferris, F.D., Krasner, D., Sibbald, R.G. "12 Toolkits for Successful Wound Care. A Case-based Approach," *Journal of Wound Care* 9:4-9, 2000.

114. Haisfield-Wolfe, M.E., and Rund, C. "Malignant Cutaneous Wounds: A Management Protocol," *Ostomy/Wound Management* 43(1):56-60, 62, 64-66, 1997.

115. Ivetic, O., and Lyne, P.A. "Fungating and Ulcerating Malignant Lesions: A Review of the Literature," *Journal of Advanced Nursing* 15(1):83-88, 1990.

116. Mortimer, P.S. "Management of Skin Problems: Medical Aspects," in Doyle, D., et al. *Oxford Textbook of Palliative Medicine,* 2nd ed. Oxford, UK: Oxford University Press, 1998.

117. Englund, F. "Wound Management in Palliative Care," *RCN Contact* 2-3, Winter 1993.

118. Hastings, D. "Basing Care on Research," *Nursing Times* 89(13):70-6, 1993.

119. McMurray, V. "Managing Patients with Fungating Malignant Wounds," *Nursing Times* 99:55-57, 2003.

120. Alexander, S. "Malignant Fungating Wounds: Key Symptoms and Psychosocial Issues," *Journal of Wound Care* 18(8):325-29, 2009.

121. Adderly, U.J., Smith, R. "Topical Agents and Dressings for Fungating Wounds," *Cochrane Database of Systematic Reviews* 2, 2007.

122. Dowsett, C. "Malignant Fungating Wounds: Assessment and Management," *British Journal of Community Nursing* 8:394-400, 2002.

123. Collier, M. "The Assessment of Patients with Malignant Fungating Wounds—A Holistic Approach: Part 1," *Nursing Times* 93(440):(Suppl) 1-4, 1997.

124. Carville, K. "Caring for Cancerous Wound in the Community," *Journal of Wound Care* 4(2):66-8, 1995.

125. Young, T. "The Challenge of Managing Fungating Wounds," *Community Nurse* 3(9):41-44, 1997.

126. Smith, S. *Skin Care Following Radiation Therapy: The Clinician's Notebook.* Carrington Laboratories, Inc. Newsletter;1(3):1-3. Available at: http://www.woundcare.org/newsvol2n2./ar3.htm. Accessed July 13, 2010.

127. Bird, C. "Managing Malignant Fungating Wounds," *Professional Nurse* 15(4):253-256, 2000.

128. Naylor, W. "Using a New Foam Dressing in the Care of Fungating Wounds," *British Journal of Nursing* 10(Suppl 6):S24-30, 2001.

129. Laverty, D. "Fungating Wounds: Informing Practice Through Knowledge/Theory," *Brit J Nurs* 12(Suppl 15):S29-40, 2003.

130. Beare, P.G., and Myers, J.L. *Adult Health Nursing,* 3rd ed. St. Louis : CV Mosby, 1998.

131. Bryant, R. "Skin Pathology," in Bryant, N., ed. *Acute and Chronic Wounds: Nursing Management.* New York: Mosby Year Book, 1992.

132. Hunter, S., Langemo, D.K., Thompson, P., Hanson, D., Anderson, J. "Radiation Wounds," *Advances in Skin & Wound Care* 20(8):438-40, 2007.

133. Black, J.M., and Black, S.B. "Surgical Wounds, Tubes, Drains," in Baranoski, S., and Ayello, E.A., eds. *Wound Care Essentials: Practice Principles.* Philadelphia: Lippincott Williams & Wilkins, 2008.

134. Williams, H.D. *Radiation Ulcers.* Available at: http://www.emedicine. com/plastic/topic 466. htm. Accessed June 17, 2010.

135. Rudolph, R. "Radiation Ulcer," in Rudolph, N., and Noe, N.M., eds. *Chronic Problem Wounds.* Boston: Little, Brown & Co., 1983.

136. Mendelsohn, E., et al. "Wound Care After Radiation Therapy," *Advances in Skin & Wound Care* 15(5):216-224, 2002.

137. Ferris, F.D., et al. *Palliative Wound Care: Managing Chronic Wounds Across Life's Continuum: A Consensus Statement from the International Palliative Wound Care Initiative, 2004.* Available at: http://www.palliativewoundcare.info. Accessed June 12, 2010.

138. Morrison, R.S. "Palliative Care Outcomes Research: The Next Steps," *Journal of Palliative Medicine* 8(1):13-15, 2005.

CHAPTER 24

Wound Care Perspectives: Present and Future

Elizabeth A. Ayello, PhD, RN, ACNS–BC, CWON, MAPWCA, FAAN, and
Sharon Baranoski, MSN, RN, CWCN, APN–CCRN, DAPWCA, FAAN

Dear Wound Care Community,

Since the the last edition of our book, we have seen the wound care community come together to provide clinical guidelines, participate in joint conferences, and treat victims of natural disasters. It seems that partnering with others to enhance wound care education and outcomes has been the underlying theme. The National Pressure Ulcer Advisory Panel (NPUAP) and the European Pressure Ulcer Advisory Panel (EPUAP) developed and released international guidelines for pressure ulcer treatment and prevention in 2009. In 2010, the Wound, Ostomy and Continence Nurses Society (WOCN) issued its updated pressure ulcer guidelines and the World Health Organization (WHO) released its document entitled "Wound and Lymphoedema Management." In the same year, the American Professional Wound Care Association (APWCA) released a position paper explaining the mnemonic SELECT, which can be used to evaluate and incorporate guidelines into clinical practice.

As more and more clinicians embrace evidence-based practice, the need for access to the current literature has become critical. Some new international wound journals have emerged in recent years, and more and more journals now provide online access for their readers as well as pre-publication notification of key articles. At the 25th Annual Clinical Symposium on Advances in Skin & Wound Care in 2010, Dr. Keith Harding reported on the significant increase in wound care articles over the past three decades (see *Table 24-1*).

Keeping up with the literature is definitely a challenge given the busy workloads of most clinicians today.

Partnering to foster worldwide education

In 2008, the World Union of Wound Healing Societies (WUWHS) held its Third Congress in Toronto, Canada, where thousands of wound care delegates convened to discuss and learn about global wound care issues. Several WUWHS position documents were released during that Congress, and the online resource WoundPedia (www.woundpedia. com) was launched. This website contains succinct summaries of evidence on focused wound care topics. We look forward to the next meeting of the world's wound societies at the fourth WUWHS conference in Yokohama, Japan in September 2012 (http:// wuwhs2012.com/).

The Wound Healing Society (WHS) and the American Academy of Wound Management (AAWM) merged their annual conferences. In 2010, the first-ever joint conference of the WOCN and the World Council of Enterostomal Therapists (WCET) was held in Phoenix, Arizona. We applaud the partnering of wound care organizations to bring education to the widest audience possible. We hope this concept of joint partnership continues in the future.

Partnering to enhance education and patient outcomes

Changing regulations in the United States have provided the impetus for yet another kind of partnership. Clinicians have partnered across disciplines as well as across care settings to enhance patient outcomes and achieve compliance with new and existing regulations.

TABLE 24-1	Increase in Wound Care Articles, 1980–2010		
Decade	**Number of articles written**		
	Venous leg ulcers	**Pressure ulcers**	**Diabetic foot ulcers**
1980-1989	517	1,874	669
1990-1999	1,115	3,472	1,191
2000-2010	1,731	5,169	4,368

The Deficit Reduction Act of 2005 requires a quality adjustment in Medicare Severity Diagnosis Related Group (MS-DRG) payments for certain hospital-acquired conditions (HAC). The Centers for Medicare and Medicaid Services (CMS) has a program on Hospital-Acquired Conditions and Present on Admission (POA) Indicator Reporting. Inpatient prospective payment system (IPPS) hospitals are now required to submit POA information regarding diagnoses for inpatient discharges. This new POA regulation added yet another concern for IPPS hospitals regarding pressure ulcers. The requirement for documentation by CMS providers so IPPS hospitals would not suffer decreased financial implications necessitated educating physicians on pressure ulcer staging. The importance of consistent, complete documentation in the medical record cannot be overemphasized.

Other CMS regulations influenced changes in the Oasis-C (for home care) and MDS 3.0 (for long-term care) documentation systems. This has provided opportunities for those care settings to take a close look at what will be required to support wound care practices in their respective settings. Long-term care facilities and home-care agencies are required to track and report on improved outcomes of care in wound patients. Outcome-based quality improvement measures and reporting have also arrived in the acute care setting. Evidence-based practice will continue to be a challenge for all healthcare providers.

Clinician competency in wound care continues to be both a challenge and a concern. A wide variety of options exist today for fostering clinical competence. Numerous certification programs are available for all levels of clinical practice, from nurses to physicians to physical therapists and other professionals. In 2010, the NPUAP released revised pressure ulcer competencies for registered nurses on its website. Professional wound care organizations will continue to research and seek advanced knowledge to benefit the health of our patients. We have only touched the tip of what we need to know about wound etiology and the healing process. The future holds much promise, and the need to learn is ever present.

Partnering to help those in need

Wound care clinicians are dedicated individuals who are willing to step in and help out when the need arises. Perhaps this is most apparent in how the wound care community has come together after the natural disasters that have occurred around the world in recent years. Whether it was the tsunami in Indonesia or Japan, or the earthquakes in China, Chile, Haiti, or Japan, the wound care community responded with compassion and expertise to provide care for those in need.

Our personal wound wish list

Personally, we have worked hard to prepare and write this third edition of *Wound Care Essentials*, spending time away from family and friends, with no shopping and not enough swimming. Instead we have been sitting at our computers, either separately in Illinois and New York or together in either Sharon's home outside Chicago or Elizabeth's condo in South Florida. Rather than reviewing wound care in the past, present, and future, we decided in this last chapter to highlight what has been happening as well as share with you our "Wound Wish List."

So what follows is Elizabeth's and Sharon's wound wish list. We have asked for some of these items before and made some new requests as well. *Can you please make our wish list come true?*

- Can interdisciplinary wound care teams become a reality in all care settings? We realize this might be asking too much, but the literature supports better outcomes for patients when an integrated team of knowledgable wound experts provide care.
- While the 1960s discovery of moist wound healing, coupled with advancements in wound dressing materials, have dramatically changed wound care practices, the reality is that these dressings are not always available for patient care. Can't we somehow create a healthcare system that allows access to—and reimbursement for—the best dressing for a particular patient's wound needs in all healthcare settings?
- Can reimbursement coverage be changed so that the emphasis is on the adequacy of debridment rather than a "number"?
- Can evidence finally provide an answer to the best turning schedule to prevent pressure ulcers?
- Can we finally have curricula in all healthcare disciplines that ensure that graduates have the wound care essentials they need to become competent practitioners? Despite the many interdisciplinary wound care conferences, interdisciplinary education still has a ways to go. As basic education courses for clinicians are built in the next decade of the 21st century, can we implement interdisciplinary and integrative education so that the team who learns together can practice together in a seamless way?
- Can we eliminate the fragmentation of wound care documentation across disciplines and across care settings? Can we please have one assessment form for both patient assessment and documentation across care settings?
- Can certification in wound care be required for designation as a wound care practitioner? We are inspired by the efforts of the WOCN, which has achieved recognization as a nursing specialty by the American Nurses Association.

- Can wound care be recognized by the American Medical Association as a medical specialty, with residency training available throughout the United States and the world?
- Can we identify which risk factors predict pressure ulcers in different care settings? Can we reach a consensus on what "skin failure," Kennedy Terminal Ulcers, and other clinical concepts mean? Can we further determine the charactertistics of suspected deep tissue injury so that the defining characteristics and interventions to prevent the evolution of these ulcers can be more apparent?
- Can we have dressings that provide pain relief in the United States?
- Can we expect more collaboration between bench scientists and clinicians that will help us address the gaps in research regarding wound care practices?
- Can we develop handheld scanning devices that will be used by healthcare providers to detect stage I pressure ulcers so that preventive measures can be implemented *before* the epidermis breaks down?
- Can we create a wound "dipstick" that would tell us a wound's pH, protease level, bacteria level, and other characteristics and be linked to the right product to use?
- Can we enhance technology to create a microphone device (maybe on our identification badges) to document wound characteristics during dressing changes, and can this documentation automatically be processed to the patient's chart and the physician's office?
- Can we expect electronic signatures that will be triggered by our fingerprints?
- Can we expect that a universal electronic medical record will soon be a reality?
- Can we learn from others: Just as our cars have climate control, can we create a wound product that could scan the wound bed and adjust for the variations in wound characteristics?
- Can we make our healthcare system borderless through more international consultation for individual patient consults, whether through telemedicine or computer technology?

- And, finally, can persons with diabetes finally have attractive designer shoes that accommodate their foot deformities? This last wish list request is so important as we both love shoes!

Future wound care challenges

As we look at the growth of wound care, we realize that much has been achieved. Of course, we have much more to learn as research continues in this field that we love. The future holds many challenges. Dr. Keith Harding addressed these challenges in his closing lecture at the 2010 Clinical Symposium in Orlando:

- Changing demographics
- Rising expectations of the services that are provided
- Demand for high quality of care within specific time frames
- An information-driven society with easy access to technological data
- A global rise in chronic disease
- Financial, moral, legal, and ethical dilemmas

We look forward in future editions of this book to seeing how many of these challenges have been addressed, and when and how many items on our wish list have come true.

Respectfully,
Elizabeth and Sharon

INDEX

i refers to an illustration; *t* refers to a table; **boldface** indicates color page.

A

Abdominal compartment syndrome (ACS), 463–464
Abdominal wounds, penetrating, treatment of, 463
Acanthosis nigricans, **C37**
Activities of daily living, restrictions in, 8–9
Activity, pressure ulcer risk and, 332*t*–333*t*, 568*t*–569*t*
Acupuncture as pain management method, 317
Acute pain, 62, 296, 571
Acute wounds
    infection and, 129, 145
        indicators of, 135*t*–136*t*
    patient response to, 5
Adjuvant pain medications, 310
Admission assessment, 45–46, 53
Agency for Healthcare Research and Quality (AHRQ),
        31, 131, 295, 326
Age, patient response and, 305
Age of wound, documenting, 106
Aging, effects of, on skin, 59, 60*i*
Aircast Diabetic Walker, 437, 437*i*
Air-fluidized support surfaces, 275–276
Alternating pressure systems as support surfaces, 277
Ambulatory Payment Classifications, 25
Amino acids, wound healing and, 248–250
Analgesic ladder for pain management, 310
Angiogenesis, wound healing and, 89, 91*i*
Ankle-brachial index (ABI), 189, 368, 406–408
Ankle-foot orthoses, 438–439
Anorexia, prescription drugs linked to, 254
Answer as pretrial step, 38
Anthropometric factors, nutritional assessment and, 246
Antimicrobial dressings, 195–196
Antimicrobial therapy, 145–148, 409, 499
Antiphospholipid antibody syndrome as wound cause, 502
Antiseptic cleaning agents, 141–142
Apligraf, 196, 232*t*
Appellate process, 41
Appetite stimulants, dietary intake and, 258
Arterial system, 360–361, 368, 398–399,
        406, 414
    femoral artery in, 399–400, 414
    perfusion in, 398
    tibial arteries in, 400
    wall architecture in, 362–363
Arterial testing, 406–407

Arterial ulcers, 398–419, *See also* Vascular ulcers
    infection indicators in, 135*i*
    pain associated with, 299
    pathophysiology of, 401–402
    patient education for, 414–415
    signs and symptoms of, 404–405, **C22**
    treatment of, 409, 411
Arteriography, 413, 451
ASSESSMENT chart, pressure ulcer, 107
ASSESSMENTS chart, wound, 108
Atypical wounds, 491–508, **C28–C35**
    Buruli ulcer, 496–497, **C29**
    drug-induced causes of, 505
    external causes of, 492, 504
    Hansen's disease, **C29**
    infectious causes of, 491, 495
    inflammatory causes of, 492
    malignancies as cause of, 492, 504, **C33**
    metabolic disorders as cause of, 502
    types of, 491–492
    vasculopathics as cause of, 501, **C28**
Autolytic debridement, 171, 183, 190–191, 345, 371
        See also Debridement

B

Bacillary angiomatosis, human immunodeficiency
        virus/acquired immunodeficiency syndrome
        population and, 538
Bacteremia, assessing, 112, 127, 138
Balanced Budget Act of 1997, 22, 25–27
Bariatric patient population, 542–550, **C36–C38**
    classifying, 543
    deep tissue injury in, 549
    as health care concern, 542, 549–550
    intertrigo in, 545–546, **C38**
    meeting needs of, 543–544
    pressure ulcers in
        characteristics of, 549
        locations of, 549
        risk factors for, 547–548
    skin assessment in, 544–545, **C36–C38**
Basement membrane zone (BMZ), 57–60
    effects of aging on, 59, 60*i*
Becaplermin gel, 206, 230, 433, 440
    diabetic foot ulcers and, 433

Bed selection, pressure ulcer risk and, 515
Biliary drainage catheters, 482
Bioburden, 126–151
  infection and, 127–129
  inflammation and, 127
  managing, 140–141
Biochemical tests, nutritional assessment
    and, 240–248
Biological therapy for debridement, 157, 346,
    See also Debridement
Bledsoe Diabetic Conformer Boot, 436–437
Blue toe syndrome, 405, 405*i*
Body mass index, nutritional assessment
    and, 246
Braden Scale for predicting pressure
    ulcer risk, 332–333, 555
  intervention recommendations based on, 335, 512
Breach of duty in malpractice claim, 41–42
Burns, infection indicators in, 135–136
Buruli ulcer as wound cause, 496–497, **C29**
BWAT tool, 116
Bypass grafting
  arterial ulcers and, 411
  venous ulcers and, 412

C

Calciphylaxis as wound cause, 502–503, **C31**
  treatment options for, 503
Calcium alginate dressings, 171, 174*i*, 193–194
Candidiasis in skin fold, 546, **C38**
Capsaicin as pain management method, 317
Carbohydrates, wound healing and, 241, 248
Caregivers, challenges for, 15–16
Carville healing sandal, 437, 438*i*
Cast walkers for diabetic foot, 434–436
CEAP classification system, 366–367
Centers for Medicare and Medicaid
    Services, 22–23
Charcot Restraint Orthotic Walker, 438, 439*i*
Charcot's foot with infection, 300, 438, **C24**
Chemical burns as wound cause, 505
Chemotaxis, wound healing in, 85–87
Chest wall reconstruction, wound care
    for, 467
Chromoblastomycosis as wound cause, 498
Chronic pain, 62, 296–297, 313–314, 570
  interventions for, 297
Chronic wounds
  associations between cytokines, undernutrition,
    and, 254–255
  geography of, 117, 495, **C3**
  infection and, 83, 85, 87, 96, 97, **C6**
  molecular and cellular abnormalities
    in, 93–95
  patient response to, 5
Civil litigation, 38, *See also* Litigation process

Cleaning agents, 141–142
Cleaning devices, 143–145
Collaboration, documenting, 50
Collagenase as debriding agent, 169, 170–171
Collagen deposition, wound healing and, 90, 92
Collagen dressings, 194–195
Colonization, infection and, 127–129, **C6**
Communication, documenting, 53
Communication tool, medical record
    as, 43–45
Community-based ethical concerns, 14
Comparison as coping strategy, 9
Complaint as pretrial step, 38–41
Complex degenerative therapy, 279
Composite dressings, 194
Compression therapy
  dressings for, 203, 204*i*
  modalities used in, 210
  as venous ulcer treatment, 29, 371
Contact layer dressings, 195
Contamination, infection and, 128, **C6**
Coordination, documenting, 50
Coping patterns, 9
Copper, wound healing and, 249, 251
Coumadin necrosis, 318
Creep phenomenon, 267, 268
Criminal litigation, 38, *See also* Litigation process
Cryofibrinogenemia as wound cause, 492, 501, **C30**
Cryoglobulinemia as wound cause, 501–502
CUA (calcific uremic arteriopathy), 503, **C32**
Cutaneous drug eruptions, human immunodeficiency
    virus/acquired immunodeficiency syndrome
    population and, 533–534
Cyclic pain, 297
  interventions for, 297
Cytokine-induced cachexia, 254
Cytokine-mediated anorexia, 254
Cytokines
  chronic wounds and, 254
  wound healing and, 85, 86*t*
Cytomegalovirus infection, human immunodeficiency
    virus/acquired immutiodefiency syndrome
    population and, 534–535

D

Daily caloric requirements, 242, 260
Damages in malpractice claim, 42–43
Debridement, 157–176, **C10, C12–C15**
  decision-making algorithm for, 185*t*
  diabetic foot ulcers and, 427
  healing process and, 157–162
  methods of, 162–173
    choosing, 172–173
  necrotic tissue removal and, 116, 157, 163, **C10**
  pain management and, 295, 297
  preparing patient and family for, 161

primary purpose of, 157
recommendations for, 159–160
venous ulcers and, 369
Deep tissue injury, pressure ulcer staging and, 106, **C19**
Defendant, 38, 39
Dehydration
    laboratory values to screen for, 247*t*
    signs of, 243
    warning signs of, 311
Deposition, 39
Depth of wound, measuring, 110–112
Dermagraft, 196
Dermis, 57–61, 58*i*, 60*i*, 63, 66, 72, 88, 105, 111, 269, 300, 327*i*
Diabetes, 241, 339, 373, 402, 404, 420–421,
    See also Diabetic foot ulcers,
    neuropathy as complication of, 296, 421–422
Diabetic foot ulcers, 420–440, **C24**. *See also* Diabetes.
    advanced technologies for treating, 435, 439
    amputation and, 421
    assessment of, 422, 424, **C24**
    care plan for, 439
    classification systems for, 431
    debridement of, 427
    as diabetes complication, 420–421, 424, 427
    diagnostic imaging for, 439
    infection and, 10, 424, 426
        indicators of, 131
    multidisciplinary strategies for, 427–431
    musculoskeletal examination for, 425–426
    neuropathy as cause of, 421–424
    offloading therapy for, 433, 434*t*
    pain and, 11
    patient teaching for, 425
    peripheral vascular disease as cause of, 427
    preventive measures for, 424, 427
    risk factors for, 421–427
    skin and nail examination for, 424–425
Digital photography as wound measurement method, 109
DIME mnemonic, 161
Direct case in trial, 40
Discharge, documenting, 52–53
Discovery as pretrial step, 38–39
Distraction as pain management method, 316
Documentation, *See also* Wound documentation
    reimbursement and, 32–33
DonJoy High-Tide Diabetic Walker, 437*i*
Doppler ultrasound, 369, 406
    handheld, 406
Drains, 477–478
Dressings, *See also* specific type
    categories of, 185
    clinician competencies for selecting, 29
    factors that influence selection of, 184
    ideal, characteristics of, 185

pain management and, 295–319
    for pressure ulcers, 302
Drugs for wound dressing, 189
Duplex ultrasound, 368, 376, 407
Durable medical equipment carriers, reimbursement and, 29–30
Duty in malpractice claim, 41

E

Edema, differential diagnosis of, 387
Edges of wound, assessing, 115
Elastic foam as support surface, 272–274
Electrical stimulation as adjuvant therapy, 200, 346–347
    diabetic foot ulcers and, 436
    pressure ulcers and, 421
Electromagnetic spectrum, **C16**
Emollients, 72, 75, 567, 570
Emotional impact of wounds, 3
Envelopment, support surface and, 270
Environment as pain management method, 317
Enzymatic debridement, 169–171, 345, 470
    See also Debridement
    agents for, l68–171
Epidermal skin stripping injuries,
    See Skin tears
Epidermis, 57–64, 58*i*, 60*i*
Episodic pain, *See* Cyclic pain
Epithelial cell migration in open wound, 182, 182*i*
Epithelialization
    assessing, 105
    wound edges with, 115, **C4**
    wound healing and, 89
Eschar, 30, 109, 115, 137–138, 158–159, 161, 169–170, 193, 411, **C10**
Ethical dilemmas in wound care, 13–14
Evisceration, 87, 98, 466
Exercise as venous ulcer treatment, 371–372
Expectation, altered, as coping strategy, 9
Expert discovery, 39
External pneumatic compression therapy, 204
Extracellular matrix, 91, 93, 266
    diabetic foot ulcers and, 423
    hemostasis and, 83
    role of, in wound healing, 87–89
Extravasation injury, 505, **C35**
Exudate
    assessing, 112
    classifying, 113
    protecting skin from, 72

F

FACES Pain Rating Scale, 303, 307–309
Factitial dermatitis as wound cause, 505, **C34**
Fats, wound healing and, 248

Fat-soluble vitamins, wound healing and, 248, 250
Fatty acids, wound healing and, 250
Feeding tubes, 477–478, 481
Fibroblasts, role of, in wound healing, 87–88, 91, 94
Financial impact, quality of life and, 12–13
Fistulas
    classifying, 482
    formation of, 112, 482
    management of, 477
Fluid and electrolyte balance as skin function, 482–483, 486
Fluid-filled support surfaces, 269, 277
Foam dressings, 68, 147, 192–193, 371, 571
Foam in support surface systems, 272
Friction as pressure ulcer cause, 338, 570
Friction reduction, support surface and, 268–269
Full-thickness wounds, healing of, 66, 105, 109, 192, 195
Fungal infections, deep, 497

G

Gangrene, 402, 405–406, 411, 414, 431, 470
Gauze dressings, 145–146, 166, 183, 316, 345, 346, 371, 517
Gender, patient response and, 5, 309
Glamorgan Scale, 555, 558
Group barriers to quality wound care, 14
Growth factors
    pressure ulcers and, 346
    wound healing and, 181, 189

H

Half-shoes for diabetic foot, 437–438, 438*i*
Hansen's disease, **C29**
Healing outcomes, patient response to, 6–8
Healing sandals for diabetic foot, 437–438, 438*i*
Health care, role of regulation in, 21
Healthcare Common Procedure Coding System, 29
Health Care Financing Administration, *See* Centers for Medicare and Medicaid Services
Health promotion, transitioning to, 14–15
Healthy feeling as coping strategy 9
Heel pressure, managing, 286
Heel protection, 284, 286–287
HEELS mnemonic for pressure ulcer risk, 329
Hemosiderin deposit, 103, **C2**
Hemostasis as wound healing phase, 83, 85
Herpes virus infection, human immunodeficiency virus/acquired immunodeficiency syndrome population and, 534
Home health agencies, reimbursement and, 27–28
Home health benefits, qualifying for, 28
Hospital Insurance trust fund, Medicare and, 22
Hospital outpatient centers, reimbursement and, 25
Hospitals, reimbursement and, 23–25

Human immunodeficiency virus/acquired immunodeficiency syndrome population, 511, 541
    cutaneous drug eruptions in, 533–534
    infectious skin disorders in, 534–539
    neoplastic disorders in, 539–540
    noninfectious skin disorders in, 538–539
    patient teaching for, 535–538
    skin alteration in, 532
Human papilloma virus infection, human immunodeficiency virus/acquired immunodeficiency syndrome population and 533–536
Humectants, 72–73
Hydration status, laboratory screening for, 246, 248*t*, 566
Hydrocolloid dressings, 191, 287, 304
Hydrofiber dressings, 226*t*
Hydrogel dressings, 171, 192, 192*i*, 225*t*
Hydrotherapy as debridement method, 164*t*, 166
Hyperbaric oxygen therapy as adjuvant therapy, 206–208, 207*i*
    diabetic foot ulcers and, 440
    pressure ulcers and, 209, 491
Hypoalbuminemic malnutrition, 380, 384, 466
Hypodermis, *See* Subcutaneous tissue,
Hysteresis, 267, 282

I

Imaging, wound documentation and, 44
Immersion, support surface and, 269–270
Impeachment, 39
Incident pain, *See* Noncyclic pain,
Individual barriers to quality wound care, 13–14
Infection, 127–140
    Centers for Disease Control and Prevention criteria for, at surgical site, 130
    defining, 127–128
    diabetic foot ulcers and, 426
    diagnosing, 139, **C6**
    identifying, 104
    indicators of, by wound type, 130
    key elements of, 128
    pressure ulcers and, 302
    progression of, in chronic wound, 85, 90, 93, 98, **C6**
    sickle cell ulcers and, 450
    signs and symptoms of, 466, 481
    treatment of, in vascular ulcers, 409
Inflammation, 127, *See also* Inflammatory phase of wound healing
Inflammatory phase of wound healing, 85, *See also* Inflammation
Injury related to breach of duty, 41
Intensive care population, 512–518
    damage related to medical devices in, 517

deep tissue injury in, 512, 518
  pressure ulcer incidence and prevalence in, 512
  risk assessment tools for, 512–514
  risk-based prevention in, 514–517
  risk factors in, 512–514
  skin assessment in, 517–518
Interface pressure
  mapping, 281, **C18**
  as tissue damage predictor, 268–269
Intermittent claudication, pain associated with, 299, 424
Intermittent compression therapy, 204
Intertrigo, 545–546, **C38**
Intestinal tubes, 479
Iron, wound healing and, 251
Isotonic saline solution as cleaning agent, 141

J

Judge as player in litigation process, 39, 40
Jury as players in litigation process, 37–39
Jury selection, 40

K

Kaposi's sarcoma, HIV/AIDS population and, 539, **C36**
Kundin gauge, 111

L

Laboratory values, nutritional assessment and, 242, 247t, 252
Lacerations, repairing, 460
Larval therapy for debridement, 171–172, *See also* Debridement
Lateral rotation as support surface feature, 275
Laughter as pain management method, 317
Leakage from wound, patient response to, 6, 517
Leg reconstruction, 472
Leg ulcers, *See also* Vascular ulcers
  infection indicators in, 134
  key themes in patients with, 11
  quality of life and, 4
Lesion, correct identification of, 48
Leukocytes, wound healing and, 95, 112, 127, 158
Levine technique for swab cultures, 137
Light therapies, 201–202, **C16**
Linear measurement of wound, 109, 110i
Litigants, 37, 39–41
Litigation process, 37–41
  medical record in, 32
  players in, 39
  pretrial, 38–41
Low-air-loss systems as support surfaces, 276–277
LOWE skin barriers for wound margins, 114t

Low-level laser therapy in wound healing, 202
Lymphatic disorder, differentiating, from venous disorder, 387
Lymphatic flow
  aspects of, 381–383
  in the leg, 383
Lymphatic system, 381–383
  lower limb anatomy of, 382
Lymphedema
  characteristic features of, 387–388, **C23**
  classes of, 387
  epidemiology of, 379
  treatment of, 388
Lymphoma, human immunodeficiency virus/acquired immunodeficiency syndrome population and, 539

M

Maceration, 98, 115, 166, 183–184, 190–192, **C3**
Maggot therapy as debridement method, 171–172, 172i, *See also* Debridement
Magnets as pain management method, 317
Malignancies as wound cause, 491–493, 504, **C33**
Malnutrition, physical signs of, 241–243, *See also* Protein-energy malnutrition
Malpractice claim
  elements of, 41–43
  initiation of, 38–39
Malpractice trials, 40, 54
Managed Care Organizations, 30
Manual lymph drainage as venous ulcer treatment, 385, 388–389
Margin of debridement, 167, 168i
Marjolin ulcer, 504, **C33**
Maturation phase of wound healing, 90–92
MDS (minimum data set), 26, 28
Meaning of wound for patient, 7–8
MEASURES acronym, 184
Mechanical debridement, 166, 169, 171, *See also* Debridement
Mechanism of wounding, patient response to, 5
Median sternotomy, wound care for, 466
Medicaid benefits provided by, 23
Medical record
  in litigation, 37–38
  purposes of, 39, 44
Medicare
  benefits provided by, 22–23
    choice program, 22
    prescription drugs and, 22–23
    reimbursement and, 23–30
Meggitt-Wagner ulcer classification, 432t
Minerals, wound healing and, 248
Minimum Data Set, 24
Mobility, pressure ulcer risk and, 514–515

Moisture, pressure ulcer risk and, 516–517
Moisture control, support surface and, 272
Moisturizers, 71
Moist wound healing, 181–184,
    See also Wound healing,
  epithelial cell migration and, 182, 182*i*
Moist wound therapy, dressing options
  for 189–190
Molluscum contragiosum, human immunodeficiencv
  virus/acquired immunodeficiency syndrome
  population and, 537–538
Motion practice as pretrial step, 39–40
Music as pain management method, 317
Mycetoma as wound cause, 499
Mycobacterial infection, atypical, as wound cause, 495–496

N

Nasogastric tubes, 478–479
Necrotic tissue
  documenting, 109
  identifying, 129
Necrotizing fasciitis, 499–501, **C30**
  conditions leading to, 500
  diagnosis of, 500–501
  signs of, 500
  treatment of, 499
Needle aspiration technique, culture specimen and, 137
Negative image of wounds, 3–4
Negative-pressure wound therapy (NPWT), 145,
  197–199, 199*i*, 484
  reimbursement for, 30
Neonatal population, 552–561
  caregiver education for 555, 560
  nutritional considerations for, 559
  pressure redistribution products for, 558–559
  pressure ulcers in
    anatomical distribution of, 553
    complications of, 553
    financial impact of, 553
    prevalence and incidence of, 552, 553*t*
    risk assessment tools for, 555–557
    risk factors far, 553–557
  skin condition scales for, 555, 559
  topical management of, 559–560
NERDS and STONES mnemonics, 133–134, **C7–C9**
Neuropathic pain, 296–297
Neuropathy
  as diabetic complication, 424
  screening methods to identify, 422, 423*i*
NICE acronym for dressing decision making, 185,
  187–188
Nociceptive pain, 296, 300
Nocturnal pain, 299
Noncyclic pain, 297–298
  interventions for, 297–298

Nonopioid analgesics, pain management
  and, 571
Nonpharmacologic treatment modalities, 314–315
Numeric pain intensity scale, 307–308
Nutrients, role of, in healing, 248–252
Nutrition
  pressure ulcers and, 242–243, 246
  wound care and, 240–261
Nutritional assessment, 242–248
  anthropometric factors and, 246
  biochemical and laboratory values
    for, 246–248
  kilocalorie needs estimation and, 247,
    249, 250
Nutritional intake, enhancing, 257–258
Nutritional interventions, 252–258
  documenting, 258
Nutritional screening, 240–242
Nutritional support, 255
  algorithm to determine need for, 256

O

OASIS, 24, 28–29
Occiput pressure ulcer, **C39**
Occlusives, 72
Occupational function, quality of life and, 4
Occupational therapy as treatment
  modality, 315–316
Odor of wound, 112
  patient response to, 5
Offloading therapy, 433, 472, 559
Opioid analgesics, pain management and, 310,
  312–313, 315

P

Pain, *See also* Wound pain
  definitions of, 295
  diabetic foot ulcers and, 306
  leg ulcers and, 10–12, 302
  managing, 11, 295–319
  patient response to, 5
  pressure ulcers and, 11–12
  quality of life and, 11
  types of, 296–297
  wound types and, 297
Pain assessment, 305–308
  elements of, 306
  guides for, 306
  intensity scales for, 304, 307
Pain impulses, skin and, 62
Pain management, 295–319
Palliative wound care, 564–578
  defining, 564
  extent of problem in, 565
  fungating wounds in, 573–574
  pain management in, 571

pressure ulcer risk assessment in, 567
protection of periwound area in, 571
radiation wounds in, 574–576
skin care needs of patient in, 566–567
wound colonization and infection in, 572–573
wound dressings in, 571–572
Pannus, **C36**
Papain-urea preparations, 169–170
Paracoccidioidomycosis as wound cause, 498–499
Partial-thickness wounds, healing of, 105–106, 182
Patient and family notification, 48–49
Patient evaluation, support surface selection and, 281, 338
Patient outcomes, documenting, 23, 44
Payne-Martin classification system for skin tears, 66, 68, **C1**
Pay-for-performance, quality improvement and, 32
Pediatric population, 552–561
nutritional considerations for, 559
patient and caregiver education for, 560
pressure redistribution products for, 558
pressure ulcers in
anatomical distribution of, 553, **C39**
complications of, 553
financial impact of, 553
prevalence and incidence of, 552
risk assessment tools for, 555
risk factors for, 553–554
skin condition scales for, 555, 556*t*
topical management of, 559–560
Peer Review Organizations, 32
Percutaneous balloon angioplasty, arterial
ulcers and, 411–412
Peripheral vascular disease, 299, 360, 398, 402
pain associated with, 299
Persistent pain, *See* Chronic pain,
Photography
wound documentation and, 49
as wound measurement method, 119
Phototherapy, 202
Physical function, quality of life and, 4–5
Physical therapy as treatment modality, 206
Physician notification and participation, 48
Plaintiff, 38–40
Planimetry for wound measurement, 110
Plantar hyperkeratosis, **C37**
Platelet-derived growth factor, 85, 168
Platelet-rich plasma, 206, 234*t*
Plethysmography, types of, 369
Podiatric physicians, callus and nails, 427
Policies and procedures, documenting, 50–52
Positioning, pressure ulcer risk and, 515–516,
See also Repositioning,
Positive outlook as coping strategy, 9
Preparedness of patient to deal with wound, 5
Preponderance of evidence standard, 41
Pressure differential, *See* Pressure gradient
Pressure gradient support surface and, 267

tissue death and, 327
Pressure redistribution
diabetic foot ulcers and, 430–431
pressure ulcer treatment and, 340–347
support surface and, 265–291, **C18**
Pressure Sore Status Tool (PSST), 116, 342
Pressure ulcers, 324–353, **C19–C21**
adjunctive therapies for, 346–347
ASSESSMENT chart for, 107
cleaning, 342
competency-based curriculum for, 350
cytokine-mediated anorexia and, 254
debridement of, 339, 345
development of, 46
discovery of, 47–48
documenting healing of, 337
ethical issues related to, 13–14
etiology of, 326–330
financial cost associated with, 326
flaps for repair of, 467
as health care problem, 324
heel pressure and, 286, 337
incidence and prevalence of, 324
infection and, 339, 341, 345
indicators of, 339–340
monitoring healing of, 342
nutrient needs for, 246, 328
nutrition care alerts for, 240
nutrition guidelines for preventing, 247
nutrition markers linked to, 482–483
nutrition therapy progress note for, 258
pain of, 12, 332*t*, 341
pitfalls to calculating, 350
prevalence by facility type, 348
preventing, 330–339, 341, 351
repairing, 468–470
reverse staging of, 340
risk assessment for, 28, 46, 50–51, 279,
331–337, 555, **C18**
importance of, 330
risk factors for development of, 268, 513
sites of, 330, **C18**
staging, 27, 109, **C20–C21**
definitions for, 339
support surfaces and, 265, **C18**
surgical closure, **C27**
tissue loading and, 267–268
tools for assessing and documenting, 117, **C18**
treatment of, 324, 340–347
Pressure Ulcer Scale for Healing (PUSH), 116, 250, 342–343
Proliferation phase of wound healing, 86–87
Prospective payment system (PPS), 23, 28
Proteases, role of, in wound healing, 92
Protection as skin function, 61–63
Protective shoes as preventive measure,
428–429

Protein
    adult need for, 243t
    wound healing and, 183
Protein, energy malnutrition, 254
    consequences of, 147
Proximate cause, 42
Prurigo nodularis, human immunodeficiency
        virus/acquired immunodeficiency syndrome
        population and, 538
Pruritus, 70, 72
    as symptom in conditions and diseases, 74
    treatment plan for, 75
Psathakis silastic sling procedure, 375
Psychological function, quality of life and, 4–13
Pulsed lavage as debridement method, 166–167
PUSH (Pressure Ulcer Scale for Healing),
        116, 250, 342–343
Pyoderma gangrenosum as wound cause,
        492–494, 504, 507, **C28**
    systemic diseases associated with, 494, 495t
    treatment options for, 495t

Q

Qualitative cultures, 138–139
Quality of care
    improving, 32
    measuring, 31–32
Quality Improvement Organization, 32
Quality of life, 4–13
    health-related, 4
Quantitative cultures, 138–140

R

Radiant heat therapy, pressure ulcers and, 346–347
Radiation dermatitis as wound cause, 505
Readiness to deal with wound, patient response to, 5
Regulation of wound care, 21
    documentation and, 32–33
    Medicaid and, 23
    Medicare and, 22–23
    quality improvement efforts and, 30–33
    reimbursement and, 23–30
    role of, 21
Reimbursement for wound care
    in complex environment, 30
    durable medical equipment carriers and, 29–30
    home health agencies and, 27–29
    hospital outpatient centers and, 25
    hospitals and, 23–25
    managed care and, 30–31
    skilled nursing facilities and, 26
Remodeling process, 90
Repositioning
    frequency of, 284
    guidelines for, 285–286
Resident Assessment Instrument, 26–27
Resident Assessment Protocols, 24

Resource utilization groups, 27
Response of others, patient response to, 5
Rest pain, 299, 404
Royce Active Hex Walker, 436–437

S

Scar management, 209, **C17**
Segmental pressures in arterial resting, 408
Self-esteem of patient, wounds and, 3
Semmes-Weinstein monofilament test to assess
        protective sensation, 403, 422–423
Senile purpura, 64, **C2**
Sensation as skin function, 61–64
Sensory perception, reduced, pressure ulcer risk and, 516
Sepsis, assessing, 112–113
Shearing force as pressure ulcer cause, 269, 328i, 329
Shear reduction, support surface and, 276
Sickle cell anemia, 446, *See also* Sickle
        cell ulcers
    blood cells in, 446
    conditions associated with, 447
    prevalence and incidence of, 446
Sickle cell ulcers, 446–456, **C25–C26**. *See also* Sickle cell
        anemia.
    assessment of, 450, **C25–C26**
    as complication of sickle cell anemia, 446
    diagnosis of, 449
    infection and, 447–448
    pain management guidelines for, 451
    pathogenesis of, 446–449
    preventing, 454
    recurrent, 449, **C26**
    treatment of, 451–454, **C25**
Significance of wound for patient, 8
Silver dressings, 192–193
Sinus tracts, documenting, 112
Skilled nursing facilities
    federal oversight of, 22
    reimbursement and, 23
Skin
    anatomy and physiology of, 57–61
    assessment of, 64–66
    effects of aging on, 60i, 63
    functions of, 61–63
    integrity and pathology of, 63–64
    tears in, 66
Skin breakdown, preventing, 265–266
Skin cleaners as cleaning agents, 141
Skin conditions, 61, 66, 70
Skin folds, in bariatric patient, **C36**
Skin Integrity Risk Assessment
        Tool, 67–68, 77
Skin substitutes, tissue-engineered,
        2, 185, 196
Skin tears, 66–70
    causes of, 66
    classifying, 68, **C1**

common sites of, 66
management of, 70
prevalence of, 66–67
prevention protocols, for, 68–70
risk assessment tool for, 67
risk factors for, 67–68
Skin trauma, 66, 377
Slough, 96, 116, 128, **C10**
differentiating tendon from, **C10**
Social interaction, limitations in, 9–10
Social supports, patient response to, 9
Societal barriers to quality wound care, 14
Soft-tissue biomechanics, 266–269
Somatic pain, 62, 296
Somatic sensation, quality of life and, 11–12
Specialty mattress selection, 279
Spider bites as wound cause, 504, **C34**
Spinal cord injury population, 520–529
incidence and prevalence of, 520–521
patient teaching for, 525
pressure ulcers in
incidence and prevalence of, 521–522
preventive strategies for, 524
recurrence of, 522
risk factors for, 523–524
treatment of, 523–524, 526
skin assessment in, 525
support surfaces for, 527
Spirituality, patient response and, 9
Sporotrichosis as wound cause, 498
Square centimeter determination as wound
measurement method, 110
Staphylococcal infection, human immunodeficiency
virus/acquired immunodeficiency syndrome
population and, 500
STAR classification of skin tears, 68, **C2**
Stereophotogrammetry, wound measurement and, 110
Stevens-Johnson syndrome (SJS), 533–534
STONES mnemonic, 133–134, **C8–C9**
Streptococcal infection, human immunodeficiency
virus/acquired immunodeficiency syndrome
population and, 493, 511
Stress-relaxation phenomenon, 267
Subcutaneous tissue, 57, 58i, 59t, 60i, 61, 63
Supplementary Medical Insurance trust fund,
Medicare and, 22
Support surfaces
characteristics of, 269–272
effectiveness of, 279, 283–284
matching, to patient needs, 278–289
materials and components used in, 266, 272–275
moisture control and, 272
performance parameters for, 266
pressure redistribution and, 269
pros and cons of, 42
shear and friction reductin, and, 270–271
standards for, 278, 281–282

temperature control and, 271–272
types of, 265, 273
Surgical dressings benefit, criteria for, 25
Surgical/sharp debridement, 167–169, **C12–C13.** *See also*
Debridement, Surgical wounds, 25, 28, 54, 97,
112–113, 120, 191, 405, 460, 465
assessment of, 460
nonhealing, causes of, 405–406, 411, 468
reconstructive ladder and, 461
tubes and drains for, 477–481
skin care around, 481
Swab culture, technique for, 133, 137, 139, 148, 426

T

Telangiectasias, 364, 365
Temperature control, support surface and, 271–272
Temperature homeostasis, 62
Thermoregulation as skin function, 61–63
Time to healing, patient response to, 5–6
TIME mnemonic, 96t, 97
Tissue bed, documenting, 107
Tissue biopsy, culture specimen and, 112
Tissue edema, pathophysiology of, in venous disease,
383–384
Toe pressures in arterial testing, 406, 409
Total contact cast for diabetic foot, 433–434, 435i
Toxic epidermal necrolysis (TEN), 473, 533–534
Traction theory, wound contraction and, 90
Transparent film dressings, 190–191
Treatment decisions, 184–189
algorithm for, 185i
economic considerations and, 189
NICE acronym for, 185, 187–188t
Treatment evaluation, documenting, 43–44
Treatment options, 166, 170–171, 181–214
Tubes
errors in, 349
types of, 478–479
Turning schedules, 285

U

Ultrasound, therapeutic, 208–209
Ultraviolet light as adjuvant therapy, 202–203
Undermining, documenting,111–112
Undernutrition
chronic wounds and, 255
effects of, 254–255
University of Texas diabetic wound
classification system, 430
University of Texas Subjective Peripheral Neuropathy
Verbal Questionnaire, 432

V

Valve transplantation, autogenous, 375
Valvuloplasty, 375
Varicose veins, 365–368, 373, 450
Vascular anatomy and physiology, 398–401

Vascular testing, 405–409
Vascular ulcers, **C22–C23.** *See also* Arterial ulcers.
  arterial, signs and symptoms in, 404–405, **C22**
  diagnosing, 402–405, **C22–C23**
  measuring healing of, 414
  patient education for, 414–415
  risk factors tot, 401, 414–415
  smoking cessation and, 402, 405, 415
  treating, 409–414
Vasculitis
  as atypical wound cause, 492–508, **C28**
  diagnostic tests for, 494–495
  potential etiologies of, 492
  treatment options for, 494–495
Venous disease
  classifying, 366, 387
  differentiating, from lymphatic
      disorder, 387
  incidence of, 365
  lymphatic failure in, 386–387
  pathophysiology of edema in, 383
  signs and symptoms of, 367–368
Venous photoplethysmography, 369
Venous system
  anatomy of, 361
  deep leg veins in, 361*i*
  superficial leg veins in, 361, 361*i*
  valve anatomy in, 362
  wall architecture in, 362
Venous testing, 369
Venous ulcers
  characteristics of, 364, **C22**
  diagnosing, 367–368
  infection indicators in, 135–136
  measuring healing of, 414
  pain associated with, 299–300
  pathogenesis of, 447–450
  pathophysiology of, 363–367
  patient education for, 414–415
  signs and symptoms of, 367–368
  treating, 369–377
Vibration perception threshold testing for sensory
      neuropathy screening, 422
Vibrio vulnificus infection as wound cause, 495, 499
Visceral pain, 296
Viscoelastic foam as support surface,
      274
Visibility of wound, patient response to, 5
Vitamin A, wound healing and, 250–251
Vitamin B, wound healing and, 243–244, 251
Vitamin C, wound healing and, 244, 249, 251
Vitamin E, wound healing and, 251

W

Walking boots, removable, for diabetic foot,
      435–436, 435*i*

Water
  as cleaning agent, 141
  wound healing and, 251–252
Water-soluble vitamins, 251
Weight loss
  classifying severity of, 246
  unintended, warning signs of, 241
Wet-to-dry dressings as debridement
      method, 166, 171
Wheelchair cushion selection, 279
Whirlpool bath
  debridement and, 166
  wound cleaning and, 144
Wound
  bioburden in, 126–151
  definition of, 2
  emotional impact of, 3
  factors that affect patient response to, 5
  patient's self-esteem and, 3, 5
  quality of life and, 2, 4–13
Wound assessment, 64–66, 101–123, *See also* Wound
      volume, measuring
  chart for, 108
  documenting, 113, 115–116, **C5**
  elements of, 103, 106
  frequency of, 104
  initial, 102–103
  nine C's of, 102
  physical examination and, 103
  repeating, 308
Wound "bar code" (gene expression pattern), **C11**
Wound bed preparation (WBP)
  best practices for, 162*t*, 196
  new model for, 97, 341
  principles of, 96, 341
Wound care
  current practices in, 172, 584–585
  decision algorithm for, 185
  documentation of, 33, 45, 584
  early practices in, 514
  ethical dilemmas in, 13–14
  future of, 583–586
  legal aspects of, 37–55
  MEASURES acronym for, 184
  nutrition and, 240–261
  palliative, 564–578
  regulation of, 21–34
  reimbursement for, 23–30
  therapeutic ultrasound and, 208
Wound cleaning, 137, 141
  agents for, 141–142
  devices for, 143–145
  pain management and, 295–319
  vascular ulcers and, 409
  venous ulcers and, 369
Wound closure, reconstructive ladder and, 461

Wound contraction, 89–90
Wound cultures and specimens, 129, 134–140
  analyzing, 138
  common types of, 135–136
  qualitative, 138–139
  quantitative, 136, 139–140
Wound dehiscence, 193, 466
Wound depth, determining, 110, 110*i*, 112, *See also*,
    Wound assessment
Wound documentation
  admission assessment and, 45–46
  collaboration, coordination, and communication
      and, 50
  correct identification of lesion and, 48
  discharge and, 52–53
  discovery of pressure ulcer and, 47–48
  guidelines for, 44
  incomplete, effect of, 43
  information flow and, 45
  legal aspects of, 44–53
  notification and participation of the
      physician and, 48
  notification of patient and family and, 48–49
  ongoing, 49
  patient outcomes and, 43–44
  photograph and imaging and, 49–50
  policies and procedures and, 50–52
  pressure ulcer development and, 46–47
  pressure ulcer risk assessment and, 46
  treatment evaluation and, 43–44
  "Turn Q 2" check box and, 47
Wound healing
  acute versus chronic, 93–97
  biology, **C16–C17**
  cytokines and, 85–86
  delayed, 93, 99
  effects of growth factors on, 88–89
  low-level laser therapy and, 202
  measuring, 110–111, 116
  moist, 145, 158, 166, 170–171, 181–184
  phases of, 86–87
  role of matrix metaloproteases in, 92–93
  sequence of events in, 83–84
  therapeutic ultrasound and, 206
Wound irrigation, 143–144, 208
Wound location, documenting, 106, 116–117
Wound pain
  cyclic, interventions for, 298
  findings of studies related to, 302
  interventions for, 297–298
  myths about, 303
  noncyclic, interventions for, 297
  preparing environment for, 302
WOUND PICTURE mnemonic, 121
Wound terminology, **C5**
Wound volume, measuring, 111
        See also Wound assessment,

X
Xerosis, 70–72, 71*i*
  causes of, 72
  classifying, 71
  itch-scratch-itch cycle in, 72
  management of, 70–72

Z
Zinc, wound healing and, 251
Z-stroke technique for swab cultures, 137